Understanding Patient Safety

Understanding Patient Safety

Third Edition

Robert M. Wachter, MD
Professor and Chair
Department of Medicine
Holly Smith Professor in Science and Medicine
Marc and Lynne Benioff Endowed Chair in Hospital Medicine
University of California, San Francisco
San Francisco, California

Kiran Gupta, MD, MPH
Assistant Professor
Department of Medicine
University of California, San Francisco
Medical Director for Patient Safety
UCSF Medical Center
San Francisco, California

Mc
Graw
Hill
Education

New York   Chicago   San Francisco   Athens   London   Madrid
Mexico City   Milan   New Delhi   Singapore   Sydney   Toronto

Understanding Patient Safety, Third Edition

1 2 3 4 5 6 7 8 9   DSS   22 21 20 19 18 17

ISBN 978-1-259-86024-9
MHID 1-259-86024-8

This book was set in Times LT Std by MPS Limited.
The editors were Amanda Fielding and Kim J. Davis.
The production supervisor was Catherine Saggese.
Project management was provided by Poonam Bisht of MPS Limited.

Library of Congress Cataloging-in-Publication Data

Names: Wachter, Robert M., author. | Gupta, Kiran, author.
  Title: Understanding patient safety / Robert M. Wachter, Kiran Gupta.
   Description: Third edition. | New York: McGraw-Hill Education, [2018] |
Includes bibliographical references and index.
Identifiers: LCCN 2017008034 | ISBN 9781259860249 (pbk. : alk. paper) | ISBN
1259860248 (pbk. : alk. paper) | ISBN 9781259860256 (Ebook) | ISBN
1259860256 (Ebook)
Subjects: | MESH: Medical Errors–prevention & control | Patient Safety |
Safety Management–methods
Classification: LCC R729.8 | NLM WB 100 | DDC 610.28/9–dc23
   LC record available at https://lccn.loc.gov/2017008034

McGraw-Hill Education Professional books are available at special quantity discounts to use as premiums and sales promotions, or for use in corporate training programs. To contact a representative, please visit the Contact Us pages at www.mhprofessional.com.

Contents

Chapter 14

Reporting Systems, Root Cause Analysis, and other Methods of Understanding Safety Issues 257

Chapter 15

Creating a Culture of Safety 281

Chapter 16

Workforce Issues 307

Preface

In late 1999, the National Academy of Medicine (NAM, then called the Institute of Medicine) published *To Err Is Human: Building a Safer Health Care System.*[1] Although the NAM has published more than 800 reports since *To Err*, none have been nearly as influential. The reason: extrapolating from data from the Harvard Medical Practice Study,[2,3] performed a decade earlier, the authors estimated that 44,000 to 98,000 Americans die each year from medical errors.* More shockingly, they translated these numbers into the now-famous "jumbo jet units," pointing out that this death toll would be the equivalent of a jumbo jet crashing each and every day in the United States.

Although some critiqued the jumbo jet analogy as hyperbolic, we like it for several reasons. First, it provides a vivid and tangible icon for the magnitude of the problem (obviously, if extended to the rest of the world, the toll would be many times higher). Second, if in fact a jumbo jet were to crash every day, who among us would even consider flying electively? Third, and most importantly, consider for a moment what our society would do—and spend—to fix the problem if there were an aviation disaster every day. The answer, of course, is that there would be no limit to what we would do to fix *that* problem. Yet prior to *To Err Is Human,* we were doing next to nothing to make patients safer.

This is not to imply that the millions of committed, hardworking, and well-trained doctors, nurses, pharmacists, therapists, and healthcare administrators *wanted* to harm people from medical mistakes. They did not—to the degree that Albert Wu has labeled providers who commit an error that causes terrible harm "second victims."[6] Yet we now understand that the problem of medical errors is not fundamentally one of "bad apples" (though there are some), but rather one of competent providers working in a chaotic system that has not prioritized safety. As Wachter and Shojania wrote in the 2004 book *Internal Bleeding*:

> *Decades of research, mostly from outside healthcare, has confirmed our own medical experience: Most errors are made by good but fallible people working in dysfunctional systems, which means that making care safer depends on buttressing the system to prevent or*

---

*A controversial 2016 study cited a death toll from medical errors of 300,000 per year in the United States.[4] We find the methods of this study to be unpersuasive, as did other experts.[5] We will return to the matter of estimating the toll from medical errors in Chapter 1.

catch the inevitable lapses of mortals. This logical approach is common in other complex, high-tech industries, but it has been woefully ignored in medicine. Instead, we have steadfastly clung to the view that an error is a moral failure by an individual, a posture that has left patients feeling angry and ready to blame, and providers feeling guilty and demoralized. Most importantly, it hasn't done a damn thing to make healthcare safer.[7]

Try for a moment to think of systems in healthcare that were truly "hardwired" for safety prior to 1999. Can you come up with any? We can think of just one: the double-checking done by nurses before releasing a unit of blood to prevent ABO transfusion errors. Now think about other error-prone areas: preventing harmful drug interactions or giving patients medicines to which they are allergic; ensuring that patients' preferences regarding resuscitation are respected; guaranteeing that the correct limbs are operated on; making sure primary care doctors have the necessary information after a hospitalization; diagnosing patients with chest pain in the emergency department correctly—none of these were organized in ways that ensured safety.

Interestingly, many of the answers were there for the taking—from industries as diverse as take-out restaurants to nuclear power plants, from commercial aviation to automobile manufacturing—and there are now dozens of examples of successes in applying techniques drawn from other fields to healthcare safety and quality (Table P-1).[8] Why does healthcare depend so much on the experiences of other industries to guide its improvement efforts? In part, it is because other industries have long recognized the diverse expertise that must be tapped to produce the best possible product at the lowest cost. In healthcare, the absence of any incentive (until recently) to focus on quality and safety, our burgeoning biomedical knowledge base, our siloed approach to training, and, frankly, professional hubris have caused us to look inward, not outward, for answers. The fact that we are now routinely seeking insights from aviation, manufacturing, education, and other industries, and embracing paradigms from engineering, sociology, psychology, and management, may prove to be the most enduring benefit of the patient safety movement.

All of this makes the field of patient safety at once vexing and exciting. To keep patients safe will take a uniquely interdisciplinary effort, one in which doctors, nurses, pharmacists, and administrators forge new types of relationships. It will demand that we look to other industries for good ideas, while recognizing that caring for patients is different enough from other human endeavors and that thoughtful adaptation is critical. It will require that we tamp down our traditionally rigid hierarchies, without forgetting the importance of leadership or compromising crucial lines of authority. It will take additional resources, although investments in safety may well pay off in new

Table P-1 EXAMPLES OF PATIENT SAFETY PRACTICES DRAWN AT LEAST IN PART FROM NONHEALTHCARE INDUSTRIES

Strategy	Nonhealthcare Example	Study Demonstrating Value in Healthcare	Impetus for Wider Implementation in Healthcare
Improved ratios of providers to "customers" (Chapter 16)	Teacher-to-student ratios (such as in class-size initiatives)	Needleman et al. (2011)	Legislation in many states mandating minimum nurse-to-patient ratios, other pressure
Decrease provider fatigue (Chapter 16)	Consecutive work-hour limitations for pilots, truck drivers	Landrigan et al. (2004)	Accreditation Council for Graduate Medical Education (ACGME) regulations limiting resident duty hours
Improve teamwork and communication (Chapter 15)	Crew resource management (CRM) in aviation	Neily et al. (2010)	Some hospitals now requiring team training for individuals who work in risky areas such as labor and delivery or surgery
Use of simulators (Chapter 17)	Simulator use in aviation and the military	Bruppacher et al. (2010)	Medical simulation now required for credentialing for certain procedures; technology improving and costs falling
Executive Walk Rounds (Chapter 22)	"Management by Walking Around" in business	Thomas et al. (2005)	Executive Walk Rounds not required, but remain a popular practice
Bar coding (Chapter 13)	Use of bar coding in manufacturing, retail, and food sales	Poon et al. (2010)	U.S. Food and Drug Administration now requires bar codes on most prescription medications; bar coding or its equivalent may ultimately be required in many identification processes

Reproduced and updated with permission from Wachter RM. Playing well with others: "translocational research" in patient safety. *AHRQ WebM&M* (serial online); September 2005. Available at: http://webmm.ahrq.gov/perspective.aspx?perspectiveID=9.

Bruppacher HR, Alam SK, LeBlanc VR, et al. Simulation-based training improves physicians' performance in patient care in high-stakes clinical setting of cardiac surgery. *Anesthesiology* 2010;112:985–992.

Landrigan CP, Rothschild JM, Cronin JW, et al. Effect of reducing interns' work hours on serious medical errors in intensive care units. *N Engl J Med* 2004;351:1838–1848.

Needleman J, Buerhaus P, Pankratz VS, et al. Nurse staffing and inpatient hospital mortality. *N Engl J Med* 2011;364:1037–1045.

Neily J, Mills PD, Young-Xu Y, et al. Association between implementation of a medical team training program and surgical mortality. *JAMA* 2010;304:1693–1700.

Poon EG, Keohane CA, Yoon CS, et al. Effect of bar-code technology on the safety of medication administration. *N Engl J Med* 2010;362:1698–1707.

Thomas EJ, Sexton JB, Neilands TB, et al. The effect of executive walk rounds on nurse safety climate attitudes: a randomized trial of clinical units. *BMC Health Serv Res* 2005;5:28.

efficiencies, lower provider turnover, and fewer expensive complications. It will require a thoughtful embrace of this new notion of systems thinking, while recognizing the absolute importance of the well-trained and committed caregiver. Again, from *Internal Bleeding*:

> *Although there is much we can learn from industries that have long embraced the systems approach, ... medical care is much more complex and customized than flying an Airbus: At 3 A.M., the critically ill patient needs superb and compassionate doctors and nurses more than she needs a better checklist. We take seriously the awesome privileges and responsibilities that society grants us as physicians, and don't believe for a second that individual excellence and professional passion will become expendable even after our trapeze swings over netting called a "safer system." In the end, medical errors are a hard enough nut to crack that we need excellent doctors and safer systems.[7]*

The first edition of *Understanding Patient Safety* was published in 2007, and the second in 2012. In preparing this third edition five years later, we were impressed by the maturation of the safety field. Between the first and second edition, for example, there were fundamental changes in our understanding of safety targets, with a shift to a focus on harm rather than errors. We saw the emergence of checklists as a key tool in safety. New safety-oriented practices, such as rapid response teams and medication reconciliation, became commonplace. The digitization of medical practice was just beginning to gain steam, but most doctor's offices and hospitals remained paper-based.

Between 2012 and today, the most impressive change has been the widespread computerization of the healthcare system. Fueled by $30 billion in incentive payments distributed under the Meaningful Use and HITECH programs, more than 90% of U.S. hospitals now have electronic health records, as do more than 70% of physician offices (in 2008, these figures were closer to one-in-ten in both hospitals and offices).[9] This means that many error types, particularly those related to handwritten prescriptions or failure to transmit information, have all but disappeared. However, they have been replaced by new classes of electronic health record–associated errors that stem from problems at the human–machine interface.[10]

In fact, mitigating the impact of unanticipated consequence has proven to be a major theme of the patient safety field. In this edition, we spend considerable time addressing such issues (Table P-2). We have learned that nearly every safety fix has a dark side. This doesn't mean that we should hesitate before implementing sensible and evidence-based safety improvements—in fact, we've seen good evidence over the past few years that our safety efforts are bearing fruit.[11] But it *does* mean that we need to improve our ability to anticipate unanticipated

Table P-2   EXAMPLES OF UNANTICIPATED CONSEQUENCES OF PATIENT SAFETY STRATEGIES*

Patient Safety Strategy	Unanticipated Consequence(s)	Comment
Computerized alerts and alarms	Alert and alarm fatigue	Clinicians often bypass alerts in electronic health record; ICU alarms often ignored because they are so frequent. Efforts underway to distinguish alarms/alerts by severity, to eliminate low yield alerts and alarms, and to use new technology tools to increase the probability that a given alert or alarm is meaningful
Computerized physician documentation	Physicians and patients no longer making eye contact, patients feeling abandoned	Many practices have hired scribes to perform data entry tasks so that the physician can concentrate on the patient and his/her problems; some emerging technologies may be able to audiotape the doctor-patient encounter and then analyze it using natural language processing
Housestaff duty hour limitations	No significant impact on patient safety, in part because of increased numbers of handoffs	Accreditation Council for Graduate Medical Education (ACGME) has relaxed some of its duty hour requirements; strong emphasis on improving handoffs
Pain as a "fifth vital sign"	Possible contribution to overuse of opiates	The growing epidemic of opiate overdoses is multifactorial, but the emphasis on measuring pain scores likely contributed to increased use of opiates in hospitalized patients. New emphasis on education about the downsides of opiates, with an emphasis on alternative modalities
Incident reporting systems	Many organizations have collected tens of thousands of incident reports, with little action	Increasing efforts to make incident reporting systems meaningful, as well as to rethink Root Cause Analyses to emphasize not just the analysis but the action (the National Patient Safety Foundation has suggested renaming them RCA^2, emphasizing both analysis and action)

*Based on authors' own analysis.

consequences, ensure that we are alert to them after we implement a safety fix, and do what we can to mitigate any harms that emerge.

This book aims to teach the key principles of patient safety to a diverse audience: physicians, nurses, pharmacists, other healthcare providers, quality and safety professionals, risk managers, hospital administrators, and others. It is suitable for all levels of readers: from the senior physician trying to learn this new way of approaching his or her work, to the medical or nursing student, to the risk manager or hospital board member seeking to get more involved in institutional safety efforts. The fact that the same book can speak to all of these groups (whereas few clinical textbooks could) is another mark of the interdisciplinary nature of this field. Although many of the examples and references are from the United States, our travels and studies have convinced us that most of the issues are the same internationally, and that all countries can learn much from each other. We have made every effort, therefore, to make the book relevant to a geographically diverse audience, and have included key references and tools from outside the United States.

Understanding Patient Safety is divided into three main sections. In Section I, we describe the epidemiology of error, distinguish safety from quality, discuss the key mental models that inform our modern understanding of the safety field, and summarize the policy environment for patient safety. In Section II, we review different error types, taking advantage of real cases to describe various kinds of mistakes and safety hazards, introduce new terminology, and discuss what we know about how errors happen and how they can be prevented. Although many prevention strategies will be touched on in Section II, more general issues regarding various strategies (from both individual institutional and broader policy perspectives) will be reviewed in Section III. After a concluding chapter, the Appendix includes a wide array of resources, from helpful Web sites to a patient safety glossary. To keep the book a manageable size, our goal is to be more useful and engaging than comprehensive—readers wishing to dig deeper will find relevant references throughout the text.

Some of the material for this book is derived or adapted from other works that we have edited or written. Specifically, some of the case presentations are drawn from *Internal Bleeding: The Truth Behind America's Terrifying Epidemic of Medical Mistakes*,[7] the "Quality Grand Rounds" series in the *Annals of Internal Medicine* (Appendix I),[12] and AHRQ WebM&M.[13] Many of the case presentations came from cases we used for the QGR series, and we are grateful to the patients, families, and caregivers who allowed us to use their stories (often agreeing to be interviewed). Of course, all patient and provider names have been changed to protect privacy.

We are indebted to our colleagues at the University of California, San Francisco, particularly Drs. Adrienne Green, Niraj Sehgal, Brad Sharpe, Urmimala Sarkar, and Sumant Ranji, for supporting our work. We are grateful to the Agency for Healthcare Research and Quality for its continued support of AHRQ Patient Safety Network, now approaching its 20th year in publication.[14] Our editorship of this widely used safety resource allows us to keep up with the safety literature each week. We are grateful to Kaveh Shojania, now of the University of Toronto, for his remarkable contributions to the safety field and for authoring the book's glossary. We thank our publisher at McGraw-Hill, Jim Shanahan, as well as our editor, Amanda Fielding. Kiran would like to thank several mentors from her time at Brigham and Women's Hospital in Boston including Drs. Tejal Gandhi, Allen Kachalia, and Joel Katz. We are also grateful to our partners in life, Katie Hafner for Bob and Manik Suri for Kiran, for their support and encouragement.

Finally, although this is not primarily a book written for patients, it is a book written *about* patients. As patient safety becomes professionalized (with "patient safety officers"), it will inevitably become jargon-heavy—"We need a root cause analysis!" "What did the Failure Mode Effects Analysis show?"— and this evolution makes it easy to take our eyes off the ball. We now know that tens of thousands of people in the United States and many times that number around the world die each year because of preventable medical errors. Moreover, every day millions of people check into hospitals or clinics worried that they'll be killed in the process of receiving chemotherapy, undergoing surgery, or delivering a baby. Our efforts must be focused on preventing these errors, and the associated anxiety that patients feel when they receive medical care in an unsafe, chaotic environment.

Some have argued that medical errors are the dark side of medical progress, an inevitable consequence of the ever-increasing complexity of modern medicine. Perhaps a few errors fit this description, but most do not. We can easily envision a system in which patients benefit from all the modern miracles available to us, and do so in reliable organizations that take advantage of all the necessary tools and systems to "get it right" the vast majority of the time. Looking back at the remarkable progress that has been made in the 17 years since the publication of *To Err Is Human*, we are confident that we can create such a system. Our hope is that this book makes a small contribution toward achieving that goal.

REFERENCES

1. Kohn L, Corrigan J, Donaldson M, eds. *To Err Is Human: Building a Safer Health System*. Committee on Quality of Health Care in America, Institute of Medicine. Washington, DC: National Academies Press; 1999.
2. Brennan TA, Leape LL, Laird NM, et al. Incidence of adverse events and negligence in hospitalized patients. Results of the Harvard Medical Practice Study I. *N Engl J Med* 1991;324:370–376.

3. Leape LL, Brennan TA, Laird N, et al. The nature of adverse events and negligence in hospitalized patients. Results of the Harvard Medical Practice Study II. *N Engl J Med* 1991;324:377–384.

4. Makary MA, Daniel M. Medical error—the third leading cause of death in the US. *BMJ* 2016;353:i2139.

5. Shojania KG, Dixon-Woods M. Estimating deaths due to medical error: the ongoing controversy and why it matters. *BMJ Qual Saf* 2017;26:423–428.

6. Wu AW. Medical error: the second victim. *West J Med* 2000;172:358–359.

7. Wachter RM, Shojania KG. *Internal Bleeding: The Truth Behind America's Terrifying Epidemic of Medical Mistakes*. New York, NY: Rugged Land; 2004.

8. Wachter RM. Playing well with others: "translocational research" in patient safety [Perspective]. *AHRQ PSNet* (serial online); September 2005. Available at: https://psnet.ahrq.gov/perspectives/perspective/9.

9. Charles D, Gabriel M, Searcy T. Adoption of Electronic Health Record Systems among U.S. Non-Federal Acute Care Hospitals: 2008-2014. ONC Data Brief, April 2015. Available at: https://www.healthit.gov/sites/default/files/data-brief/2014HospitalAdoptionDataBrief.pdf.

10. Sittig DF, Singh H. Defining health information technology–related errors. New developments since *To Err Is Human*. *Arch Intern Med* 2011;171:1281–1284.

11. Saving Lives and Saving Money: Hospital-Acquired Conditions Update. December 2015. Agency for Healthcare Research and Quality, Rockville, MD. Available at: https://www.ahrq.gov/professionals/quality-patient-safety/pfp/interimhacrate2014.html.

12. Wachter RM, Shojania KG, Saint S, et al. Learning from our mistakes: Quality Grand Rounds, a new case-based series on medical errors and patient safety. *Ann Intern Med* 2002;136:850–852.

13. Available at: https://psnet.ahrq.gov/webmm.

14. Available at: https://psnet.ahrq.gov.

AN INTRODUCTION TO PATIENT SAFETY AND MEDICAL ERRORS

THE NATURE AND FREQUENCY OF MEDICAL ERRORS AND ADVERSE EVENTS

1

ADVERSE EVENTS, PREVENTABLE ADVERSE EVENTS, AND ERRORS

Although the four words well known to every physician—"first, do no harm"—date back to Hippocrates over 2000 years ago, and many hospitals continue the time-honored tradition of hosting Morbidity and Mortality, or "M&M," conferences to discuss errors, medical errors have long been considered an inevitable by-product of modern medicine or the unfortunate detritus of bad providers. The dialogue around medical error only began to change in the past generation, most dramatically in late 1999, with the National Academy of Medicine's (NAM, formerly the Institute of Medicine, IOM) publication of the landmark report *To Err Is Human: Building a Safer Health System*.[1] This report, which estimated that 44,000 to 98,000 Americans die each year from medical mistakes, generated tremendous public and media attention, and set the stage for unprecedented efforts to improve patient safety. Of course, these seminal works built on a rich tapestry of inquiry and leadership in the field of patient safety (Appendix III), familiar to a small group of devotees but generally unknown to mainstream providers, administrators, policymakers, and patients.

The NAM death estimate, which was drawn from thousands of chart reviews in New York,[2,3] Colorado, and Utah[4] in the late 1980s and early 1990s, was followed by studies that showed huge numbers of medication errors, communication problems in intensive care units (ICUs), gaps in the discharge process, retained sponges in the operating room—in short, everywhere one looked there was evidence of major problems in patient safety. Moreover, accompanying this information in the professional literature were scores of dramatic reports in the lay media: errors involving the wrong patient going to a procedure, surgery on the wrong limb, chemotherapy overdoses, botched transplants, patients released from the emergency department (ED) only to die later from myocardial infarction or septic shock, and more (Table 1-1).

The patient safety literature contains many overlapping terms to describe safety-related issues. Although the terms sometimes confuse more than clarify, two key distinctions underlie most of the terminology and allow one to keep it relatively straight. First, because patients commonly experience adverse outcomes, it is important to distinguish adverse outcomes as a result of medical care from morbidity and mortality that patients suffer as a consequence of their underlying medical conditions. The former are known as *adverse events* or *harm* (the two terms are generally used interchangeably) and have been defined by the Institute for Healthcare Improvement as follows:

> *Unintended physical injury resulting from or contributed to by medical care (including the absence of indicated medical treatment) that requires additional monitoring, treatment, or hospitalization, or that results in death.*[5]

Second, because patients may experience harm from their medical care in the absence of any errors (i.e., from accepted complications of surgery or medication side effects), the patient safety literature separates *preventable adverse events* from *nonpreventable* ones. Figure 1-1 shows a Venn diagram depicting these various terms.

Now, where do *errors* or *mistakes* fit in? The safety literature commonly defines an error as "an act of commission (doing something wrong) or omission (failing to do the right thing) leading to an undesirable outcome or significant potential for such an outcome."[6] Note that many errors do not result in adverse events (Figure 1-1)—we generally characterize the more serious ones as "near misses" or "close calls." Note too that some errors involve care that falls below a professional standard of care—these are called *negligence* and may create legal liability or a duty to compensate the patient in some systems (Chapter 18). Finally, although most preventable adverse events involve errors, not all of them do (see "The Challenges of Measuring Errors and Safety," below).

In the early days of the patient safety movement, most of the focus was on measuring and decreasing the incidence of errors. Increasingly, safety experts prefer to highlight preventable adverse events or preventable harm—rather than errors—as the main target of the field. Framing this issue in the language of the Donabedian process–outcome–structure triad (Chapter 3),[7] one might think about harm as the "outcome" and errors as the "process." Advocates

Table 1-1	SELECTED MEDICAL ERRORS THAT GARNERED EXTENSIVE MEDIA ATTENTION IN THE UNITED STATES*		
Error	**Institution**	**Year**	**Impact**
An 18-year-old woman, Libby Zion, daughter of a prominent reporter, dies of a medical mistake, partly due to lax resident supervision	Cornell's New York Hospital	1984	Public discussion regarding resident training, supervision, and work hours. Led to New York law regarding supervision and work hours, ultimately culminating in ACGME duty hour regulations (Chapter 16)
Betsy Lehman, a *Boston Globe* healthcare reporter, dies of a chemotherapy overdose	Harvard's Dana-Farber Cancer Institute	1994	New focus on medication errors, role of ambiguity in prescriptions, and possible role of computerized prescribing and decision support (Chapters 4 and 13)
Willie King, a 51-year-old diabetic, has the wrong leg amputated	University Community Hospital, Tampa, Florida	1995	New focus on wrong-site surgery, ultimately leading to Joint Commission's Universal Protocol, and later the surgical checklist, to prevent these errors (Chapter 5)
18-month-old Josie King dies of dehydration	Johns Hopkins Hospital	2001	Josie's parents form an alliance with Johns Hopkins' leadership (leading to the Josie King Foundation and catalyzing Hopkins' safety initiatives), demonstrating the power of institutional and patient collaboration
Jesica Santillan, a 17-year-old girl from Mexico, dies after receiving a heart–lung transplant of the wrong blood type	Duke University Medical Center	2003	New focus on errors in transplantation, and on enforcing strict, high reliability protocols for communication of crucial data (Chapters 2 and 8)
The twin newborns of actor Dennis Quaid are nearly killed by a large heparin overdose	Cedars-Sinai Medical Center	2007	Renewed focus on medication errors and the potential value of bar coding to prevent prescribing errors (Chapters 4 and 13)
Rory Staunton, a 12-year-old boy, is readmitted and ultimately dies of septic shock after initially being sent home from the emergency department	New York University Langone Medical Center	2012	Emphasis on early detection and treatment of sepsis
Joan Rivers, a famous comedian, suffers cardiac arrest while undergoing laryngoscopy and endoscopy under sedation at an ambulatory center; she dies a week later	Yorkville Endoscopy LLC	2014	Raises concerns regarding the safety of performing certain procedures in the ambulatory setting as well as the need to appropriately consent patients for procedures

ACGME, Accreditation Council for Graduate Medical Education.

*Other countries have had similar errors that also helped catalyze the safety field. For example, in the United Kingdom the 2001 publication of a national inquiry into childhood deaths after surgery at the Bristol Royal Infirmary was a defining event for the patient safety movement. See Walshe K, Offen N. A very public failure: lessons for quality improvement in healthcare organizations from the Bristol Royal Infirmary. *Qual Saf Health Care* 2001;10:250–256.

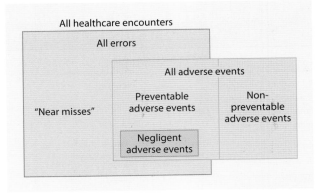

Figure 1-1 ■ Venn diagram depicting patient safety terminology.

of this approach see several advantages to it. First, focusing on adverse events removes the implication that a specific provider was responsible for the harm, which may generate defensiveness by caregivers or an inordinate focus by the organization on dealing with the individual rather than the system (Chapter 2).[8–10] Moreover, patients, quite naturally, care more about what happened to them than whether their doctor or nurse made a mistake.

Although these advocates make a valid argument, it is worth appreciating that the terms "preventable adverse events" or "preventable harm" are perhaps a bit too politically correct, lacking the visceral punch of "error" or "mistake" that helped launch the safety field. One can be sure that this vigorous debate—which has been with us since the early days of the field[11,12]—will continue. For now, patient safety's center of gravity remains adverse events/harm as the focus of measurements and interventions.

These distinctions are important to understand as one tries to wade through the safety literature or interpret individual cases. To help illustrate the point, let's consider three scenarios involving a patient with a prosthetic joint infection, who is placed appropriately on a prolonged course of intravenous vancomycin but who develops renal failure. If the renal dysfunction began while the patient's vancomycin level was being monitored at appropriate intervals and the level was felt to be in the therapeutic range, he would be said to be the victim of an adverse event (often called a *side effect* when caused by a medication), but not a preventable adverse event or a medical error. Such cases should prompt us to reevaluate the benefit-to-risk ratio of the intervention (in this patient and others like him) and to try to improve the science (i.e., identify a strategy with a comparable benefit but lower risk), but not to infer that there was a mistake in the patient's care or that the harm was preventable.

If, on the other hand, the patient developed renal failure because the vancomycin level was too high, but there was no overt error on the part of the physician (she was following standard guidelines for dosing and monitoring), the patient would be said to have suffered a *preventable adverse event*, but the case would still not be characterized as having been caused by an error. Here too, the focus should be on reassessing the benefit-to-risk ratio in this and similar patients and on improving the science, although it is worth considering systems changes (such as more frequent monitoring) that might have made a difference in this case and ones like it.

Finally, it would be a preventable adverse event *and an error* if the patient developed renal failure because the physician prescribed another antibiotic that increases the risk of nephrotoxicity in patients already on vancomycin without checking for possible drug interactions. As we'll see, rather than focusing on the failures of the individual caregiver (unless such carelessness is habitual or willful), the more productive stance will likely be to consider systems changes (a computerized order entry system with robust decision support[13]) that might prevent such errors and harm in the future.

Before leaving the area of patient safety terminology, we should add that some safety experts bristle at the distinction between preventable and nonpreventable adverse events, reminding us that certain types of harm previously thought unpreventable are now known to be preventable with better systems. Some even contend that labeling such events "nonpreventable" is defeatist and self-fulfilling. Probably the strongest support for this argument comes from the story of central line–associated bloodstream infections, which were once felt to be an inevitable by-product of modern medicine but are now known to be largely preventable with the consistent application of a "bundle" of safety practices[14] (Chapter 10). Although this point of view has considerable merit, the distinction between preventability and nonpreventability permeates the literature, and blurring it risks a public perception that all adverse events result from errors, which they do not. As one point of reference, studies of cases of harm in hospitalized patients generally find about half to have been preventable.[9,10]

This debate is likely to continue because measurement is so fundamental to our efforts to improve safety. Robust and reliable measurement is the cornerstone for conducting sound research about patient safety practices, prioritizing areas of focus for study and implementation, holding individuals and institutions accountable for performance, and assessing how we are faring in our efforts to improve safety.[8] Indeed, some literature indicates that the overall trend in adverse events has remained stable over time, despite large-scale efforts to improve safety.[15] So, although matters of terminology and measurement might seem arcane and of only marginal relevance to patients, caregivers, administrators, and policymakers, they are really quite central to the field.

THE CHALLENGES OF MEASURING ERRORS AND SAFETY

At Douglastown Hospital, the Patient Safety Officer has become concerned about the frequency of medication errors. One patient received a 10-fold overdose of insulin when the order "please give 10U regular insulin" was interpreted as "100 regular insulin." Another patient received a cephalosporin antibiotic for pneumonia, despite being allergic to this class of drugs. A third suffered a cardiac arrest due to an opioid overdose.

In response to these incidents, the hospital invested in a $50 million computerized provider order entry system. This expense meant that the hospital had to forego its planned purchase of a new 256-slice computed tomography scanner and the construction of two new operating rooms (investments with near-guaranteed positive returns on investment). The Chief Financial Officer (CFO) asks the safety officer, "How will we know that we've made a difference?"

The CFO's question seems relatively straightforward, but is much harder to answer than you might think. Let's consider various ways of measuring errors.

The most common method is through self-reports of errors by providers, usually referred to as *incident reports*. While these reports were initially completed on paper forms, they are increasingly inputted through computerized systems to facilitate aggregation of data, management of follow up, and identification of themes. Incident reports (see also Chapter 14) might seem like a reliable way of tracking errors, but there are several problems with using them to measure the frequency of errors.[16] First, although nurses tend to report errors through incident reporting systems, few doctors do,[17] either not reporting at all or reporting through informal channels (such as, in teaching programs, telling the chief residents). Second, as most reporting systems are voluntary, the frequency of reports will be influenced by many factors other than the number of errors. Let's say the institution has improved its safety culture (Chapter 15) such that reporting of errors is now strongly encouraged by local leaders and incident reports result in tangible action. Under these circumstances, an increase in incident reports might well reflect the same number of, or even fewer, errors that are simply being reported more diligently. This conundrum distinguishes measuring patient safety from measuring the quality of care, which is less dependent on voluntary reporting and thus can be done more reliably (Chapter 3).

Another method of measuring safety is through a series of *patient safety indicators* gleaned from large administrative data sets. The most widely used indicator set is the Agency for Healthcare Research and Quality's (AHRQ) Patient Safety Indicators (PSIs), comprised of 26 outcomes or processes that are plausibly related to safety[18] (Appendix V). Although AHRQ has cautioned that these indicators should only be used as clues for identifying safety problems (because they are derived from administrative data, they produce results that may be inaccurate or do not correlate very well to actual safety[19–21]), they are increasingly publicly reported, carry financial consequences for hospitals, and may impact hospital rankings and subject hospitals to media scrutiny that may not be warranted.[22–24]

Given the problem in using incident reports and administrative data to measure the frequency of errors or harm, are there other ways? One could *review charts* for evidence of errors. This, in fact, is what the Harvard Medical Practice Study investigators did as they searched for "preventable adverse events."[2–4] (Their numbers served as the foundation for the NAM's estimate of 44,000 to 98,000 deaths per year from medical error reported in *To Err Is Human*.) Unfortunately, chart review is expensive and labor intensive (this burden may be eased somewhat by electronic medical record systems, particularly if they capture data in organized ways rather than as free text or if natural language processing improves; Chapter 13), poor charting may be on the same gene as the propensity to commit errors (thus penalizing institutions and providers who document well), the medicolegal climate almost certainly induces some "buffing of the chart" after an error, and chart review is simply not a very reliable way to determine whether an error has occurred.[25] The latter problem is partly due to the inevitability of hindsight bias, in which knowledge of the final outcome influences the reviewer's determination regarding whether a given act was an error, a problem that also bedevils many malpractice investigations.[26]

Over the past several years, the use of *trigger tools* has emerged as a favored method to measure the incidence of adverse events in many healthcare settings. The most popular of these is the *Global Trigger Tool*, developed by the Institute for Healthcare Improvement. The premise behind trigger tools is that some errors in care will engender a response that can be tracked—in essence, a clue that an adverse event, or an error, may have occurred.[27] For example, the patient with a warfarin overdose may be given a dose of Vitamin K or fresh frozen plasma to counteract the excess anticoagulant, or a patient who has received too much morphine may be treated with an opiate antagonist such as naloxone. Or, a patient insufficiently observed on the medical ward may need to be transferred urgently to the ICU, another event captured by the Global Trigger Tool.

Although trigger tools can identify cases of medical errors that incident reporting- or administrative data-based systems miss, their overall effectiveness remains uncertain. While one study demonstrated reasonably good interrater reliability,[28] a more recent study found poor interrater reliability when the Global Trigger Tool was employed by five teams across five hospitals.[29]

Because many triggers do not represent errors or even true harm, they are best used as a screen, followed by more detailed chart review. The use of the Global Trigger Tool currently involves significant labor costs (largely for the follow-up chart reviews), but some of this effort may eventually be automated. It is also important to keep in mind that most of the literature on trigger tools has focused on the hospital setting; their use in the outpatient world will need further study. Selected triggers from the Global Trigger Tool are shown in Table 1-2.

Several studies have utilized the IHI Global Trigger Tool to assess the state of patient safety. The results are sobering. Landrigan and colleagues tracked the rates of adverse events of nine hospitals in North Carolina from 2003 to 2008, and found no significant improvement in harm rates during these years, despite major efforts to improve safety.[9] A study by the U.S. Office of the Inspector General (OIG) of the Department of Health and Human Services found that one in eight Medicare patients experienced a significant adverse event during their hospitalization.[10] Finally, Classen and colleagues found that approximately one in three hospitalized patients experienced an adverse event of some kind.[8] This study, which compared the test characteristics of the Global Trigger Tool with that of voluntary incident reports and the AHRQ Patient Safety Indicators, found that the former was far more sensitive and specific (Table 1-3). Table 1-4 highlights some of the advantages and disadvantages of the most common methods of measuring errors and adverse events.[30]

There are two other assessment methods that bear mention. First published in 2001 in the United Kingdom, the *hospital standardized mortality ratios* (HSMR)—a method pioneered by Professor Brian Jarman of Imperial College London—has generated significant enthusiasm. At first glance, a single risk-adjusted mortality statistic is an intuitively appealing "roll-up" measure that seems to capture many aspects of safety and quality and can be trended over time. In part because of this natural appeal to policymakers, this measure became a major focus of quality and safety efforts in the United Kingdom, and the finding of high HSMR triggered several hospital investigations.[31]

However, the HSMR was eventually criticized heavily due to inadequate risk adjustment methods as well as the low number of deaths thought to be truly preventable; indeed, Lilford and Pronovost called its use a "bad idea that won't go away."[32,33] Moreover, a 2010 study found that four different popular methods of measuring hospital mortality rates came to wildly different conclusions about hospital quality.[34]

A recent trend has been to *ask patients themselves to identify instances of harm or errors*. This too is an appealing idea, in that it grows out of a broader movement to engage patients in their own safety and respect their roles as active participants in care. Early studies demonstrated that patients are able to identify some errors missed by other assessment methods.[35,36] That said, the

Table 1-2   SELECTED TRIGGERS FROM THE INSTITUTE FOR HEALTHCARE IMPROVEMENT'S (IHI) GLOBAL TRIGGER TOOL
Care module triggers
Any code or arrest
Abrupt drop of >25% in haematocrit
Patient fall
Readmission within 30 days
Transfer to higher level of care
Surgical module triggers
Return to surgery
Intubation/reintubation in postanesthesia care unit
Intra- or postoperative death
Postoperative troponin level >1.5 ng/mL
Medication module triggers
PTT >100 s
INR >6
Rising BUN or creatinine >2 times baseline
Vitamin K administration
Narcan (Naloxone) use
Abrupt medication stop
Intensive care module triggers
Pneumonia onset
Readmission to intensive care
Intubation/reintubation
Perinatal module
Third- or fourth-degree lacerations
ED module
Readmission to ED within 48 h
Time in ED >6 h

BUN, blood urea nitrogen; ED, emergency department; PTT, partial thromboplastin time.
Reproduced with permission from Griffin FA, Resar RK. *IHI Global Trigger Tool for Measuring Adverse Events*. Cambridge, MA: Institute for Healthcare Improvement; 2009. Available at: www.IHI.org.

overall utility of this strategy, including whether placing patients in this position compromises their sense of trust in their caregivers, has not yet been fully defined. Chapter 21 delves more deeply into the role of patients in protecting their own safety.

As we've seen, there are many ways to try to measure the number of errors and cases of harm. The key point is that the frequency will vary markedly depending on the method used,[37] and a robust institutional or external

Table 1-3 SENSITIVITY AND SPECIFICITY OF THREE METHODS OF MEASURING ADVERSE EVENTS		
Method	**Sensitivity (%)**	**Specificity (%)**
Global Trigger Tool	94.9	100
AHRQ Patient Safety Indicators	5.8	98.5
Voluntary Error Reporting	0	100

From Classen DC, Resar R, Griffin F, et al. 'Global Trigger Tool' shows that adverse events in hospitals may be ten times greater than previously measured. *Health Aff (Millwood)* 2011;30:581–589.

Table 1-4 ADVANTAGES AND DISADVANTAGES OF VARIOUS STRATEGIES FOR MEASURING SAFETY AND HARM		
Measurement Strategies	**Advantages**	**Disadvantages**
Retrospective Chart Review (by itself or after use of a trigger tool)	Considered the "gold standard," contains rich detailed clinical information	Costly, labor-intensive, data quality variable due to incomplete clinical information, retrospective review only. Efficiency improved by focusing chart reviews on cases identified by a reliable trigger tool
Voluntary Incident Reporting Systems	Useful for internal quality improvement and case-finding, highlights adverse events that providers perceive as important	Capture small fraction of adverse events, retrospective review only based on provider self-reports, no standardization or uniformity of adverse events reported
Automated Surveillance	Can be used retrospectively or prospectively, helpful in screening patients who may be at high risk for adverse events using standardized protocols	Need electronic data to run automated surveillance, high proportion of "triggered" cases are false positives
Administrative/Claims Data (e.g., AHRQ Patient Safety Indicators)	Low-cost, readily available data, useful for tracking events over time across large populations, can identify "potential" adverse events	Lack detailed clinical data, concerns over variability and inaccuracy of *ICD-9-CM* codes across and within systems, may detect high proportion of false positives

Reprinted with permission from AHRQ Patient Safety Network: Rosen AK. Are we getting better at measuring patient safety? *AHRQ WebM&M* [serial online]; November 2010. Available at: https://psnet.ahrq.gov/perspectives/perspective/94.

program to assess the state of patient safety and learn from errors and adverse events will need to integrate several of these methods (Chapters 20 and 22). Shojania calls this the "elephant of patient safety," in that what you see depends on what part of the animal you're looking at.[38]

THE FREQUENCY AND IMPACT OF ERRORS

In part because of different definitions and assessment methods, various studies have shown differing rates of adverse events. Overall, while early studies[2–4] identified adverse events in approximately 1 in 10 admissions, recent ones, using the Global Trigger Tool, have found rates ranging from 1 in 8 (the OIG study[10]) to 1 in 3 (Classen et al.[8]). Whether this change represents a true increase in harm or more sensitive measures is unknown. (Interestingly, overall hospital mortality rates have fallen markedly in recent years, further highlighting the "elephant" of safety measurement.) In any case, given the substantial efforts that have gone into improving safety over the past decade, the adverse event figures remain sobering, and should cause us to redouble our efforts and to make sure that we are on the correct path.

Of course, not all adverse events are created equal: we are more concerned about adverse events that result in death or disability than those that lead to an extra day in the hospital or a delay in a test or a medication. (The caveat here, as always, is that some near misses—cases in which there was no harm at all—illustrate important systems problems and have tremendous learning value for organizations.[39]) Many safety studies use the National Coordinating Council for Medication Error Reporting and Prevention's Index for Categorizing Errors (*NCC MERP Index*), which grades errors on a scale of A to I (Figure 1-2). Most published studies focus on cases in which errors reached patients and caused harm: labeled "E" (temporary harm that requires intervention) through "I" (death). Most healthcare systems that use trigger tools or similar methods to analyze their own adverse events do the same.

Overall, although about two-thirds of adverse events cause little or no patient harm, about one-third do—ranging from minor harm (such as a prolonged hospitalization) to permanent disability (Figure 1-3). This risk is not evenly distributed—some unfortunate patients have a far higher chance of suffering a significant adverse event, and as one classic study demonstrated, these patients often experience multiple events.[40] For example, it has been estimated that the average patient in the ICU has 1.7 errors in his or her care per ICU day[41] and the average hospitalized medical patient experiences one medication error per day![42] Patients on multiple medications or on particularly risky medications (e.g., anticoagulants, opiates, insulin, and sedatives)[43,44] are more likely to be harmed, as are older patients (Figure 1-3).

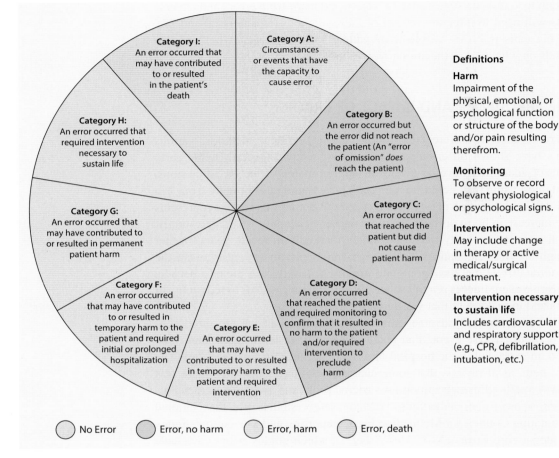

Figure 1-2 ■ The NCC MERP Index for categorizing errors. (Reprinted with permission from the National Coordinating Council for Medication Error Reporting and Prevention, © 2001. Available at: http://www.nccmerp.org/sites/default/files/indexColor2001-06-12.pdf.)

The financial impact of medical errors and adverse events is enormous. The NAM report estimated that the overall national (U.S.) cost for preventable adverse events (in the late 1990s) was between 17 billion and 29 billion dollars;[1] this estimate was essentially stable in a 2011 study.[45] Including "nonpreventable" adverse events would double these figures. As these numbers come exclusively from hospital-based studies, adding in the impact of adverse events in ambulatory clinics,[46] nursing homes and assisted living facilities,[47] and other settings would drive them still higher.

When viewed this way, it becomes difficult to argue that we cannot afford to fix the problem of medical errors. Historically, widespread fee-for-service payment systems in the United States have been part of the problem—both

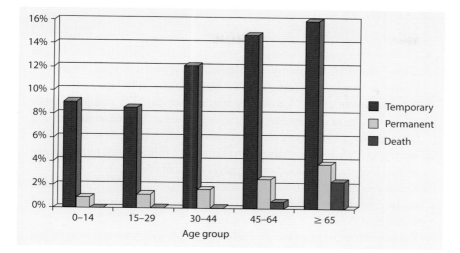

Figure 1-3 ▪ Proportion of patients experiencing an adverse event who suffer temporary (<1 year) disability, permanent disability, or death, by age group. Note that not only does the severity of harm go up with age, but so does the chance of an adverse event (in this Australian study it was approximately 10% per admission in younger patients, up to nearly 25% per admission in patients over 65). (Reproduced with permission from Weingart SN, Wilson RM, Gibberd RW, Harrison B. Epidemiology of medical error. *BMJ* 2000;320:774–777; Wilson RM, Runciman WB, Gibberd RW, Harrison BT, Newby L, Hamilton JD. The quality in Australian health care study. *Med J Aust* 1995;163:458–471.)

providers and institutions have generally been compensated (often quite handsomely) for unsafe care, with little financial incentive to make the requisite investments in safer systems. The advent of accountable care organizations (ACOs) and focus on population health management—caring for the patient across the continuum—may shift financial incentives in a way that prompts providers and institutions to invest in safety. Even in countries and organizational structures that *do* lose money from errors and harm (e.g., capitated systems such as Kaiser Permanente or the Veterans Affairs system in the United States, or the United Kingdom's National Health Service), doing the accounting to determine the "return on investment" from spending on safety is tricky.[48] Many recent policy initiatives are designed to increase the cost of errors and harm to systems, in an effort to promote investment in safety.

Yet, the largest impact of medical errors and adverse events remains the toll they take on patients and their loved ones—best measured in anxiety, harm, and deaths. Moreover, in so many cases, providers are "second victims" of unsafe systems that let them down when they most needed the support.[49] For all these reasons, the moral and ethical case for patient safety remains the most powerful motivator of all.

KEY POINTS

- The modern patient safety movement began with the publication of the National Academy of Medicine's report on medical errors, *To Err Is Human: Building a Safer Health System*, in late 1999.
- Adverse events (also known as harms) are injuries resulting from medical care, as opposed to adverse outcomes arising from underlying disease. Not all adverse events are preventable—those that are usually involve errors. In many cases, preventability relies on system changes that reduce the likelihood of the adverse events in question.
- Errors are acts of commission (doing something wrong) or omission (failing to do the right thing) leading to an undesirable outcome or significant potential for such an outcome.
- Measuring errors remains challenging. Many systems depend on voluntary reports by providers (incident reports), which detect only a small fraction of errors. Other methods, such as patient safety indicators drawn from administrative data sets, may be overly sensitive and should be augmented by detailed chart review.
- The use of the Global Trigger Tool—seeking clues about a possible adverse event, followed by detailed chart review—has become increasingly popular in recent years, in keeping with a shift in focus from errors to adverse events as targets for measurement and interventions.
- From a variety of studies, at least 1 in 10 (perhaps as high as 1 in 3) hospital admissions is marred by an adverse event, and about half of these are preventable. About one-third of these adverse events cause true patient harm.

| REFERENCES

1. Kohn L, Corrigan J, Donaldson M, eds. *To Err Is Human: Building a Safer Health System*. Washington, DC: Committee on Quality of Health Care in America, Institute of Medicine: National Academies Press; 1999.
2. Brennan TA, Leape LL, Laird NM, et al. Incidence of adverse events and negligence in hospitalized patients. Results of the Harvard Medical Practice Study I. *N Engl J Med* 1991;324:370–376.
3. Leape LL, Brennan TA, Laird N, et al. The nature of adverse events and negligence in hospitalized patients. Results of the Harvard Medical Practice Study II. *N Engl J Med* 1991;324:377–384.
4. Thomas EJ, Studdert DM, Burstin HR, et al. Incidence and types of adverse events and negligent care in Utah and Colorado. *Med Care* 2000;38:261–271.

5. Available at: http://www.IHI.org.

6. Available at: https://psnet.ahrq.gov/glossary/e.

7. Donabedian A. The quality of care. How can it be assessed? *JAMA* 1988;260:1743–1748.

8. Classen DC, Resar R, Griffin F, et al. 'Global Trigger Tool' shows that adverse events in hospitals may be ten times greater than previously measured. *Health Aff (Millwood)* 2011;30:581–589.

9. Landrigan CP, Parry GJ, Bones CB, Hackbarth AD, Goldmann DA, Sharek PJ. Temporal trends in rates of patient harm resulting from medical care. *N Engl J Med* 2010;363:2124–2134.

10. Levinson DR. *Adverse Events in Hospitals: National Incidence Among Medicare Beneficiaries.* Washington, DC: US Department of Health and Human Services, Office of the Inspector General; November 2010. Report No. OEI-06-09-00090.

11. Layde PM, Maas LA, Teret SP, et al. Patient safety efforts should focus on medical injuries. *JAMA* 2002;287:1993–1997.

12. McNutt RA, Abrams R, Aron DC, et al. Patient safety efforts should focus on medical errors. *JAMA* 2002;287:1997–2001.

13. Classen DC, Phansalkar S, Bates DW. Critical drug–drug interactions for use in electronic health records systems with computerized physician order entry: review of leading approaches. *J Patient Saf* 2011;7:61–65.

14. Latif A, Halim MS, Pronovost PJ. Eliminating infections in the ICU: CLABSI. *Curr Infect Dis Rep* 2015;17:491.

15. Shojana KG, Thomas EJ. Trends in adverse events over time: why are we not improving? *BMJ Qual Saf* 2013;22:273–277.

16. Shojania KG. The frustrating case of incident-reporting systems. *Qual Saf Health Care* 2008;17:400–402.

17. Rowin EJ, Lucier D, Pauker SG, et al. Does error and adverse event reporting by physicians and nurses differ? *Jt Comm J Qual Patient Saf* 2008;34:537–545.

18. Available at: http://www.qualityindicators.ahrq.gov/Modules/PSI_TechSpec.aspx.

19. Isaac T, Jha AK. Are Patient Safety Indicators related to widely used measures of hospital quality? *J Gen Intern Med* 2008;23:1373–1378.

20. Romano PS, Mull HJ, Rivard PE, et al. Validity of selected AHRQ Patient Safety Indicators based on VA National Surgical Quality Improvement program data. *Health Serv Res* 2009;44:182–204.

21. White RH, Sadeghi B, Tancredi D, et al. How valid is the ICD-9-CM based AHRQ Patient Safety Indicator for postoperative venous thromboembolism? *Med Care* 2009;47:1237–1243.

22. Kubasiak JC, Francescatti AB, Behal R, Myers JA. Patient Safety Indicators for judging hospital performance: still not ready for prime time. *Am J Med Qual* 2017;32:129–133.

23. Winters BD, Bharmal A, Wilson RF, et al. Validity of the Agency for Health Care Research and Quality Patient Safety Indicators and the Centers for Medicare and Medicaid Hospital-acquired Conditions: a systematic review and meta-analysis. *Med Care* 2016;54:1105–1111.

24. Rajaram R, Barnard C, Bilimoria KY. Concerns about using the patient safety indicator-90 composite in pay-for-performance programs. *JAMA* 2015;313:897–898.

25. Thomas EJ, Lipsitz SR, Studdert DM, Brennan TA. The reliability of medical record review for estimating adverse event rates. *Ann Intern Med* 2002;136:812–816.

26. Caplan RA, Posner KL, Cheney FW. Effect of outcome on physician judgments of appropriateness of care. *JAMA* 1991;265:1957–1960.

27. Classen DC, Lloyd RC, Provost L, Griffin FA, Resar R. Development and evaluation of the Institute for Healthcare Improvement global trigger tool. *J Patient Saf* 2008;4:169–177.

28. Sharek PJ, Parry G, Goldmann D, et al. Performance characteristics of a methodology to quantify adverse events over time in hospitalized patients. *Health Serv Res* 2011;46:654–678.

29. Schildmeijer K, Nilsson L, Arestedt K, Perk J. Assessment of adverse events in medical care: lack of consistency between experienced teams using the global trigger tool. *BMJ Qual Saf* 2012;21:307–314.

30. Rosen AK. Are we getting any better at measuring patient safety? *AHRQ WebM&M* [serial online]; November 2010. Available at: http://webmm.ahrq.gov/perspective. aspx?perspectiveID=94.

31. Bottle A, Jarman B, Aylin P. Strengths and weaknesses of hospital standardised mortality ratios. *BMJ* 2011;342:c7116.

32. Lilford R, Pronovost P. Using hospital mortality rates to judge hospital performance: a bad idea that just won't go away. *BMJ* 2010;340:955–957.

33. Hogan H, Zipfel R, Neuburger J, Hutchings A, Darzi A, Black N. Avoidability of hospital deaths and association with hospital-wide mortality ratios: retrospective case record review and regression analysis. *BMJ* 2015;351:h3239.

34. Shahian DM, Wolf RE, Iezzoni LI, Kirle L, Normand SL. Variability in the measurement of hospital-wide mortality rates. *N Engl J Med* 2010; 363:2530–2539.

35. Weissman JS, Schneider EC, Weingart SN, et al. Comparing patient-reported hospital adverse events with medical record review: do patients know something that hospitals do not? *Ann Intern Med* 2008;149:100–108.

36. Zhu J, Stuver SO, Epstein AM, Schneider EC, Weissman JS, Weingart SN. Can we rely on patients' reports of adverse events? *Med Care* 2011; 49:948–955.

37. Levtzion-Korach O, Frankel A, Alcalai H, et al. Integrating incident data from five reporting systems to assess patient safety: making sense of the elephant. *Jt Comm J Qual Patient Saf* 2010;36:402–410.

38. Shojania KG. The elephant of patient safety: what you see depends on how you look. *Jt Comm J Qual Patient Saf* 2010;36:399–401, AP1–AP3.

39. Wu AW, ed. *The Value of Close Calls in Improving Patient Safety*. Oakbrook Terrace, IL: Joint Commission Resources; 2011.

40. Weingart SN, Wilson RM, Gibberd RW, Harrison B. Epidemiology of medical error. *BMJ* 2000;320:774–777.

41. Donchin Y, Gopher D, Olin M, et al. A look into the nature and causes of human errors in the intensive care unit. *Crit Care Med* 1995;23:294–300.

42. Aspden P, Wolcott J, Bootman JL, et al., eds. *Preventing Medication Errors: Quality Chasm Series. Committee on Identifying and Preventing Medication Errors*. Washington, DC: National Academies Press; 2007.

43. Kanjanarat P, Winterstein AG, Johns TE, Hatton RC, Gonzalez-Rothi R, Segal R. Nature of preventable adverse drug events in hospitals: a literature review. *Am J Health Syst Pharm* 2003;60:1750–1759.

44. Bates DW, Boyle D, Vander Vliet M, Schneider J, Leape L. Relationship between medication errors and adverse drug events. *J Gen Intern Med* 1995;10:199–205.

45. Van Den Bos J, Rustagi K, Gray T, Halford M, Ziemkiewicz E, Shreve J. The $17.1 billion problem: the annual cost of measurable medical errors. *Health Aff (Millwood)* 2011;30:596–603.

46. Sarkar U, Wachter RM, Schroeder SA, Schillinger D. Refocusing the lens: patient safety in ambulatory chronic disease care. *Jt Comm J Qual Patient Saf* 2009;35:377–383.

47. Young HM, Gray SL, McCormick WC, et al. Types, prevalence, and potential clinical significance of medication administration errors in assisted living. *J Am Geriatr Soc* 2008;56:1199–1205.

48. Weeks WB, Bagian JP. Making the business case for patient safety. *Jt Comm J Qual Saf* 2003;29:51–54.

49. Wu AW. Medical error: the second victim. *West J Med* 2000;172:358–359.

ADDITIONAL READINGS

Advances in Patient Safety: New Directions and Alternative Approaches. Rockville, MD: Agency for Healthcare Research and Quality; July 2008. AHRQ Publication Nos. 080034 (1–4).

Hilfiker D. Facing our mistakes. *N Engl J Med* 1984;310:118–122.

Howell AM, Burns EM, Hull L, Mayer E, Sevdalis N, Darzi A. International recommendations for national patient safety incident reporting systems: an expert Delphi consensus-building process. *BMJ Qual Saf* 2017;26:150–163.

Jha A, Pronovost P. Toward a safer health care system: the critical need to improve measurement. *JAMA* 2016;315:1831–1832.

Macrae C. The problem with incident reporting. *BMJ Qual Saf* 2016;25:71–75.

Millman EA, Pronovost PJ, Makary MA, Wu AW. Patient-assisted incident reporting: including the patient in patient safety. *J Patient Saf* 2011;7:106–108.

Mitchell I, Schuster A, Smith K, Pronovost P, Wu A. Patient safety incident reporting: a qualitative study of thoughts and perceptions of experts 15 years after 'To Err is Human.' *BMJ Qual Saf* 2016;25:92–99.

Murff HJ, FitzHenry F, Matheny ME, et al. Automated identification of postoperative complications within an electronic medical record using natural language processing. *JAMA* 2011;306:848–855.

Parry G, Cline A, Goldmann D. Deciphering harm measurement. *JAMA* 2012;307: 2155–2156.

Pronovost PJ, Cleeman JI, Wright D, Srinivasan A. Fifteen years after To Err is Human: a success story to learn from. *BMJ Qual Saf* 2016;25:396–399.

Pronovost PJ, Colantuoni E. Measuring preventable harm: helping science keep pace with policy. *JAMA* 2009; 301:1273–1275.

Pronovost PJ, Lilford R. Analysis and commentary: a road map for improving the performance of performance measures. *Health Aff (Millwood)* 2011;30:569–573.

Rosenthal MM, Sutcliffe KM, eds. *Medical Error: What Do We Know? What Do We Do?* San Francisco, CA: Jossey-Bass; 2002.

Spath PL, ed. *Error Reduction in Health Care: A Systems Approach to Improving Patient Safety.* 2nd ed. San Francisco, CA: Jossey-Bass; 2011.

Stavropoulou C, Doherty C, Tosey P. How effective are incident-reporting systems for improving patient safety? *Milbank Quarterly* 2015;93:826–866.

Thomas EJ, Classen DC. Patient safety: let's measure what matters. *Ann Intern Med* 2014;160:642–643.

Thomas EJ, Studdert DM, Newhouse JP, et al. Costs of medical injuries in Utah and Colorado. *Inquiry* 1999;36:255–264.

Vincent C. *Patient Safety*. 2nd ed. London: Elsevier; 2010.

Vincent C, Amalberti R. *Safer Healthcare: Strategies for the Real World*. New York, NY: SpringerOpen; 2016.

BASIC PRINCIPLES OF PATIENT SAFETY | 2

THE MODERN APPROACH TO PATIENT SAFETY: SYSTEMS THINKING AND THE SWISS CHEESE MODEL

Historically, the approach to medical errors had been to blame the provider delivering care to the patient, the one acting at what is sometimes called the "sharp end" of care: the surgeon performing the transplant operation or the internist working up a patient's chest pain, the nurse hanging the intravenous medication bag, or the pharmacist preparing the chemotherapy. Over the last two decades, we have recognized that this approach overlooks the fact that most errors are committed unintentionally by hardworking, well-trained individuals, and such errors are unlikely to be prevented by simply admonishing people to be more careful, or worse, by shaming, firing, or suing them.

The current approach to patient safety replaces "the blame and shame game" with *systems thinking*—a paradigm that acknowledges the human condition—namely, that humans err—and concludes that safety depends on creating systems that anticipate errors and either prevent or catch them before they cause harm. While such an approach has long been the cornerstone of safety improvements in other high-risk industries, systems thinking had been ignored in medicine until more recently.

British psychologist James Reason's "Swiss cheese model" of organizational accidents has been widely embraced as a mental model for system safety[1,2] (Figure 2-1). This model, drawn from innumerable accident investigations in fields such as commercial aviation and nuclear power, emphasizes that in complex organizations, a single "sharp-end" (the person in the control booth in the nuclear plant, the surgeon making the incision) error is rarely enough to cause harm. Instead, such errors must penetrate multiple incomplete layers of protection ("layers of Swiss cheese") to cause a devastating result. Reason's model highlights the need to focus less on the (futile) goal of trying to perfect human behavior and suggests that greater effort be directed at shrinking the holes in the Swiss cheese (sometimes referred to as

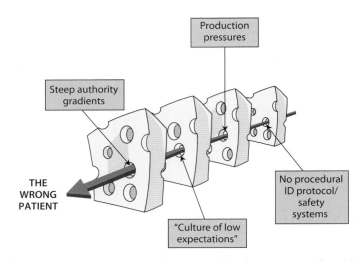

Figure 2-1 ■ James Reason's Swiss cheese model of organizational accidents. The analysis is of "The Wrong Patient" case in Chapter 15. (Reproduced with permission from Reason JT. *Human Error*. New York, NY: Cambridge University Press; 1990. Copyright © 1990 Cambridge University Press.)

latent errors) by creating multiple overlapping layers of protection to decrease the probability that the holes will ever align and allow an error to result in harm.

The Swiss cheese model emphasizes that analyses of medical errors need to focus on their "root causes"—not just the smoking gun, sharp-end error, but all the underlying conditions that made an error possible (or, in some situations, inevitable) (Chapter 14). A number of investigators have developed schema for categorizing the root causes of errors; the most widely used, by Charles Vincent, is shown in Table 2-1.[3,4] The schema explicitly forces those reviewing the error to think about contributing factors and to ask, for example, whether there should have been a checklist or read back required for a particular process, whether the resident was too fatigued to think clearly, or whether the young nurse was too intimidated to speak up when she suspected an error.

ERRORS AT THE SHARP END: SLIPS VERSUS MISTAKES

Even though we now understand that the root cause of hundreds of thousands of errors each year lies at the "blunt end," the proximate cause *is* often an act committed (or neglected, or performed incorrectly) by a provider. Even as we continue to embrace the systems approach as the most useful paradigm, it would be shortsighted not to tackle these human errors simultaneously. After all, even a room filled with flammable gas will not explode unless someone strikes a match.

Table 2-1	CHARLES VINCENT'S FRAMEWORK FOR CATEGORIZING THE ROOT CAUSES OF ERRORS	
Framework	**Contributory Factors**	**Examples of Problems That Contribute to Errors**
Institutional	Regulatory context Medicolegal environment	Insufficient priority given by regulators to safety issues; legal pressures against open discussion, preventing the opportunity to learn from adverse events
Organization and management	Financial resources and constraints Policy standards and goals Safety culture and priorities	Lack of awareness of safety issues on the part of senior management; policies leading to inadequate staffing levels
Work environment	Staffing levels and mix of skills Patterns in workload and shifts Design, availability, and maintenance of equipment Administrative and managerial support	Heavy workloads, leading to fatigue; limited access to essential equipment; inadequate administrative support, leading to reduced time with patients
Team	Verbal communication Written communication Supervision and willingness to seek help Team leadership	Poor supervision of junior staff; poor communication among different professions; unwillingness of junior staff to seek assistance
Individual staff member	Knowledge and skills Motivation and attitude Physical and mental health	Lack of knowledge or experience; long-term fatigue and stress
Task	Availability and use of protocols Availability and accuracy of test results	Unavailability of test results or delay in obtaining them; lack of clear protocols and guidelines
Patient	Complexity and seriousness of condition Language and communication Personality and social factors	Distress; language barriers between patients and caregivers

Reproduced with permission from Vincent C. Understanding and responding to adverse events. *N Engl J Med* 2003;348:1051–1056; Vincent C, Taylor-Adams S, Stanhope N. Framework for analysing risk and safety in clinical medicine. *BMJ* 1998; 316:1154–1157.

When analyzing human errors, it is useful to distinguish "slips" from "mistakes." To do so, one must appreciate the difference between *conscious* behavior and *automatic* behavior. Conscious behavior is what we do when we "pay attention" to a task, and is especially important when we are doing something new, like learning to play the piano for the first time. On the other hand, automatic behaviors are the things we do almost unconsciously. While these tasks may have required a lot of thought initially, after a while we do them virtually "in our sleep." Humans prefer automatic behaviors because they take less energy, have predictable outcomes, and allow us to "multitask"—like drinking coffee while driving a car. However, some behaviors that feel automatic may require conscious thought. For example, when a doctor tries to write a "routine" prescription while simultaneously pondering the differential diagnosis for a challenging patient, he is at risk, both for making errors in the routine, automatic process of writing the prescription ("slips") and in the conscious process of determining the diagnosis ("mistakes").

Now that we've distinguished the two types of tasks, let's turn to slips versus mistakes. *Slips* are inadvertent, unconscious lapses in the performance of some automatic task: you absently drive to work on Sunday morning because your automatic behavior kicks in and dictates your actions. Slips occur most often when we put an activity on "autopilot" so we can manage new sensory inputs, think through a problem, or deal with emotional upset, fatigue, or stress (a pretty good summing up of most healthcare environments). *Mistakes*, on the other hand, result from incorrect choices. Rather than blundering into them while we are distracted, we usually make mistakes because of insufficient knowledge, lack of experience or training, inadequate information (or inability to interpret available information properly), or applying the wrong set of rules or algorithms to a decision (we'll delve into this area more deeply when we discuss diagnostic errors in Chapter 6).

When measured on an "errors per action" yardstick, conscious behaviors are more prone to mistakes than automatic behaviors are prone to slips. However, slips probably represent the greater threat to patient safety because so much of what healthcare providers do is automatic. Doctors and nurses are most likely to slip while doing something they have done correctly a thousand times: asking patients if they are allergic to any medications before prescribing an antibiotic, remembering to verify a patient's identity before sending her off to a procedure, or loading a syringe with heparin (and not insulin) before flushing an IV line (the latter two cases are described in Chapters 15 and 4, respectively).

The complexity of healthcare work adds to the risks. Like pilots, soldiers, and others trained to work in high-risk occupations, doctors and nurses are programmed to do many specific tasks, under pressure, with a high degree of accuracy. But unlike most other professions, medical jobs typically combine three very different types of tasks: lots of conscious behaviors (complex decisions, judgment calls), many "customer" interactions, and innumerable automatic behaviors. Physician training, in particular, has traditionally emphasized the highly cognitive aspects of clinical practice, has focused less on the human interactions, and, until recently, has completely ignored the importance and riskiness of automatic behaviors.

With all of this in mind, how then should we respond to the inevitability of slips? Historically, the typical response would have been to reprimand (if not fire) a nurse for giving the wrong medication, admonishing her to "be more careful next time!" Even if the nurse tried to be more careful, she would be just as likely to commit a different error while automatically carrying out a different task in a different setting. As James Reason reminds us, "Errors are largely unintentional. It is very difficult for management to control what people did not intend to do in the first place."[2]

And it is not just managers whose instinct is to blame the provider at the sharp end—we providers blame ourselves! When we make a slip—a stupid error in something that we usually do perfectly "in our sleep"—we feel embarrassed. We chastise ourselves harder than any supervisor could, and swear we'll never make a careless mistake like that again.[5] Realistically, though, such promises are almost impossible to keep.

Whatever the strategy employed to prevent slips (and they will be discussed throughout the book), a clear lesson is that boring, repetitive tasks can be dangerous and are often performed better by machines. In medicine, these tasks include monitoring a patient's oxygen level during a long surgery, suturing large wounds, holding surgical retractors steady for a long time, and scanning mountains of data for significant patterns. As anesthesiologist Alan Merry and legal scholar and novelist Alexander McCall Smith have observed:

> *people have no need to apologize for their failure to achieve machine-like standards in those activities for which machines are better suited. They are good at other things—original thought, for one, empathy and compassion for another . . . It is true that people are distractible—but in fact this provides a major survival advantage for them. A machine (unless expressly designed to detect such an event) will continue with its repetitive task while the house burns down around it, whereas most humans will notice that something unexpected is going on and will change their activity . . .*[6]

COMPLEXITY THEORY AND COMPLEX ADAPTIVE SYSTEMS

The decisions made and actions taken by individual doctors and nurses occur in the context of the structure, policies, and culture of their organizations and healthcare systems. We will explore these issues later in this book because appreciating this context is often the key to improving safety. For now, as we think about mental models relevant to safety, it is worth introducing the topic of complexity theory.[7]

You'll recall that we referred to complexity earlier when discussing many of the decisions that frontline caregivers need to make every day. But another type of complexity—that of the entire ecosystem of care—is also at play when we consider patient safety. *Complexity theory* is a branch of management thinking which holds that large organizations don't operate like predictable and static machines, in which Inputs A and B predictably lead to Result C. Rather, they operate as *complex adaptive systems*, with elements of unpredictability, codependancy, and nonlinearity that must be appreciated as we try to make them work better.[8]

Complexity theory divides decisions and problems into three general categories: simple, complicated, and complex.[9] *Simple* problems are ones in which the inputs and outputs are known and the inherent risk is minimal; solutions can be achieved by following a recipe or a set of rules. Baking a cake is a simple problem, as is choosing the right antibiotics to treat pyelonephritis. *Complicated* decisions involve substantial uncertainties and increased risk: the solutions may not be readily apparent, but they are potentially knowable. An example is designing a rocket ship to fly to the moon—if you were working for NASA in 1962 and heard President Kennedy declare this as a national goal, you probably believed it was not going to be easy but, with enough brainpower and resources, it could be done. Finally, *complex* decisions are likened to raising a child; they bear the highest level of risk. Although we may have a general sense of what works, the actual formula for success is, alas, unknowable (or certainly seems so most days!).

In a recent book, safety experts Charles Vincent and Rene Amalberti present a model describing three contrasting approaches to safety based on the inherent risk within a particular industry[10] (Figure 2-2). For example, "ultra safe" industries, such as civil aviation and certain areas of medicine (e.g., blood transfusions), are characterized as avoiding risk. These industries tend to grant significant authority to regulatory bodies and supervisors, leaving little room for frontline workers to deviate from routine operations. In the middle are "high reliability" industries. Examples here include oil, marine, and shipping, as well as elective surgery within medicine, areas that involve some degree of risk but achieve safety by granting authority to the groups and teams directly responsible for the work who "prepare and rehearse flexible routines for the management of hazards."

Finally, the third approach to safety is seen in industries the authors term "ultra adaptive"—ones in which embracing risk is the essence of what the professionals in the industry do. Examples here include deep-sea fishing, the military during times of war, and, within healthcare, the treatment of rare cancers and trauma. These industries grant significant authority to experts who rely on personal knowledge and experience and must be aware of their own limitations. Vincent and Amalberti acknowledge that, while the model described in

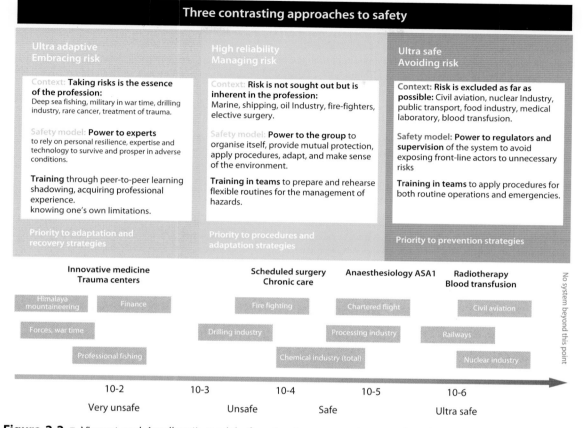

Three contrasting approaches to safety

Ultra adaptive
Embracing risk

Context: **Taking risks is the essence of the profession:**
Deep sea fishing, military in war time, drilling industry, rare cancer, treatment of trauma.

Safety model: **Power to experts** to rely on personal resilience, expertise and technology to survive and prosper in adverse conditions.

Training through peer-to-peer learning shadowing, acquiring professional experience.
knowing one's own limitations.

Priority to adaptation and recovery strategies

High reliability
Managing risk

Context: **Risk is not sought out but is inherent in the profession:**
Marine, shipping, oil Industry, fire-fighters, elective surgery.

Safety model: **Power to the group** to organise itself, provide mutual protection, apply procedures, adapt, and make sense of the environment.

Training in teams to prepare and rehearse flexible routines for the management of hazards.

Priority to procedures and adaptation strategies

Ultra safe
Avoiding risk

Context: **Risk is excluded as far as possible:** Civil aviation, nuclear Industry, public transport, food industry, medical laboratory, blood transfusion.

Safety model: **Power to regulators and supervision** of the system to avoid exposing front-line actors to unnecessary risks

Training in teams to apply procedures for both routine operations and emergencies.

Priority to prevention strategies

Innovative medicine
Trauma centers

Scheduled surgery
Chronic care

Anaesthesiology ASA1

Radiotherapy
Blood transfusion

No system beyond this point

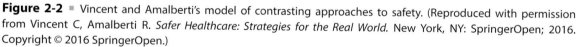

Himalaya mountaineering | Finance

Fire fighting | Chartered flight | Civil aviation

Forces, war time | Drilling industry | Processing industry | Railways

Professional fishing | Chemical industry (total) | Nuclear industry

| 10-2 | 10-3 | 10-4 | 10-5 | 10-6 |

Very unsafe | Unsafe | Safe | Ultra safe

Figure 2-2 ■ Vincent and Amalberti's model of contrasting approaches to safety. (Reproduced with permission from Vincent C, Amalberti R. *Safer Healthcare: Strategies for the Real World.* New York, NY: SpringerOpen; 2016. Copyright © 2016 SpringerOpen.)

Figure 2-2 presents neatly divided categories, the reality is that many industries have some tasks and jobs that are ultra safe and others that are extremely risky. Perhaps no industry illustrates this level of variation more than healthcare.[10]

Understanding the differences in risk is vital because to achieve safety we need to match our approaches to the types of problems at hand. A checklist may be a wonderful solution for a simple problem, but a distraction for a complex one. Enacting a series of rules and policies may seem like progress, but may actually set us back if doing so stifles innovation and collegial exchange among frontline workers. Sometimes the best approach to a complex problem is to test an intervention that seems sensible, to measure the impact (making sure workers feel able to speak truthfully and staying attuned to unanticipated consequences), and to repeat this cycle many times.

Table 2-2	SOME KEY PRINCIPLES AND ASSUMPTIONS DRAWN FROM COMPLEXITY THEORY AND THE STUDY OF COMPLEX ADAPTIVE SYSTEMS

- Relationships between parts are more important than the parts themselves.
- Neither the system nor its external environment is, or ever will be, constant—emergence and natural creativity are the norm. Equilibrium is actually an unhealthy state.
- Individuals within a system are independent and creative decision makers and highly interdependent.
- Uncertainty and paradox are inherent within the system.
- Problems cannot be solved like a machine can solve something, but they can nevertheless be "moved forward" if you understand the patterns that are creating them.
- Effective solutions can emerge from minimum specifications or simple rules rather than overspecification.
- Small changes can have big effects (nonlinearity).
- Behavior exhibits patterns (that can be termed "attractors").
- Change is more easily adopted when it taps into attractor patterns.

Reproduced with permission from Tamarack—an institute for community engagement. Complexity—a conversation with Brenda Zimmerman. Available at: http://webcache.googleusercontent.com/search? q=cache:PWV-ns_hMtcJ:www.outcomemapping.ca/download/simonhearn_en_Complexity__a_conversation_with_Brenda_Zimmerman__2005_155.doc+&cd=1&hl=en&ct=clnk&gl=us.

But, as organizational expert Paul Plsek points out, our recognition of the complexity of healthcare systems is not a call for chaos. "A somewhat surprising finding from research on complex adaptive systems," he writes, "is that relatively simple rules can lead to complex, emergent, innovative system behavior."[8] Atul Gawande expands on this point in *The Checklist Manifesto*.[9] By specifying a few behaviors and encouraging cross-talk among frontline caregivers, a good checklist can lead to remarkable improvements that go well beyond adherence to the items on the list (Chapter 15).

Table 2-2 presents a distillation of some of the key lessons from studies of complex adaptive systems. We'll return to these issues several times over the course of the book, such as when we discuss culture and High Reliability Organizations (Chapter 15) and consider how to build strong institutional patient safety programs (Chapter 22).

GENERAL PRINCIPLES OF PATIENT SAFETY IMPROVEMENT STRATEGIES

Drawing on these mental models, today's patient safety field emphasizes the need to shore up systems to prevent or catch errors rather than to create "goof-proof" individual providers. For example, errors in routine behaviors ("slips") can best be prevented by *building in redundancies and cross checks*, in the form of checklists, read backs ("let me read your order back to you"), and other standardized safety practices (e.g., signing the surgical site prior to an operation, asking patients their name before medication administration). These models also emphasize the need for *standardization and simplification*. For example, standardizing the process of taking a patient to the magnetic resonance imaging scanner makes it far easier to "bake in" the correct safety procedures.

Recently, there has been increased emphasis on decreasing errors at the person–machine interface through the use of *forcing functions*—engineering solutions that lower the probability of human error. The classic example outside medicine was the 1980s-era modifications to automobile braking systems that rendered it impossible to place a car in reverse when the driver's foot is off the brake. In healthcare, one famous forcing function was to change the gas nozzles and connectors so that anesthesiologists could not mistakenly hook up the wrong gas to a patient. Given the ever-increasing complexity of modern medicine, building in such forcing functions in devices and technologies such as intravenous pumps, cardiac defibrillators, mechanical ventilators, and computerized order entry systems is crucial to safety (Chapter 7).

In addition to systems enhancements, there has been a growing recognition of the importance of improving communication and teamwork. Commercial pilots all participate in "crew resource management" courses in which they train for emergencies with other crew, learning to encourage open dialogue, communicate clearly using standard language, and utilize checklists, debriefings, and other systemic approaches. The evidence that such training enhances patient safety is persuasive.[11] The term "culture of safety" is used as shorthand to describe an environment in which teamwork, clear communication, and openness about errors (both to other healthcare professionals and to patients) are operative (Chapter 15).

Another key patient safety principle is to *learn from one's mistakes*. This may take multiple forms. Safe systems have a culture in which errors are openly discussed, often in morbidity and mortality (M&M) conferences. There is a new push to make sure that such discussions include members of the appropriate disciplines (such as nursing and hospital administration, not just physicians), point out errors rather than gloss over them in the name of avoiding a punitive atmosphere, and emphasize systems thinking and solutions.[12,13] In addition to open discussions at conferences, safe organizations build in mechanisms to hear about errors from frontline staff, often via incident reporting systems or unit-based safety teams,[13,14] and to perform detailed ("root cause") analyses[15] of major errors ("sentinel events") in an effort to define all the "layers of Swiss cheese" that need attention (Chapter 14). They also recognize the realities of complex adaptive systems: overmanaging workers through boatloads of top-down, prescriptive rules and directives may be more unsafe than tolerating some degree of flexibility and experimentation on the frontlines. In recent years, organizations that excel in learning from their experience are often described as *Learning Healthcare Systems*.

Finally, there is increasing appreciation of the importance of a *well-trained, well-staffed, and well-rested workforce* in delivering safe care. There is now evidence linking low nurse-to-patient ratios, long work hours, and lack of board certification to poor patient outcomes (Chapter 16).[16–20] Such research is catalyzing a more holistic view of patient safety, recognizing that the implementation of "safer systems" will not create safe patient care if the providers are overextended, poorly trained, or undersupervised. Nor is "systems thinking" an excuse to allow caregivers or their leaders to remain unaccountable for failing to follow appropriate and well-vetted safety rules (Chapter 19).[21]

This long list of potential approaches to improving safety (each of which will be discussed in greater detail later) highlights one of the great challenges in the field: in the absence of comparative evidence, and in light of the high cost of some of the interventions (e.g., improved staffing, computerized order entry, simulation, teamwork training), even organizations committed to safety can become bewildered as they consider which approach to emphasize.[22] Institutions quite naturally focus on the practices that are measured, publicly reported, and compensated. As the next chapter will show, such a prioritization scheme will tend to elevate quality improvement strategies over those focused on patient safety because the results of the former are easier to measure. Thankfully, many of the approaches to improving quality, such as computerization and standardization, should also yield safety benefits.

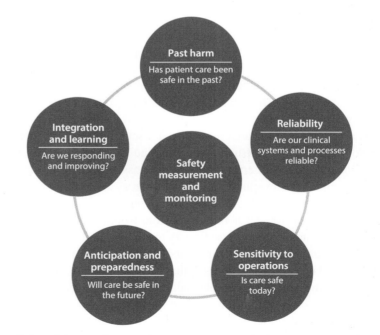

Figure 2-3 ▪ Framework to guide organizations seeking to measure and improve patient safety. (Reproduced with permission from Vincent C, Burnett S, Carthey J. Safety measurement and monitoring in healthcare: a framework to guide clinical teams and healthcare organisations in maintaining safety. *BMJ Qual Saf* 2014;23:670–677.)

On the other hand, because improving culture is both difficult and hard to measure, it risks being shuffled to the bottom of the deck, notwithstanding its importance to patient safety. Acknowledging that measurement of harm is flawed, Vincent, Burnett, and Carthey have outlined a framework for organizations to assess patient safety across five dimensions[23] (Figure 2-3 and Table 2-3).

Table 2-3 ASSESSING THE FIVE DIMENSIONS OF SAFETY	
Dimension	**Illustrative Measures and Assessments**
Harm	Case record review Global trigger tool National audits Patient safety indicators Rates of surgical complications Incidence of falls Incidence of pressure ulcers Mortality and morbidity
Reliability of safety critical processes	Observation of safety critical behavior Audit of equipment availability Monitoring of vital signs Monitoring of stroke care bundles Venous thromboembolism risk assessment Assessment of suicide risk
Sensitivity to operations	Safety walk-rounds and conversations Talking to patients Ward rounds and routine reviews of patients and working conditions Briefings and debriefings Observation and conversations with clinical teams Real-time monitoring and feedback in anesthesia
Anticipation and preparedness	Structured reflection Risk registers Human reliability analysis Safety cases Safety culture assessment Anticipated staffing levels and skill mix
Integration and learning	Aggregate analysis of incidents and complaints Feedback and implementation of safety lessons by clinical teams Regular integration and review by clinical teams and general practice Whole system suites of safety metrics, for example, web-enabled portal's clinical unit level Population level analyses of safety metrics

Reproduced with permission from Vincent C, Burnett S, Carthey J. Safety measurement and monitoring in healthcare: a framework to guide clinical teams and healthcare organisations in maintaining safety. *BMJ Qual Saf* 2014;23:670–677.

KEY POINTS

- The modern approach to patient safety is based on "systems thinking"— a recognition that most errors are made by competent, careful, and caring providers, and preventing these errors often involves embedding providers in a system that anticipates glitches and catches them before they do harm.
- James Reason's "Swiss cheese model" is the dominant paradigm for understanding the relationship between active ("sharp end") errors and latent ("blunt end") errors; it is important to resist the temptation to focus solely on the former and neglect the latter.
- A variety of strategies should be employed to create safer systems, including simplification, standardization, building in redundancies, improving teamwork and communication, and learning from past mistakes.
- There is a growing appreciation of the complexity of healthcare delivery organizations, which are vivid examples of complex adaptive systems. Such systems rarely respond in linear, predictable ways to prescriptive policies. This means that efforts to improve safety must combine rules and standards with messier activities that account for the importance of culture, innovation, and iterative learning.

REFERENCES

1. Reason JT. *Human Error*. New York, NY: Cambridge University Press; 1990.
2. Reason JT. *Managing the Risks of Organizational Accidents*. Aldershot, Hampshire, England: Ashgate; 1997.
3. Vincent C. Understanding and responding to adverse events. *N Engl J Med* 2003;348:1051–1056.
4. Vincent C, Taylor-Adams S, Stanhope N. Framework for analysing risk and safety in clinical medicine. *BMJ* 1998;316:1154–1157.
5. Harrison R, Lawton R, Perlo J, Gardner P, Armitage G, Shapiro J. Emotion and coping in the aftermath of medical error: a cross-country exploration. *J Patient Saf* 2015;11:28–35.
6. Merry A, Smith AM. *Errors, Medicine, and the Law*. Cambridge, England: Cambridge University Press; 2001.
7. Plsek P, Greenhalgh T. The challenge of complexity in health care. *BMJ* 2001;323:625–628.
8. Plsek P. Redesigning health care with insights from the science of complex adaptive systems. Appendix B in: Committee on Quality Health Care in America, Institute of Medicine. *Crossing the Quality Chasm: A New Health System for the 21st Century*. National Academies Press: Washington, DC; 2001:309–322.

9. Gawande A. *The Checklist Manifesto: How to Get Things Right.* New York, NY: Metropolitan Books; 2009.

10. Vincent C, Amalberti R. *Safer Healthcare: Strategies for the Real World.* New York, NY: SpringerOpen; 2016.

11. Weaver SJ, Dy SM, Rosen MA. Team-training in healthcare: a narrative synthesis of the literature. *BMJ Qual Saf* 2014;23:359–372.

12. Katz D, Detsky AS. Incorporating metacognition into morbidity and mortality rounds: the next frontier in quality improvement. *J Hosp Med* 2016;11:120–122.

13. Kwok ES, Calder LA, Barlow-Krelina E, et al. Implementation of a structured hospital-wide morbidity and mortality rounds model. *BMJ Qual Saf* 2017;26:439–448.

14. Timmel J, Kent PS, Holzmueller CG, Paine L, Schulick RD, Pronovost PJ. Impact of the Comprehensive Unit-Based Safety Program (CUSP) on safety culture in a surgical inpatient unit. *Jt Comm J Qual Patient Saf* 2010;36:252–260.

15. Wu AW, Lipshutz AKM, Pronovost PJ. Effectiveness and efficiency of root cause analysis in medicine. *JAMA* 2008;299:685–687.

16. Shekelle PG. Nurse-patient ratios as a patient safety strategy: a systematic review. *Ann Intern Med* 2013;158:404–409.

17. Clendon J, Gibbons V. 12 h shifts and rates of error among nurses: a systematic review. *J Nurs Stud* 2015;52:1231–1242.

18. Lipner RS, Hess BJ, Phillips RL Jr. Specialty board certification in the United States: issues and evidence. *J Contin Educ Health Prof* 2013;33(suppl 1):S20–S35.

19. Wingo MT, Halvorsen AJ, Beckman TJ, Johnson MG, Reed DA. Associations between attending physician workload, teaching effectiveness and patient safety. *J Hosp Med* 2016;11:169–173.

20. Ball JE, Murrells T, Rafferty AM, Morrow E, Griffiths P. 'Care left undone' during nursing shifts: associations with workload and perceived quality of care. *BMJ Qual Saf* 2014;23:116–125.

21. Wachter RM. Personal accountability in healthcare: searching for the right balance. *BMJ Qual Saf* 2013;22:176–180.

22. Wachter RM. Patient safety at ten: unmistakable progress, troubling gaps. *Health Aff (Millwood)* 2010;29:165–173.

23. Vincent C, Burnett S, Carthey J. Safety measurement and monitoring in healthcare: a framework to guide clinical teams and healthcare organisations in maintaining safety. *BMJ Qual Saf* 2014;23:670–677.

ADDITIONAL READINGS

Berwick DM. The science of improvement. *JAMA* 2008;299:1182–1184.

Dixon-Woods M, Bosk CL, Aveling EL, Goeschel CA, Pronovost PJ. Explaining Michigan: developing an ex post theory of a quality improvement program. *Milbank Q* 2011;89:167–205.

Garvin DA, Edmondson AC, Gino F. Is yours a learning organization? *Harv Bus Rev* 2008;86:109–116.

Helmreich RL. On error management: lessons from aviation. *BMJ* 2000;320:781–785.

Jha A, Pronovost PJ. Toward a safer health care system: the critical need to improve measurement. *JAMA* 2016;315:1831–1832.

Kapur N, Parand A, Soukup T, Reader T, Sevdalis N. Aviation and healthcare: a comparative review with implications for patient safety. *JRSM Open* 2015;7:2054270415616548.

Kronick R, Arnold S, Brady J. Improving safety for hospitalized patients: much progress but many challenges remain. *JAMA* 2016;316:489–490.

Leape LL. Error in medicine. *JAMA* 1994;272:1851–1857.

Rogers J, Gaba DM. Have we gone too far in translating ideas from aviation to patient safety? *BMJ* 2011;342:c7309–c7310.

Sturmberg JP, Martin CM. *Handbook of Systems and Complexity in Health.* New York, NY: Springer Science & Business Media; 2013.

Wachter RM, Shojania KG. *Internal Bleeding: The Truth Behind America's Terrifying Epidemic of Medical Mistakes.* New York, NY: Rugged Land; 2004.

Watson SR, Pronovost PJ. Building a highway to quality health care. *J Patient Saf* 2016;12:165–166.

Weick KE, Sutcliffe KM. *Managing the Unexpected: Assuring High Performance in an Age of Complexity.* 2nd ed. San Francisco, CA: John Wiley & Sons; 2007.

Woods DD, Dekker S, Cook R, Johannesen L, Sarter N. *Behind Human Error.* 2nd ed. Burlington, VT: Ashgate; 2010.

SAFETY, QUALITY, AND VALUE | 3

WHAT IS QUALITY?

The National Academy of Medicine (NAM, formerly the Institute of Medicine, IOM) defines quality of care as "the degree to which health services for individuals and populations increase the likelihood of desired health outcomes and are consistent with current professional knowledge." In its seminal 2001 report, *Crossing the Quality Chasm,* the NAM advanced six aims for a quality healthcare system (Table 3-1): patient safety, patient-centeredness, effectiveness, efficiency, timeliness, and equity.[1] Note that this framework depicts safety as one of these six components, in essence making it a subset of quality. Note also that, though many clinicians tend to think of quality as being synonymous with the delivery of evidence-based care, the NAM's definition is much broader and includes matters that are of particular importance to patients (patient-centeredness and timeliness) and to society (equity).

Although the NAM makes clear that quality is more than the provision of care supported by science, evidence-based medicine *does* provide the foundation for much of quality measurement and improvement. For many decades, the particular practice style of a senior clinician or a prestigious medical center determined the standard of care, and variation in treatment approach for the same condition was widespread. Without discounting the value of experience and mature clinical judgment, the modern paradigm for identifying optimal practice has changed, driven by the explosion in clinical research over the past two generations (the number of randomized clinical trials has grown from less than 500 per year in 1970 to almost 25,000 per year in 2015). This research has helped define "best practices" in many areas of medicine, ranging from preventive strategies for a 64-year-old woman with diabetes to the treatment of the patient with acute myocardial infarction and cardiogenic shock.

Health services researcher Avedis Donabedian's taxonomy is widely used for measuring the quality of care. "Donabedian's Triad" divides quality measures into *structure* (how is care organized), *process* (what was done), and

Table 3-1	**THE NAM'S SIX AIMS FOR A QUALITY HEALTHCARE SYSTEM**
Healthcare must be safe	
Healthcare must be effective	
Healthcare must be patient-centered	
Healthcare must be timely	
Healthcare must be efficient	
Healthcare must be equitable	

Reproduced with permission from Committee on Quality of Health Care in America, Institute of Medicine. *Crossing the Quality Chasm: A New Health System for the 21st Century.* Washington, DC: National Academies Press; 2001.

outcomes (what happened to the patient).[2] When used to assess the quality of care, each element of this framework has important advantages and disadvantages[3] (Table 3-2). The growth in clinical research has established the link between certain processes of care and improved health outcomes; because of this, process measures have frequently been used as proxies for quality. Examples include measuring whether hospitalized patients with pneumonia received influenza and pneumococcal vaccinations, and measuring glycosylated hemoglobin (hemoglobin A1c) at appropriate intervals in outpatients with diabetes. While there is still value in using process measures to assess quality in certain circumstances, the field's focus is shifting toward the use of outcome measures such as 30-day risk-standardized mortality and 30-day readmissions.

The difference between process and outcome measures is worth clarifying. If the focus of measurement was on whether or not the physician *checked* the hemoglobin A1c (or the blood pressure or cholesterol) at appropriate intervals, that measure would be considered a classic process measure. On the other hand, if the focus was on the *actual value* of the hemoglobin A1c (i.e., fraction of patients with hemoglobin A1c below 7%), that would be considered an outcome—more specifically, an *intermediate outcome,* as it is really a proxy for outcomes we care about, such as mortality, kidney function, or retinopathy.[4] Although such intermediate outcomes may seem like attractive hybrids between process measures and true outcomes, it is important to appreciate that intermediate outcomes, like true outcome measures (see below), may require case-mix adjustment to fairly assess the quality of care. More importantly, the medical literature is replete with cautionary reports on the results of interventions that improved plausible intermediate outcomes (such as suppression of premature ventricular contractions or raising levels of HDL cholesterol) but had no effect—or even increased risk of harm—on the main outcomes of interest.[5,6]

Table 3-2 ADVANTAGES AND DISADVANTAGES OF USING STRUCTURE, PROCESS, AND OUTCOME (THE "DONABEDIAN TRIAD") TO MEASURE THE QUALITY OF CARE

Measure	Simple Definition	Advantages	Disadvantages
Structure	How was care organized?	May be highly relevant in a complex health system	May fail to capture the quality of care by individual physicians Difficult to determine the "gold standard"
Process	What was done?	More easily measured and acted upon than outcomes May not require case-mix adjustment May directly reflect quality (if carefully chosen) No time lag—can be measured when care is provided	A proxy for outcomes All may not agree on "gold standard" processes May promote "cookbook" medicine, especially if physicians and health systems try to "game" their performance
Outcome	What happened to the patient?	What we really care about	May take years to occur May not reflect quality of care Requires case-mix and other adjustment to prevent "apples-to-oranges" comparisons

Reproduced with permission from Shojania KG, Showstack J, Wachter RM. Assessing hospital quality: a review for clinicians. *Eff Clin Pract* 2001;4:82–90.

Where the science of case-mix adjustment is suitably advanced (e.g., in cardiac bypass surgery[7]), measures of outcomes such as mortality rates are often used. The caveat is crucial: if case-mix adjustment is not done well, the surgeon or hospital that accepts (or is referred) the sickest patients may appear to be worse than the lesser surgeon or institution that takes only easy cases. Furthermore, case-mix adjustment is often based on administrative data. If care is not documented and coded adequately, case-mix adjustment is not a reliable reflection of the true severity of illness.[8]

Finally, when the processes are quite complex and the science of case-mix adjustment is immature, structural measures are often used as proxies for quality. As with process measures, using structural measures in this way assumes that good research has linked such elements to overall quality. Examples of such structural measures supported by strong evidence include the presence of intensivists in critical care units, a dedicated stroke service, nurse-to-patient ratios, and computerized provider order entry (CPOE).

It is worth highlighting another special kind of outcome measure. As we've seen, the NAM appropriately considers patient experience to be one of the key dimensions of quality. Accordingly, assessments of such experience—generally collected through patient satisfaction surveys administered after hospitalizations and ambulatory visits—have become important quality measures, both because they reflect an outcome that we intrinsically care about, and because they may be associated with higher quality care.[9,10] The growing emphasis placed on patient experience metrics is reflected in the Affordable Care Act (ACA) of 2010, which established Medicare's "value-based purchasing" (VBP) program—a pay-for-performance (P4P) initiative that financially rewards or penalizes hospitals based on how well they do on a mix of process and outcome measures. In its first few years, VBP placed significant emphasis on process measures (e.g., administration of aspirin and beta-blockers to patients with myocardial infarction). More recent versions of VBP have focused more on outcome measures (e.g., 30-day risk-adjusted mortality for patients with acute myocardial infarction, pneumonia, and heart failure), as well as patient experience, safety, cost, and efficiency[11] (Figure 3-1).

Harvard Business School professor Michael Porter argues that we should focus our attention on outcome measures, as they are what matter to patients.[12] Although we agree in theory, as the Chapter 1 discussion of the problems with using hospital mortality rates as a measure of the quality and safety of care made clear (and at the risk of being obvious),[8] validated process measures are more useful for assessing the quality of care than bad outcome measures.[13]

Moreover, good outcome measures don't obviate the need for process and structural measurement. Let's say we find that our readmission rates for heart failure patients or our mortality rates for stroke admissions are higher

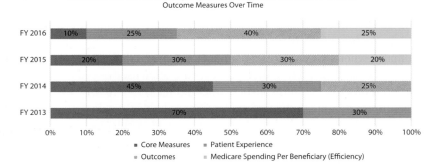

Figure 3-1 ▪ The figure shows the shift in domain weights from process to outcome measures over time within Medicare's Value-Based Purchasing Program.

than we would like. The next step, of course, is to examine our processes and structures and compare them to those of our peers or to known best practices. This is what we mean when we say that one of the downsides of outcome measures is that they are not directly actionable.[3] In the end, it is clear that a thoughtful mix of all elements of the Donabedian Triad—process, structure, and outcome—is essential for developing a sound program of quality measurement and improvement.

THE EPIDEMIOLOGY OF QUALITY PROBLEMS

In a series of pioneering studies, Wennberg and colleagues demonstrated large and clinically indefensible variations in care from one city to another for the same problem or procedure.[14] Despite efforts, research demonstrates that variations in the quality of care for patients based on race, income, and gender (*healthcare disparities*) persist.[15] These findings hint at a fundamental flaw in modern medical practice: after seeing such profound variations in common processes and procedures, as well as in the outcomes of comparable patient groups, we can only conclude that care is often inconsistent with evidence.

Stimulated by early studies on disparities and variations, researchers have more directly measured the frequency with which clinicians and healthcare organizations deliver care that comports with the best evidence available. McGlynn and colleagues studied more than 400 evidence-based measures of quality, and found that practice was consistent with the evidence *only 54% of the time*.[16] Although adherence to evidence-based processes generally correlates with improved clinical outcomes,[17] sustaining adherence after implementing necessary changes in practices remains challenging.[18] These large differences between best and actual practice have caused patients, providers, and policymakers to seek methods to drive and support quality improvement (QI) activities.

CATALYSTS FOR QUALITY IMPROVEMENT

The problems described above have exposed several impediments to the reliable delivery of high-quality care, including the lack of information regarding provider or institutional performance (although this is changing with the growth of public reporting for certain metrics), the weakness of incentives for QI, the difficulty for practicing physicians to stay abreast of evidence-based medicine, and, until recently, the absence of system support (such as information technology) for quality. Each will need to be addressed in order to make substantial gains in the quality of care.

The first step in QI begins with *measurement.* Initially, there were only a handful of generally accepted quality measures, and most focused on processes of care, such as whether patients with acute myocardial infarction received aspirin or beta-blockers. Over time, the number of metrics which healthcare organizations are responsible for has grown rapidly, promulgated by a variety of organizations, including payers (such as the Centers for Medicare & Medicaid Services [CMS]), accreditors and regulators (such as the Joint Commission), as well as medical societies. (In the United States, an organization called the National Quality Forum exists largely to review proposed measures and endorse those that meet prespecified validity criteria.[19]) By the end of 2013, CMS had developed 25 different measurement programs with over 822 discrete metrics, a massive increase compared to 2006, when there were only five programs with 119 measures[20] (some are displayed in Table 3-3). While these measures have identified many opportunities for improvement among individual physicians, practices, hospitals, and post-acute care centers, institutions face tremendous challenges developing the infrastructure needed to actually measure and transmit the required data back to CMS.

Given the enormous amount of new literature published each year, no individual physician can possibly remain abreast of all the evidence-based advances in a given field. *Practice guidelines,* such as those for the care of community-acquired pneumonia or for deep venous thrombosis prophylaxis, aim to synthesize evidence-based practices into sets of summary recommendations. Although some providers deride guidelines as "cookbook medicine," there is increasing agreement that standardizing best practices is ethically and clinically appropriate; in fact, so-called *High Reliability Organizations* "hard wire" such practices whenever possible (Chapter 15). The major challenges for guideline developers are updating them as new knowledge accumulates and designing them so they can be easily implemented at the point of care.[21] *Clinical pathways* are similar to guidelines, but attempt to articulate a series of steps, usually temporal (on day 1, do the following; on day 2; and so on). They are most useful for relatively straightforward and predictable processes such as the postoperative management of patients after cardiac bypass surgery or hip replacement.

| THE CHANGING QUALITY LANDSCAPE

Although one could argue that professionalism should be sufficient incentive to provide high-quality care, providing such care depends on building a system to reliably translate research into practice—which takes significant investments (i.e., in developing guidelines, physician education, hiring case managers or clinical pharmacists, building information systems, and more).

Table 3-3   EXAMPLES OF PUBLICLY REPORTED QUALITY MEASURES

Acute cardiovascular condition measures

Hospital 30-day all-cause risk standardized readmission rate following acute myocardial infarction

Hospital 30-day, all-cause, risk standardized mortality rate following acute myocardial infarction hospitalization for patients 18 and older

Outpatients with chest pain or possible heart attack who received fibrinolytics within 30 minutes of arrival

Outpatients with chest pain or possible heart attack who received aspirin within 24 hours of arrival or before transferring from the emergency department

Heart failure measures

Hospital 30-day, all-cause, risk standardized readmission rate following heart failure hospitalization

Hospital 30-day, all-cause, risk-standardized mortality rate following heart failure hospitalization for patients 18 and older

Pneumonia measures

Hospital 30-day, all-cause, risk-standardized readmission rate following pneumonia hospitalization

Hospital 30-day, all-cause, risk-standardized mortality rate following pneumonia hospitalization for patients 18 and older

Stroke

Hospital 30-day, all-cause, risk-standardized readmission rate following stroke hospitalization

Hospital 30-day, all-cause, risk-standardized mortality rate following stroke hospitalization for patients 18 and older

Patient experience

Patients who reported that their nurses and doctors "always" communicated well

Patients who reported that they "always" received help as soon as they wanted

Patients who gave their hospital a rating of 9 or 10 on a scale from 0 (lowest) to 10 (highest)

Patients who reported YES, they would definitely recommend the hospital

Healthcare-associated infections

Central line-associated bloodstream infections (CLABSI) in ICUs

Catheter-associated urinary tract infections (CAUTI) in ICUs and select wards

Surgical site infections from colon surgery

Surgical site infections from abdominal hysterectomy

Methicillin-resistant *Staphylococcus aureus* (MRSA) bloodstream infections

Clostridium difficile (*C. difficile*) infections

Available at: https://www.medicare.gov/hospitalcompare/search.html?

Historically, payers compensated physicians and hospitals the same, regardless of whether or not the quality of care delivered was superb or appalling, providing little incentive to make the requisite investments.

This is changing rapidly, with a blizzard of initiatives and metrics—including P4P programs under which providers and healthcare organizations are paid based on quality—to support and catalyze QI activities. Virtually all involve several steps: defining reasonable quality measures (evidence-based measures that capture appropriate structures, processes, or outcomes), measuring the performance of providers or systems, and using these results to promote change. Although each of these steps comes with its own challenges, the final one has probably created the greatest degree of uncertainty and been the subject of the most experimentation.

The first step in activities designed to promote QI involves *selecting appropriate measures.* For local QI activities, it may be fine to use process measures that seem plausibly connected to an outcome of interest, even if the evidence connecting the two is not bulletproof. It is also often appropriate to use measures captured through self-reporting by the involved providers while acknowledging the inherent biases in such data. Although we all aspire to perfect measurement, "don't let the perfect be the enemy of the good" is a reasonable rule for many local QI projects.

On the other hand, it makes sense to insist on higher standards for measures that are being used for public reporting or P4P programs. Chassin and colleagues have called these high-stake assessments "Accountability Measures" and proposed four criteria that they should meet (Table 3-4).[22]

This distinction is of more than academic interest. Jha and colleagues have shown that even if a provider checks a box attesting that he or she provided discharge counseling to patients with heart failure (the process measure), there is no correlation to readmission rates (the outcome), probably because the quality of such counseling and individual patient comprehension vary widely.[23] Moreover, after Medicare instituted a quality measure assessing the timing of initial antibiotic administration for patients with pneumonia

---

Table 3-4   **PROPOSED CRITERIA FOR "ACCOUNTABILITY MEASURES" ADDRESSING PROCESSES OF CARE**
1. There is a strong evidence base showing that the care process leads to improved outcomes
2. The measure accurately captures whether the evidence-based care process has, in fact, been provided
3. The measure addresses a process that has few intervening care processes that must occur before the improved outcome is realized
4. Implementing the measure has little or no chance of inducing unintended adverse consequences

Reproduced with permission from Chassin MR, Loeb JM, Schmaltz SP, Wachter RM. Accountability measures—using measurement to promote quality improvement. *N Engl J Med* 2010;363:683–688.

(the "Four Hour Rule"), subsequent studies demonstrated that many emergency department (ED) patients who were given antibiotics by rushed physicians later proved not to have pneumonia, or any infection, at all.[24] As another example, although postoperative venous thromboembolism (VTE) rates have been incorporated into several pay-for-performance quality improvement initiatives including Medicare's VBP program, evidence suggests that the measure may be flawed due to surveillance bias and that hospitals with higher rates of VTE may simply spend more time and resources doing unnecessary imaging.[25] It is clear that we have much to learn about which measures to target, how to collect the data, and how to promote improvement at a reasonable cost and with a minimum of unanticipated consequences.

Once we settle on appropriate measures, the next steps involve *promoting and supporting improvement* to make it stick. Although one might hope that clear feedback will generate meaningful improvement in a provider's performance, experience has shown that this strategy leads to only modest change. Increasingly, a strategy directed at *transparency* (disseminating the results of quality measures to key stakeholders) is becoming the norm. With simple transparency, the hope is that providers will find the public dissemination of their quality gaps to be sufficiently concerning to motivate improvement. Further, many believe that patients (or their proxies, such as third-party payers) will begin to use such data to make choices about where patients receive care. To date, although there is little evidence that patients are using such data to make purchasing decisions, studies *have* shown impressive improvements in some publicly reported quality measures, supporting the premise that transparency itself may generate change.[22] Berwick, James, and Coye's framework (Figure 3-2) is useful for considering the two interwoven pathways—selection by patients or purchasers, and change undertaken by the provider organization—through which measurement and transparency can stimulate improvement.[26]

Increasingly, programs that tie payments for service to quality performance (*Pay for Performance,* or "P4P") are being utilized to motivate improvement.[27] Although P4P is conceptually attractive, it raises a number of questions: Are quality data accurate? Should payments go to best performers or to those with the greatest improvements? Do existing measures adequately assess quality in patients with complex, multisystem disease? And does P4P erode professionalism or create undue focus on measurable practices and relative inattention to other important processes that are not being compensated?[28] P4P, in its current form, has yielded only a marginal change in quality beyond that generated by public reporting alone (Figure 3-3). Some suggest that to make a real difference, these programs require larger financial incentives and improved program design.[29,30] There are numerous P4P programs currently in existence[11,31–34] (Table 3-5).

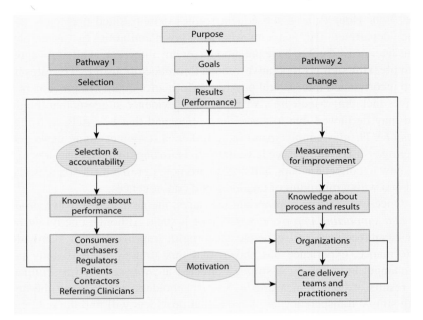

Figure 3-2 ▪ The figure demonstrates the two interwoven pathways (selection and change) by which measurement of performance measures can lead to improvement. (Reproduced with permission from Berwick DM, James B, Coye MJ. Connections between quality measurement and improvement. *Med Care* 2003;41:I30–I38.)

Notwithstanding the mixed evidence of effectiveness, the emphasis on P4P is continuing to grow, especially at the individual physician level. The Medicare Access and CHIP Reauthorization Act (MACRA) was passed by the U.S. Congress in 2015 and targets Medicare payments to physicians. Combining several existing quality reporting programs into one framework (Physician Quality Reporting System, Medicare's Electronic Health Record [EHR] Incentive Program, and Value-Based Payment Modifier), the Merit-based Incentive Payment System (MIPS) under MACRA incentivizes physicians to provide higher quality care and facilitates the Department of Health and Human Services' (HHS) goal of tying the majority of Medicare payments to value and increasing the amount of Medicare payments associated with alternative payment models. While the details of this program are still being worked out at the time of this writing, it is clear that pay-for-performance is here to stay and physicians will need to focus on building the infrastructure necessary to succeed under value-based models of care. The jury is still out on whether the benefits are enough to overcome the concerns raised above.[28,35]

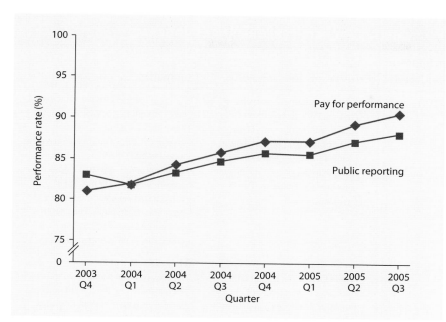

Figure 3-3 ▪ Relative performance in two groups of hospitals that either participated in a pay-for-performance program (in addition to having their data publicly reported) versus those hospitals subject to public reporting alone. The rate is the percentage of patients given the specified care on 10 process measures in three conditions (acute myocardial infarction, congestive heart failure, and pneumonia). (Reproduced with permission from Lindenauer PK, Remus D, Roman S, et al. Public reporting and pay for performance in hospital quality improvement. *N Engl J Med* 2007;356:486–496.)

QUALITY IMPROVEMENT STRATEGIES

Whether the motivation is ethics, embarrassment, or economics, the next question is how to actually improve the quality of care. There is no simple answer. Most institutions and physicians with success in this area use a variation of the "Plan-Do-Study-Act" (PDSA) cycle (Figure 3-4), recognizing that QI activities must be carefully planned and implemented, that their impact needs to be measured, and that the results of these activities need to be fed back into the system in a continuously iterative process of improvement. A number of more complex and sophisticated methods (Lean, Six Sigma, Toyota Production System) have been developed in the business, manufacturing, and engineering industries, and have been adapted to healthcare, often (but not always) successfully.[36,37] A detailed discussion of these methods is

Table 3-5   **VARIOUS PAY-FOR-PERFORMANCE PROGRAMS**[*]

Program	Location: Sponsor (Year Introduced)	Criteria for Bonus/Penalty	Comments
MACRA	U.S.: CMS (2015)	Under MACRA, most independent physician practices will see an adjustment in payment. Those not performing at or above the national threshold will face up to a maximum of −9% payment adjustment in Medicare Part B payments in 2020	Drives providers to provide value-based care through two payments options: merit-based incentive payment system (MIPS) or alternative payment model (APM). MIPS combines the meaningful use, physician quality reporting system (PQRS), and value-based payment modifier (VM) programs. Each physician's MIPS composite score will be posted on CMS' physician compare website
Value-based Purchasing[11]	U.S.: CMS (2012)	Up to 2% of hospital reimbursement withheld, and can be earned back, based on mixture of clinical processes/outcomes and patient satisfaction scores	Weight given to various categories of metrics changes annually with focus increasingly moving toward outcome measures, patient satisfaction, cost and efficiency
Meaningful Use[30]	U.S.: CMS (2011–12)	Approximately $25 billion in payments were offered to hospitals and physicians for implementing IT systems that met certain initial standards; within several years, this changed to reimbursement penalties for those lacking IT	Initial meaningful use criteria included using computerized order entry, performing drug–drug interaction and drug-allergy checks, and maintaining up-to-date problem lists (Table 13–6)
Readmission Penalties[31]	U.S.: CMS (2012)	Hospitals with excess numbers of readmissions will see their reimbursements cut	As of 2015, up to 3% of Medicare payments are withheld for those in highest quartile of readmissions
"No Pay for Errors"[32]	U.S.: CMS and some private payers (2009)	Hospitals that previously received extra payments for certain complicating conditions no longer receive these payments if these conditions are deemed preventable	Examples of these conditions are certain hospital-associated infections, pressure ulcers, and retained surgical objects. Relatively small amount of money at risk
Primary Care Pay-for-Performance Program[33]	UK: National Health Service (2004)	GPs received bonuses based on performance on more than 100 ambulatory quality measures	GPs could earn approximately 25% bonus based on performance

CMS, Centers for Medicare & Medicaid Services; GP, general practitioners; IT, information technology; UK, United Kingdom; U.S., United States.

[*]In 2019, several of these programs will be folded into MACRA including PQRS, VM, and meaningful use.

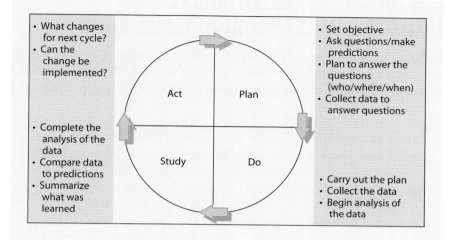

- What changes for next cycle?
- Can the change be implemented?

- Complete the analysis of the data
- Compare data to predictions
- Summarize what was learned

Act

Plan

Study

Do

- Set objective
- Ask questions/make predictions
- Plan to answer the questions (who/where/when)
- Collect data to answer questions

- Carry out the plan
- Collect the data
- Begin analysis of the data

Figure 3-4 ▪ The PDSA cycle.

beyond the scope of this book; interested readers are referred to several excellent resources.[38–40]

In addition to the PDSA cycle, several other tactics are useful. For QI practices that require predictable repetition, efforts to "hard wire" the practice or use alternative providers who focus on the activity are often beneficial. For example, the strategy most likely to increase the rate of pneumococcal vaccination of hospitalized patients with pneumonia is to embed it in a standard computerized order set.[41] Having a nurse remove the patient's shoes before the doctor enters the room can increase rates of diabetic foot examinations in outpatient practice. Empowering critical care nurses or respiratory therapists to follow a weaning protocol safely shortens the time patients with respiratory failure spend on mechanical ventilators.[42]

In some areas, though, QI involves much more complex and interdependent activities. In these circumstances, bringing teams together to examine their practices and participate in a PDSA cycle is the most likely path to success. For example, two hospitals participated in peer-to-peer assessments, sending teams from one institution to the other to observe differences in organizational approaches to safety and quality and in reducing specific aspects of patient harm. The result: each institution issues a report to the other with recommendations and both developed plans for improvement.[43] This kind of approach is likely to be facilitated by team training and is in keeping with what we have come to understand about improvement in complex adaptive systems of care (Chapters 2 and 15).[44]

COMMONALITIES AND DIFFERENCES BETWEEN QUALITY AND PATIENT SAFETY

Although patient safety is a subset of healthcare quality, it is important to appreciate the sometimes subtle differences between the two areas, particularly when it comes to measuring performance and changing practices and systems.

Mr. S, a 74-year-old man, is admitted to the hospital with severe substernal chest pain. In the ED, his electrocardiogram (ECG) shows an ST elevation pattern typical of a large, anterior myocardial infarction. In this hospital, which has a cardiac catheterization lab, ST-elevation myocardial infarctions are managed with primary percutaneous coronary intervention (PCI). There is strong evidence linking "door-to-balloon time" to a patient's ultimate outcome. In this case, there is a delay in reaching the cardiologist on call; when he finally arrives an hour later, the cardiac catheterization lab is not prepared for the procedure, leading to another delay. The cardiologist, Dr. G, orders metoprolol, a beta-blocker. The pharmacist is concerned that the dose ordered seems high but is reluctant to page the doctor, who is known for his "difficult personality." So the pharmacist fills the metoprolol as ordered by the cardiologist. Luckily, the mistake is recognized by the ED nurse who questions Dr. G and the correct dose is administered as the patient is being wheeled up for his angioplasty. The higher dose could have dropped the patient's blood pressure to dangerous levels. As a result of the delays, the door-to-balloon time is 150 minutes, well above the established standard of care of 90 minutes or less. The patient survives, but is left with a moderate amount of heart damage (ejection fraction 35%, normal 55%–70%) and symptomatic heart failure.

This case illustrates both quality and safety problems. Placing the order for the wrong dose of medication is clearly an error. Approaches to preventing such errors include computerization, standardization of common doses, and changes in culture to ensure that the pharmacist would promptly call the physician to clarify an ambiguous order. But the prolonged door-to-balloon time also represents a quality problem, a failure in the process of care. There were no overt errors in this process, it just took far longer than it should have because of lack of coordination, planning, and training. The combined result of both kinds of problems was a poor outcome for the patient.

Differentiating quality and safety problems is important as we consider their causes and how best to prevent them. Let's assume that the patient's insurer was interested in measuring the quality and safety of care in this hospital. It would be relatively easy to implement a transparent, auditable process to document the door-to-balloon time. Ditto for whether the patient received an aspirin, a beta-blocker, or a flu shot at discharge. Turning to outcomes, it would be straightforward to figure out whether Mr. S and similar patients were alive or dead at the time of discharge (though remember that we'd need some pretty sophisticated case-mix adjustment to be sure that our outcome assessment wasn't unfairly disadvantaging hospitals or doctors that attract sicker patients). Public reporting of door-to-balloon times, perhaps accompanied by higher reimbursement for better performance (via P4P), would likely spur improved performance.

But how could this insurer learn that Dr. G ordered the wrong dose of beta-blocker? It is difficult to imagine a transparent, auditable, and efficient system that does not depend on self-reporting by the nurse, pharmacist, or physician to capture the error. Moreover, a strategy of public reporting (or P4P) for medication errors might leave providers reluctant to report them, causing the system to be unaware that such errors were occurring and ill prepared to generate the shared knowledge—as well as the money and will—to fix them.

The process of fixing both problems (door-to-balloon times and medication errors) might be relatively similar, in that both are likely to require changes in core processes, thoughtful implementation of technology (perhaps an automatic ECG reader for the chest pain protocol; CPOE with standardized auto-populated doses for the medication error), and changes in culture (an unwavering commitment to change by system leaders; simulation training to improve door-to-balloon time performance; teamwork training to improve physician–pharmacist communication and dampen down hierarchies in order to mitigate medication errors).[45]

The bottom line is that patients have a right to expect care that is *both* high quality and safe. The IOM (now NAM) report on medical errors, *To Err Is Human,* helped catalyze a national push to improve safety, and has led to important changes in culture, training, regulation, and technology.[46] However, because measuring safety tends to depend so often on providers reporting and retrospective chart review (perhaps using trigger tools described in Chapter 1), the twin strategies of transparency and differential payment are more likely to improve quality than safety.[47] Happily, the two endeavors have enough commonalities (the need for improved information systems, standardization, and simplification, use of multidisciplinary teams, and improvement cycles) that QI initiatives will often result in better safety. Other cornerstones of patient safety, such as the creation of a safety culture (Chapter 15), may be largely independent of QI efforts and will require a distinct focus. And all of these quality and safety improvement activities are relevant to the increasingly important work of removing waste and unnecessary cost from our healthcare system.

VALUE: CONNECTING QUALITY (AND SAFETY) TO THE COST OF CARE

Outside the world of healthcare, we base most of our purchasing decisions on our perception of *value*: quality divided by cost. Who among us is rich enough to always buy the very best thing, or frugal enough to always buy the least expensive one? Much of the focus of our lives as consumers is spent trying to determine the value of the things we're considering buying—whether it's a car, a house, a café mocha, or a college education—by weighing the measured (or perceived) quality against the cost. As we do this, we ask a simple question: is the item or service worth the price?

Healthcare decisions have traditionally not been made this way, partly because of the limited ability of patients (and their doctors, for that matter) to make rational judgments about the quality of a given physician, surgeon, or hospital, and partly because one of the functions of healthcare insurance is to shield patients from shouldering the full cost of their purchasing decisions. In other words, when you're buying your Starbucks coffee or an Audi sedan, you're well aware of the price and are in a perfect position to judge whether the quality (and safety, in the case of the car) is worth it. But in healthcare, the service is often "covered," or the patient is responsible for only a portion of the cost. With the advent of population health programs such as Accountable Care Organizations (ACOs), this may be slowly changing.

Much of the decade-long revolution in quality measurement and reporting can be seen as an effort to provide patients (or other interested parties, such as, in the United States, employers or insurers or, in countries with single-payer systems, the government) with the information they need to make rational decisions about healthcare value. This framework becomes even more important as the costs of healthcare continue to rise, crowding out resources for other worthwhile private and public pursuits. Increasingly, efforts to improve quality, safety, and patient satisfaction are not taking place in a cost-agnostic vacuum. Rather, healthcare providers and organizations will be pushed relentlessly to improve both the numerator *and the denominator* of the value equation.[12]

In this environment, we can already see the incentives shifting, from promoting the best care to promoting the best care *at the lowest cost*. In both Medicare's "value-based purchasing" and "no pay for errors" initiatives, anything but perfect performance leads to reimbursement cuts rather than additional payments for top performers.[11,33] The proportion of payments tied to some type of P4P initiative—for both hospitals and individual physicians—will undoubtedly continue to increase in the years to come.

KEY POINTS

- Safety is usually considered a subset of quality, but it is more difficult to measure, in part because identification of incidents often depends on self-reports by caregivers.
- Quality measurement is best thought of in terms of "Donebedian's Triad": structure, process, or outcomes. Each type of measure has advantages and disadvantages when compared with the others.
- Measures being employed for public reporting and pay for performance ("Accountability Measures") must meet a higher standard than those used for internal QI.
- There is tremendous activity in the healthcare marketplace promoting transparency (i.e., public reporting) and differential payments based on performance ("pay for performance"). The latter efforts are taking on multiple forms, including so-called "value-based purchasing" and "no pay for errors" initiatives.
- Cost pressures in the United States and elsewhere mean that the healthcare system's target will no longer be quality or safety alone, but value—quality (including safety, access, and the patient's experience) divided by cost.

REFERENCES

1. Committee on Quality of Health Care in America, Institute of Medicine. *Crossing the Quality Chasm: A New Health System for the 21st Century.* Washington, DC: National Academies Press; 2001.
2. Donabedian A. The quality of care. How can it be assessed? *JAMA* 1988;260:1743–1748.
3. Shojania KG, Showstack J, Wachter RM. Assessing hospital quality: a review for clinicians. *Eff Clin Pract* 2001;4:82–90.
4. Kerr EA, Krein SL, Vijan S, Hofer TP, Hayward RA. Avoiding pitfalls in chronic disease quality measurement: a case for the next generation of technical quality measures. *Am J Manag Care* 2001;7:1033–1043.
5. Echt D, Liebson P, Mitchell L, et al. Mortality and morbidity in patients receiving encainide, flecainide, or placebo: The Cardiac Arrhythmia Suppression Trial. *N Engl J Med* 1991;324:781–788.
6. The AIM-HIGH Investigators. Niacin in patients with low HDL cholesterol levels receiving intensive statin therapy. *N Engl J Med* 2011;365:2255–2267.
7. Ferris TG, Torchiana DF. Public release of clinical outcomes data—online CABG report cards. *N Engl J Med* 2010;363:1593–1595.

8. Gupta K, Wachter RM, Kachalia A. Financial incentives and mortality: taking pay for performance a step too far. *BMJ Qual Saf* 2017;26(2):164–168.

9. Wang DE, Tsugawa Y, Figueroa JF, Jha AK. Association between the Centers for Medicare and Medicaid Services hospital star rating and patient outcomes. *JAMA Intern Med* 2016;176:848–850.

10. Kemp KA, Santana MJ, Southern DA, McCormack B, Quan H. Association of inpatient hospital experience with patient safety indicators: a cross-sectional, Canadian study. *BMJ Open* 2016;6e011242.

11. Hospital Value-Based Purchasing. Available at: https://www.cms.gov/Outreach-and-Education/Medicare-Learning-Network-MLN/MLNProducts/downloads/Hospital_VBPurchasing_Fact_Sheet_ICN907664.pdf.

12. Porter ME, Larsson S, Lee TH. Standardizing patient outcomes measurement. *N Engl J Med* 2016;374:504–506.

13. Kubasiak JC, Francescatti AB, Behal R, Myers JA. Patient safety indicators for judging hospital performance: still not ready for prime time. *Am J Med Qual* 2017;32:129–133.

14. Wennberg JE, Freeman JL, Culp WJ. Are hospital services rationed in New Haven or over-utilised in Boston? *Lancet* 1987;1:1185–1189.

15. *National Healthcare Quality and Disparities Reports*. Rockville, MD: Agency for Healthcare Research and Quality; April 2015. AHRQ Publication No. 15-0007.

16. McGlynn EA, Asch SM, Adams J, et al. The quality of health care delivered to adults in the United States. *N Engl J Med* 2003;348:2635–2645.

17. Higashi T, Shekelle PG, Adams JL, et al. Quality of care is associated with survival in vulnerable older patients. *Ann Intern Med* 2005;143:274–281.

18. Ament SM, de Groot JJ, Maessen JM, Dirksen CD, van der Weijden T, Kleijnen J. Sustainability of professionals' adherence to clinical practice guidelines in medical care: a systematic review. *BMJ Open* 2015;5:e008073.

19. In conversation with … Janet Corrigan [Perspective]. *AHRQ PSNet* [serial online]; April 2010. Available at: https://psnet.ahrq.gov/perspectives/perspective/85/in-conversation-with-janet-corrigan-phd-mba?q=corrigan.

20. Centers for Medicare and Medicaid Services. *2015 National Impact Assessment of the Centers for Medicare &Medicaid Services (CMS) Quality Measures Report*. Baltimore, MD: Centers for Medicare and Medicaid Services. Available at: https://www.cms.gov/medicare/quality-initiatives-patient-assessment-instruments/qualitymeasures/downloads/2015-national-impact-assessment-report.pdf.

21. Pronovost P. Enhancing physicians' use of clinical guidelines. *JAMA* 2013;310:2501–2502.

22. Chassin MR, Loeb JM, Schmaltz SP, Wachter RM. Accountability measures—using measurement to promote quality improvement. *N Engl J Med* 2010;363:683–688.

23. Jha AK, Orave EJ, Epstein AM. Public reporting of discharge planning and rates of readmissions. *N Engl J Med* 2009;361:2637–2645.

24. Wachter RM, Flanders SA, Fee C, Pronovost PJ. Public reporting of antibiotic timing in patients with pneumonia: lessons from a flawed performance measure. *Ann Intern Med* 2008;149:29–32.

25. Minami CA, Bilimoria KY. Are higher hospital venous thromboembolism rates an indicator of better quality?: evaluation of the validity of a hospital quality measure. *Adv Surg* 2015;49:185–204.

26. Berwick DM, James B, Coye MJ. Connections between quality measurement and improvement. *Med Care* 2003;41:I-30–I-38.

27. Kahn CN 3rd, Ault T, Potetz L, Walke T, Chambers JH, Burch S. Assessing Medicare's hospital pay-for-performance programs and whether they are achieving their goals. *Health Aff (Millwood)* 2015;34:1281–1288.

28. Epstein A. Pay for performance at the tipping point. *N Engl J Med* 2007;356:515–517.

29. McKethan A, Jha AK. Designing smarter pay for performance programs. *JAMA* 2014;213:1617–1618.

30. Jha AK. Time to get serious about pay for performance. *JAMA* 2013;309:347–348.

31. Blumenthal D, Tavenner M. The "Meaningful Use" regulation for electronic health records. *N Engl J Med* 2010;363:501–504.

32. Epstein AM. Revisiting readmissions—changing the incentives for shared accountability. *N Engl J Med* 2009;360:1457–1459.

33. Wachter RM, Foster NE, Dudley RA. Medicare's decision to withhold payment for hospital errors: the devil is in the details. *Jt Comm J Qual Patient Saf* 2008; 34:116–123.

34. Ryan AM, Burgess JF Jr, Pesko MF, Borden WB, Dimick JB. The early effects of Medicare's mandatory hospital pay-for-performance program. *Health Serv Res* 2015;50:81–97.

35. Lindenauer PK, Remus D, Roman S, et al. Public reporting and pay for performance in hospital quality improvement. *N Engl J Med* 2007;356:486–496.

36. D'Andreamatteo A, Ianni L, Llega F, Sargiacomo M. Lean in healthcare: a comprehensive review. *Health Policy* 2015;119:1197–1209.

37. Kelly EW, Kelly JD, Hiestand B, Wells-Kiser K, Starling S, Hoekstra JW. Six Sigma process utilization in reducing door-to-balloon time at a single academic tertiary care center. *Prog Cardiovasc Dis* 2010;53:219–226.

38. Arthur J. *Lean Six Sigma for Hospitals: Improving Patient Safety, Patient Flow and the Bottom Line*. 2nd ed. New York, NY: McGraw-Hill Education; 2016.

39. Liker J, Ross K. *The Toyota Way to Service Excellence: Lean Transformation in Service*. New York, NY: McGraw-Hill Education; 2016.

40. Butler G, Caldwell C, Poston N. *Lean-Six Sigma for Healthcare: A Senior Leader Guide to Improving Cost and Throughput*. 2nd ed. Milwaukee: ASQ Quality Press; 2009.

41. Schedlbauer A, Prasad V, Mulvaney C, et al. What evidence supports the use of computerized alerts and prompts to improve clinicians' prescribing behavior? *J Am Med Inform Assoc* 2009;16:531–538.

42. Danckers M, Grosu H, Jean R, et al. Nurse driven, protocol-directed weaning from mechanical ventilation improves clinical outcomes and is well accepted by intensive care unit physicians. *J Crit Care* 2013;28:433–441.

43. Mort E, Bruckel J, Donelan K, et al. Improving health care quality and patient safety through peer-to-peer assessment: demonstration project in two academic medical centers. *Am J Med Qual* October 23, 2016. [Epub ahead of print].

44. Plsek P. Redesigning health care with insights from the science of complex adaptive systems. Appendix B in: *Committee on Quality Health Care in America, Institute of Medicine. Crossing the Quality Chasm: A New Health System for the 21st Century*. Washington, DC: National Academies Press; 2001:309–322.

45. Curry LA, Spatz E, Cherlin E, et al. What distinguishes top-performing hospitals in acute myocardial infarction mortality rates? A qualitative study. *Ann Intern Med* 2011;154:384–390.

46. Kohn LT, Corrigan JM, Donaldson MS, eds. *To Err Is Human: Building a Safer Health System*. Washington, DC: National Academies Press; 1999.

47. Pronovost PJ, Miller MR, Wachter RM. Tracking progress in patient safety: an elusive target. *JAMA* 2006;296:696–699.

ADDITIONAL READINGS

Austin JM, McGlynn EA, Pronovost PJ. Fostering transparency in outcomes, quality, safety, and costs. *JAMA* 2016;316:1661–1662.

Bilimoria KY, Barnard C. The new CMS hospital quality star ratings: the stars are not aligned. *JAMA* 2016;316:1761–1762.

Blumenthal D, Abrams M, Nuzum R. The Affordable Care Act at 5 Years. *N Engl J Med* 2015;373:1580.

Burstin H, Leatherman S, Goldmann D. The evolution of healthcare quality measurement in the United States. *J Intern Med* 2016;279:154–159.

Christensen CM, Grossman JH, Hwang J. *The Innovator's Prescription: A Disruptive Solution for Health Care*. New York, NY: McGraw-Hill; 2009.

Eddy DM. Clinical decision making: from theory to practice. Connecting value and costs: whom do we ask, and what do we ask them? *JAMA* 1990;264:1737–1739.

Friebel R, Steventon A. The multiple aims of pay-for-performance and the risk of unintended consequences. *BMJ Qual Saf* 2016;25:827–831.

Gawande A. Annals of medicine: the cost conundrum—what a Texas town can teach us about health care. *New Yorker* June 1, 2009: Reporting & Essays.

Horn SD. Performance measures and clinical outcomes. *JAMA* 2006;296:2731–2732.

Hota B, Webb TA, Stein BD, Gupta R, Ansell D, Lateef O. Consumer rankings and health care: toward validation and transparency. *Jt Comm J Qual Patient Saf* 2016;42:439–446.

Joshi MS, Ransom ER, Nash DB, Ransom SB, eds. *The Healthcare Quality Book*. 3rd ed. Chicago, IL: Health Administration Press; 2014.

McClellan M, McKethan AN, Lewis JL, Roski J, Fisher ES. A national strategy to put accountable care into practice. *Health Aff (Millwood)* 2010;29:982–990.

Mechanic RE. When new Medicare payment systems collide. *N Engl J Med* 2016; 374:1706–1709.

Moriates C, Arora V, Shah N. *Understanding Value-Based Healthcare*. New York, NY: McGraw-Hill Education; 2015.

TYPES OF MEDICAL ERRORS

MEDICATION ERRORS | 4

SOME BASIC CONCEPTS, TERMS, AND EPIDEMIOLOGY

In June 1995, a middle-aged man named Ramon Vasquez went to see his physician in Odessa, Texas, for chest pain. His physician, suspecting angina, prescribed a medication in addition to ordering further testing. The actual handwritten prescription is reproduced in Figure 4-1.

Despite the advent of electronic prescribing, millions of prescriptions each year, particularly in ambulatory settings, are still handwritten. In 1995, of course, handwritten prescriptions were the norm—and a major source of medical error. From the figure, can you determine whether the prescription is for Plendil (a calcium channel blocker that can be used to treat angina), Isordil (another anti-anginal that works through a different mechanism), or Zestril (an ACE inhibitor used to treat high blood pressure and heart failure)?

The physician actually intended to prescribe 120 tablets of Isordil at its typical dose of 20 mg by mouth (po) every (Q) 6 hours. Ramon Vasquez's pharmacist read the prescription as Plendil and instructed the patient to take a 20-mg pill every 6 hours. Unfortunately, the usual starting dose of Plendil is 10 mg/day, making this an eightfold overdose. A day later, Mr. Vasquez's blood pressure dropped to critically low levels, leading to heart failure. He died within the week.

The modern pharmaceutical armamentarium represents one of health-care's great advances. There are now highly effective agents to treat or mitigate the effects of most common medical conditions: hypertension, hyperlipidemia, diabetes, heart disease, cancer, stroke, acquired immunodeficiency syndrome (AIDS), and more. Taken correctly, the benefits of these medications far outweigh their side effects, though the latter remains a concern even when medications are prescribed and taken correctly.

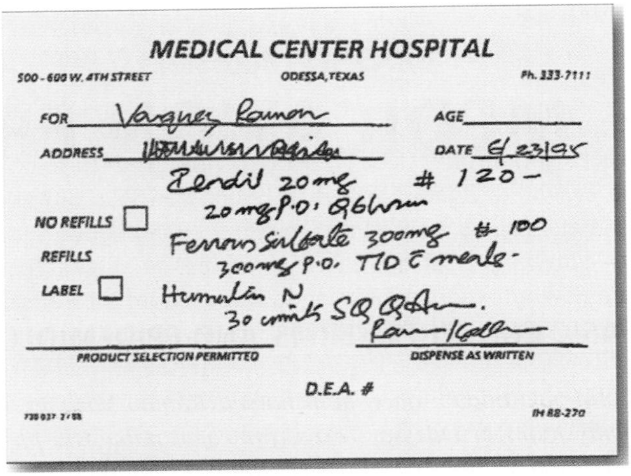
MEDICAL CENTER HOSPITAL
500 - 600 W. 4TH STREET ODESSA, TEXAS Ph. 333-7111
FOR Vasquez Ramon AGE
ADDRESS DATE 6/23/95
Zendil 20 mg # 120 -
NO REFILLS 20 mg P.O. Q6h
Ferrous Sulfate 300mg # 100
REFILLS 300mg P.O. TID c meals.
LABEL Humulin N
30 units SQ
PRODUCT SELECTION PERMITTED DISPENSE AS WRITTEN
D.E.A. #

Figure 4-1 ▪ Ramon Vasquez's prescription.

But the growth in medications (there are now more than 10,000 prescription drugs and biologicals—and 300,000 over-the-counter products—available in the United States[1]) and prescriptions (approximately 60% of American adults are taking some type of prescription medication[2]) has led to a huge increase in the complexity of the medication prescribing and administration process. It has been estimated that at least 5% of hospitalized patients experience an *adverse drug event* (ADE; harm experienced by a patient as a result of a medication, from either a side effect or the consequence of an error) at some point during their stay. Another 5% to 10% experience a potential ADE, meaning that they nearly took the wrong medicine or the wrong dose but didn't, often thanks to a last minute catch or sheer luck.[3] Elderly patients are particularly vulnerable; almost half of all nursing home residents are exposed to inappropriate medications.[4] The cost of preventable medication errors in U.S. hospitals was estimated at $16.4 billion annually in 2010.[5]

Things are no safer outside the hospital. One surveillance study estimated that four emergency department visits for ADEs occurred per 1000 patients annually and over 25% of these visits required hospital admission.[6] In addition, approximately 4.5 million ambulatory visits occur annually due to ADEs.[7] The cost of preventable medication errors in the ambulatory setting is significant, bumping the total cost of medication errors to over $20 billion each year.[5]

Historically, many discussions about medication errors focused on the famous illegibility of physicians' handwriting, but as a result of the rapid uptake of computerized provider order entry (CPOE) and electronic prescribing (stimulated by the 2009 Health Information Technology for Economic and Clinical Health Act, or HITECH, under which the federal government provided funds to expand the use of health information technology) bad handwriting is becoming a less important source of error. Unfortunately, medication errors remain distressingly common.

There are many steps along the medication prescribing and administration pathway that are vulnerable to mistakes. To illustrate these steps, let's follow the life of an inpatient prescription, in a hospital without CPOE and bar code medication administration (BCMA)[1]:

- A physician handwrites a prescription in the "Doctors' Orders" section of the chart.
- A clerk removes a carbon copy of the order and faxes it to the pharmacy, while a nurse transcribes the order into the Medication Administration Record (MAR).
- A pharmacist receives the faxed copy, reads it, and retypes the medication, dose, and frequency into the pharmacy's computer system, which generates labels, a bill, and an electronic trail that facilitates tracking of inventory.
- A pharmacist manually transfers the medication (if a pill) from a large bottle into "unit doses"—either cups or a shrink-wrapped container. Intravenous medication may require specialized mixing.
- The medication is delivered to the patient's floor; the label includes the name of the medication and the patient's name. The medicine may be delivered to the floor on a cart, via a manual transport system, or a pneumatic tube system.
- The nurse goes to the MAR, sees that the patient is due for a medication, searches the medication cart for it, and walks to the patient's room with the medication (along with different medications for her other patients).
- The nurse enters the patient's room, confirms the patient's identity, checks the medication, and administers it.

Believe it or not, this is a simplified version of the actual process. Several hospitals have described about *50 to 100 distinct steps* that take place between the time a doctor decides to order a medicine and the time that medicine is delivered to the patient.

The outpatient process is simpler, but only by a bit. Before the advent of electronic prescribing, the doctor traditionally gave the patient a paper prescription to carry to a pharmacy. Not only might the prescription itself be prone to errors (wrong medicine, wrong dose, illegibility, failure on the part of the physician to account for allergies or drug–drug, drug–disease, or drug–diet

---

[1]While the medication process is now digital in most U.S. hospitals, this is not invariably so, particularly in small and rural hospitals. And, lest you think that CPOE and BCMA eliminate the possibility of medication errors, in Chapter 13 we'll describe a major medication error that occurred in a fully wired hospital.

interactions), but the administration of the medication (generally a mistake in the pharmacy), the need for proper monitoring (forgetting to check electrolytes and kidney function in a patient started on a diuretic and/or angiotensin-converting enzyme inhibitor), the patient's ability to take the medication correctly (e.g., failure to follow instructions properly or storing the medications in incorrect bottles; Chapter 21), the caregiver's ability to administer the medication correctly,[8] or the patient's ability to take the medication at all,[9] for that matter, are all vulnerable to error. In such a complex system, statistical law inevitably takes its toll: in a 50-step process in which each step is done correctly 99% of the time, the chance that at least one error will occur is a staggering 39%!

> *Sarah Geller was a 68-year-old woman who had undergone a cardiac bypass operation. After a stormy postoperative course she seemed to be on the road to recovery. However, on the morning of her planned transfer out of the intensive care unit (ICU), she suffered a grand mal seizure. This shocked her caregivers. She had no seizure history and was not on any medications known to lower the seizure threshold. They drew some blood tests, and emergently wheeled her to the computed tomography (CT) scanner to rule out the possibility of a stroke or intracerebral hemorrhage. While she was in transit, the lab paged the doctors to report that Geller's serum glucose was undetectable. Despite multiple infusions of glucose, she never recovered from her coma. In the subsequent investigation, it was determined that her bedside tray in the ICU contained vials of both heparin (used to "flush" her intravenous lines to keep them open) and insulin. The vials were of similar size and shape (Figure 4-2). The nurse, intending to flush Ms. Geller's line with heparin, had inadvertently administered a fatal dose of insulin.[10]*

As this case demonstrates, mitigating the problem of medication errors requires solutions that address the steps involved in both the prescribing and administration phases[1,2] (Figure 4-3). Many of the solutions that have been increasingly adopted over the last decade are technological: the role of CPOE, electronic prescribing, computerized decision support, and bar coding and/or radio-frequency identification (RFID) systems will be discussed in greater detail in Chapter 13. The remainder of this chapter will focus on solutions more specific to the medication prescribing and administration process: standardization, vigilance and the "Five Rights," double-checks, preventing interruptions and distractions, unit dosing, removal of risky medications from certain settings, the role of clinical pharmacists, and meeting the challenges of look-alike, sound-alike medications. A final section will review the main strategy to avoid medication errors at the time of care transitions: medication reconciliation.

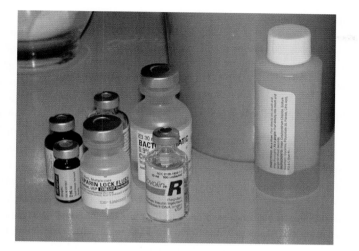

Figure 4-2 ▪ Heparin and insulin vials on a bedside tray.

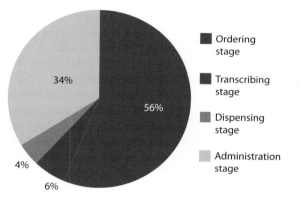

- Ordering stage
- Transcribing stage
- Dispensing stage
- Administration stage

34%

56%

4%

6%

Figure 4-3 ▪ Medication errors, by stage of the medication process. (Adapted from Bates DW, Cullen DJ, Laird N, et al. Incidence of adverse drug events and potential adverse drug events. Implications for prevention. ADE Prevention Study Group. *JAMA* 1995;274:29–34.)

STRATEGIES TO DECREASE MEDICATION ERRORS

Standardization and decreasing ambiguity

In 1994, Betsy Lehman, a popular Boston Globe health columnist, was hospitalized for recurrent breast cancer at Dana-Farber Cancer Institute. Her experimental protocol called for her to receive an unusually high dose of cyclophosphamide (a chemotherapy agent), followed by a bone marrow transplant. The ordering physicians wrote a prescription: "cyclophosphamide 4 g/sq m over four days," intending that she receive a total of 4 g/m² of body surface area spread out over 4 days. Instead, the nurses administered the total dose (4 g/m²) on each of the 4 days, a fourfold overdose. She died within a month.

The highly publicized death of Betsy Lehman helped catalyze the modern patient safety movement (Table 1-1), supporting the case for computerization and decision support. It is easy to envision how a computer system preprogrammed with the chemotherapy protocol that either presented the correct dose as a default option to the ordering clinician or automatically alarmed when someone prescribed an out-of-range dose might have prevented the error that killed Betsy Lehman.[11] But Lehman's death also underscored the need for standardization: general agreements on inviolable ways of communicating certain medication orders that would be understandable to everyone involved in a patient's care.[12] For example, a hospital could mandate that all medications given over multiple days *must* have the daily dose written each day. Or that high-risk medications could only be ordered for one day at a time.

One source of ambiguity has been the long-standing use of abbreviations for certain medications. In 2004, the Joint Commission prohibited hospitals from using a group of "high-risk abbreviations" (Table 4-1), insisting

Table 4-1 THE JOINT COMMISSION'S "DO NOT USE" LIST		
Do Not Use	**Potential Problem**	**Use Instead**
U (unit)	Mistaken for "0" (zero), the number "4" (four), or "cc"	Write "unit"
IU (International Unit)	Mistaken for IV (intravenous) or the number 10 (ten)	Write "International Unit"
Q.D., QD, q.d., qd (daily)	Mistaken for each other	Write "daily"
Q.O.D., QOD, q.o.d, qod (every other day)	Period after the Q mistaken for "I" and the "O" mistaken for "I"	Write "every other day"
Trailing zero (*X*.0 mg)	Decimal point is missed	Write *X* mg
Lack of leading zero (. *X* mg)		Write 0. *X* mg
MS	Can mean morphine sulfate or magnesium sulfate	Write "morphine sulfate"
MSO_4 and $MgSO_4$	Confused for one another	Write "magnesium sulfate"

© The Joint Commission, 2017. Reprinted with permission. Available at: https://www.jointcommission.org/facts_about_do_not_use_list/.

that the full name of these medications and instructions ("morphine sulfate," not "MS04"; "Insulin 10 Units," not "Insulin 10 U") be spelled out. One of the advantages of CPOE has been its ability to further standardize nomenclature and markedly limit the use of abbreviations. However, as will be further discussed in Chapter 13, CPOE has the capacity to create new classes of medication errors if it is not well designed and implemented.[13–15]

Vigilance and the "Five Rights" of medication administration

While many advances in medication safety have come from system changes such as automation and double-checks, individual caregivers are responsible for doing what they can to ensure the safety of their patients. One long-standing nursing principle is known as the "Five Rights" (Table 4-2), highlighting the five checks that a nurse is expected to make before administering a medication to a patient. Some have argued for additional checks, including right documentation, right action (i.e., the medication is being given for the correct indication), right form (i.e., oral vs. intravenous, can the pill be safely crushed?), and right response (i.e., the nurse should monitor the patient's response to the medication).[16] Some add still another: the right of a patient to refuse a medication. Although these additional rights have not yet become standard practice, they further illustrate the tremendous challenges of correct medication administration and the limitations of human vigilance as a safety bulwark.

Double-checks

Other high-risk industries (nuclear power, aviation, the armed services) have long used double, and even triple, checks to ensure that critical processes are executed correctly. Patient safety, for its part, has come a long way relatively

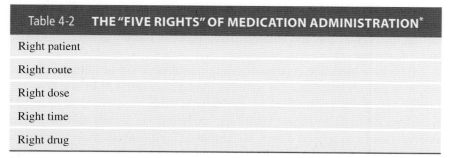

Table 4-2	THE "FIVE RIGHTS" OF MEDICATION ADMINISTRATION*
Right patient	
Right route	
Right dose	
Right time	
Right drug	

*Some have suggested additions to the original list of "Five Rights," including right documentation, right action, right form, right response, and the right of a patient to refuse a medication.[16]

quickly. Fifteen years ago, the only process with standardized and inviolable independent double-checks in most hospitals was that of blood administration (in which two nurses confirm ABO blood types prior to a transfusion). Thankfully, most hospitals now have built-in double checks for chemotherapy[12] and other high-risk medications. However, even when double-checks are required by policy, it is critical to ensure that they are truly independent. It is very easy (natural, in fact) for the second check to become lackadaisical, in essence a rubber stamp, thereby providing false reassurance rather than truly increased safety.

Preventing interruptions and distractions

Each step in the medication prescribing, preparation, and administrative process is subject to error. While automation has been introduced into every phase, the vast majority of medication deliveries still involve humans in each of those phases. For example, even in a hospital with computerized order entry, the physician still needs to decide on the medication and dosage, a pharmacist needs to take the order and dispense the medication to the floor, and the nurse needs to collect the correct medication from a dispensing machine and deliver it to the patient.

Each of these steps is subject to mistakes, and recent research has quantified the extent to which distractions and interruptions increase the probability of errors (see also Chapter 7).[17] Most of the research has focused on the nursing portion of this chain, although there is little reason to believe that prescribing physicians[18] or pharmacists are any less susceptible to the hazards of interruptions and distractions.[19]

One time–motion study of nurses preparing and administering medications found an average of 1.2 interruptions during every medication pass.[20] In a memorable example, it took over 2 hours for a nurse to retrieve one particular medication from a storage device, because the device forced the nurse to close all 25 drawers each time she wanted to retrieve the medication. Even the process of administering high-risk medications, such as chemotherapy, is frequently interrupted.[21] In one study, every time a nurse was interrupted during the preparation and administration process, there was a 12% increase in clinical errors.[22]

Emerging evidence is demonstrating that decreasing or eliminating distractions and interruptions can improve medication safety.[23] In one hospital, nurses were given a protected hour during which they were not to be disturbed by telephone calls or pages. While the study did not isolate this particular intervention from several others, it did find a significant decrease in medication errors.[24] Another hospital created a "No Interruption Zone" (marked off by red tape on the floor) to indicate that a critical care nurse was not to be interrupted. The establishment of the No Interruption Zone was associated with a reduction in both interruptions and administration errors.[25]

Before we get too excited about such interventions, it's worth heeding the cautionary note of Rivera-Rodriguez and Karsh, who point out that certain interruptions are crucial to the delivery of high-quality and safe care.[26] They argue against banning interruptions outright, as interventions need to account for the complexity of healthcare systems. This is an important argument to consider—it's easy to see how certain strategies to eliminate interruptions could lead to unintended consequences and "squeezed balloons." A 2014 systematic review of the value of reducing interruptions during medication administration found weak evidence in support of this strategy.[27]

Obviously, one cure for interruptions and distractions would be to remove humans from the medication prescribing/delivery process. While automation is likely to do that to some degree, people will remain active and necessary participants in the medication prescribing and administration pathway for the foreseeable future. This makes continued attention to, and innovations in, this area essential.

Unit dosing

This refers to the packaging of medications in ready-to-use units that are prepared in the pharmacy and then delivered to the clinical floor. Unit dosing was developed in the 1960s, replacing the old method in which the pharmacy sent large bottles of pills or intravenous medications to a floor, expecting that the nurses would perform the mixing or dispensing. Studies have generally found that unit-dose administration is associated with fewer medication errors, and the practice has now become nearly ubiquitous in American hospitals.[28] Many pharmacy systems now include automatic dispensing machines, which are usually computerized and often linked to centralized inventory control systems and have been showed to reduce errors associated with medication administration and provide a sound return on investment.[29,30]

Removal of medications from certain settings

The most widely cited example of this strategy is the removal of concentrated potassium from patient care areas. Because of the lethality associated with intravenous potassium overdoses (as when intravenous potassium is used in cases of capital punishment), such removal seems like a good idea. Rather than having the nurses add potassium to their intravenous solutions on the floor, the new system depends on potassium being added to intravenous bags by pharmacists before the premixed bags are sent to the ward.

This approach is an example of a more general strategy called *forcing functions* (Chapters 2 and 7): technical or physical obstacles designed to decrease the probability of error in error-prone circumstances or environments. Forcing functions are designed to anticipate common human errors and make harm from them impossible by blocking either the error or its consequences. As mentioned in Chapter 2, the most widely cited example of a forcing function was the reengineering of automobile braking systems in the 1980s to make it impossible to shift a car into reverse when the driver's foot was off the brake.

The removal of concentrated potassium from clinical settings would seem to be such a forcing function, and thus a logical safety solution. Yet even this seemingly simple strategy was beset by unintended consequences, as many nurses found that it took too long for their intravenous drips to arrive from the pharmacy. Because potassium was still allowed in the ICUs (it often needs to be given emergently there), floor nurses began pilfering potassium from ICU stashes and hoarding it, creating an even more chaotic and potentially unsafe situation.[31] The lesson from this experience is not that keeping dangerous medications such as potassium on the floor is a good idea (it probably isn't), but rather that frontline workers often thwart apparently "commonsensical safety fixes" when the fixes get in the way of their perceived ability to do their jobs efficiently, a process known as a "workaround."[32,33] Safety planners need to seek out such actual or potential workarounds through focus groups and observations of providers doing their daily work, lest they create an "underground economy" in unsafe practices (Chapter 7).

The use of clinical pharmacists

Of all the strategies employed to try to decrease medication errors, the insertion of clinical pharmacists into the medication prescribing and administration processes is one of the most powerful (of course, this is in addition to having pharmacists read prescriptions and dispense medications, both core functions). For example, in one classic study, clinical pharmacists became part of an ICU team in an academic medical center. They educated the physicians and trainees, rounded with the teams, and intervened when they saw a medication error in the making. The intervention resulted in a nearly threefold decrease in the frequency of ADEs, which reduced patient harm and yielded significant cost savings.[34] Other studies have found impressive reductions in preventable ADEs and inappropriate medication use when pharmacists assisted with medication reconciliation and pharmacy technicians were integrated into emergency departments.[35–37] Unfortunately, in the United States, the high cost and a national shortage of pharmacists have led these strategies to be relatively underemployed.

Meeting the challenge of look-alike, sound-alike medications

Although the U.S. Food and Drug Administration (FDA) now tries, during its drug approval process, to minimize the possibility that a new medication name will be confused with an old one, with 10,000 agents in the pharmacopoeia some problems are inevitable. Among the most confusing examples: the opioid hydromorphone and the anti-hypertensive hydralazine and the antidepressant clomipramine and the fertility agent clomiphene.

There are a number of strategies to help minimize the risk of confusion, including the user of "tall man" lettering for the suffixes of drugs that begin with the same prefix, such as "clomiPHENE" and "clomiPRAMINE"[38] (Table 4-3 shows some examples of FDA-approved generic drugs' names with "tall man" lettering). But eradicating this problem entirely will require technological help, including bar coding administration systems[39] and computerized order entry with decision support.[40] For example, one can imagine a system that would ask for each medication's indication, and balk if the indication was "seizures" and the chosen medication was Celebrex (instead of Cerebyx; see Chapter 13).

Medication reconciliation

This chapter has emphasized medication safety when the patient is static: in an ICU bed, on a medical floor, or visiting a doctor in a clinic. But the greatest opportunities for errors in the medication process likely come when patients are transitioning from one setting to another (see also Chapter 8): being admitted to or discharged from the hospital, going from their primary care physician's office to that of a specialist, transferring out of the ICU to the floor, or going from the floor to the operating room. Studies have shown that unintended medication discrepancies are common, occurring in about 30% of patients at the time of admission[41] (about 40% of these have moderate or severe potential for harm[42]), a similar percentage when they transfer from one hospital site to another,[43] and in 14% of cases at hospital discharge.[44]

Medication reconciliation is the process of reviewing a patient's complete medication regimen on both ends of a care transition in an effort to avoid unintended inconsistencies.[45] While many physicians have for long asked their patients to bring their "old meds" to their clinic appointments

Table 4-3 EXAMPLES FROM FDA-APPROVED LIST OF GENERIC DRUG NAMES WITH TALL MAN LETTERS*	
Drug Name with Tall Man Letters	**Confused with**
aceta**ZOLAMIDE**	aceto**HEXAMIDE**
bu**PROP**ion	bus**PIR**one
chlorpro**MAZINE**	chlorpro**PAMIDE**
clomi**PHENE**	clomipramine
cyclo**SERINE**	cyclosporine
DAUNOrubicin	**DOXO**rubicin
dimenhy**DRINATE**	diphenhydramine
DOBUTamine	**DOP**amine
glipi**ZIDE**	glyburide
hydr**ALAZINE**	hydr**OXY**zine-**HYDRO**morphone
medroxy**PROGESTER**one	methyl**PREDNIS**olone-methyl**TESTOSTER**one
ni**CAR**dipine	**NIFE**dipine
predniso**LONE**	prednisone
risperi**DONE**	r**OPINIR**ole
sulf**ADIAZINE**	sulfi**SOXAZOLE**
TOLAZamide	**TOLBUT**amide
vin**BLAS**tine	vincristine

*In 2001, the U.S. FDA began requiring the manufacturers of many of these products to use "tall man" lettering (e.g., clomiPHENE and clomiPRAMINE) on their labels. A link to the FDA and ISMP lists of look-alike drug names with recommended tall man letters is provided in Reference 38.

(often called a "brown bag review"), medication reconciliation has become formalized relatively recently. The search for optimal methods of performing reconciliation gained considerable momentum when, in 2004, the Institute for Healthcare Improvement included it among the recommended practices in its 100,000 Lives Campaign (Table 20-2).[46] The following year, the Joint Commission named "med rec" as one of its National Patient Safety Goals, and in 2006 the organization added it as a requirement for hospital accreditation.

Unfortunately, while medication reconciliation has great face validity, the methods for accomplishing it have varied widely and research on it has produced mixed results. The methods have included having pharmacists perform the entire process, involving patients (particularly ambulatory patients) in their own reconciliation, and embedding the process in electronic systems. While one study involving pharmacists demonstrated improved clinical outcomes and reductions in ADEs,[47] a subsequent randomized controlled trial showed that about half of the adult patients who received a pharmacist-driven intervention involving medication reconciliation at the time of hospital discharge still experienced a clinically significant medication error.[48] Nevertheless, the literature generally seems to suggest that integrating pharmacists into the medication reconciliation process is helpful and may even be cost-effective.[49]

While research is beginning to illustrate some best practices in medication reconciliation, uncertainty about what really works remains and most successful studies illustrate beneficial effects on potential ADEs rather than true patient harm. Indeed, two reviews on inpatient medication reconciliation concluded that, although pharmacist-led interventions could mitigate medication discrepancies and potential ADEs after discharge, the clinical impact of these discrepancies was small and therefore medication reconciliation by itself may not significantly reduce adverse events or readmissions.[50,51] Many institutions have seen their medical reconciliation initiatives stall because of disagreements on crucial issues, such as whose job it is to perform the reconciliation.[52] In light of this uncertainty, the Joint Commission has gone back and forth on its medical reconciliation requirements, softening its enforcement in 2009 but tightening it in 2011. The challenges of medication reconciliation vividly illustrate how difficult it is to implement even relatively "simple" fixes in highly complex systems of care (Chapter 2).

Conservative prescribing

It is worth emphasizing one final point. One key to minimizing medication errors is to limit the use of medications to situations in which they are truly indicated—in other words, when the potential benefit to the patient exceeds the risk of harm. As one example of this principle, elderly hospitalized patients who received medications considered inappropriate (such as prolonged use of proton pump inhibitors, aspirin in patients without a history of cardiovascular disease, or sedatives and opiates in patients with a history of falls) have a nearly twofold increase in their odds of an adverse event during the hospitalization.[53] Schiff et al. have outlined a series of principles for *conservative prescribing* (Table 4-4), and they are well worth following.[54]

Table 4-4   PRINCIPLES OF CONSERVATIVE PRESCRIBING

Think beyond drugs

Seek nondrug alternatives first

Consider potentially treatable underlying causes of problems rather than just treating the symptoms with a drug

Look for opportunities for prevention rather than focusing on treating symptoms or advanced disease

Use the test of time as a diagnostic and therapeutic trial whenever possible

Practice more strategic prescribing

Use only a few drugs and learn to use them well

Avoid frequent switching to new drugs without clear, compelling evidence-based reasons

Be skeptical about individualizing therapy

Whenever possible, start treatment with only one drug at a time

Maintain heightened vigilance regarding adverse effects

Have a high index of suspicion for adverse drug effects

Educate patients about possible adverse effects to ensure that they are recognized as early as possible

Be alert to clues that you may be treating or risking withdrawal symptoms

Approach new drugs and new indications cautiously and skeptically

Learn about new drugs and new indications from trustworthy, unbiased sources

Do not rush to use newly marketed drugs

Be certain that the drug improves actual patient-centered clinical outcomes rather than just treating or masking a surrogate marker

Be vigilant about indications creep

Do not be seduced by elegant molecular pharmacology or drug physiology

Beware of selective reporting of studies

Work with patients for a more deliberative shared agenda

Do not hastily or uncritically succumb to patient requests for drugs, especially drugs that they have heard advertised

Avoid mistakenly prescribing additional drugs for refractory problems, failing to appreciate the potential for patient nonadherence

Avoid repeating prescriptions for drugs that a patient has previously tried unsuccessfully or that caused an adverse reaction

Discontinue treatment with drugs that are not working or are no longer needed

Work with patients' desires to be conservative with medications

Consider longer-term, broader effects

Think beyond short-term beneficial drug effects to consider longer-term benefits and risks

Look for opportunities to improve prescribing systems, changes that can make prescribing and medication use safer

KEY POINTS

- With the explosive growth in available medications, ADEs (both side effects and medication errors) are one of the most common threats to patient safety.
- Errors can occur at any point in the medication chain, particularly in the prescribing and administration stages. For medications prescribed in the ambulatory environment, patient-related errors and inadequate monitoring are also common.
- Information technology has been shown to decrease medication errors, including prescribing errors (through CPOE and computerized decision support) and administration errors (through bar coding and other identification techniques). Unintended consequences are common, however, and need to be anticipated.
- In addition to these information technology-related solutions, other important medication safety strategies include standardization, checking the "Five Rights," double-checks, preventing unnecessary distractions and interruptions, unit dosing, removal of high-risk medications from certain settings, engaging clinical pharmacists, specific strategies to mitigate the risks of look-alike, sound-alike medications, and performing medication reconciliation at the time of care transitions.
- Another important way to avoid medication errors is to follow principles of conservative prescribing: avoiding the inappropriate use of medications.

REFERENCES

1. Aspden P, Wolcott J, Bootman JL, Cronenwett LR, eds. Committee on Identifying and Preventing Medication Errors. *Preventing Medication Errors: Quality Chasm Series.* Institute of Medicine. Washington, DC: National Academies Press; 2007.
2. Kantor ED, Rehm CD, Haas JS, Chan AT, Giovannucci EL. Trends in prescription drug use among adults in the United States. *JAMA* 2015;314:1818–1831.
3. Bates DW, Cullen DJ, Laird N, et al. Incidence of adverse drug events and potential adverse drug events. Implications for prevention. ADE Prevention Study Group. *JAMA* 1995;274:29–34.
4. Morin L, Laroche ML, Texier G, Johnell K. Prevalence of potentially inappropriate medication use in older adults living in nursing homes: a systematic review. *J Am Med Dire Assoc* 2016;17:862.e1–e9.
5. *Preventing Medication Errors: A $21 Billion Opportunity.* Washington, DC: National Priorities Partnership and National Quality Forum; December 2010. Available at: www.qualityforum.org/NPP/docs/Preventing_Medication_Error_CAB.aspx.

6. Shehab N, Lovegrove MC, Geller AI, Rose KO, Weidle NJ, Budnitz DS. US emergency visits for outpatient adverse drug events, 2013–2014. *JAMA* 2016;316:2115–2125.

7. Sarkar U, López A, Masselli JH, Gonzales R. Adverse drug events in U.S. adult ambulatory medical care. *Health Serv Res* 2011;46:1517–1533.

8. Berthe-Aucejo A, Girard D, Lorrot M, et al. Evaluation of frequency of paediatric oral liquid medication dosing errors by caregivers: amoxicillin and josamycin. *Arch Dis Child* 2016;101:359–364.

9. Sidorkiewicz S, Tran VT, Cousyn C, Perrodeau E, Ravaud P. Discordance between drug adherence as reported by patients and drug importance as assessed by physicians. *Ann Fam Med* 2016;14:415–421.

10. Bates DW. Unexpected hypoglycemia in a critically ill patient. *Ann Intern Med* 2002;137:110–116.

11. Aziz MT, Ur-Rehman T, Qureshi S, Bukhari NI. Reduction in chemotherapy order errors with computerized physician order entry and clinical decision support systems. *HIM J* 2015;44:13–22.

12. Neuss MN, Gilmore TR, Belderson KM, et al. 2016 Updated American Society of Clinical Oncology/Oncology Nursing Society chemotherapy administration safety standards, including standards for pediatric oncology. *J Oncol Pract* 2016;12:1262–1271.

13. Brown CL, Mulcaster HL, Triffitt KL, et al. A systematic review of the types and causes of prescribing errors generated from using computerized provider order entry systems in primary and secondary care. *J Am Med Inform Assoc* 2017;24:432–440.

14. Slight SP, Eguale T, Amato MG, et al. The vulnerabilities of computerized physician order entry systems: a qualitative study. *J Am Med Inform Assoc* 2016;23:311–316.

15. Schiff GD, Hickman TT, Volk LA, Bates DW, Wright A. Computerised prescribing for safer medication ordering: still a work in progress. *BMJ Qual Saf* 2016;25:315–319.

16. Elliott M, Liu Y. The nine rights of medication administration: an overview. *Br J Nurs* 2010;19:300–305.

17. Hayes C, Jackson D, Davidson PM, Power T. Medication errors in hospitals: a literature review of disruptions to nursing practice during medication administration. *J Clin Nurs* 2015;24:3063–3076.

18. Magrabi F, Li SY, Day RO, Coiera E. Errors and electronic prescribing: a controlled laboratory study to examine task complexity and interruption effects. *J Am Med Inform Assoc* 2010;17:575–583.

19. Raimbault M, Guérin A, Caron E, Lebel D, Bussiéres JF. Identifying and reducing distractions and interruptions in a pharmacy department. *Am J Health Syst Pharm* 2013;70:186–190.

20. Elganzouri ES, Standish CA, Androwich I. Medication Administration Time Study (MATS): nursing staff performance of medication administration. *J Nurs Adm* 2009;39:204–210.

21. Trbovich P, Prakash V, Stewart J, Trip K, Savage P. Interruptions during the delivery of high-risk medications. *J Nurs Adm* 2010;40:211–218.

22. Westbrook JI, Woods A, Rob MI, Dunsmuir WT, Day RO. Association of interruptions with an increased risk and severity of medication administration errors. *Arch Intern Med* 2010;170:683–690.

23. Prakash V, Koczmara C, Savage P, et al. Mitigating errors caused by interruptions during medication verification and administration: interventions in a simulated ambulatory chemotherapy setting. *BMJ Qual Saf* 2014;23:884–892.

24. Kliger J. Giving medication administration the respect it is due. Comment on: "Association of interruptions with an increased risk and severity of medication administration errors". *Arch Intern Med* 2010;170:690–692.

25. Anthony K, Wiencek C, Bauer C, Daly B, Anthony MK. No interruptions please: impact of a no interruption zone on medication safety in intensive care units. *Crit Care Nurse* 2010;30:21–29.

26. Rivera-Rodriguez AJ, Karsh BT. Interruptions and distractions in healthcare: review and reappraisal. *Qual Saf Health Care* 2010;19:304–312.

27. Raban MZ, Westbrook JI. Are interventions to reduce interruptions and errors during medication administration effective?: a systematic review. *BMJ Qual Saf* 2014;23:414–421.

28. Murray MD, Shojania KG. Unit-dose drug distribution systems. In: Shojania KG, Duncan BW, McDonald KM, et al., eds. *Making Health Care Safer: A Critical Analysis of Patient Safety Practices*. Evidence Report/Technology Assessment No. 43, AHRQ Publication No. 01-E058. Rockville, MD: Agency for Healthcare Research and Quality; 2001.

29. Chapuis C, Roustit M, Bal G, et al. Automated drug dispensing system reduces medication errors in an intensive care setting. *Crit Care Med* 2010;38:2275–2281.

30. Fanning L, Jones N, Manias E. Impact of automated dispensing cabinets on medication selection and preparation error rates in an emergency department: a prospective and direct observational before-and-after study. *J Eval Clin Pract* 2016;22:156–163.

31. Potassium may no longer be stocked on patient care units, but serious threats still exist! ISMP Medication Safety Alert! Acute care ed. October 4, 2007;12:1–2.

32. Seaman JB, Erlen JA. Workarounds in the workplace: a second look. *Orthop Nurs* 2015;34:235–240.

33. Tucker AL, Heisler WS, Janisse LD. Designed for workarounds: a qualitative study of the causes of operational failures in hospitals. *Perm J* 2014;18:33–41.

34. Leape LL, Cullen DJ, Clapp MD, et al. Pharmacist participation on physician rounds and adverse drug events in the intensive care unit. *JAMA* 1999;282:267–270.

35. Tong EY, Roman C, Mitra B, et al. Partnered pharmacist charting on admission in the general medical and emergency short-stay unit—a cluster-randomised controlled trial in patients with complex medication regimens. *J Clin Pharm Ther* 2016;41:414–418.

36. Buckley MS, Harinstein LM, Clark KB, et al. Impact of a clinical pharmacy admission medication reconciliation program on medication errors in "high-risk" patients. *Ann Pharmacother* 2013;47:1599–1610.

37. Rubin EC, Pisupati R, Nerenberg SF. Utilization of pharmacy technicians to increase the accuracy of patient medication histories obtained in the emergency department. *Hosp Pharm* 2016;51:396–404.

38. ISMP updates its list of drug name pairs with tall man letters. FDA and ISMP Lists of Look-Alike Drug Names with Recommended Tall Man Letters. Institute for Safe Medication Practices; June 2016. Available at: http://www.ismp.org/Tools/tallman letters.pdf.

39. Poon EG, Keohane CA, Yoon CS, et al. Effect of bar-code technology on the safety of medication administration. *N Engl J Med* 2010;362:1698–1707.

40. Ranji SR, Rennke S, Wachter RM. Computerised provider order entry combined with clinical decision support systems to improve medication safety: a narrative review. *BMJ Qual Saf* 2014;23:773–780.

41. Tam VC, Knowles SR, Cornish PL, Fine N, Marchesano R, Etchells EE. Frequency, type and clinical importance of medication history errors at admission to hospital: a systematic review. *CMAJ* 2005;173:510–515.

42. Bishop MA, Cohen BA, Billings LK, Thomas EV. Reducing errors through discharge medication reconciliation by pharmacy services. *Am J Health Syst Pharm* 2015;72:S120–S126.

43. Bell CM, Rahimi-Darabad P, Orner AI. Discontinuity of chronic medications in patients discharged from the intensive care unit. *J Gen Intern Med* 2006; 21:937–941.

44. Forster AJ, Murff HJ, Peterson JF, Gandhi TK, Bates DW. The incidence and severity of adverse events affecting patients after discharge from the hospital. *Ann Intern Med* 2003;138:161–167.

45. Patient safety primers: medication reconciliation. AHRQ Patient Safety Network. Available at: https://psnet.ahrq.gov/primers/primer/1/medication-reconciliation.

46. Berwick DM, Calkins DR, McCannon CJ, Hackbarth AD. The 100,000 Lives Campaign: setting a goal and a deadline for improving health care quality. *JAMA* 2006;295:324–327.

47. Schnipper JL, Kirwin JL, Cotugno MC, et al. Role of pharmacist counseling in preventing adverse drug events after hospitalization. *Arch Intern Med* 2006;166:565–571.

48. Kripalani S, Roumie CL, Dalal AK, et al. Effect of a pharmacist intervention on clinically important medication errors after hospital discharge: a randomized trial. *Ann Intern Med* 2012;157:1–10.

49. Najafzadeh M, Schnipper JL, Shrank WH, Kymes S, Brennan TA, Choudhry NK. Economic value of pharmacist-led medication reconciliation for reducing medication errors after hospital discharge. *Am J Manag Care* 2016;22:654–661.

50. Mueller SK, Sponsler KC, Kripalani S, Schnipper JL. Hospital-based medication reconciliation practices: a systematic review. *Arch Intern Med* 2012;172:1057–1069.

51. Kwan JL, Lo L, Sampson M, Shojania KG. Medication reconciliation during transitions of care as a patient safety strategy: a systematic review. *Ann Intern Med* 2013;158:397–403.

52. Poon EG. Medication reconciliation: whose job is it? [Spotlight]. *AHRQ WebM&M* [serial online]; September 2007. Available at: http://webMM.ahrq.gov/case.aspx? caseID=158.

53. Hamilton H, Gallagher P, Ryan C, Byrne S, O'Mahony D. Potentially inappropriate medications defined by STOPP criteria and the risk of adverse drug events in older hospitalized patients. *Arch Intern Med* 2011;171:1013–1019.

54. Schiff GD, Galanter WL, Duhig J, Lodolce AE, Koronkowski MJ, Lambert BL. Principles of conservative prescribing. *Arch Intern Med* 2011;171:1433–1440.

ADDITIONAL READINGS

Bates DW, Spell N, Cullen DJ, et al. The costs of adverse drug events in hospitalized patients. *JAMA* 1997;277:307–311.

Ferrah N, Lovell JJ, Ibrahim JE. Systematic review of the prevalence of medication errors resulting in hospitalization and death of nursing home residents. *J Am Geriatr Soc* 2017;65(2):433–442.

Mansur JM. Medication safety systems and the important role of pharmacists. *Drugs Aging* 2016;33:213–221.

Marien S, Krug B, Spinewine A. Electronic tools to support medication reconciliation—a systematic review. *J Am Med Inform Assoc* 2017;24(1):227–240.

McDowell SE, Mt-Isa S, Ashby D, Ferner RE. Where errors occur in the preparation and administration of intravenous medicines: a systematic review and Bayesian analysis. *Qual Saf Health Care* 2010;19:341–345.

Polinski JM, Moore JM, Kyrychenko P, et al. An insurer's care transition program emphasizes medication reconciliation, reduces readmissions and costs. *Health Aff (Millwood)* 2016;35:1222–1229.

Renaudin P, Boyer L, Esteve MA, Bertault-Peres P, Auquier P, Honore S. Do pharmacist-led medication reviews in hospitals help reduce hospital readmissions? A systematic review and meta-analysis. *Br J Clin Pharmacol* 2016;82(6):1660–1673.

Weingart SN, Wilson RM, Gibberd RW, Harrison B. Epidemiology of medical error. *BMJ* 2000;320:774–777.

Zhong W, Feinstein JA, Patel NS, Dai D, Feudtner C. Tall Man lettering and potential prescription errors: a time series analysis of 42 children's hospitals in the USA over 9 years. *BMJ Qual Saf* 2016;25:233–240.

SURGICAL ERRORS | 5

SOME BASIC CONCEPTS AND TERMS

More than 20 million people undergo surgery every year in the United States alone. Historically, surgery was considered extremely dangerous, in part because of the risks associated with the surgery itself (bleeding, infection), and in part because of the risks of anesthesia. Because of safety advances in both of these fields, surgeries today are extremely safe, and anesthesia-related deaths are rare.[1] Advances in surgery, anesthesia, and postoperative care have led to major declines in surgical mortality.[2]

Nevertheless, a number of troubling surgical safety issues persist. This chapter will address some of the more problematic issues directly related to surgery: anesthesia-related safety complications, wrong-site and wrong-patient surgery, retained foreign bodies, and surgical fires. The chapter will conclude with a brief discussion of nonsurgical procedural safety.

Of course, the field of surgery is not immune to medication errors (Chapter 4), diagnostic errors (Chapter 6), teamwork and communication errors (Chapter 9), and nosocomial infections, including surgical site infections (Chapter 10). These issues are covered in their respective chapters, although some elements that are more specific to surgery—such as the use of the surgical checklist—will be touched on here.

As with medication errors, in which problems from the intervention are grouped under a broad term ("adverse drug events") that includes both errors and side effects (Chapter 4), some surgical complications occur despite impeccable care, while others are caused by errors. Surgeries account for a relatively high percentage of both adverse events and preventable adverse events. For example, one of the major chart review studies of adverse events (the Utah–Colorado study) found that 45% of all adverse events were in surgical patients; of these, 17% resulted from negligence and 17% led to permanent disability. Looked at another way, 3% of patients who underwent an operation suffered an adverse event, and half of these were preventable.[3] Another systematic review estimates that about 1 in 20 surgical patients experiences a preventable adverse event, most of which were related to perioperative care.[4]

The field of surgery has always taken safety extremely seriously. In the early twentieth century, Boston surgeon Ernest Codman was among the first people in healthcare to measure complications of care and approach them scientifically. Codman's "End-Result Hospital"—following every patient for evidence of errors in treatment and disseminating the results of this inquiry—was both revolutionary and highly controversial[5–7] (Appendix III). Nevertheless, in 1918 the American College of Surgeons began inspecting hospitals, an effort that foreshadowed the Joint Commission (Chapter 20). Dr. Lucian Leape, a pediatric surgeon, is largely responsible for bringing the issue of patient safety to the fore of medical practice.[8,9] In addition, the field of surgery has pioneered the use of comparative data (most prominently in the form of the National Surgical Quality Improvement Program[10]) and regional collaboratives (such as in the Northern New England Cardiovascular Disease Study Group[11]) to promote performance improvement.

Despite these remarkable contributions, surgery, like the rest of medicine, has traditionally approached safety as a matter of individual excellence: a complication was deemed to represent a personal failing on the part of the surgeon. The shift in focus to systems improvement has catalyzed major advances in surgical safety.

VOLUME–OUTCOME RELATIONSHIPS

Beginning with a 1979 study by Luft et al. that demonstrated a relationship between higher volumes and better outcomes for certain surgeries, a substantial literature has generally supported the commonsensical notion that when it comes to procedures, "practice makes perfect."[12] The precise mechanism of this relationship has not been elucidated, but it seems to hold for both the volume of individual operators (e.g., the surgeon, the interventional cardiologist) and the institution (e.g., the hospital or surgicenter).[13]

Although much of the volume–outcome relationship probably owes to the fact that teams take time to gel—learning to anticipate each others' reactions and preferences—there also seems to be a learning curve for procedural competence. One of the best-studied examples is that of laparoscopic cholecystectomy, a technique that essentially replaced the more dangerous and costly open cholecystectomy in the early 1990s. As "lap choley" emerged as the preferred procedure for gallbladder removal, tens of thousands of practicing surgeons needed to learn the procedure well after the completion of their formal training, providing an organic test of the volume–outcome curve.

The findings were sobering. One early study of lap choleys showed that injuries to the common bile duct dropped almost 20-fold once surgeons had at least a dozen cases under their belts.[14] After that, the learning curve flattened, but not by much: the rate of common bile duct injury on the 30th case was still 10 times higher than the rate after 50 cases.

Patients can be confident that graduates of today's surgical residencies are well trained in the techniques of laparoscopic surgery. But in the early days of a new procedure, patients have no such reassurance. A 1991 survey found that only 45% of 165 practicing surgeons who had participated in a 2-day practical course on laparoscopic cholecystectomy felt the workshop had left them adequately prepared to start performing the procedure. Yet, three-quarters of these surgeons reported that they implemented the new procedure immediately after returning to their practices.[15]

Obviously, part of the solution to the volume–outcome and learning curve conundrums lies in the development of innovative training models, including the use of medical simulation (Chapter 17). In fact, one study found that surgical residents who underwent simulation training until they reached a predefined level of proficiency were one-third as likely to commit technical errors during laparoscopic cholecystectomy as those who received traditional training.[16] In addition, some surgical and procedural specialties are now requiring minimum volumes for privileging and board certification, and a major coalition of payers (the Leapfrog Group) promotes high-volume centers as one of its safety standards under the banner of "evidence-based hospital referral" and at the time of this writing (2017) is asking hospitals to report on their annual hospital and surgeon volume for ten volume-sensitive surgeries (Table 5-1) to better inform minimum hospital and surgeon volume standards. Certain states or insurers are insisting on minimum volumes or channeling patients to higher volume providers; institutions that achieve good outcomes and have high volumes are sometimes dubbed "Centers of Excellence."

Although such policies appear attractive at first, they are not without their own risks. First, patients may not be anxious to travel long distances to receive care from high-volume providers or institutions. Second, volumes that are *too* high may actually compromise quality by overtaxing institutions or physicians. Finally, many of the procedures being discussed, such as cardiac or transplant surgery, are relatively lucrative. Losing them could threaten the economic viability of low-volume institutions, which often cross-subsidize nonprofitable services (e.g., care of the uninsured, trauma care) with profits from the well-reimbursed surgeries. This is not to say that channeling patients to high-volume (or better yet, demonstrably safer or higher quality) doctors and practices is a mistake, but rather that it is a complex maneuver that requires thoughtful consideration of both expected and unforeseen consequences.[17]

With all of the discussion regarding safe systems, it is important to remember that procedural skills still matter. In a remarkable study published in 2013, Birkmeyer and colleagues asked bariatric surgeons to submit videotapes of one of their operations. A panel of at least 10 peers, blinded to the identity

Table 5-1   LIST OF 10 SURGICAL PROCEDURES FOR WHICH THE LEAPFROG GROUP IS SEEKING TO ESTABLISH MINIMUM VOLUME STANDARDS FOR SAFETY*
Bariatric surgery for weight loss
Esophageal resection
Lung resection
Pancreatic resection
Rectal cancer surgery
Carotid endarterectomy
Open aortic aneurysm repair
Mitral valve repair and replacement
Hip replacement
Knee replacement

*In 2017, the Leapfrog Group is asking hospitals to report on their annual hospital and surgeon volume for the above volume-sensitive surgeries to inform the minimum hospital and surgeon volume standards for safety as recommended by Leapfrog's national expert panel.

More information is available at: http://www.leapfroggroup.org/ratings-reports/surgeon-volume-and-surgical-appropriateness.

of the surgeon and the patient outcomes, reviewed each videotape and rated the surgical technique. The ratings varied tremendously, with some surgeons deemed to have stellar technique while others were judged to be mediocre. In an analysis blinded to the procedural technique scores, the scores were found to be highly correlated to a series of key surgical outcomes, including mortality, complications, infections, and re-operations.[18] In keeping with the "practice makes perfect" theme, while surgical skill was not related to years in practice, fellowship training, or teaching hospital practice site, it was strongly related to procedural volume.

PATIENT SAFETY IN ANESTHESIA

Although it is often stated that the modern patient safety movement began in late 1999 with the publication of *To Err Is Human* by the National Academy of Medicine (NAM, formerly the Institute of Medicine),[19] the field of anesthesia is a noteworthy exception. Anesthesia began focusing on safety a generation earlier, and its success holds lessons for the rest of the patient safety field.

In 1972, a young engineer named Jeff Cooper began work at the Anesthesia Bioengineering Unit at Massachusetts General Hospital (MGH). Similar to Codman 60 years before him, he was troubled by what he saw at MGH: mistakes were common, cover-ups were the norm, and systems to prevent errors were glaringly absent. Even worse, numerous procedures and processes appeared error-prone in their design. For example, he noticed that turning the dial clockwise increased the dose of anesthetic in some anesthesia machines, and decreased it in others. After delivering a lecture entitled, "The Anesthesia Machine: An Accident Waiting to Happen," Cooper and his colleagues began analyzing procedures and equipment from a human factors perspective (Chapter 7), using the technique of "critical incident analysis" to explore all causative factors for mistakes.[20–22]

Around the same time, anesthesiology was in the midst of a malpractice crisis characterized by acrimony and skyrocketing insurance premiums. Other researchers, recognizing the possibility that there might be error patterns, embarked on a detailed review of settled malpractice cases for themes and lessons ("closed-case analysis").[23] Indeed, common themes were identified, including poor machine design, a lack of standardization, lax policies and procedures, and inadequate education.

Though the research and insights from Cooper's work and the closed-case analyses were crucial, improving safety in practice would not be possible without widespread engagement of physicians. Luckily, as so often happens, the right person emerged at the right time. Ellison "Jeep" Pierce assumed the presidency of the American Society of Anesthesiologists in 1983. Motivated by the experience of a friend's daughter who died under anesthesia during a routine dental procedure, Pierce conceived of a foundation to help support work to make care safer—in fact, he probably coined the term "patient safety" in founding the Anesthesia Patient Safety Foundation (APSF).[24] The APSF, working closely with other professional, healthcare, and industry groups, helped propel the field forward, first by convincing caregivers that the safety problem was real and that it was soluble with the right approach.[25,26]

The lessons from the anesthesia safety movement are broadly applicable to efforts directed at improving overall patient safety.[1,27,28] First, safety requires strong leadership, characterized by a commitment to openness and a willingness to embrace change. Second, learning from past mistakes is an essential part of patient safety. In the case of anesthesia, the closed-case reviews produced key insights. Third, although technology is not the complete answer to safety, it is an essential part of the solution. In anesthesia, the thoughtful application of oximetry, capnography, and automated blood pressure monitoring has proven vital to saving lives. Fourth, where applicable, the use of human factors engineering and forcing functions can markedly enhance safety (Chapter 7). For example, changing the anesthesia tubing so that the incorrect gases could not be hooked up was crucial; this was a far more effective maneuver than trying to educate or remind anesthesiologists about the possibility of mix-ups.

Finally, anesthesia found itself in the throes of a malpractice crisis and simultaneously had to grapple with a number of highly visible errors reported in the media. Sparks like these are often necessary to disrupt the inertia and denial that can undermine many safety efforts. And it worked: in the 1980s, anesthesiologists paid exorbitant rates for malpractice insurance—among the highest in the medical profession. Now that errors causing patient harm are so unusual in the field of anesthesia, current malpractice premiums fall in the midrange of all specialties, a good example of the "business case for safety."

WRONG-SITE/WRONG-PATIENT SURGERY

In 1995, Willie King, a 51-year-old diabetic man with severe peripheral vascular disease, checked into a hospital in Tampa, Florida, for amputation of a gangrenous right leg. The admitting clerk mistakenly entered into the computer system that Mr. King was there for a left below-the-knee amputation. An alert floor nurse caught the error after seeing a printout of the day's operating room (OR) schedule; she called the OR to correct the mistake. A scrub nurse made a handwritten correction to the printed schedule, but the computer's schedule was not changed. Since this computer schedule was the source of subsequent printed copies, copies of the incorrect schedule were distributed around the OR and hospital. King's surgeon entered the OR, read the wrong procedure off one of the printed schedules, prepped the wrong leg, and then began to amputate it. The error was discovered partway through the surgery, too late to save the left leg. Of course, the gangrenous right leg still needed to be removed, and a few weeks later it was, leaving King a double amputee.

Events like these are so egregious that they have been dubbed "Never Events"—meaning that they should never occur under any circumstances (Appendix VI). And who could possibly disagree? A recent systematic review of surgical never events suggests that there is one wrong-site surgery event per 100,000 surgical procedures.[29] Studies that also considered outpatient surgery and nonsurgical procedures have given higher estimates.[30,31] A published review suggests that wrong site surgery in head and neck surgery is common, with events in otolaryngology procedures accounting for 0.3% to 4.5%

of all wrong site surgeries.[32] In 2010, an MGH surgeon publicly disclosed performing the wrong surgical procedure on a patient's hand in a prominent medical journal.[33]

When one hears of wrong-site or wrong-patient procedures, it is difficult to resist the instinct to assign blame, usually to the operating surgeon. Yet we know there must be something more at play than simply a careless surgeon or nurse. The answer, as usual, is Swiss cheese (Chapter 2) and bad systems. Appreciating this makes clear the need for a multidimensional approach aimed at preventing the inevitable human slips from causing irrevocable harm.

The Joint Commission has promoted the use of the *Universal Protocol* to prevent wrong-site and wrong-patient surgery and procedures (Table 5-2). In essence, the protocol acknowledges that single solutions to this problem are destined to fail, and that robust fixes depend on multiple overlapping layers of protection. Several elements of the Universal Protocol merit further comment.

At first glance, *sign-your-site*—the surgeon marks the surgical site in indelible ink after verifying the correct site—would appear to be a particularly strong solution. But the early history of sign-your-site demonstrates that even reasonable safety solutions can fail without strong standard policies and enforcement protocols. In the mid-1990s, before the Joint Commission or surgical professional societies entered the fray, a number of well-meaning orthopedic surgeons began to use markings to help ensure that they operated on the correct surgical site. Unfortunately, without a standardized approach, the result would have been nearly comical if it wasn't so scary: some surgeons placed an "X" on the surgical site (as in "X marks the spot"), while others placed an "X" on the *opposite* limb (as in "don't cut here"). Although there were no documented cases of wrong-site surgery resulting from this anarchy, the implementation of standard rules was crucial (under the Universal Protocol, the surgical site is the only one to be marked). Even today, the effectiveness of site marking depends on its correct implementation (Figure 5-1).[34] We have also learned that the strategies that help prevent laterality errors (right vs. left arm) may not work for other types of wrong-site surgery, such as incorrect spinal level errors.[35]

Another key element in the Universal Protocol is the *time out*, during which the entire surgical team is supposed to huddle and briefly discuss and agree upon the patient's name and intended procedure. This too seems like a robust safety solution, a fail-safe step sure to catch any errors that eluded prior protections. Yet we have come to recognize how dependent this step is on having a culture of safety (Chapters 9 and 15), one in which all those involved in caring for the patient are comfortable raising their concerns "up the authority gradient." Without a safe culture and good communication, interventions such as time outs can be robotic and perfunctory, providing the illusion, rather than the reality, of safety.[30]

Table 5-2   THE JOINT COMMISSION'S "UNIVERSAL PROTOCOL FOR PREVENTING WRONG-SITE, WRONG-PROCEDURE, AND WRONG-PERSON SURGERY"

Conduct a preprocedure verification process

1. Implement a preprocedure process to verify the correct procedure, for the correct patient, at the correct site.
   Note: The patient is involved in the verification process when possible
2. Identify the items that must be available for the procedure and use a standardized list to verify their availability. At a minimum, these items include the following:
   - Relevant documentation (e.g., history and physical, signed procedure consent form, nursing assessment, and preanesthesia assessment)
   - Labeled diagnostic and radiology test results (e.g., radiology images and scans, or pathology and biopsy reports) that are properly displayed
   - Any required blood products, implants, devices, and/or special equipment for the procedure
     Note: The expectation of this element of performance is that the standardized list is available and is used consistently during the preprocedure verification. It is not necessary to document that the standardized list was used for each patient
3. Match the items that are to be available in the procedure area to the patient

Mark the procedure site

1. Identify those procedures that require marking of the incision or insertion site. At a minimum, sites are marked when there is more than one possible location for the procedure and when performing the procedure in a different location would negatively affect quality or safety
   Note: For spinal procedures, in addition to preoperative skin marking of the general spinal region, special intraoperative imaging techniques may be used for locating and marking the exact vertebral level
2. Mark the procedure site before the procedure is performed and, if possible, with the patient involved
3. The procedure site is marked by a licensed independent practitioner who is ultimately accountable for the procedure and will be present when the procedure is performed. In limited circumstances, the licensed independent practitioner may delegate site marking to an individual who is permitted by the organization to participate in the procedure and has the following qualifications:
   - An individual in a medical postgraduate education program who is being supervised by the licensed independent practitioner performing the procedure, who is familiar with the patient, and who will be present when the procedure is performed
   - A licensed individual who performs duties requiring a collaborative agreement or supervisory agreement with the licensed independent practitioner performing the procedure (i.e., an advanced practice registered nurse [APRN] or physician assistant [PA]), who is familiar with the patient, and who will be present when the procedure is performed
     Note: The hospital's leaders define the limited circumstances (if any) in which site marking may be delegated to an individual meeting these qualifications
4. The method of marking the site and the type of mark is unambiguous and is used consistently throughout the hospital
   Note: The mark is made at or near the procedure site and is sufficiently permanent to be visible after skin preparation and draping. Adhesive markers are not the sole means of marking the site
5. A written, alternative process is in place for patients who refuse site marking or when it is technically or anatomically impossible or impractical to mark the site (e.g., mucosal surfaces or perineum)

(continued)

Table 5-2   THE JOINT COMMISSION'S "UNIVERSAL PROTOCOL FOR PREVENTING WRONG-SITE, WRONG-PROCEDURE, AND WRONG-PERSON SURGERY" *(continued)*

Mark the procedure site

Note: Examples of other situations that involve alternative processes include:

- Minimal access procedures treating a lateralized internal organ, whether percutaneous or through a natural orifice
- Teeth
- Premature infants, for whom the mark may cause a permanent tattoo

A time out is performed before the procedure

1. Conduct a time out immediately before starting the invasive procedure or making the incision
2. The time out has the following characteristics:
   - It is standardized, as defined by the hospital
   - It is initiated by a designated member of the team
   - It involves the immediate members of the procedure team, including the individual performing the procedure, the anesthesia providers, the circulating nurse, the operating room technician, and other active participants who will be participating in the procedure from the beginning
3. When two or more procedures are being performed on the same patient, and the person performing the procedure changes, perform a time out before each procedure is initiated
4. During the time out, the team members agree, at a minimum, on the following:
   - Correct patient identity
   - The correct site
   - The procedure to be done
5. Document the completion of the time out
   Note: The hospital determines the amount and type of documentation

Reprinted with permission from the Joint Commission. Available at: https://www.jointcommission.org/assets/1/18/UP_Poster1.PDF. © The Joint Commission, 2017.

While the components of the Universal Protocol made sense and likely led to some improvements in surgical safety, this is yet another example (like medication reconciliation, discussed in Chapter 4) in which a more holistic approach, one that respected the challenges of achieving meaningful changes within complex adaptive systems (Chapter 2), was needed.[34] The past several years have seen a number of successful experiments that embedded the core processes (such as sign-your-site and preoperative time outs and briefings[36]) within a broader set of activities designed to create a culture of safety, encourage communication, increase situational awareness, and focus all of the members of the surgical team on the task at hand.[37,38]

The first such effort was an eight-hospital international study that combined the use of the World Health Organization's Surgical Safety Checklist (Figure 5-2) with a variety of other activities designed to improve teamwork and communication.[39] While its results—a nearly 50% decrease in deaths and

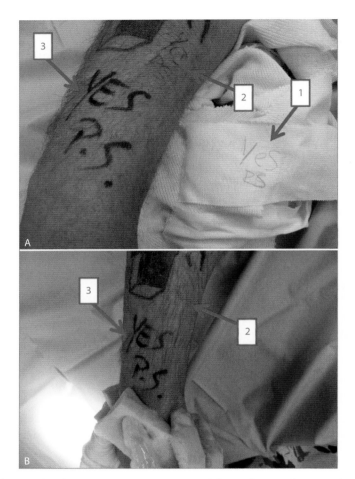

Figure 5-1 ▪ Clinical example of correct versus incorrect modalities of surgical site marking. **(A)** This patient was scheduled for a surgical procedure on his right forearm. The intern marked and initialed the site on the dressing, which came off prior to surgery (1). The resident corrected the mistake by marking the surgical site on skin, using a regular pen (2). Neither the marking nor the initials are legible (2). Finally, the site was again marked and initialed by the attending surgeon with a permanent marker (3). **(B)** During the surgical preparation, the site marking with the regular pen was washed off immediately (2), whereas the permanent marker remained visible throughout the surgical preparation (3). This example emphasizes the crucial importance of using a permanent marker and large and legible letters, and signing the marking with the surgeon's initials. "YES" is the designated, standardized identifier for the correct surgical site at Denver Health Medical Center. (Reproduced with permission from Stahel PF, Mehler PS, Clarke TJ, Varnell J. The 5th anniversary of the "Universal Protocol": pitfalls and pearls revisited. *Patient Saf Surg* 2009;3:14. [Original figure available from PubMed Central at: http://www.ncbi.nlm.nih.gov/pmc/articles/PMC2712460/figure/F1/.])

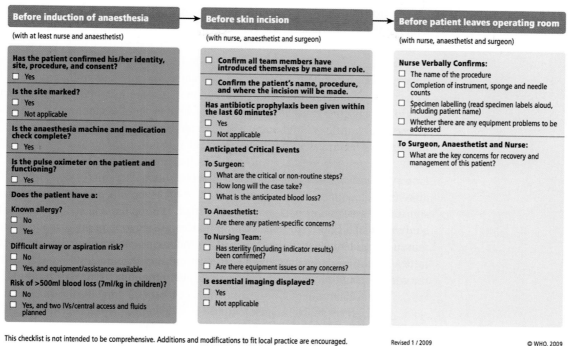

Figure 5-2 ■ The World Health Organization's surgical safety checklist. (Available at: http://apps.who.int/iris/ bitstream/10665/44186/2/9789241598590_eng_Checklist.pdf. Reproduced with permission.)

complications, at both well and poorly resourced hospitals—were impressive, the study's validity has been questioned in light of the before-and-after design, the absence of controls for confounding variables, and the fact that the outcomes did not correlate with the degree of compliance with the intervention.[40]

Reassuringly, an even more comprehensive surgical safety intervention (this one involved 11 distinct checklists applied by caregivers along the surgical continuum) was implemented at six teaching hospitals in the Netherlands.[41] Patients at participating hospitals had 30% fewer complications and a nearly 50% lower mortality rate than those at control institutions. As in the seminal study in Michigan ICUs (Chapter 10)—in which a checklist-based intervention resulted in major decreases in central line–associated bloodstream infections, leading many people to focus on the checklist as a magic bullet[42,43]—both the WHO and the Netherlands study authors emphasized the importance of culture change and teamwork as key success factors.[39,41] In fact, the WHO investigators subsequently demonstrated that improvements in safety culture correlated with the improved surgical outcomes.[44] Moreover, a study of the implementation of teamwork training (along with checklists) in 74 Veterans

Affairs hospitals found a striking improvement in surgical mortality, along with evidence of a dose–response curve.[45]

Soberingly, a more recent study looking at the impact of a mandatory surgical safety checklist at 101 hospitals in Ontario, Canada did not find any improvement in mortality, surgical complications, readmissions, and length of stay.[46] Commenting on the study, Dr. Lucian Leape suggests that in order for checklists to achieve the desired effect of improved safety outcomes, implementation, workflow, and local culture need to be carefully considered.[47] Dr. Atul Gawande, an author of the original WHO study, critiqued the Ontario study design, noting that it might not have been adequately powered.[48] However, another study of Medicare patients undergoing surgery in Michigan also found no improvements with the use of the surgical checklist.[49] One reason for the variable impact may have been elucidated by an English checklist study, which found implementation practices varied widely.[50] This literature makes it clear that checklists are part of the answer, but only part. Because issues related to checklists, teamwork, and culture have become so central to the entire field of patient safety, we will discuss them more fully in Chapter 15.

RETAINED SPONGES AND INSTRUMENTS

In October 2002, a Canadian woman repeatedly tripped the alarm on a metal detector as she attempted to board a flight in Regina, Saskatchewan. On a closer search, the detector wand continued to bleep as it was passed over her abdomen. Since security personnel were unable to identify anything metallic on her person, they let her board her flight to Calgary. The woman wondered whether the episode was related to the recurrent stomach pain she'd been experiencing since her abdominal surgery four months earlier. After her trip, she saw her doctor, who ordered an abdominal x-ray. Shockingly, it showed the outline of a metal retractor, a tool used by the surgical team months earlier. The surgeons had inadvertently left the object behind when they sutured her incision, which was no small feat—the retractor was a foot long and 2 inches wide, practically the size of a crowbar.

The term "retained sponge" (also called "gossypibomas," from the Latin "gossypium" [cotton] and "boma" [place of concealment][51]) is often used as a catchall phrase for all manner of surgical paraphernalia left behind after surgery. A review by Gawande et al. of 54 patients with retained foreign bodies over a 16-year period found that roughly two-thirds were actual sponges—square or rectangular bits of absorbent gauze designed to soak up blood in the operative field—while the remaining one-third were surgical instruments.[52] This frequency corresponds to an overall "retained sponge" rate of about 1 per 10,000 surgeries,[53] which works out to at least one case each year for a typical large hospital in the United States. Because the study drew its sample from malpractice cases, the problem is undoubtedly more common than this published estimate. In fact, a more recent study found a retained foreign object rate of one per 5500 operations.[54] Determining actual incidence is made more challenging by the fact that the average retained surgical sponge is discovered seven years after the surgery.[55]

Unlike many other safety problems, the retained sponge/instrument problem would seem to be preventable by the thoughtful implementation of systematic, mechanical solutions. In the 1940s, manufacturers produced sponges with loops that were attached to a 2-in. metal ring. The ring then hung outside the operative field while the sponges were placed inside the field. When the operation was over, the nurse simply harvested the sponges by gathering the rings—the way a trail of fishing hooks is pulled out of the water by reeling in the line. Clever as this sounds, surgeons found the ring system unwieldy, and many simply cut the rings off: a classic example of a *routine rule violation* (Chapter 15).[56] By the 1960s, manufacturers tried another approach, producing surgical sponges with an embedded radiopaque thread (Figure 5-3A) meant to show up on x-rays (Figure 5-3B). But obtaining a postoperative x-ray on every patient is impractical. In most cases, the x-ray is done months later, when a patient experiences persistent postoperative pain and the doctors are trying to figure out why.

To laypeople, leaving a sponge or tool behind may seem like a particularly boneheaded error—until you remember that complex or emergency surgeries often require dozens, even hundreds, of sponges (along with scores of

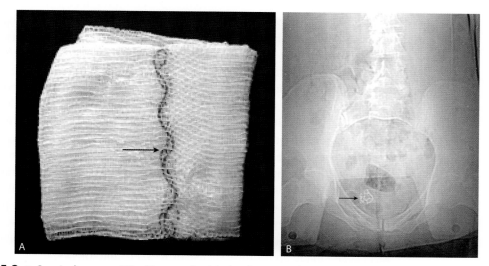

Figure 5-3 ▪ Surgical sponge **(A)** with an embedded radiopaque thread, shown on x-ray **(B)**.

other instruments and needles), inserted and removed under considerable time pressure. This is one reason surgical teams have long used "sponge, sharp, and instrument counts." The standard protocol requires four separate counts: when the instruments are set up and the sponges are unpacked, when the surgery begins and the items are called for and used, at the time of closure, and during external suturing. Unfortunately, the chaotic and pressured circumstances in most busy ORs and the frequent changes in personnel,[57] coupled with the reluctance of the nurses to admit (consciously or not) to the fallacy of an earlier count, create situations in which the counts fail. In the most startling finding of Gawande et al.'s study, while one-third of the retained sponge cases had not been subject to a documented count, two-thirds of the cases were.[52] In about half the cases, there were actually *multiple counts documented to be in agreement.* This means that every sponge and instrument was accounted for, despite the fact that one would turn up later—rather inconveniently—in a patient's abdomen.

The real lesson from all of this is that what initially appears to be a perfectly logical safety practice often turns out to be highly flawed when implemented. Because sponge counts of any kind are inherently unreliable, some experts have recommended taking an x-ray of every surgical site before the field is sutured. Even if x-rays were free and patients and staff were willing to put up with the procedure and additional radiation exposure, keeping anesthetized surgical patients on the table any longer than strictly necessary is not without its own risks. Partly for this reason, Gawande and his colleagues recommend x-rays only in high-risk cases: those involving emergency surgery, prolonged surgery, surgery that required a real-time change in clinical strategy, and surgery on obese patients. Even this plan has gaps, because radiopaque markers are subtle and can be overlooked on x-rays.[54]

Ultimately, the best solution to the retained foreign object problem probably lies in new technology. Some companies have developed bar-coded sponges,[57] while others have embedded their sponges with radio-frequency ID (RFID) tags that cause a detector wand to *beep* when the surgeon waves it over the field before closure.[58] Still others have built automatic "sponge counters," resembling tollbooth coin machines, which can be loaded up and checked after every surgery. Although the experience with these technologies is still limited, institutions utilizing them have reported positive results. In a decision-analytic model, both the bar-coded sponge and radio-frequency-tagged sponge systems appear to be more cost-effective than either sponge counting or programs of universal or selective postprocedure radiographs (bar coding is less expensive than radio-frequency tagging, but probably takes more nursing time to use).[59] One study showed that organizations implementing RFID technology had fewer retained surgical sponges than those that did not. Reassuringly, the cost savings (fewer x-rays, less OR time, and lower legal costs) made up for the expense of RFID technology.[60]

SURGICAL FIRES

Surgical fires are unusual but frightening and potentially deadly. It has been estimated that there are between 50 and 200 such fires annually in the United States, leading to morbidity in 20% of cases (often severe, including tracheal or pulmonary burns) and one or two deaths.[51,61]

The genesis of surgical fires, one-third of which involve the airway, is the confluence of what has been called the *fire safety triangle*: an ignition source (such as electrocautery and lasers), a fuel source (e.g., gauze, drapes, even endotracheal tubes [Figure 5-4]), and oxidizers (usually oxygen but sometimes nitrous oxide). There is some evidence that the incidence of surgical fires is increasing, probably owing to the more frequent use of cautery and lasers in the OR, and more aggressive use of oxygen in anesthetized patients.[62]

A series of prevention maneuvers has been recommended, addressing all three elements of the triangle.[61] They include the following: ignition sources should be stored away from the patients and their tips should be visualized while hot, time should be allowed for alcohol-based prep solutions to dry prior to draping patients, oxygen concentrations should be kept to the lowest safe amount, and cautery around the airway should be used sparingly and only after the anesthesiologist is warned so that he or she can turn down the oxygen.

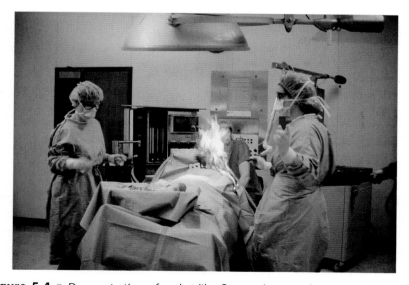

Figure 5-4 ■ Demonstration of rocket-like flames shooting from an endotracheal tube caused by laser ignition of the tube with 100% oxygen flowing. (Courtesy of ECRI Institute; reproduced with permission. Figure available at: https://psnet.ahrq.gov/webmm/case/346/fire-in-the-hole-an-or-fire. Copyright 2011 ECRI Institute. www.ecri.org. 5200 Butler Pike, Plymouth Meeting, PA 19462. 610–825–6000.)

In case of a fire in the OR or procedural suite, all personnel should be immediately notified. For fires involving the airway, the flow of gas should be turned off and the airway cooled with normal saline. For fires in other locations, smothering with water, saline, or by physical means is advised; use of a carbon dioxide fire extinguisher should be reserved for persistent flames.

SAFETY IN NONSURGICAL BEDSIDE PROCEDURES

While most of the attention regarding procedural safety has focused on the OR, there is growing recognition that nonsurgical procedures carry risks as well. As we turn our attention to bedside procedures, it is worth appreciating some differences between the two domains. One big one: the OR is (on a good day) an organized system of care, where policies and procedures can be enacted and measured, and individual participants can be given responsibility for compliance (i.e., "The circulating nurse will not allow the procedure to begin until the time out has been completed"). On the other hand, some procedures (such as thoracentesis and central line placement) may involve only a single physician and his or her patient, offering fewer opportunities for independent double-checks.

Complication rates for certain bedside procedures are surprisingly high. For example, 6% of thoracenteses result in a pneumothorax, one-third of which require chest tube placement.[63] Central venous catheter placement can be very risky, with complication rates (arterial laceration, pneumothorax, thrombosis, and infection) exceeding 15%.[64] Paracentesis, lumbar puncture, and arthrocentesis are somewhat safer, but all have significant risks.[65,66]

Strategies to decrease the risks of procedures fall into several categories: education and skill building, policies and practices to decrease overall process risks such as wrong-patient and wrong-site procedures, adjunctive technologies, and organizational changes.

There is abundant evidence that our traditional academic strategy of "see one, do one, teach one" is both ineffective and unethical (Chapter 17). As one window into this, studies have shown that many residents remain uncomfortable with certain procedures even after being charged with supervising them for their junior colleagues.[67] Most of the advances in the area of *education and skill building* have come through the development of formal curricula and competency-based assessment strategies including forbidding learners from performing procedures independently until they have been deemed competent.[68,69] (The use of simulation to enhance both teaching and assessment of procedures is further discussed in Chapter 17.) There are now a number of Web-based aids (the videos produced by the *New England Journal of Medicine* are some of the best available[70]) that demonstrate correct technique and pitfalls far better than a static textbook chapter or monograph ever could.

Bedside procedures are at risk for the same kinds of *wrong-site and wrong-patient errors* that we discussed earlier. In fact, a study of 132 self-reported wrong-site or wrong-patient events found that similar numbers came from nonoperative procedures as formal surgeries.[71] One study examined lessons learned from wrong-side thoracenteses and determined that contributing factors included lack of site marking, failure to perform a time out, inadequate consent, and failure to verify appropriate side with existing radiologic studies. The authors suggested that errors might be prevented by adhering to the Universal Protocol for bedside procedures.[72] Indeed, the Joint Commission requires the bedside proceduralist to perform the same Universal Protocol for bedside procedures as is required for major surgical operations.[73,74] While it is permissible for an individual proceduralist to go through the protocol alone, bringing another person in the room for an independent check is a sound practice. Barsuk et al. reengineered the procedure process—including adding requirements for procedural kits (which included relevant checklists) to be signed out by nurses from locked storage cabinets (a forcing function, Chapter 7) and that nurses be present at all procedures—and found that compliance with the Universal Protocol skyrocketed, from 16% to 94%.[75]

Adjunctive technologies can be quite helpful. The most important is *bedside ultrasound*, whose use drastically lowers the rates of pneumothorax after thoracentesis and adverse events after central line placement.[76,77] Learning to use bedside ultrasound correctly is not trivial, and teaching this skill should be integrated into the educational program described above.[68,69] Of course, other technologies may more directly improve the safety of certain procedures. For example, the availability of peripherally inserted central catheters (*PICC lines*) has obviated the need for subclavian or jugular puncture in many patients who require access to the central circulation.

Finally, some hospitals have developed dedicated *procedure services* to improve the safety of procedures. These services are staffed by a limited number of physicians (frequently hospitalists) who receive additional training in the relevant procedures and commit to spending significant time on the service. The premise behind these services was that they would enhance safety and patient satisfaction[78–80] via several mechanisms: narrowing the number of providers and thereby ensuring that those performing procedures are skilled and have high volumes, allowing for implementation of standard policies and protocols, and freeing clinicians from other distractions while performing procedures. Although one study found no difference in the rate of major complications between procedures performed by a dedicated procedure service and primary medical teams, it did show that procedures performed by the procedure service were more likely to comply with patient safety best practices.[81] Another study showed that a teaching procedure service improved residents' confidence and experience in performing common bedside procedures.[82]

In teaching hospitals, the procedure service not only ensures the safety of individual procedures but also takes on responsibility for educating trainees, in matters ranging from the angle of insertion of the needle to correct hygiene practices, and from the proper use of ultrasound to when a procedure is *not* indicated or too risky and needs to be referred to a more specialized provider (i.e., the interventional radiologist). We believe that these services represent a major advance in patient safety and should be implemented widely.

KEY POINTS

- Patient safety issues in surgery include those common to other fields (e.g., medication errors, healthcare-associated infections, readmissions, communication mishaps), and also several specific to surgery (e.g., wrong-site surgery, retained sponges, OR fires).
- Evidence for a volume–outcome relationship in many surgical areas and for a tight relationship between surgical technique and patient outcomes argue for new types of simulator training.
- Anesthesia embraced the importance of many patient safety principles (systems thinking, human factors engineering, learning from mistakes, standardization) earlier than any other field in medicine, and has amassed the most impressive safety record.
- A comprehensive application of the "Universal Protocol" (including "sign-your-site" and the preprocedural "time out"), coupled with teamwork training and the use of checklists, is currently the best strategy to prevent wrong-site and wrong-patient errors and has been demonstrated to improve surgical outcomes.
- Retained sponges and other surgical instruments are an uncommon safety hazard. Sponge counts and x-rays have traditionally been the main preventive strategies, but the use of more robust detection technologies such as RFID is increasing.
- Surgical fires result from the interaction of the elements of the fire safety triangle (ignition source, fuel source, and oxidizers). They can be prevented with adherence to a series of safety maneuvers addressing each element of the triangle.
- Nonsurgical procedures, such as thoracentesis and central line placement, carry significant risks. Robust competency-based training, proper adjunctive use of bedside ultrasound, implementing checklists and time outs, and a dedicated procedure service can decrease these risks significantly.

REFERENCES

1. Gaba DM. Anaesthesiology as a model for patient safety in health care. *BMJ* 2000;320:785–788.
2. Bainbridge D, Martin J, Arango M, Cheng G; Evidence-based Peri-operative Clinical Outcomes Research (EPiCOR) Group. Perioperative and anaesthetic-related mortality in developed and developing countries: a systematic review. *Lancet* 2012;380:1075–1081.
3. Thomas EJ, Studdert DM, Burstin HR, et al. Incidence and types of adverse events and negligent care in Utah and Colorado. *Med Care* 2000;38:261–271.
4. Anderson O, Davis R, Hanna GB, Vincent CA. Surgical adverse events: a systematic review. *Am J Surg* 2013;206:253–262.
5. Sharpe VA, Faden AI. *Medical Harm: Historical, Conceptual and Ethical Dimensions of Iatrogenic Illness.* Cambridge, England: Cambridge University Press; 1998.
6. Neuhauser D. John Williamson and the terrifying results of the medical practice information demonstration project. *Qual Saf Health Care* 2002;11:387–389.
7. Vincent C. *Patient Safety.* 2nd ed. London: Elsevier; 2010.
8. Leape LL. Error in medicine. *JAMA* 1994;272:1851–1857.
9. Leape LL. An interview with Lucian Leape. *Jt Comm J Qual Saf* 2004;30:653–658.
10. Maggard-Gibbons M. The use of report cards and outcome measurements to improve the safety of surgical care: the American College of Surgeons National Surgical Quality Improvement Program. *BMJ Qual Saf* 2014;23:589–599.
11. O'Connor GT, Plume SK, Olmstead EM, et al. A regional intervention to improve the hospital mortality associated with coronary artery bypass graft surgery. The Northern New England Cardiovascular Disease Study Group. *JAMA* 1996;275:841–846.
12. Luft HS, Bunker JP, Enthoven AC. Should operations be regionalized? The empirical relation between surgical volume and mortality. *N Engl J Med* 1979;301:1364–1369.
13. Reames BN, Ghaferi AA, Birkmeyer JD, Dimick JB. Hospital volume and operative mortality in the modern era. *Ann Surg* 2014;260:244–251.
14. Moore MJ, Bennett CL. The learning curve for laparoscopic cholecystectomy. The Southern Surgeons Club. *Am J Surg* 1995;170:55–59.
15. Morino M, Festa V, Garrone C. Survey on Torino courses. The impact of a two-day practical course on apprenticeship and diffusion of laparoscopic cholecystectomy in Italy. *Surg Endosc* 1995;9:46–48.
16. Ahlberg G, Enochsson L, Gallagher AG, et al. Proficiency-based virtual reality training significantly reduces the error rate for residents during their first 10 laparoscopic cholecystectomies. *Am J Surg* 2007;193:797–804.
17. Sade RM, ed. *The Ethics of Surgery: Conflicts and Controversies.* Oxford: Oxford University Press; 2015.
18. Birkmeyer JD, Finks JF, O'Reilly A, et al. Surgical skill and complication rates after bariatric surgery. *N Engl J Med* 2013;369:1434–1442.
19. Kohn L, Corrigan J, Donaldson M, eds. *To Err Is Human: Building a Safer Health System.* Committee on Quality of Health Care in America, Institute of Medicine. Washington, DC: National Academies Press; 1999.
20. Cooper JB, Newbower RS, Long CD, McPeek B. Preventable anesthesia mishaps: a study of human factors. *Anesthesiology* 1978;49:399–406.

21. Cooper JB, Long CD, Newbower RS, Philip JH. Critical incidents associated with intraoperative exchanges of anesthesia personnel. *Anesthesiology* 1982;56:456–461.

22. Cooper JB, Newbower RS, Kitz RJ. An analysis of major errors and equipment failures in anesthesia management: considerations for prevention and detection. *Anesthesiology* 1984;60:34–42.

23. Caplan RA, Posner KL, Ward RJ, Cheney FW. Adverse respiratory events in anesthesia: a closed claims analysis. *Anesthesiology* 1990;72:828–833.

24. Pierce EC. 40 years behind the mask: safety revisited. *Anesthesiology* 1996;29: 965–975.

25. Gawande A. *Complications: A Surgeon's Notes on an Imperfect Science.* New York, NY: Metropolitan Books; 2002.

26. Eichhorn JH. The Anesthesia Patient Safety Foundation at 25: a pioneering success in safety, 25th anniversary provokes reflection, anticipation. *Anesth Analg* 2012;114:791–800.

27. Lagasse RS. Anesthesia safety: model or myth? A review of the published literature and analysis of current original data. *Anesthesiology* 2002;97:1609–1617.

28. Cooper JB. Getting into patient safety: a personal story. [Perspective]. *AHRQ PSNet* [serial online]; August 2006. Available at: https://psnet.ahrq.gov/perspectives/perspective/29.

29. Hempel S, Maggard-Gibbons M, Nguyen DK, et al. Wrong-site surgery, retained surgical items, and surgical fires: a systematic review of surgical never events. *JAMA Surg* 2015;150:796–805.

30. Seiden SC, Barach P. Wrong-side/wrong-site, wrong-procedure, and wrong-patient adverse events: are they preventable? *Arch Surg* 2006;141:931–939.

31. Neily J, Mills PD, Eldridge N, et al. Incorrect surgical procedures within and outside of the operating room. *Arch Surg* 2009;144:1028–1034.

32. Liou TN, Nussenbaum B. Wrong-site surgery in otolaryngology—head and neck surgery. *Laryngoscope* 2014;124:104–109.

33. Ring DC, Herndon JH, Meyer GS. Case records of the Massachusetts General Hospital: case 34-2010: a 65-year-old woman with an incorrect operation on the left hand. *N Engl J Med* 2010;363:1950–1957.

34. Stahel PF, Mehler PS, Clarke TJ, Varnell J. The 5th anniversary of the "Universal Protocol": pitfalls and pearls revisited. *Patient Saf Surg* 2009;3:14.

35. Mody MG, Nourbakhsh A, Stahl DL, Gibbs M, Alfawareh M, Garges KJ. The prevalence of wrong level surgery among spine surgeons. *Spine* 2008;33:194–198.

36. Allard J, Bleakley A, Hobbs A, Coombes L. Pre-surgery briefings and safety climate in the operating theater. *BMJ Qual Saf* 2011;20:711–717.

37. Weick KE. The collapse of sensemaking in organizations: the Mann Gulch disaster. *Adm Sci Q* 1993;38:628–652.

38. Healey AN, Nagpal K, Moorthy K, Vincent CA. Engineering the system of communication for safer surgery. *Cogn Tech Work* 2011;13:1–10.

39. Haynes AB, Weiser TG, Berry WR, et al. Safe Surgery Saves Lives Study Group. A surgical safety checklist to reduce morbidity and mortality in a global population. *N Engl J Med* 2009;360:491–499.

40. Birkmeyer JD. Strategies for improving surgical quality—checklists and beyond. *N Engl J Med* 2010;363:1963–1965.

41. de Vries EN, Prins HA, Crolla RM, et al. SURPASS Collaborative Group. Effect of a comprehensive surgical safety system on patient outcomes. *N Engl J Med* 2010;363:1928–1937.

42. Pronovost P, Needham D, Berenholtz S, et al. An intervention to decrease catheter-related bloodstream infections in the ICU. *N Engl J Med* 2006;355:2725–2732.

43. Bosk CL, Dixon-Woods M, Goeschel CA, Pronovost PJ. Reality check for checklists. *Lancet* 2009;374:444–445.

44. Haynes AB, Weiser TG, Berry WR, et al. Safe Surgery Saves Lives Study Group. Changes in safety attitude and relationship to decreased postoperative morbidity and mortality following implementation of a checklist-based surgical safety intervention. *BMJ Qual Saf* 2011;20:102–107.

45. Neily J, Mills PD, Young-Xu Y, et al. Association between implementation of a medical team training program and surgical mortality. *JAMA* 2010;304:1693–1700.

46. Urbach DR, Govindarajan A, Saskin R, Wilton AS, Baxter NN. Introduction of surgical safety checklists in Ontario, Canada. *N Engl J Med* 2014;370:1029–1038.

47. Leape LL. The checklist conundrum. *N Engl J Med.* 2014;370:1063–1064.

48. Gawande A. When checklists work and when they don't. Web blog post. The Health Services Research Blog. The Incidental Economist, 2015. Available at: http://the incidentaleconomist.com/wordpress/when-checklists-work-and-when-they-dont/.

49. Reames BN, Scally CP, Thumma JR, Dimick JB. Evaluation of the effectiveness of a surgical checklist in Medicare patients. *Med Care* 2015;53:87–94.

50. Russ SJ, Sevalis N, Moorthy K, et al. A qualitative evaluation of the barriers and facilitators toward implementation of the WHO surgical safety checklist across hospitals in England: lessons from the "surgical checklist implementation project". *Ann Surg* 2015;261:81–91.

51. Zahiri HR, Stromberg J, Skupsky H, et al. Prevention of 3 "never events" in the operating room: fires, gossypiboma, and wrong-site surgery. *Surg Innov* 2011;18:55–60.

52. Gawande AA, Studdert DM, Orav EJ, Brennan TA, Zinner MJ. Risk factors for retained instruments and sponges after surgery. *N Engl J Med* 2003;348:229–235.

53. Hempel S, Maggard-Gibbons M, Nguyen DK, et al. Wrong-site surgery, retained surgical items, and surgical fires: a systematic review of surgical never events. *JAMA Surg* 2015;150:796–805.

54. Cima RR, Kollengode A, Garnatz J, Storsveen A, Weisbrod C, Deschamps C. Incidence and characteristics of potential and actual retained foreign object events in surgical patients. *J Am Coll Surg* 2008;207:80–87.

55. Wan W, Le T, Riskin L, Macario A. Improving safety in the operating room: a systematic literature review of retained surgical sponges. *Curr Opin Anaesthesiol* 2009;22:207–214.

56. de Saint Maurice G, Auroy Y, Vincent C, Amalberti R. The natural lifespan of a safety policy: violations and system migration in anaesthesia. *Qual Saf Health Care* 2010;19:327–331.

57. Greenberg CC, Diaz-Flores R, Lipsitz SR, et al. Bar-coding surgical sponges to improve safety: a randomized controlled trial. *Ann Surg* 2008;247:612–616.

58. Inaba K, Okoye O, Aksoy H, et al. The role of radio frequency detection system embedded surgical sponges in preventing retained surgical sponges: a prospective evaluation in patients undergoing emergency surgery. *Ann Surg* 2016;264:599–604.

59. Regenbogen SE, Greenberg CC, Resch SC, et al. Prevention of retained surgical sponges: a decision-analytic model predicting relative cost-effectiveness. *Surgery* 2009;145:527–535.

60. Williams TL, Tung DK, Steelman VM, Chang PK, Szekendi MK. Retained surgical sponges: findings from incident reports and a cost-benefit analysis of radiofrequency technology. *J Am Coll Surg* 2014;219:354–364.

61. Caplan RA, Barker SJ, Connis RT, et al. American Society of Anesthesiologists Task Force on Operating Room Fires. Practice advisory for the prevention and management of operating room fires. *Anesthesiology* 2013;118:271–290.

62. Landro L. In just a flash, simple surgery can turn deadly. *Wall Street Journal* February 18, 2009:D1.

63. Gordon CE, Feller-Kopman D, Balk EM, Smetana GW. Pneumothorax following thoracentesis: a systematic review and meta-analysis. *Arch Intern Med* 2010;170:332–339.

64. Parienti JJ, Mongardon N, Mégarbane B, et al. Intravascular complications of central venous catheterization by insertion site. *N Engl J Med* 2015;373:1220–1229.

65. Sharzehi K, Jain V, Naveed A, Schreibman I. Hemorrhagic complications of paracentesis: a systematic review of the literature. *Gastroenterol Res Pract* 2014:2014. Article ID 985151.

66. Sempere AP, Berenguer-Ruiz L, Lezcano-Rodas M, Mira-Berenguer F, Waez M. Lumbar puncture: its indications, contraindications, complications and technique. *Rev Neurol* 2007;45:433–436.

67. Mourad M, Kohlwes J, Maselli J; MERN Group, Auerbach AD. Supervising the supervisors—procedural training and supervision in internal medicine residency. *J Gen Intern Med* 2010;25:351–356.

68. Dong Y, Suri HS, Cook DA, et al. Simulation-based objective assessment discerns clinical proficiency in central line placement: a construct validation. *Chest* 2010;137:1050–1056.

69. Barsuk JH, McGaghie WC, Cohen ER, Balachandran JS, Wayne DB. Use of simulation-based mastery learning to improve the quality of central venous catheter placement in a medical intensive care unit. *J Hosp Med* 2009;4:397–403.

70. Available at: http://www.nejm.org/multimedia/medical-videos.

71. Stahel PF, Sabel AL, Victoroff MS, et al. Wrong-site and wrong-patient procedures in the universal protocol era: analysis of a prospective database of physician self-reported occurrences. *Arch Surg* 2010;145:978–984.

72. Miller KE, Mims M, Paull DE, et al. Wrong-side thoracentesis: lessons learned from root cause analysis. *JAMA Surg* 2014;149:774–779.

73. The Joint Commission. Universal Protocol; 2010. Available at: https://www.joint commission.org/assets/1/18/UP_Poster1.PDF.

74. Norton E. Implementing the universal protocol hospital-wide. *AORN J* 2007; 85:1187–1197.

75. Barsuk JH, Brake H, Caprio T, Barnard C, Anderson DY, Williams MV. Process changes to increase compliance with the Universal Protocol for bedside procedures. *Arch Intern Med* 2011;171:947–949.

76. Mercaldi CJ, Lanes SF. Ultrasound guidance decreases complications and improves the cost of care among patients undergoing thoracentesis and paracentesis. *Chest* 2013;143:532–538.

77. Lalu MM, Fayad A, Ahmed O, et al. Ultrasound-guided subclavian vein catheterization: a systematic review and meta-analysis. *Crit Care Med* 2015;43:1498–1507.

78. Mourad M, Auerbach AD, Maselli J, Sliwka D. Patient satisfaction with a hospitalist procedure service: is bedside procedure teaching reassuring to patients? *J Hosp Med* 2011;6:219–224.

79. Smith CC, Gordon CE, Feller-Kopman D, et al. Creation of an innovative inpatient medical procedure service and a method to evaluate house staff competency. *J Gen Intern Med* 2004;19:510–513.

80. Lucas BP, Asbury JK, Wang Y, et al. Impact of a bedside procedure service on general medicine inpatients: a firm-based trial. *J Hosp Med* 2007;2:143–149.

81. Tukey MH, Wiener RS. The impact of a medical procedure service on patient safety, procedure quality and resident training opportunities. *J Gen Intern Med* 2015;29:485–490.

82. Mourad M, Ranji S, Sliwka D. A randomized controlled trial of the impact of a teaching procedure service on the training of internal medicine residents. *J Grad Med Educ* 2012;4:170–175.

ADDITIONAL READINGS

Ali M, Osborne A, Bethune R, Pullyblank A. Preoperative surgical briefings do not delay operating room start times and are popular with surgical team members. *J Patient Saf* 2011;7:138–142.

Birkmeyer JD. Strategies for improving surgical quality—checklists and beyond. *N Engl J Med* 2010;363:1963–1965.

Birkmeyer NJ, Dimick JB, Share D, et al. Hospital complication rates with bariatric surgery in Michigan. *JAMA* 2010;304:435–442.

Bock M, Doz P, Fanolla A, et al. A comparative effectiveness analysis of the implementation of surgical safety checklists in a tertiary care hospital. *JAMA Surg* 2016;151:639–644.

Encinosa WE, Hellinger FJ. The impact of medical errors on ninety-day costs and outcomes: an examination of surgical patients. *Health Serv Res* 2008;43:2067–2085.

Fan CJ, Pawlik TM, Daniels T, et al. Association of safety culture with surgical site infection outcomes. *J Am Coll Surg* 2016;222:122–128.

Gawande A. *Better: A Surgeon's Notes on Performance.* New York, NY: Metropolitan Books; 2007.

Gawande A. *The Checklist Manifesto: How to Get Things Right.* New York, NY: Metropolitan Books; 2009.

Spruce L. Back to basics: preventing surgical fires. *AORN J* 2016;104:217–224.

DIAGNOSTIC ERRORS | 6

SOME BASIC CONCEPTS AND TERMS

Since its inception, the patient safety movement has emphasized medication errors, handoff errors, communication and teamwork errors, healthcare-associated infections, and surgical errors; all of these areas are amenable to technological (e.g., computerized order entry), procedural (e.g., double checks), and policy (e.g., "sign-your-site") solutions. Until recently, diagnostic errors have been less well emphasized, in part because they are more difficult to measure and to fix.

Interestingly, diagnostic errors were underemphasized from the very beginning of the patient safety movement.[1] In the landmark Institute of Medicine (IOM) report *To Err Is Human*,[2] the term "medication errors" is mentioned 70 times, while the phrase "diagnostic errors" comes up only twice. This is ironic, since diagnostic errors accounted for 17% of preventable errors in the Harvard Medical Practice Study,[3] the source of the IOM estimate of 44,000 to 98,000 yearly deaths from medical mistakes (the "jumbo jet a day" figure that helped launch the safety movement; Chapter 1) and continue to account for a significant amount of preventable harm to patients. A review of malpractice claims data in the United States for the period from 1986 through 2010 found that out of 350,706 paid claims, diagnostic errors accounted for almost one-third of claims and the highest amount of total payments.[4] Another estimate suggests that diagnostic error affects 12 million adult outpatients every year in the United States.[5]

As the field of patient safety evolves, the momentum for addressing the problem of diagnostic error—now viewed as a critical patient safety issue—is growing.[6,7] In response, in 2015 the National Academy of Medicine (NAM, formerly the IOM) released another landmark report entitled *Improving Diagnosis in Health Care*. The report concludes that the vast majority of patients will experience a diagnostic error at some point and suggests that greater collaboration among stakeholders is required to mitigate the problem.[8] The report also emphasizes the need for accurate measurement of diagnostic error and outlines opportunities to improve the diagnostic process and reduce error.

At first glance, diagnostic errors would seem to represent human failings—pure lapses in cognition. And it is true that, perhaps more than any other area in patient safety, the training and skills of the clinician remain of paramount importance. However, in keeping with our modern understanding of patient safety, there *are* system fixes that can decrease the frequency and consequences of diagnostic mistakes. In this chapter, we will discuss the cognitive as well as the process failures (such as failure to transfer the results of a crucial laboratory or radiologic study to the correct provider in a timely way) that give rise to diagnostic errors.

MISSED MYOCARDIAL INFARCTION: A CLASSIC DIAGNOSTIC ERROR

Annie Jackson, a 68-year-old African-American woman with mild diabetes, high blood pressure, and elevated cholesterol, presented to the emergency department after 30 minutes of squeezing chest discomfort. An ECG was quickly obtained. The ER physician, Dr. Zoe Bennett, studied the tracing and saw some nonspecific changes in the ST and T segments—not entirely normal but not the ST-segment elevations that are classic for acute myocardial infarction (MI). On exam, she found mild tachycardia, clear lungs, and mild tenderness over the lower part of the patient's sternum. She considered the latter discovery quite reassuring (after all, such tenderness would be more characteristic of a musculoskeletal process than a heart attack), but also ordered a troponin (a biomarker released by damaged heart cells). It came back mildly elevated, again not in the range specific for MI but not normal either. Nevertheless, she made a diagnosis of costochondritis (inflammation of the sternum–rib joint), prescribed an anti-inflammatory agent and bed rest, and released Ms. Jackson from the emergency department. The patient died later that night, a victim of an undiagnosed and untreated MI.

We can only guess which cognitive error caused Dr. Bennett to release Annie Jackson from the ER.[9] Perhaps because Ms. Jackson was a woman, the ER doctor underestimated her chance of having a heart attack. Dr. Bennett almost certainly relied too heavily on chest wall tenderness for her diagnosis—it is unusual, but not unheard of, in MI patients. She also overemphasized the lack of clear evidence on the ECG and troponin tests. Although they were "nonspecific," both were clearly abnormal and thus justified admitting Ms. Jackson or placing her in an observation unit for cardiac monitoring as well as a repeat ECG and troponin. Perhaps Dr. Bennett was just exhausted after a long day at work.[10]

We do know, however, that this particular error—sending patients home with heart attacks—is distressingly common and frequently lethal. Approximately 1% of admissions for acute MI represent a prior missed diagnosis.[11] Because missed MI is the best-studied diagnostic error, we will use it to make several broader points about these errors.

In the 1970s, researchers began studying the problem of missed MIs and quickly concluded that many errors were related to patient characteristics. Physicians were more likely to send patients home despite worrisome histories or abnormal data when the patients were in groups traditionally believed to be at lower risk for MI, such as younger patients (under age 55) and women. Nonwhites were also mistakenly sent home more often, raising the question of racial bias, conscious or unconscious, among caregivers.[12] In one particularly sobering study, 720 physicians were shown videotapes of actors playing patients with chest pain that could have been cardiac in etiology.[13] Four actors, each speaking precisely the same script, appeared on the videos: a white man, a white woman, a black man, and a black woman. Regardless of their own race and ethnicity, the physicians were far more likely to recommend cardiac catheterization for the white male than for the black female. Similar variations in diagnostic and therapeutic practices have been seen elsewhere in medicine, catalyzing efforts to address these "*healthcare disparities*."[14]

Researchers found that physician-specific differences were also at play. For example, one study showed that senior physicians were significantly more likely than their younger colleagues to correctly hospitalize chest pain patients (those with real MIs).[15] Were the older physicians better diagnosticians? Perhaps not—the older physicians were also more likely to hospitalize patients *without* heart attacks. In other words, with experience came risk aversion. Another study showed that risk aversion was not simply a function of age. One hundred and nineteen physicians completed a questionnaire assessing their attitudes toward risk. Doctors who appeared to be risk seekers (e.g., those who like fast cars and sky diving) were four times more likely to send the same chest pain patient home than the risk avoiders.[16]

One could easily look at cases like Annie Jackson's and vilify Dr. Bennett for careless doctoring, an egregious misdiagnosis, and a fatal mistake. But by now, hopefully, you're approaching this case with a more systems-focused mindset, thinking: How can we improve our ability to diagnose patients who come to the ER or the outpatient clinic with a constellation of symptoms, findings, and risk factors that may yield ambiguous results but can be life-threatening? Too often, without a systematic approach, the clinical decision—to admit or discharge the patient or to provide a particular intervention or treatment—is based on the physician's faulty reasoning, which in turn may be traced to poor training, inadequate experience, personal and professional bias, fuzzy thinking brought on by overwork and fatigue, or even the physician's own tolerance for risk.

COGNITIVE ERRORS: ITERATIVE HYPOTHESIS TESTING, BAYESIAN REASONING, AND HEURISTICS

As cognitive psychologists began to study how physicians think, they found that even well-trained doctors engage in faulty thinking because they take cognitive shortcuts, reinforced by a professional culture that rewards the appearance of certainty.[17,18] This means that preventing diagnostic errors is likely to depend on understanding how physicians approach diagnostic decisions, and providing them with tools (either cognitive or adjunctive, such as information technology) to help them make correct decisions more often.

Beginning in the 1970s, several researchers began to try to understand how great diagnosticians think. Led by Dr. Jerome Kassirer (later the editor of the *New England Journal of Medicine*), they observed the diagnostic reasoning of dozens of clinicians, and found that the good ones naturally engaged in a process called *iterative hypothesis testing*.[19] This means that, after hearing the initial portion of a case, they immediately began thinking about possible scenarios to explain the facts, modifying their opinions as more information became available. For example, a skilled physician presented with the case of a 57-year-old man with three days of chest pain, shortness of breath, and light-headedness responds by thinking, "The worst thing this could be is a heart attack or pulmonary embolism. I need to ask a few more questions to see if the chest pain bores through to the back, which would make me worry about an aortic dissection. I'll also ask about typical cardiac symptoms, such as sweating and nausea, and see if the pain is squeezing or radiates to the left arm or jaw. But even if it doesn't, I'll certainly get an ECG to be sure no cardiac event has occurred. If he also reports a fever or cough, I might begin to suspect pneumonia or pleurisy. The chest x-ray should help sort that out."

Every answer the patient gives and each positive or negative finding on the physical examination (*yes, there is a fever*; *no, the spleen is not enlarged*) triggers an automatic, almost intuitive recalibration of the probability of the various alternatives. The skilled diagnostician does this so effortlessly that novices often struggle as they try to understand the science that underlies the expert's decision to embrace certain facts (the clear lung fields in the patient with dyspnea markedly elevate the probability of pulmonary embolism since this would be highly unusual in severe heart failure) while discarding others (the lack of an S_3 gallop—a subtle and often absent finding—does little to dissuade the expert from the possibility of heart failure).

We now recognize that much of this art consists of applying an unconscious, intuitive version of *Bayes' theorem*, developed by the eighteenth-century British theologian-turned-mathematician Thomas Bayes.[20] In essence, Bayes' theorem says that any medical test must be interpreted from two perspectives. The first is: How accurate is the test? That is, how often does it give right or wrong answers? The second is: How likely is it that this patient has the disease the test is looking for? Bayesian reasoning is why it is foolish to screen apparently healthy 35-year-old executives with a cardiac treadmill test (or, for that matter, a "heart scan"), because positive results will mostly be false positives. Conversely, a 65-year-old smoker with high cholesterol who develops squeezing chest pain when shoveling snow has about a 95% chance of having significant coronary artery disease. In this case, a negative treadmill test lowers this probability to only about 80%, so the clinician who reassures the patient that the normal treadmill means his heart is fine is making a terrible, and potentially fatal, mistake.

In addition to misapplications of iterative hypothesis testing and failure to appreciate the implications of Bayesian reasoning, we now understand that many diagnostic errors are caused by cognitive shortcuts ("*heuristics*") that clinicians take, often in the name of efficiency.[21] For example, many errors occur when clinicians are too quick to pronounce judgment, and then defend that turf too vigorously despite the emergence of contradictory evidence.[17,18] This is human nature, of course; we tend to see what we expect to see rather than than what's actually in front of our eyes. By the way, did you notice the word "than" used twice in a row in the previous sentence? Even when we don't intend to do it, our brains can take cognitive shortcuts to get us to our goal—whether it's finishing a sentence or discharging a patient from the ER.

This particular cognitive bias, known as "anchoring" (or "premature closure"), is only one of the many pitfalls that underlie many diagnostic errors. Other common biases include affective bias, availability bias, context errors, and premature closure (Table 6-1).[8] Practicing physicians were first introduced to these concepts in the past 15 years (many through a bestselling 2011 book by Daniel Kahneman, who won a Nobel Prize for helping to elucidate many of these biases[22]), although the concepts have long been applied to other domains in which decisions need to be made under conditions of uncertainty, ranging from battlefields to Wall Street.

Empirical research has contributed to our understanding of the impact of cognitive biases in healthcare. In one interesting study, internal medicine residents were presented with a series of cases in which the diagnosis was known.[23] The researchers then presented additional cases with similar symptoms but different correct diagnoses. The residents were more likely to offer (mistaken) diagnoses drawn from the first cases in the subsequent cases, clear evidence of availability bias. The researchers repeated the exercise after asking residents to engage in *reflective practice*, a process that lies at the core of a skill known as *metacognition* (thinking about one's own thinking).[24] The impact of availability bias fell sharply, offering hope that some errors related to faulty application of heuristics can be prevented.

Table 6-1	**EXAMPLES OF HEURISTICS AND BIASES THAT INFLUENCE DECISION MAKING**	
Heuristic or Bias	**Medical Example**	**Nonmedical Example**
Anchoring is the tendency to lock onto salient features in the patient's initial presentation and failing to adjust this initial impression in the light of later information.	A patient is admitted from the emergency department with a diagnosis of heart failure. The hospitalists who are taking care of the patient do not pay adequate attention to new findings that suggest another diagnosis.	We buy a new car based on excellent reviews and tend to ignore or downplay negative features that are noticed.
Affective bias refers to the various ways that our emotions, feelings, and biases affect judgment.	New complaints from patients known to be "frequent flyers" in the emergency department are not taken seriously.	We may have the belief that people who are poorly dressed are not articulate or intelligent.
Availability bias refers to our tendency to more easily recall things that we have seen recently or things that are common or that impressed us.	A clinician who just recently read an article on the pain from aortic aneurysm dissection may tend toward diagnosing it in the next few patients he sees who present with nonspecific abdominal pain, even though aortic dissections are rare.	Because of a recent news story on a tourist kidnapping in Country "A," we change the destination we have chosen for our vacation to Country "B."
Context errors reflect instances where we misinterpret the situation, leading to an erroneous conclusion.	We tend to interpret that a patient presenting with abdominal pain has a problem involving the gastrointestinal tract, when it may be something else entirely: for example, an endocrine, neurologic, or vascular problem.	We see a work colleague picking up two kids from an elementary school and assume he or she has children, when they are instead picking up someone else's children.
Search satisficing, also known as **premature closure**, is the tendency to accept the first answer that comes along that explains the facts at hand, without considering whether there might be a different or better solution.	The emergency department clinician seeing a patient with recent onset of low back pain immediately settles on a diagnosis of lumbar disc disease without considering other possibilities in the differential diagnosis.	We want a plane ticket that costs no more than $1000 and has no more than one connection. We perform an online search and purchase the first ticket that meets these criteria without looking to see if there is a cheaper flight or one with no connections.

Reproduced with permission from Balogh E, Miller B, Ball J, eds. *Improving Diagnosis in Health Care.* Committee on Diagnostic Error in Health Care, National Academy of Medicine. Washington, DC: National Academies Press; 2015.

There is also evidence that experienced clinicians are more likely to avoid premature closure than inexperienced ones,[25] which gives hope that this competency can be inculcated (although it seems unlikely that classroom training will ever match the impact of receiving feedback about a missed diagnosis in a real patient).[26] There is also evidence that a clinician's emotional state can influence the risk of committing diagnostic errors[27] and that providing an opportunity for reflection might help mitigate such risk.[28] While few of us are able to change our emotional state at will, helping clinicians become more aware of their state of mind and its potential impact on clinical care (*I realize that I'm angry. I'd better slow down and rethink this or ask a colleague for help*) may also help prevent some errors.

IMPROVING DIAGNOSTIC REASONING

In Chapter 13, we will explore the role of computerized decision support and more general use of information technology in helping physicians to be smarter diagnosticians. At this juncture, suffice it to say that such computerized adjuncts are likely to help clinicians make better, more evidence-based decisions, but will not for the foreseeable future replace the clinician's mind as the main diagnostic workhorse.

Can our cognitive biases be overcome? Perhaps more than any area in clinical medicine, when diagnosing patients we need to learn from our mistakes and to deepen our understanding of clinical reasoning. As with most errors, the answer will come through systems thinking, but here this means better systems for training physicians to avoid common diagnostic speed bumps (Table 6-1). As Canadian safety expert and emergency medicine physician Pat Croskerry puts it:

> One uniquely distinguishing characteristic of those who make high-quality decisions is that they can largely free themselves from the common pitfalls to which novices are vulnerable. A rite of passage in all disciplines of medicine is learning about clinical pitfalls that have been identified by the discipline's experts. This [says] in effect, "Here is a typical error that will be made, and here is how to avoid it."[21]

Interestingly, in the case of the chest pain triage decision (a decision that early researchers hoped to perfect through a combination of electronic decision support and a better appreciation of diagnostic pitfalls), most experts concluded that the quest for diagnostic certainty is futile. In a number of research studies, even the best algorithms could not reliably identify patients whose actual risk of MI was so low that it was safe to send them home—especially when the penalty for even occasional failure might be a tragic death and a

Table 6-2   TWELVE TIPS FOR TEACHING AVOIDANCE OF DIAGNOSTIC ERRORS
1. Explicitly describe heuristics and how they affect clinical reasoning
2. Promote the use of "diagnostic time outs"
3. Promote the practice of "worst-case scenario medicine"
4. Promote the use of a systematic approach to common problems
5. Ask why
6. Teach and emphasize the value of the clinical exam
7. Teach Bayesian theory as a way to direct the clinical evaluation and avoid premature closure
8. Acknowledge how the patient makes the clinician feel
9. Encourage learners to find clinical data that don't fit with a provisional diagnosis; ask "What can't we explain?"
10. Embrace zebras
11. Encourage learners to slow down
12. Admit one's own mistakes

Reproduced with permission from Trowbridge RL. Twelve tips for teaching avoidance of diagnostic errors. *Med Teach* 2008;30:496–500.

multimillion-dollar lawsuit. So the real progress in chest pain triage has come not from honing our diagnostic abilities, but rather from developing ways (usually involving repeated cardiac biomarker tests and a predischarge stress test) to "rule out MI" inexpensively over a reasonably short (6–12 hours) observational period. In essence, we have abandoned our quest for diagnostic perfection and accepted instead the more mundane task of managing our uncertainty safely by resolving it quickly and inexpensively.

Yet the studies cited earlier offer some hope that clinicians' cognitive abilities can be improved—by teaching trainees about heuristics and providing opportunities for reflective practice, giving physicians feedback about diagnoses they got right and wrong, and encouraging participation in M&M and similar conferences in which diagnostic errors are dissected and reviewed. Trowbridge's 12 tips for teaching avoidance of diagnostic errors (Table 6-2) seem like a useful starting point for these educational efforts.[29]

In light of the emerging popularity of checklists in other parts of the safety field (Chapters 5 and 15), some authorities have even advocated the use of diagnostic checklists—both general checklists that prompt clinicians to collect complete data and engage in metacognition (Table 6-3) and specific ones that force consideration of "do not miss" diagnoses when faced with certain symptoms or signs such as chest pain or tachycardia.[30] Some groups have even developed patient-oriented "checklists" to help patients become better stewards of their own health information and aid in the diagnostic process (Table 6-4).

Table 6-3	**PROPOSED GENERAL DIAGNOSTIC CHECKLIST**

- ❑ Obtain your own complete medical history
- ❑ Perform a focused and purposeful physical exam
- ❑ Generate initial hypotheses and differentiate these with additional history, physical exam, and diagnostic tests
- ❑ Pause to reflect—take a diagnostic "time out"
  - ○ Was I comprehensive?
  - ○ Did I consider the inherent flaws of heuristic thinking?
  - ○ Was my judgment affected by any other bias?
  - ○ Do I need to make the diagnosis now, or can I wait?
  - ○ What is the worst-case scenario?
- ❑ Embark on a plan, but acknowledge uncertainty and ensure a pathway for follow-up

Reproduced with permission from Ely JW, Graber ML, Croskerry P. Checklists to reduce diagnostic error. *Acad Med* 2011;86:307–313. © 2011 Association of American Medical Colleges. Published by Lippincott Williams & Wilkins, Inc.

Table 6-4	**CHECKLIST DESIGNED FOR PATIENTS TO FACILITATE GETTING THE RIGHT DIAGNOSIS**

- ❑ Tell your story well: be clear, complete, and accurate when you tell your clinician about your illness
- ❑ Be a good historian
- ❑ Be a good record keeper
- ❑ Be an informed consumer
- ❑ Take charge of managing your health
- ❑ Know your test results
- ❑ Follow-up
- ❑ Make sure it is the right diagnosis

Adapted with permission from the National Patient Safety Foundation. Available at: www.npsf.org/?page=rightdiagnosis.

The theory behind diagnostic checklists emerges out of cognitive psychology's "dual-process" model of thinking and reasoning (Figure 6-1), which states that clinicians engage in both Type 1 (fast, reflexive, intuitive, and largely subconscious) and Type 2 (analytic, slow, deliberate, and requiring focused attention) thinking.[31] Checklists might help prevent Type 1 errors by forcing physicians to slow down and overcome their innate diagnostic overconfidence.[17,18] While this is an elegant model and an appealing idea, a randomized trial found that the use of diagnostic checklists in the emergency room did not improve error rates.[32] Further research to understand the full potential of such interventions is needed.

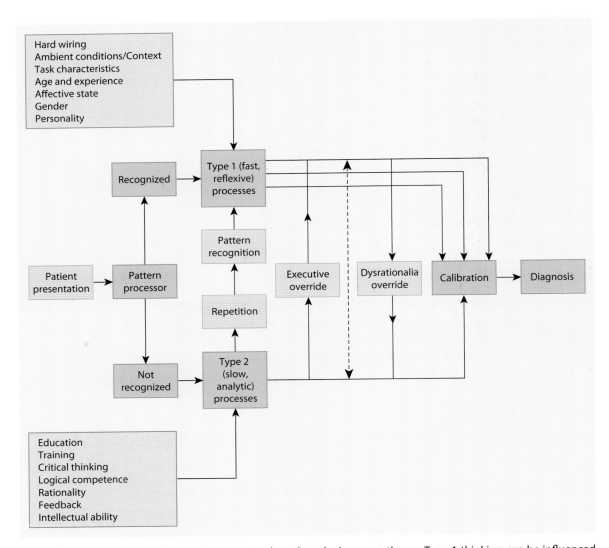

Figure 6-1 ■ A model for diagnostic reasoning based on dual-process theory. Type 1 thinking can be influenced by multiple factors, many of them subconscious (specific biases, emotional reaction toward or previous experiences with the patient or any of the diagnoses being considered), and is therefore represented as multiple channeled. On the other hand, Type 2 processes are single channeled and linear. Type 2 override of Type 1 ("executive override") occurs when physicians take a time out to reflect on their thinking, possibly with the help of checklists. In contrast, Type 1 thinking may irrationally override Type 2 ("dysrationalia override") when physicians insist on going their own way, such as when they ignore evidence-based clinical decision rules that can usually outperform them. "Calibration" represents the degree to which the perceived and actual diagnostic accuracy correspond. (Adapted with permission from Croskerry P, Singhal G, Mamede S. Cognitive debiasing 1: origins of bias and theory of debiasing. *BMJ Qual Saf* 2013;22:ii58–ii64.)

SYSTEM, COMMUNICATION, AND INFORMATION FLOW ISSUES IN DIAGNOSTIC ERRORS

While the discussion thus far has emphasized the cognitive aspects of diagnostic errors, many such errors owe to more classic systems problems such as poor communication and inadequate information transfer. Singh et al. usefully break these problems down into five domains: provider-patient encounters, diagnostic testing, follow-up, provider-provider interactions, and patient-specific factors (e.g., adherence).[33] Table 6-5 and Figure 6-2[34] illustrate this taxonomy. Figure 6-3 from the NAM report on diagnostic error shows places in the diagnostic process where failures may occur and contribute to diagnostic error.[8]

These system and informational problems are likely to be more easily addressed than the cognitive ones described earlier. For example, electronically prompting clinicians to follow-up on laboratory tests and x-rays should improve diagnostic accuracy, as should providing better access to specialty

Table 6-5	TAXONOMY OF DIAGNOSTIC ERROR DIMENSIONS	
Process Dimension	**Description**	**Example**
Provider-patient encounter	Problems with history, physical exam, or ordering diagnostic tests for further workup	Significant symptoms are not noted or acted upon at the time of the encounter
Diagnostic tests	Problems with ordered tests either not performed or performed/interpreted incorrectly	Incorrect laboratory test result due to mislabeled specimen
Follow-up and tracking	Problems with follow-up of abnormal diagnostic test results or scheduling of follow-up visits	No follow-up of abnormal x-ray despite suspicious finding
Referrals	Lack of appropriate actions on requested consultation or communication breakdown from consultant to referring provider	Consultant requests additional information from referring provider, but referring provider does not respond to the enquiry
Patient-related issues	Low adherence to following physician recommendations and/or seeking care, failure to provide critical history information	Patient does not show up for a scheduled diagnostic test

Reproduced with permission from Singh H, Graber ML, Kissam SM, et al. System-related interventions to reduce diagnostic errors: a narrative review. *BMJ Qual Saf* 2012;21:160–170.

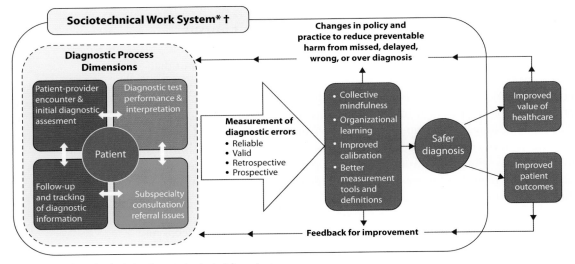

* Includes eight technological and non-technological dimensions
† Includes external factors affecting diagnostic performance and measurement such as payment systems, legal factors, national quality
measurement initiatives, accreditation, and other policy and regulatory requirements.

Figure 6-2 ■ A framework for diagnostic error depicting the sociotechnical system in which diagnosis takes place as well as ways to learn from errors to improve the diagnostic process. (Reproduced with permission from Singh H, Sittig DF. Advancing the science of measurement of diagnostic errors in healthcare: the Safer Dx framework. *BMJ Qual Saf* 2015;24:103–110.)

consultation, online evidence-based resources, and up-to-date problem lists. One organization successfully leveraged its electronic health record to proactively identify patients at risk for diagnostic error.[35] Schiff and Bates have chronicled the many ways that advanced information systems might help prevent diagnostic errors (Table 6-6).[36] Additional discussion of these issues can be found in Chapters 8 and 13.

OVERDIAGNOSIS

Most of the emphasis in the area of diagnostic errors has been in missed diagnoses or wrong diagnoses. But there is a problem with overdiagnosis as well—the detection of abnormalities that will never cause symptoms or death during a patient's lifetime if left alone. This problem may be accelerating because of the growing availability of highly sensitive diagnostic tests to identify small lesions (tumors mostly, but also partial vascular blockages, blood clots, and other lesions) whose clinical importance is unknown. "Because doctors don't know which patients are overdiagnosed," writes Gilbert Welch of Dartmouth,

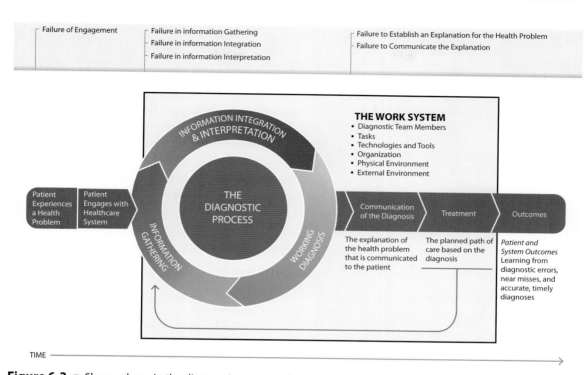

Figure 6-3 ▪ Shows places in the diagnostic process where failures can happen that may lead to diagnostic errors. (Reproduced with permission from Balogh E, Miller B, Ball J, eds. *Improving Diagnosis in Health Care.* Committee on Diagnostic Error in Health Care, National Academy of Medicine. Washington, DC: National Academies Press; 2015.)

whose work has helped put this issue on the patient safety map, "we tend to treat them all."[37]

For example, we are diagnosing many more cases of prostate and breast cancer than in the past, due to the widespread use of highly sensitive PSA screening and mammography. While it is not certain that aggressive treatment of these early cancers is leading to improved overall outcomes, it is undoubtedly leading to some cases of harm.[38,39] Similarly, the incidence of pulmonary embolism is rising, probably due to the remarkable ability of computed tomographic pulmonary angiography to find small, and potentially clinically unimportant, emboli.[40]

There is another issue at play as well. Diagnoses that previously were largely unknown—restless leg syndrome, fibromyalgia, and low testosterone, for example—became commonplace after pharmaceutical companies with potentially effective treatments began to beseech patients to "ask your doctor" about them. Woloshin and Schwartz call this "disease mongering" and it is likely that it adds to the toll of overdiagnosis and overtreatment.[41]

Table 6-6   LEVERAGING ELECTRONIC CLINICAL DOCUMENTATION TECHNOLOGY TO DECREASE DIAGNOSTIC ERROR RATES

Role for Electronic Documentation	Goals and Features of Redesigned Systems
Providing access to information	Ensure ease, speed, and selectivity of information searches; aid cognition through aggregation, trending, contextual relevance, and minimizing of superfluous data
Recording and sharing assessments	Provide a space for recording thoughtful, succinct assessments, differential diagnoses, contingencies, and unanswered questions; facilitate sharing and review of assessments by both patient and other clinicians
Maintaining dynamic patient history	Carry forward information for recall, avoiding repetitive patient querying, and recording while minimizing copying and pasting
Maintaining problem lists	Ensure that problem lists are integrated into workflow to allow for continuous updating
Tracking medications	Record medications patient is actually taking, patient responses to medications, and adverse effects to avert misdiagnoses and ensure timely recognition of medication problems
Tracking tests	Integrate management of diagnostic test results into note workflow to facilitate review, assessment, and responsive action as well as documentation of these steps
Ensuring coordination and continuity	Aggregate and integrate data from all care episodes and fragmented encounters to permit thoughtful synthesis
Enabling follow-up	Facilitate patient education about potential red flag symptoms; track follow-up
Providing feedback	Automatically provide feedback to clinicians upstream, facilitating learning from outcomes of diagnostic decisions
Providing prompts	Provide checklists to minimize reliance on memory and directed questioning to aid in diagnostic thoroughness and problem solving
Providing placeholder for resumption of work	Delineate clearly in the record where clinician should resume work after interruption, preventing lapses in data collection and thought process
Calculating Bayesian probabilities	Embed calculator into notes to reduce errors and minimize biases in subjective estimation of diagnostic probabilities

(continued)

Table 6-6 LEVERAGING ELECTRONIC CLINICAL DOCUMENTATION TECHNOLOGY TO DECREASE DIAGNOSTIC ERROR RATES (*continued*)	
Role for Electronic Documentation	**Goals and Features of Redesigned Systems**
Providing access to information sources	Provide instant access to knowledge resources through context-specific "infobuttons" triggered by keywords in notes that link user to relevant textbooks and guidelines
Offering second opinion or consultation	Integrate immediate online or telephone access to consultants to answer questions related to referral triage, testing strategies, or definitive diagnostic assessments
Increasing efficiency	More thoughtful design, workflow integration, and distribution of documentation burden could speed up charting, freeing time for communication and cognition

Reproduced with permission from Schiff GD, Bates DW. Can electronic clinical documentation help prevent diagnostic errors? *N Engl J Med* 2010;362:1066–1069.

THE POLICY CONTEXT FOR DIAGNOSTIC ERRORS

Since diagnostic reasoning is so central to many physicians' own notion of professionalism, there is a lot of activity (keeping up with the literature, attending courses, tracking down follow-up on patients) that, at its core, focuses on improving diagnostic effectiveness. The fact that these activities are often undertaken voluntarily (although sometimes promoted by board certification or continuing education requirements) is impressive.

But the kinds of pressures for quality and safety that are now marbled through the rest of the healthcare system (Chapter 3)—accreditation standards, public reporting, and pay for performance—largely bypass the issue of diagnostic errors. For example, none of the Agency for Healthcare Research and Quality's 26 Patient Safety Indicators (Appendix V), nor the 34 Safe Practices recommended by the National Quality Forum (Appendix VII), assess diagnostic accuracy.[42] Of course, this is linked to the reasons that diagnostic errors received so little attention in the first decade of the safety movement: these errors are difficult to measure and fix.[1]

The growing literature on preventable harm associated with diagnostic error, coupled with the 2015 NAM report, may well create a burning platform that will spark policy changes that stimulate improvement in diagnosis. The NAM concluded its report with eight goals for improving diagnosis and reducing diagnostic error (Table 6-7).[8] Achieving these goals will require the collaboration of multiple stakeholders, including providers, patients, healthcare organizations, professional societies, and policymakers.

Table 6-7   **GOALS FOR IMPROVING DIAGNOSIS AND REDUCING DIAGNOSTIC ERROR**
Facilitate more effective teamwork in the diagnostic process among healthcare professionals, patients, and their families
Enhance healthcare professional education and training in the diagnostic process
Ensure that health information technologies support patients and healthcare professionals in the diagnostic process
Develop and deploy approaches to identify, learn from, and reduce diagnostic errors and near misses in clinical practice
Establish a work system and culture that supports the diagnostic process and improvements in diagnostic performance
Develop a reporting environment and medical liability system that facilitates improved diagnosis by learning from diagnostic errors and near misses
Design a payment and care delivery environment that supports the diagnostic process
Provide dedicated funding for research on the diagnostic process and diagnostic errors

Reproduced with permission from Balogh E, Miller B, Ball J, eds. *Improving Diagnosis in Health Care.* Committee on Diagnostic Error in Health Care, National Academy of Medicine. Washington, DC: National Academies Press; 2015.

Some of the urgency to find robust measures of and solutions to diagnostic errors comes because healthcare organizations and providers find themselves increasingly assessed based on their adherence to a variety of quality and safety measures that are based on the presumption that the diagnosis is correct (*in a patient with heart failure, did the doctor prescribe an ACE inhibitor?*). In such an environment, hospitals, clinics, and providers may be compensated handsomely for giving the "right treatment" for the wrong diagnoses.

KEY POINTS

- Despite advances in laboratory testing, clinical imaging, and information technology, diagnostic errors remain commonplace. Despite their frequency, because they are more difficult to measure and fix than other adverse events, they have been relatively neglected in the patient safety movement.
- A landmark 2015 report by the National Academy of Medicine was commissioned, in part, to elevate the status of diagnosis errors in the field of patient safety.
- Clinicians' diagnostic and therapeutic actions are influenced by both patient-related (e.g., age, gender, race) and clinician-related (e.g., fatigue, past experience, risk tolerance) factors.

- Good diagnosticians correctly apply iterative hypothesis testing and Bayesian reasoning, and avoid cognitive pitfalls and biases, such as anchoring (getting stuck on initial impressions) and the availability heuristic (being unduly influenced by prior cases).
- Improving diagnostic reasoning will involve both computerized decision support and training clinicians to be more effective diagnostic thinkers. Electronic tools that allow for accurate, timely flow of key information will also help.
- Although not traditionally emphasized in the patient safety field, overdiagnosis—prompted by both increasingly sensitive screening tests and corporate marketing—is an important safety problem as well.

REFERENCES

1. Wachter RM. Why diagnostic errors don't get any respect—and what can be done about them. *Health Aff (Millwood)* 2010;29:1605–1610.
2. Kohn L, Corrigan J, Donaldson M, eds. *To Err Is Human: Building a Safer Health System.* Committee on Quality of Health Care in America, Institute of Medicine. Washington, DC: National Academies Press; 1999.
3. Leape LL, Brennan TA, Laird N, et al. The nature of adverse events in hospitalized patients. Results of the Harvard Medical Practice Study II. *N Engl J Med* 1991;324:377–384.
4. Saber Tehrani AS, Lee H, Mathews SC, et al. 25-year summary of US malpractice claims for diagnostic errors 1986–2010: an analysis from the National Practitioner Data Bank. *BMJ Qual Saf* 2013;22:672–680.
5. Sing H, Meyer AN, Thomas EJ. The frequency of diagnostic errors in outpatient care: estimations from three large observational studies involving US adult populations. *BMJ Qual Saf* 2014;23:727–731.
6. Graber ML, Wachter RM, Cassel CK. Bringing diagnosis into the quality and safety equations. *JAMA* 2012;308:1211–1212.
7. Schiff GD, Leape LL. Commentary: how can we make diagnosis safer? *Acad Med* 2012;87:135–138.
8. Balogh E, Miller B, Ball J, eds. *Improving Diagnosis in Health Care.* Committee on Diagnostic Error in Health Care, National Academy of Medicine. Washington, DC: National Academies Press; 2015.
9. Croskerry P. The importance of cognitive errors in diagnosis and strategies to minimize them. *Acad Med* 2003;78:775–780.
10. Welp A, Meier LL, Manser T. The interplay between teamwork, clinicians' emotional exhaustion and clinician-rated patient safety: a longitudinal study. *Crit Care* 2016;20:110.

11. Moy E, Barrett M, Coffey R, Hines AL, Newman-Toker DE. Missed diagnoses of acute myocardial infarction in the emergency department: variation by patient and facility characteristics. *Diagnosis* 2015;2:29–40.

12. Lee TH, Rouan GW, Weisberg MC, et al. Clinical characteristics and natural history of patients with acute myocardial infarction sent home from the emergency room. *Am J Cardiol* 1987;60:219–224.

13. Schulman KA, Berlin JA, Harless W, et al. The effect of race and sex on physicians' recommendations for cardiac catheterization. *N Engl J Med* 1999;340:618–626.

14. Agency for Healthcare Research and Quality. *National Healthcare Disparities Report: Summary*. Rockville, MD: Agency for Healthcare Research and Quality; 2014. Available at: http://www.ahrq.gov/sites/default/files/wysiwyg/research/findings/nhqrdr/nhqdr14/2014nhqdr.pdf.

15. Ting HH, Lee TH, Soukup JR, et al. Impact of physician experience on triage of emergency room patients with acute chest pain at three teaching hospitals. *Am J Med* 1991;91:401–408.

16. Pearson SD, Goldman L, Orav EJ, et al. Triage decisions for emergency department patients with chest pain: do physicians' risk attitudes make the difference? *J Gen Intern Med* 1995;10:557–564.

17. Brezis M, Orkin-Bedolach Y, Fink D, Kiderman A. Does physician's training induce overconfidence that hampers disclosing errors? *J Patient Saf* January 11, 2016. [Epub ahead of print].

18. Meyer AN, Payne VL, Meeks DW, Rao R, Singh H. Physicians' diagnostic accuracy, confidence, and resource requests: a vignette study. *JAMA Intern Med* 2013;173:1952–1958.

19. Kassirer JP. Teaching clinical medicine by iterative hypothesis testing—let's preach what we practice. *N Engl J Med* 1983;309:921–923.

20. Wachter RM, Shojania KG. Diagnostic errors. In: *Internal Bleeding: The Truth behind America's Terrifying Epidemic of Medical Mistakes*. New York, NY: Rugged Land; 2004.

21. Croskerry P. Achieving quality in clinical decision making: cognitive strategies and detection of bias. *Acad Emerg Med* 2002;9:1184–1204.

22. Kahneman D. *Thinking Fast and Slow*. New York, NY: Farrar, Straus and Giroux; 2011.

23. Mamede S, van Gog T, van den Berge K, et al. Effect of availability bias and reflective reasoning on diagnostic accuracy among internal medicine residents. *JAMA* 2010;304:1198–1203.

24. Mamede S, Schmidt HG, Rikers R. Diagnostic errors and reflective practice in medicine. *J Eval Clin Pract* 2007;13:138–145.

25. Eva KW, Link CL, Lutfey KE, McKinlay JB. Swapping horses midstream: factors related to physicians' changing their minds about a diagnosis. *Acad Med* 2010;85:1112–1117.

26. Trowbridge RL, Dhaliwal G, Cosby KS. Educational agenda for diagnostic error reduction. *BMJ Qual Saf* 2013;22:ii28–ii32.

27. Croskerry P, Abbass A, Wu AW. Emotional influences in patient safety. *J Patient Saf* 2010;6:199–205.

28. Hess BJ, Lipner RS, Thompson V, Holmboe ES, Graber ML. Blink or think: can further reflection improve initial diagnostic impressions? *Acad Med* 2015;90:112–118.

29. Trowbridge RL. Twelve tips for teaching avoidance of diagnostic errors. *Med Teach* 2008;30:496–500.
30. Ely JW, Graber ML, Croskerry P. Checklists to reduce diagnostic error. *Acad Med* 2011;86:307–313.
31. Croskerry P, Singhal G, Mamede S. Cognitive debiasing 1: origins of bias and theory of debiasing. *BMJ Qual Saf* 2013;22:ii58–ii64.
32. Ely JW, Graber MA. Checklists to prevent diagnostic errors: a pilot randomized controlled trial. *Diagnosis* 2015;2:163–169.
33. Singh H, Graber ML, Kissam SM, et al. System-related interventions to reduce diagnostic errors: a narrative review. *BMJ Qual Saf* 2012;21:160–170.
34. Singh H, Sittig DF. Advancing the science of measurement of diagnostic errors in healthcare: the Safer Dx framework. *BMJ Qual Saf* 2015;24:103–110.
35. Graber ML, Trowbridge R, Myers JS, Umscheid CA, Strull W, Kanter MH. The next organizational challenge: finding and addressing diagnostic error. *Jt Comm J Qual Patient Saf* 2014;40:102–110.
36. Schiff GD, Bates DW. Can electronic clinical documentation help prevent diagnostic errors? *N Engl J Med* 2010;362:1066–1069.
37. Welch HG. Overdiagnosis and mammography screening. *BMJ* 2009;339:b1425.
38. Welch HG, Schwartz LM, Woloshin S. *Overdiagnosed. Making People Sick in the Pursuit of Health.* Boston, MA: Beacon Press; 2011.
39. Esserman L. When less is better, but physicians are not afraid to intervene. *JAMA Intern Med* 2016;176(7):888–889.
40. Wiener RS, Schwartz LM, Woloshin S. When a test is too good: how CT pulmonary angiograms find pulmonary emboli that do not need to be found. *BMJ* 2013;347:f3368.
41. Woloshin S, Schwartz LM. Giving legs to restless legs: a case study of how the media helps make people sick. *PLoS Med* 2006;3:e170.
42. Newman-Toker DE, Pronovost PJ. Diagnostic errors—the next frontier for patient safety. *JAMA* 2009;301:1060–1062.

ADDITIONAL READINGS

Ely JW, Graber ML. Preventing diagnostic errors in primary care. *Am Fam Physician* 2016;94:426–432.
Gandhi TK, Lee TH. Patient safety beyond the hospital. *N Engl J Med* 2010;363:1001–1003.
Gladwell M. *Blink: The Power of Thinking Without Thinking.* New York, NY: Little, Brown and Company; 2005.
Groopman J. *How Doctors Think.* Boston, MA: Houghton Mifflin; 2007.
Haskell HW. What's in a story? Lessons from patients who have suffered diagnostic failure. *Diagnosis* 2014;1:53–54.
Hoffmann TC, Del Mar C. Clinicians' expectations of the benefits and harms of treatments, screening, and tests: a systematic review. *JAMA Intern Med* 2017;177:407–419.
Jørgensen KJ, Gøtzsche PC, Kalager M, Zahl PH. Breast cancer screening in Denmark: a cohort study of tumor size and overdiagnosis. *Ann Intern Med* 2017;166:313–323.
Kahneman D, Lovallo D, Sibony O. Before you make that big decision …. *Harv Bus Rev* 2011;89:50–60, 137.

Kahneman D, Slovic P, Tversky A. *Judgment under Uncertainty: Heuristics and Biases.* Cambridge, England: Cambridge University Press; 1987.

Kassirer JP, Kopelman RI. Cognitive errors in diagnosis: instantiation, classification, and consequences. *Am J Med* 1989;86:433–441.

Klein G. *Sources of Power: How People Make Decisions.* Cambridge, MA: Massachusetts Institute of Technology; 1999.

Lewis M. *The Undoing Project: A Friendship that Changed Our Minds.* New York: W.W. Norton & Co.; 2016.

Norman GR, Monteiro SD, Sherbino J, Ilgen JS, Schmidt HG, Mamede S. The causes of errors in clinical reasoning: cognitive biases, knowledge deficits, and dual process thinking. *Acad Med* 2017;92:23–30.

Ofri D. *What Doctors Feel: How Emotions Affect the Practice of Medicine.* Boston, MA: Beacon Press; 2013.

Pauker SG, Wong JB. How (should) physicians think? A journey from behavioral economics to the bedside. *JAMA* 2010;304:1233–1235.

Saposnik G, Redelmeier D, Ruff CC, Tobler PN. Cognitive biases associated with medical decisions: a systematic review. *BMC Med Inform Decis Mak* 2016;16:138.

Schmidt T, Maag R, Foy AJ. Overdiagnosis of coronary artery disease detected by coronary computed tomography angiography: a teachable moment. *JAMA Intern Med* 2016;176:1747–1748.

Singh H. Diagnostic errors: moving beyond "no respect" and getting ready for prime time. *BMJ Qual Saf* 2013;22:789–792.

Vaughn VM, Chopra V, Howell JD. War games and diagnostic errors. *BMJ* 2016;355:i6342.

Weingart SN, Saadeh MG, Simchowitz B, et al. Process of care failures in breast cancer diagnosis. *J Gen Intern Med* 2009;24:702–709.

Welch HG. *Less Medicine More Health: 7 Assumptions that Drive too Much Medical Care.* Boston, MA: Beacon Press; 2013.

Zwaan L, Singh H. The challenges in defining and measuring diagnostic error. *Diagnosis* 2015;2:97–103.

HUMAN FACTORS AND ERRORS AT THE PERSON–MACHINE INTERFACE

7

INTRODUCTION

Until now, we have discussed several paradigm shifts required to improve patient safety. The dominant one, of course, is replacing an environment based on "blame and shame" with one in which safety is viewed as a top priority and systems thinking is employed effectively. Second is an awareness of the impact of culture and relationships on communication and the exchange of information. This chapter* will introduce another lens through which to view safety problems: how human factors engineering (HFE) can improve the safety of person–machine interactions and the environment in which healthcare providers work.

To prime ourselves for a discussion of HFE, let us consider the following scenarios:

- An obstetric nurse inadvertently connects an opiate pain medication intended for an epidural catheter into a mother's intravenous (IV) line, leading to the patient's death.[1] A subsequent review demonstrated that the bags and lines used for epidural and IV infusions were similar in size and shape, leaving nothing but human vigilance to prevent a bag intended for epidural use from connecting to an IV catheter or hub.
- A hospitalized elderly man dies after a heart attack suffered while in a monitored bed in one of America's top hospitals. A later investigation reveals that the main crisis monitor had been turned off, and multiple lower level

---

*A previous version of this chapter was coauthored by Bryan Haughom, MD.

alarms—including ones that showed that the patient's heart rate was slowing dangerously for nearly half an hour before his heart stopped—weren't noticed by the busy nursing staff, who had become so inured to frequent false alarms that they suffered from "alarm fatigue."[2]

- Modern multichannel infusion pumps are routinely used in the ICU to administer multiple medications and fluids through a single central line (Figure 7-1). This often results in a confusing tangle of tubes that cannot be easily differentiated. No surprise, then, that a busy ICU nurse might adjust the dose of the wrong medication.
- Medications are often stored in vials in doses that are highly concentrated. This means that they frequently need to be carefully diluted before being administered. For example, a vial of phenylephrine contains 10 mg/mL, while the usual IV dose administered to patients is

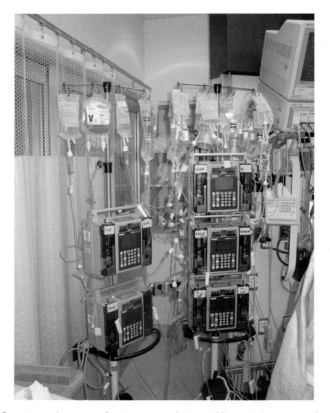

Figure 7-1 ■ A modern sea of intravenous drips and lines. Is it any wonder that there are sometimes errors when incorrect medications or rates are administered to a desperately ill patient? (Courtesy of Michael Gropper, MD, PhD, with permission.)

0.1 mg—one-hundredth of the dose in the vial! Inadvertent administration of full strength phenylephrine can cause a stroke.

- An elderly patient dies when a Code Blue team—responding to the call for help after a cardiac arrest—is unable to connect the defibrillator pads to the defibrillator.[3] A subsequent analysis showed that over the years the hospital had accumulated more than a dozen defibrillator models on its floors, so providers were often unfamiliar with the models at hand and incompatibilities were common.[4]

In each of these examples, significant hazards resulted from people interacting with products, tools, procedures, and processes in the clinical environment. One could argue that these errors could have been prevented by more careful clinicians or more robust training. However, as we have already learned, to minimize the chances that fallible humans (in other words, all of us) will cause patient harm, it is critical to apply systems thinking. In the case of person–machine interfaces, this systems focus leads us to consider issues around device design, the environment, and the care processes that accompany device use. The field of HFE provides the tools to accomplish this.

HUMAN FACTORS ENGINEERING

Human factors engineering is an applied science of systems design that is concerned with the interplay between humans, machines, and their work environments.[5] Its goal is to assure that devices, systems, and working environments are designed to minimize the likelihood of error and optimize safety. As one of its central tenets, the field recognizes that humans are fallible, they often overestimate their abilities, and they underestimate their limitations. Human factors engineers strive to understand the strengths and weaknesses of our physical and mental abilities and use that information to design safer devices, systems, and environments.

HFE is a hybrid field, mixing various engineering disciplines, design, and cognitive psychology. Its techniques have long been used in the highly complex and risky fields of aviation, electrical power generation, and petroleum refining, but its role in patient safety has only recently been appreciated and some would say that progress has been slow.[6–8] In applying HFE to healthcare, there has been a particular emphasis on the design and use of devices such as IV pumps, catheters, computer software and hardware, and the like.

Many medical devices and electronic health record systems have poorly designed user interfaces that are confusing and clumsy to use.[9,10] According to the U.S. Food and Drug Administration (FDA), approximately half of all medical device recalls between 1985 and 1989 stemmed from poor design. FDA officials, along with other human factors experts, now recognize the importance of integrating human factors principles into the design of medical equipment.[11,12]

In Chapter 2, we introduced the concept of *forcing functions*, design features that prevent the user from taking an action without deliberately considering information relevant to that action. The 1980s-era redesign of automobiles to make it impossible to place a car in reverse if the driver's foot is off the brake provides a classic example of a forcing function. In healthcare, forcing functions have been developed to make it impossible to connect the wrong gas canisters to an anesthetized patient or to prevent patients from overdosing themselves while receiving patient-controlled analgesia (PCA). Although forcing functions are the most straightforward application of HFE, it is important to appreciate other healthcare applications, ranging from improving device design to aiding in device procurement decisions to evaluating processes within the care environment.

For example, many hospitals are now approaching the challenge of increasing the frequency with which providers clean their hands partly as a human factors problem (Chapter 10).[13,14] While these institutions continue to work on education and observation, they also ensure that cleaning gel dispensers are easy to use and strategically located throughout the hospital wards. In fact, a whole field of patient safety–centered hospital and clinic design has emerged, and some buildings have been constructed using human factors principles.[15,16]

Despite these early success stories, HFE remains conspicuously underused as a patient safety tool, for reasons ranging from the lack of well-defined avenues to report and correct design or process flaws within hospitals to the natural tendency of highly trained caregivers to feel that they can outsmart or work around problems. With the dramatic growth in the volume and complexity of man–machine clinical interactions, the probability that human workers will make mistakes has escalated, as has the importance of considering HFE approaches.

USABILITY TESTING AND HEURISTIC ANALYSIS

One of the key tools in HFE is *usability testing*, in which experts observe frontline workers engaging in their task under realistic conditions—either actual patient care, or simulated environments that closely resemble reality. Users are observed, videotaped, and asked to "talk through" their thought processes, explaining their actions as well as their difficulties with a given application or device. Engineers then analyze the data in order to fine-tune their design for the users, the chosen tasks, and the work environment.[17]

Software engineers and design firms now see usability testing as an indispensable part of their work, preferring to make modifications at the design stage instead of waiting until errors have become apparent after real-world implementation. Similarly, many equipment manufacturers and a growing number of healthcare organizations now employ individuals with human factors expertise to advise them on equipment purchasing decisions, modify existing equipment to prevent errors, or identify error-prone equipment and environmental situations. These trained individuals instinctively approach errors with a human factors mindset, asking questions about usability and possible human factors solutions before considering fixes involving retraining and incentives, interventions that may seem easier than device or environmental redesign but are generally far less effective.

Usability testing can be a complex process, requiring not only human factors experts but also extensive investigatory time and cooperation from users. A less resource-intensive alternative is known as *heuristic analysis*.[18] The term heuristics was first mentioned in Chapter 6 in reference to the cognitive shortcuts that clinicians often take during diagnostic reasoning, shortcuts that can lead to errors. In the context of HFE, though, heuristics have a different connotation: "rules of thumb" or governing principles for device or system design. In heuristic evaluations, the usability of a particular system or device is assessed by applying established design fundamentals such as visibility of system status, user control and freedom, consistency and standards, flexibility, and efficiency of use (Table 7-1).[19,20]

During a heuristic evaluation, experts navigate the user interface searching for usability issues. In essence, analysts try to put themselves in the shoes of the end user, looking for error-prone functions or designs that might ultimately compromise safety. The information gleaned from these analyses becomes feedback to the design teams, who iteratively update and refine the design of prototypes. The ultimate shortcoming of heuristics, however, is that they are only as good as the analyst performing the evaluation. Without putting end users in real-time situations and observing their work, it is difficult to fully unearth problematic design issues. Nevertheless, heuristic evaluations can provide valuable information to a design team, or even to a hospital looking to review devices or systems they already own or are looking to purchase.[18,21]

Inability to truly stand in for the novice is only one problem that designers and engineers have in anticipating all the safety hazards of complex systems. During an interview, Donald Norman, the author of the best-selling book, *The Design of Everyday Things*,[22] reflected on another real-world human factors issue:

> *[As an engineer], you focus too much, and don't appreciate that all the individual elements of your work, when combined together, create*

Table 7-1 **EXAMPLES OF HEURISTIC PRINCIPLES**	
Visibility of system status	Users should be aware of system status
	System should provide appropriate feedback as well as appropriate instructions to complete a task
User control and freedom	Users should feel "in control" of a system
	System should provide clear exits at every step of a task, supply undo as well as redo functions, and avoid irreversible actions
Match between system and world	Language utilized by the system should be that of the end user
	System should fit within the mental model of the end user
Consistency and standards	User interface and system functions should be consistent
Recognition rather than recall	Users' memory load should be minimized
	Systems should take advantage of user's inherent tendency to process information in "chunks" as opposed to by rote memory
Flexibility and efficiency of use	Interfaces should be designed to accommodate customizability
Error recovery and prevention	Systems should be designed to prevent errors before they occur
	If errors do occur, users should be able to recover from them via reversible actions
	The system should also provide clear steps detailing how to recover
Help and documentation	Help and documentation should be available to users
	The language used should be appropriate for the end user, avoid jargon

Adapted from Ginsburg G. Human factors engineering: a tool for medical device evaluation in hospital procurement decision-making. *J Biomed Inform* 2005;38:213–219; Zhang J, Johnson TR, Patel VL, Paige DL, Kubose T. Using usability heuristics to evaluate patient safety of medical devices. *J Biomed Inform* 2003;36:23–30; Kushniruk AW, Patel VL. Cognitive and usability engineering methods for the evaluation of clinical information systems. *J Biomed Inform* 2004;37:56–76.

a system—one that might be far more error-prone than you would have predicted from each of the individual components. For example, the anesthesiologist may review beforehand what is going to be needed. And so he or she picks up the different pieces of equipment that measure the different things, like the effects of the drugs on the patient. Each instrument actually may be designed quite well, and it may even have been rigorously tested. But each instrument works differently. Perhaps each has an alarm that goes off when something's wrong. Sounds good so far. But when you put it together as a system it's a disaster. Each alarm has a different setting, and the appropriate response to one may be incredibly dangerous for another. When things really go wrong, all the alarms are beeping and the resulting cacophony of sounds means nobody can get any work done. Instead *of tending to the patient, you're spending all of your time turning off the alarms. So part of the problem is not seeing it as a system, that things have to work in context. And that these items actually should be talking to each other so that they can help the anesthesiologist prioritize the alarms.*[23]

The difficulty of anticipating all these interactions and dependencies is yet another powerful argument for usability testing, not only of individual devices but also of multiple devices as they interact in actual systems.

In addition to their use in the design and purchase of medical devices such as ventilators, programmable IV pumps, defibrillators, and anesthesia equipment, human factors principles should also be utilized in the design and implementation of advanced information technology systems (Chapter 13). With the increasing computerization of healthcare, this interface—between HFE and information technology—is becoming ever more critical, and the growing list of unintended consequences of information technology systems is partly an indictment of our lack of focus on this area.[24,25]

The consequences go well beyond inefficiency and workarounds. One prominent pediatric teaching hospital reported an increase in mortality rates after a commercial computerized provider order entry (CPOE) system went live.[26] Although the findings are controversial and a subsequent study at another hospital (using the same CPOE system) found improved mortality,[27] the authors' description of the problems is a useful cautionary note regarding the hazards of poor design and implementation. For example, they observed:

Before CPOE implementation, physicians and nurses converged at the patient's bedside to stabilize the patient. After CPOE implementation, while one physician continued to direct medical management, a second physician was often needed solely to enter orders into the computer during the first 15 minutes to one hour if a patient arrived in extremis. Downstream from order entry, bedside nurses were no longer allowed to grab critical medications from a satellite medication dispenser located in the ICU because as part of CPOE implementation, all medications, including vasoactive agents and antibiotics, became centrally located within the pharmacy department. The priority to fill a medication order was assigned by the pharmacy department's algorithm. Furthermore, because pharmacy could not process medication orders until they had been activated, ICU nurses also spent significant amounts of time at a separate computer terminal and away from the bedside. When the pharmacist accessed the CPOE system to process an order, the physician and the nurse were "locked out," further delaying additional order entry.[26]

Human factors techniques can also be used to increase the safety of a working environment, such as by standardizing devices within a hospital to make training easier and increase reliability, carefully designing equipment and processes in a pharmacy to ensure that pharmacists always dispense the right drug in the correct dose, and optimizing a clinical work environment by providing adequate lighting, eliminating distractions (including excess noise), and ensuring that care providers receive adequate rest.

APPLYING HUMAN FACTORS ENGINEERING PRINCIPLES

In the end, usability testing and heuristic analysis can be used together or separately to design safe, effective, and intuitive devices for use in complex clinical care situations. Let's now return to the clinical scenarios outlined at the beginning of the chapter. How could HFE principles be applied to prevent these unsafe conditions? Here are some approaches human factors engineers might consider for each scenario:

- To prevent an epidural–intravenous mix-up, a forcing function could ensure that medications intended for epidural use are physically incapable of connecting to IV hubs.[28,29] An effective bar-coding system is another obvious solution. (Tragically—and ironically—the hospital where this error occurred *had* a bar-coding system, but its usability and reliability problems were well known and the nurses had learned to use workarounds, particularly in urgent situations.[1,30])
- Alarm fatigue can be mitigated by careful selection of equipment and by implementing policies and procedures developed after consultation with nurses and other caregivers and detailed observations of workflow.[2,31] This issue will be further discussed in Chapter 13.
- By employing standardized color coding and other techniques, nurses using multichannel infusion pumps can more easily differentiate IV lines.[32]
- Pharmacies can be equipped with high-reliability robotic systems that produce bar-coded unit-dose medications that can be double-checked using bar-coding devices at the bedside before they are administered to the patient. Multidose vials are inherently risky and should be avoided where possible.[33]
- The hospital where this error occurred standardized its defibrillators (buying more simple, "goof-proof" ones) and increased the frequency of testing.[3,4,34]

A classic case study in the application of HFE to another patient safety problem, adapted from the book *Set Phasers on Stun*,[35] is described in Box 7-1.

Box 7-1 A CASE STUDY OF A FATAL ERROR THAT MIGHT HAVE BEEN PREVENTED BY AN HFE APPROACH

HM was a 4-year-old girl with a complex history, including birth defects and cardiac problems. She was no stranger to the hospital, to the telemetry unit, or to its nurses. Nurse K carefully attended to her fragile patient, ensuring that each of the six ECG leads was properly placed on HM's small body. As soon as they were all in place, Nurse K gently folded the bed sheet over HM's frail torso, and tucked her into bed. After properly connecting the ECG leads to the patient, the final step was to plug them into the heart monitor, which would allow the nurses to observe HM's heart rhythm at the nursing station down the hall.

After Nurse K lifted the guardrail on the side of the bed, she grabbed the ECG cord and scanned the head of the bed for the connection to the monitor. As was typical in this unit, there were several machines at the bedside—in this case, including an ECG machine and an IV infusion pump. The cord connected to the ECG leads in her hand had a characteristic six-pin connector at the end. It was designed such that it would fit perfectly with its counterpart. She grabbed the cord that was dangling down next to the heart monitor, lined up the two ends and pushed them together. It didn't even

cross her mind that the cord she had just connected could potentially be from something other than the ECG machine. After all, she was a seasoned nurse who handled these machines every day, and they all seemed to have different connecting pins.

Unbeknownst to her she had connected the ECG leads to the IV infusion pump. The cord from the infusion pump matched the size and shape of the six-pin ECG cord reasonably well. The similarity might not have been so dangerous had the infusion pump not been a battery powered portable model. Nurse K had no way to know she had been holding a live electrical wire, with the full electrical current of the IV pump. Connecting the cords delivered a direct shock to the little girl's chest, from which she could not be revived.

Though it may be easy simply to claim that Nurse K should have paid closer attention to the situation, it would be an incomplete analysis. Even if she had been paying attention, would she have avoided this fateful error? We may never know. However, looking at this case through a human factors lens reveals a number of potential pitfalls to which Nurse K fell victim. The most glaring is

(continued)

Box 7-1   A CASE STUDY OF A FATAL ERROR THAT MIGHT HAVE BEEN PREVENTED BY AN HFE APPROACH (*continued*)

the similarity between the ECG and IV pump cord. Despite the fact that they weren't perfect matches, they matched closely enough that one could connect the two. The most powerful HFE solution might be designing the two connections to have unique colors or shapes—the ECG cord round and the IV pump cord square, for example. Perhaps the device industry might be willing to subscribe to a set of standards such that all ECG cords have the same color and shape (ditto for pump cords). Another solution might be to have a warning label on the infusion pump's cord, alerting that it can deliver a direct and potentially fatal current.

Even beyond the design of the devices, what other problems may have led to this child's death? Could the conditions of the room—the setup, the lighting, the ambient noise, or the nurse's workload—have played a role in the outcome? Maybe Nurse K wasn't used to seeing these particular device models in the same room. Maybe the demands of her job and the busy environment of a hospital floor were taking their toll. We'll never know for sure. But it is certain that the thoughtful application of HFE principles to this situation would have made it a safer environment.

Reproduced with permission from Casey S. *Set Phasers on Stun: And Other True Tales of Design, Technology, and Human Error*. 2nd ed. Santa Barbara, CA: Aegean Publishing; 1998.

KEY POINTS

- HFE is the applied science of systems design. It is concerned with the interplay of humans, machines, and their work environments.
- Thoughtful application of HFE principles can help prevent errors at the person–machine interface.
- Usability testing and heuristic analysis aim to identify error-prone devices or systems before they lead to harm.
- The initial focus of HFE in healthcare was on the design of medical devices. Today it is broader, with efforts to try to create safe environments of care (i.e., designing hospital rooms around safety principles) and to decrease errors associated with poorly designed clinical information systems.

REFERENCES

1. Smetzer J, Baker C, Byrne FD, Cohen MR. Shaping systems for better behavioral choices: lessons learned from a fatal medication error. *Jt Comm J Qual Patient Saf* 2010;36:152–163, 1AP–2AP.

2. Kowalczyk L. Boston Medical Center reduces monitor alarms. *Boston Globe.* December 23, 2013. Available at: https://www.bostonglobe.com/lifestyle/health-wellness/2013/12/23/boston-medical-center-reduces-monitor-alarms-says-care-safer-for-patients-less-stressful-for-staff/szqFan1sE7CgHnfsuT2fEL/story.html.

3. Resuscitation errors: a shocking problem. *AORN J* 2013;98:49, 98.

4. Fairbanks RJ, Caplan SH, Bishop PA, Marks AM, Shah MN. Usability study of two common defibrillators reveals hazards. *Ann Emerg Med* 2007;50:424–432.

5. Human Factors Engineering. July 2016. Available at: https://psnet.ahrq.gov/primers/primer/20/human-factors-engineering.

6. Kohn LT, Corrigan JM, Donaldson MD. *To Err Is Human—Building a Safer Health System.* Washington, DC: National Academy Press; 1999.

7. Gurses AP, Ozok AA, Pronovost PJ. Time to accelerate integration of human factors and ergonomics in patient safety. *BMJ Qual Saf* 2012;21:347–351.

8. Waterson P, Catchpole K. Human factors in healthcare: welcome progress, but still scratching the surface. *BMJ Qual Saf* 2016;25:480–484.

9. Mattox E. Medical devices and patient safety. *Crit Care Nurse* 2012;32:60–68.

10. Schiff GD, Amato MG, Eguale T, et al. Computerised physician order entry-related medication errors: analysis of reported errors and vulnerability testing of current systems. *BMJ Qual Saf* 2015;24:264–271.

11. Food and Drug Administration. *Human Factors.* Available at: http://www.fda.gov/MedicalDevices/DeviceRegulationandGuidance/HumanFactors/default.htm.

12. Weinger MB, Wiklund M, Gardner-Bonneau D. *Handbook of Human Factors in Medical Device Design.* Boca Raton, FL: CRC Press, 2011.

13. Gawande A. *Better: A Surgeon's Notes on Performance.* New York, NY: Metropolitan Books; 2007.

14. Aboumatar H, Ristaino P, Davis RO, et al. Infection prevention promotion program based on the PRECEDE model: improving hand hygiene behaviors among healthcare personnel. *Infect Control Hosp Epidemiol* 2012;33:144–151.

15. Facilities Guidelines Institute, AIA Academy of Architecture for Health. 2006 *Guidelines for Design and Construction of Health Care Facilities.* Washington, DC: The American Institute of Architects; 2006.

16. Birnbach DJ, Nevo I, Scheinman SR, Fitzpatrick M, Shekhter I, Lombard JL. Patient safety begins with proper planning: a quantitative method to improve hospital design. *Qual Saf Health Care* 2010;19:462–465.

17. Chan J, Shojania KG, Easty AC, Etchells EE. Usability evaluation of order sets in a computerized provider order entry system. *BMJ Qual Saf* 2011;20:932–940.

18. Zhang J, Johnson TR, Patel VL, Paige DL, Kubose T. Using usability heuristics to evaluate patient safety of medical devices. *J Biomed Inform* 2003;36:23–30.

19. Kushniruk AW, Patel VL. Cognitive and usability engineering methods for the evaluation of clinical information systems. *J Biomed Inform* 2004;37:56–76.

20. Nielsen J. *Usability Engineering*. New York, NY: Academic Press; 1993.

21. Ginsburg G. Human factors engineering: a tool for medical device evaluation in hospital procurement decision-making. *J Biomed Inform* 2005;38:213–219.

22. Norman DA. *The Design of Everyday Things: Revised and Expanded Edition*. New York, NY: Basic Books; 2013.

23. Norman DA. In conversation with… Donald A. Norman. [Perspective]. *AHRQ PSNet* [serial online]; November 2006. Available at: https://psnet.ahrq.gov/perspectives/perspective/33.

24. Sittig DF, Singh H. Defining health information technology–related errors: new developments since 'to err is human'. *Arch Intern Med* 2011;171:1281–1284.

25. Coiera E, Ash J, Berg M. The unintended consequences of health information technology revisited. *Yearb Med Inform* 2016;(1):163–169.

26. Han YY, Carcillo JA, Venkataraman ST, et al. Unexpected increased mortality after implementation of a commercially sold computerized physician order entry system. *Pediatrics* 2005;116:1506–1512.

27. Longhurst CA, Parast L, Sandborg CI, et al. Decrease in hospital-wide mortality rate after implementation of a commercially sold computerized physician order entry system. *Pediatrics* 2010;126:14–21.

28. Epidural-IV route mix-ups: reducing the risk of deadly errors. *ISMP Medication Safety Alert! Acute Care Edition*. July 3, 2008;13:1–3.

29. Simmons D, Symes L, Guenter P, Graves K. Tubing misconnections: normalization of deviance. *Nutr Clin Pract* 2011;26:286–293.

30. Voshall B, Piscotty R, Lawrence J, Targosz M. Barcode medication administration work-arounds: a systematic review and implications for nurse executives. *J Nurs Adm* 2013;43:530–535.

31. Paine CW, Goel VV, Ely E, et al. Systematic review of physiologic monitor alarm characteristics and pragmatic interventions to reduce alarm frequency. *J Hosp Med* 2016;11:136–144.

32. Porat N, Bitan Y, Shefi D, Donchin Y, Rozenbaum H. Use of colour-coded labels for intravenous high-risk medications and lines to improve patient safety. *Qual Saf Health Care* 2009;18:505–509.

33. Vanderveen T. Vial mistakes involving heparin [Spotlight]. *AHRQ WebM&M* [serial online]; May 2009. Available at: https://psnet.ahrq.gov/webmm/case/201.

34. Karsh BT, Scanlon M. When is a defibrillator not a defibrillator? When it's like a clock radio…. The challenge of usability and patient safety in the real world. *Ann Emerg Med* 2007;50:433–435.

35. Casey SM. *Set Phasers on Stun: And Other True Tales of Design, Technology, and Human Error*. Santa Barbara, CA: Aegean Publishing Company; 1998.

ADDITIONAL READINGS

Cooper JB, Newbower RS, Long CD, McPeek B. Preventable anesthesia mishaps: a study of human factors. *Anesthesiology* 1978;49:399–406.

Decker S. *Patient Safety: A Human Factors Approach*. New York, NY: CRC Press; 2011.

France DJ, Throop P, Walczyk B, et al. Does patient-centered design guarantee patient safety? Using human factors engineering to find a balance between provider and patient needs. *J Patient Saf* 2005;1:145–153.

Gosbee J. Human factors engineering can teach you how to be surprised again. *AHRQ WebM&M* (serial online); November 2006. Available at: http://webmm.ahrq.gov/perspective.aspx?perspectiveID=32.

Hignett S, Jones EL, Miller D, et al. Human factors and ergonomics and quality improvement science: integrating approaches for safety in healthcare. *BMJ Qual Saf* 2015;24:250–254.

Maughan BC, Lei L, Cydulka RK. ED handoffs: observed practices and communication errors. *Am J Emerg Med* 2011;29:502–511.

Russ AL, Fairbanks RJ, Karsh BT, Militello LG, Saleem JJ, Wears RL. The science of human factors: separating fact from fiction. *BMJ Qual Saf* 2013;22:802–803.

Simmons D. Central, not epidural. *AHRQ WebM&M* (serial online): September 2011. Available at: https://psnet.ahrq.gov/webmm/case/250/central-not-epidural.

Slight SP, Eguale T, Amato MG, et al. The vulnerabilities of computerized physician order entry systems: a qualitative study. *J Am Med Inform Assoc* 2016;23:311–316.

Spath PL, ed. *Error Reduction in Health Care: A Systems Approach to Improving Patient Safety*. 2nd ed. San Francisco, CA: Jossey-Bass; 2011.

Spear SJ, Schmidhofer M. Ambiguity and workarounds as contributors to medical error. *Ann Intern Med* 2005;142:627–630.

Tonks A. Safer by design. *BMJ* 2008;336:186–188.

Weinger MB, Gaba DM. Human factors engineering in patient safety. *Anesthesiology* 2014;120:801–806.

TRANSITION AND HANDOFF ERRORS | 8

An 83-year-old man with a history of chronic obstructive pulmonary disease (COPD), gastroesophageal reflux disease, and paroxysmal atrial fibrillation with sick sinus syndrome was admitted to the cardiology service of a teaching hospital for initiation of an antiarrhythmic medication and placement of a permanent pacemaker.

The patient underwent pacemaker placement via the left subclavian vein at 2:30 PM. A routine postoperative single-view radiograph was taken and showed no pneumothorax. The patient was sent to the recovery unit for overnight monitoring. At 5:00 PM, the patient stated he was short of breath and requested his COPD inhaler. He also complained of new left-sided back pain. The nurse found that the patient's room air oxygen saturation had dropped from 95% to 88% and placed him on supplemental oxygen. She then paged the covering physician to come and assess the patient. The patient had been admitted to the nurse practitioner (NP)-run cardiology service earlier in the day (a non-house staff service), but at night, the on-call intern provided nighttime coverage for this service.

The intern, who had never met the patient before, examined him and found that he was already feeling better and that his oxygenation had improved after receiving the supplemental oxygen. The nurse suggested ordering a stat x-ray in light of the recent surgery. The intern concurred and the portable x-ray was completed within 30 minutes. About an hour later, the nurse wondered about the x-ray result and asked the covering intern if he had looked at it. The intern stated that he was signing out follow-up of the x-ray results to the night float resident, who was coming on duty at 8:00 PM.

Meanwhile, the patient continued to feel well except for mild back pain. The nurse gave him analgesics and continued to monitor his heart rate and respirations. At 10:00 PM, the nurse still hadn't heard anything about the x-ray, so she called the night float resident.

The night float had been busy with an emergency but promised to look at the x-ray and advise the nurse if there was any problem. Finally at midnight, the evening nurse signed out to the night shift nurse, mentioning the patient's symptoms and noting that the night float intern had not yet called about the x-ray results.

The next morning, the radiologist read the x-ray performed at 6:00 PM the previous evening and notified the NP that it showed a large left pneumothorax. A chest tube was placed at 2:30 PM—nearly a full day after the x-ray was performed. Luckily, the patient suffered no long-lasting harm from the delay, but could have deteriorated rapidly.[1]

SOME BASIC CONCEPTS AND TERMS

In a perfect world, patients would stay in one place and be cared for by a single set of doctors and nurses. But, come to think of it, who would want such a world? Patients get sick, and then get better. Doctors and nurses work shifts, and then go home. Residents graduate from their programs and enter practice. So handoffs—the process of transferring primary authority and responsibility for clinical care from a departing caregiver to an incoming one[2]—and transitions are facts of medical life.

As we all learned when we played the game of "telephone" as kids, every handoff and transition comes with the potential for a "voltage drop" in information. (While it's possible that a fresh set of eyes or circumstances might offer a new perspective that will benefit the patient, our purpose here is not to explore that optimistic scenario.) In fact, handoff and transitional errors are among the most common and consequential errors in healthcare. The 2003 limitation in residency duty hours, and the further tightening of these restrictions in 2011, markedly increased the number of handoffs in the inpatient setting in teaching hospitals in the United States. Perhaps as a result, the last several years have seen a growing body of literature focused on ways to mitigate the harm that has historically accompanied handoffs and care transitions.

Healthcare is chock-full of two kinds of transitions and handoffs.[3] The first are *patient-related*, as a patient moves from place to place within the healthcare system, either within the same building or from one location to another (Table 8-1). The second are *provider-related*, which occur even when patients are stationary (Table 8-2).

Both kinds of handoffs are fraught with hazards. For example, one study found that 12% of patients experienced preventable adverse events after hospital discharge, most commonly medication errors (Chapter 4).[4] Part of the problem is that nearly half of all discharged patients have test results that

Table 8-1	**EXAMPLES OF PATIENT-RELATED TRANSITIONS**

❑ Patient referred from primary care provider to subspecialty consultant
❑ Patient is admitted from the emergency department to the ICU
❑ Patient leaves the ICU to obtain a computed tomography (CT) scan
❑ Patient is discharged from the hospital to go to a skilled nursing facility

Table 8-2	**EXAMPLES OF PROVIDER-RELATED TRANSITIONS (WHEN PATIENT IS STATIONARY)**

❑ Daytime resident signs out to night float resident and leaves the hospital
❑ Oncologist's partner covers the hospitalized patients over a weekend
❑ Night shift nurse leaves and the morning nurse takes over
❑ Recovery room nurse goes on break and another nurse covers the patients

are pending at discharge, and many of them (more than half in one study) fall through the cracks.[5] In another study, researchers surveyed medical and surgical residents, most of whom cited inadequate signouts and non-standard signout practices as causing patient harm, especially when these handoffs took place over the phone or with frequent interruptions.[6] One multicenter study demonstrated that the implementation of a standardized handoff bundle across nine residency programs resulted in a 23% decrease in medical errors and a 30% decrease in preventable adverse events.[7] Further supporting the importance of standardization, a prospective cohort study found that the use of a web-based handover tool led to a statistically significant decrease in medical errors, especially those caused by failures in communication and inadequate handoffs.[8,9]

Even if we grant that some transitions are necessary, one might reasonably ask whether healthcare needs to have quite so many of them. The answer is probably yes. Research has demonstrated that patients appeared to suffer more harm when their nurses work shifts longer than 10 hours, as compared to when nurses work 8 to 9 hour shifts.[10] The issue may be more complicated than shift length alone. Although one classic study showed that intensive care unit (ICU) residents make fewer errors when they work shifts averaging 16 hours instead of the traditional 30 to 36 hours (Chapter 16),[11] a more recent study of surgical residents showed improved satisfaction with continuity of patient care and handoffs in the group that did not have to adhere to strict limitations on shift length and time off between shifts (although both groups in the study were limited to the same number of total hours per workweek).[12] Unfortunately, in a 24/7 hospital, shift limits, and their associated handoffs,

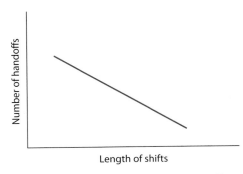

Figure 8-1 ▪ The trade-off between shift length and handoffs.

are a necessity (Figure 8-1), such as many of the ones in the case described at the beginning of this chapter (Figure 8-2).

Although some might wistfully long for the day when the family doctor cared for patients in the office, the emergency room, the hospital, and possibly the operating and delivery room as well, most patients now expect care to be provided by a variety of physicians, such as emergency room providers, surgeons, and hospitalists, depending on the site of care.[13] As these specialists become involved in a patient's care, they create transitions and the need for accurate information transfer. So too does a patient's clinical need to escalate the level of care (such as transitioning from hospital floor to step-down unit) or the economic realities that often drive de-escalation (hospital to skilled nursing facility).

The presence of all these handoffs and transitions makes it critical to consider how information is passed between providers and places. Catalyzed in part by the mandated reduction in resident work hours in the United States that began in 2003 (with further restrictions in 2011, accompanied that year by a mandate that residency programs establish formal curricula around handoffs [Chapter 16]), there has been far more attention paid to handoffs in recent years.

There is increased pressure coming from the policy arena as well. In 2006, the Joint Commission issued National Patient Safety Goal 2E (Appendix IV), which required healthcare organizations to "implement a standardized approach to handoff communications including an opportunity to ask and respond to questions." Spurred on by studies demonstrating staggeringly high 30-day readmission rates in Medicare patients (20% overall, nearly 30% in patients with heart failure),[14] Medicare began financially penalizing hospitals with high readmission rates in 2012.[15] All of this attention has prompted research and improvement efforts focused on handoffs and transitions, giving us a deeper understanding of best practices, which have both structural and interpersonal components.

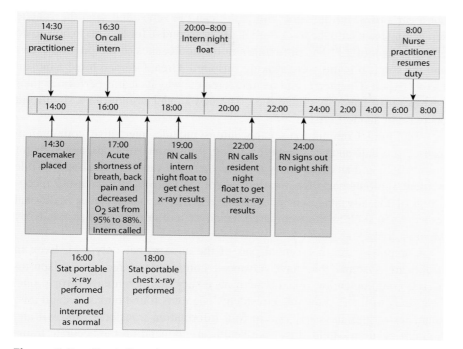

Figure 8-2 ■ Handoffs in the case that begins this chapter. (Reprinted with permission from AHRQ Patient Safety Network: Vidyarthi A. Triple handoff [Spotlight]. *AHRQ WebM&M* [serial online]; September 2006. Available at: https://psnet.ahrq.gov/webmm/case/134.)

This chapter will provide a general overview of best practices for person-to-person handoffs and patient transitions, and then focus on one particularly risky transition: hospital discharge. Additional information about handoffs and transitions can be found in the discussion of medication reconciliation (Chapter 4), information technology tools (Chapter 13), and resident duty hours (Chapter 16).

BEST PRACTICES FOR PERSON-TO-PERSON HANDOFFS

Like many other areas of patient safety, the search for best practices in handoffs has led us to examine how other industries and organizations move information around. This search has revealed several elements of effective handoffs: an information system, a predictable and standardized structure, and robust interpersonal communication. In one particularly memorable example, physicians at London's Great Ormond Street Children's Hospital studied Formula 1 motor racing, particularly the pit-stop crews (who switch out a car's tires, fill the tank with gas, clean the vents, and send the vehicle screeching back onto the track—all in seven seconds), for lessons in how to do effective handoffs.[16] The differences in the approaches of the pit-stop crews and the surgical teams were striking. Inspired, Great Ormond hired a human factors expert (Chapter 7) and reengineered the way its teams performed their postoperative handoffs (Table 8-3). The new model resulted in a significant decrease in handoff errors.[17,18]

The Joint Commission's expectations include interactive communications, up-to-date and accurate information, limited interruptions, a process for verification, and an opportunity to review any relevant historical data. While written sign-outs can take a variety of forms, there is an increasing recognition of the advantages of *computerized sign-out systems* over traditional index cards, such as the web-based handover tool described in the study by Mueller et al.[8]

Computers are an essential part of the answer, but only part. Even in healthcare systems that have advanced computerized records, person-to-person communication remains both necessary and potentially error prone. One study of internal medicine residents' signouts found omissions and mischaracterizations in nearly one in four information transfers.[19] In civil and military aviation—fields that, like healthcare, depend on the accurate transmission of information—the so-called *phonetic alphabet* is often used during voice communications. In this system, a standardized word substitutes for a single letter (such as *Alpha* for "A," *Bravo* for "B," *Charlie* for "C," and so on), which permits one person to clarify a bit of information, such as the spelling of a name, without wasting time thinking of words that might have a common reference. Using this same system in a hospital, "Oscar Romeo" for operating room (OR) would never be confused with "Echo Romeo" for emergency room (ER).

Read backs are also commonly used in aviation and other industries to prevent improperly received messages. For example, a pilot receiving flight plan clearance over the radio from Air Traffic Control always reads it back. In healthcare, we have long used read-back procedures to verify the identity of blood transfusion recipients, but, remarkably, no tradition of read backs for other transfers of risky information existed until the process was mandated by the Joint Commission in 2004 (Appendix IV). It is one measure of our inattention to patient safety that until recently a physician would have been far more likely to hear the words, "Let me read your order back to you," when calling her local Chinese takeout restaurant than when she called the nurses' station of virtually any American hospital.[20] In one study, read back improved the transfer of critical clinical information during simulated emergencies.[21]

Safety Theme	Practice	Establishment of Handover Protocol
Table 8-3 LESSONS LEARNED FROM FORMULA 1 MOTOR RACING AND AVIATION INDUSTRIES FOR IMPROVING PATIENT HANDOVER FROM SURGERY TO INTENSIVE CARE		
Leadership	**Formula 1**: the "lollipop" man coordinates the pit stop. **Aviation**: the captain has command and responsibility	**Old**: unclear who was in charge. **New**: anesthetist given overall responsibility for coordinating team, transferred to the intensivist at the end of the handover
Task sequence	**Formula 1 and aviation**: there is a clear rhythm and order to events	**Old**: inconsistent and nonsequential. **New**: three phases defined: (1) equipment and technology handover; (2) information handover; (3) discussion and plan
Task allocation	**Formula 1**: each team member has only one to two clearly defined tasks. **Aviation**: explicit acknowledged allocation of tasks for emergencies	**Old**: informal and erratic. **New**: people allocated tasks: ventilation—anesthetist; monitoring—operating room assistant; drains—nurses. The anesthetist identified and handed information over to the key receiving people
Predicting and planning	**Formula 1**: failure modes and effects analysis (FMEA) used to break down pit stops into individual tasks and risks. **Aviation**: pilots are trained to anticipate the expected, and to plan contingencies	**Old**: risks identified informally and often not acted upon. **New**: a modified FMEA was conducted and senior representatives commented on highest areas of risk. Safety checks were introduced, and the need for a ventilation transfer sheet was identified
Discipline and composure	**Formula 1**: very little verbal communication during a pit stop. **Aviation**: explicit communication strategies used to ensure a calm and organized atmosphere	**Old**: ad hoc and unstructured, with several simultaneous discussions in different areas of the ICU and theaters. **New**: communication limited to the essential during equipment handover. During information handover, the anesthetist and then the surgeon speak alone and uninterrupted, followed by discussion and agreement of the recovery plan
Checklists	**Formula 1 and aviation**: a well-established culture of using checklists	**Old**: none. **New**: a checklist was defined and used as the admission note by the receiving team
Involvement	**Aviation**: crew members of all levels are encouraged and trained to speak up	**Old**: communications primarily within levels (e.g., consultant to consultant or junior to junior). **New**: all team members and grades encouraged to speak up. Built into discussions in phase 3

(continued)

Safety Theme	Practice	Establishment of Handover Protocol
	Table 8-3 LESSONS LEARNED FROM FORMULA 1 MOTOR RACING AND AVIATION INDUSTRIES FOR IMPROVING PATIENT HANDOVER FROM SURGERY TO INTENSIVE CARE (*continued*)	
Briefing	**Formula 1 and aviation**: well-established cultures of briefing even on race day, and before every flight	**Old and new** (process already in place): planning begins in a regular multidisciplinary meeting, reconfirmed the week before surgery, with further problems highlighted on the day
Situation awareness	**Formula 1**: the "lollipop man" has overall situation awareness at pit stops. **Aviation**: pilots are trained for situation awareness. In difficult circumstances the senior pilot manages the wider aspects of the flight while the other pilot controls the aircraft	**Old**: not previously identified as being important. **New**: the consultant anesthetist and intensivist have responsibility for situation awareness at handover, and regularly stand back to make safety checks
Training	**Formula 1**: a fanatical approach to training and repetition of the pit stop. **Aviation**: training and assessment are regularly conducted in high-fidelity simulators	**Old**: no training existed. **New**: a high turnover of staff requires an alternative approach. The protocol could be learned in 30 minutes. Formal training introduced; laminated training sheets detailing the process are provided at each bedside
Review meetings	**Formula 1**: regular team meetings to review events. **Aviation**: crew are encouraged to debrief after every flight	**Old and new** (already in place): a weekly well-attended clinical governance meeting, where problems/solutions openly discussed

Adapted with permission from Catchpole KR, de Leval MR, McEwan A, et al. Patient handover from surgery to intensive care: using Formula 1 pit-stop and aviation models to improve safety and quality. *Paediatr Anaesth* 2007;17:470–478.

The bottom line is that having a standardized process for provider-to-provider signout is essential.[22,23] Signouts should take place in a standard place and at a standard time, and the incoming and outgoing personnel must overlap to the degree needed to transmit the relevant information. Ensuring that signouts occur in a quiet room, free of distractions, is critical, as is ensuring that both parties have access to the hospital's information system during the process. Increasingly, the I-PASS mnemonic (**I**llness Severity, **P**atient Summary, **A**ction List, **S**ituation Awareness and Contingency Planning, **S**ynthesis by Receiver) is being implemented, particularly in teaching hospitals, to standardize signout (Table 8-4).[24] Several studies have

Table 8-4	THE MNEMONIC "I-PASS," HIGHLIGHTING THE ELEMENTS OF A SAFE AND EFFECTIVE HANDOFF
Illness severity of patient	Stable, "watcher," unstable
Patient summary	Summary statement Events leading up to admission Hospital course Ongoing assessment Plan
Action list	To do list Time line and ownership
Situation awareness and contingency planning	Know what's going on Plan for what might happen
Synthesis by receiver	Receiver summarized what was heard Asks questions Restates key action/to do items

Reproduced with permission from Starmer AJ, Spector ND, Srivastava R, et al. I-PASS, a mnemonic to standardize verbal handoffs. *Pediatrics* 2012;129:201–204.

shown that implementation of I-PASS improves safety.[25,26] (On the UCSF medical service, we insist that shift change handoffs occur face-to-face, while end of rotation handoffs, such as when one hospitalist is signing out to another after a 1- to 2-week stint, may take place by telephone, with both parties simultaneously reviewing the electronic health record, sometimes via remote access.)

Beyond these "must do's," there are many variations on the theme. One study showed that the use of *daily event reports*—key overnight incidents automatically emailed to the daytime team by the nighttime coverage—reduced the duration of signout and improved the quality of handoffs.[27] In a pediatric ICU, the use of a daily *goal sheet*—a simple device to ensure that physicians, nurses, and patients focused on the same limited set of goals—and standardized bedside rounds led to improved communication, shorter ICU lengths of stay, decreased healthcare-associated infections, and mortality.[28] A dry erase *whiteboard* in patients' rooms can promote communication and teamwork among all of the involved providers.[29] While all of these interventions seem intuitively sensible and relatively straightforward to implement, by now it will not surprise you to learn that they are actually complex changes that should be viewed through a human factors lens (Chapter 7) to be sure they meet their purpose and don't create unintended consequences.[17]

SITE-TO-SITE HANDOFFS: THE ROLE OF THE SYSTEM

Joe Benjamin, a 43-year-old mechanic, came to his local ER with chest pain, and was admitted to the hospital to "rule out MI." Benjamin's ER physician ordered a chest x-ray in addition to the cardiac enzymes and serial electrocardiograms. Since nobody expected Benjamin's x-ray to show anything exciting, and since there was no checklist or protocol to remind anyone to check it, it was forgotten as soon as it was taken. Twelve hours later, after all of the heart attack tests proved negative, Benjamin was discharged. The discharging hospitalist, unaware of the chest x-ray, didn't think to follow-up the results. Meanwhile, the radiologist had reviewed the x-ray and noticed a small lung nodule. He filed a report in the patient's record. Although a final discharge summary from the emergency visit was faxed to the patient's primary care physician's office, it was lost and never read.

Two years later, Joe Benjamin developed a chronic cough and a repeat chest x-ray revealed an obvious lung nodule. The radiologist's report read, "The nodule is markedly enlarged compared to prior imaging." That was the first Benjamin's primary physician had heard of the prior x-ray, and it was too late. Eighteen months later, Joe Benjamin was dead of lung cancer.[20]

In its 2001 report, *Crossing the Quality Chasm: A New Health System for the 21st Century*, the Institute of Medicine (now the National Academy of Medicine, NAM) compared the U.S. healthcare delivery system to a railroad whose tracks change gauge every few miles:

Healthcare is composed of a large set of interacting systems— paramedic, emergency, ambulatory, inpatient, and home healthcare; testing and imaging laboratories; pharmacies; and so forth—that are connected in loosely coupled but intricate networks of individuals, teams, procedures, regulations, communications, equipment, and devices. These systems function within such diverse and diffuse management, accountability, and information structures that the overall term health system is today a misnomer.[30]

Historically, the major potential failure point in all of these interlocking systems was the piece of paper, the basic unit of medical record keeping for centuries. Moving paper across healthcare transitions is inherently risky, as it can easily get lost. Unfortunately, although the vast majority of U.S. hospitals and a substantial fraction of outpatient providers are using electronic record systems, discharge summaries and other records are often still printed and faxed to providers practicing in other systems! Moreover, several people, separated by place and function, often need to see patient data simultaneously, and each may create new data and observations that must be added to the record. Neither paper nor disconnected electronic systems provide the ideal medium for seamless care transitions and information transfer.

Many of the handoff techniques discussed earlier can help here as well, including the use of read backs, standard communication protocols, and checklists (such as for hospital discharge) for patients/families (Table 8-5) and providers (Table 8-6). But part of the problem relates to the absence of integration in most of American medicine. Take, for example, hospital discharge—an inherently risky transition. In the United States, the hospital discharging the patient and the physician receiving the patient are usually not part of the same organization (in most cases, the physician is an independent practitioner). Therefore, the physician's office information system, even if it is computerized, will rarely communicate effectively with the hospital's system, and vice versa. This is a set up for a voltage drop at a most critical time.

Integrated systems of care—in which the same organization owns or runs the doctor's office, the nursing home, and the hospital—have great advantages in this regard. Patients who leave a U.S. Veterans Affairs (VA) hospital for a nursing home generally go to a VA-owned facility; the same is true for patients in the huge Kaiser Permanente system and other large integrated delivery systems. The reason these handoffs generally go better is partly organizational,

Table 8-5   **A PATIENT/FAMILY DISCHARGE CHECKLIST**
You are about to be discharged from the hospital. Please be sure you and/or your family members know the answer to these questions BEFORE you leave:
Do you understand why you were hospitalized, what your diagnosis is, and what treatments you received?
Are there any test results you are still waiting for? Who should you contact for those results?
Has a provider reviewed your medications with you? Do you know which of your home medications to continue, what the current doses are, and which you should stop taking?
Where and when are your follow-up appointments?
What are the warning signs of relapse or medication side effects you should look for?
Who should you contact if you are having difficulties?
Does your primary care physician know you were here and that you are leaving?

Reprinted with permission from AHRQ Patient Safety Network: Forster A. Discharge fumbles [Spotlight]. *AHRQ WebM&M* [serial online]; December 2004. Available at: https://psnet.ahrq.gov/webmm/case/84.

Table 8-6　　**A CLINICIAN DISCHARGE CHECKLIST**

Discharge medications
Review with the patient
Highlight changes from hospital
Specifically inform patient about side effects

Discharge summaries
Dictate in a timely fashion
Include discharge medications (highlight changes from admission)
List outstanding tests and reports that need follow-up
Give copies to all providers involved in the patient's care

Communication with patient/family
Provide patient with medication instructions, follow-up details, and clear instructions
　on warning signs and what to do if things are not going well
Confirm that patient comprehends your instructions
Include a family member in these discussions if possible

Communication with the primary physician
Make telephone contact with primary care physician prior to discharge

Follow-up plans
Discharge clinic
Follow-up phone calls
Appointments or access to primary providers

Reprinted with permission from AHRQ Patient Safety Network: Forster A. Discharge fumbles
　[Spotlight]. *AHRQ WebM&M* [serial online]; December 2004. Available at: https://psnet.ahrq.gov/
　webmm/case/84.

partly psychological, and partly informational. Organizationally, when a single system is responsible for care on both sides of a specialty or facility gap, they collaborate on smoothing the transition and bear the consequence of any problems. Psychologically, human beings simply communicate better with colleagues than with strangers. Finally, from an informatics standpoint, large integrated systems tend to devote more resources to constructing, maintaining, and improving the computerized linkages so critical to optimal communication.

In the United States, there is considerable policy pressure designed to prod healthcare delivery systems and physicians to higher levels of integration. Payment changes such as bundling[31] (a single payment for an episode of care lasting weeks or months) and the promotion of Accountable Care Organizations[32,33] (a delivery system that includes the physicians and facilities [i.e., hospitals, clinics, skilled nursing facilities], is at risk for its cost and quality outcomes, and can receive a bonus for high-value care) are, at their core, efforts to promote integration (Chapter 3). Whether they will succeed remains to be seen, but they are promising initiatives, and current plans call for them to grow over time.

Recognizing that most of the American healthcare system remains fragmented, much of the federal effort to computerize U.S. healthcare—backed up by nearly $30 billion in incentive payments—has been focused on creating a set of standards and protocols to promote *interoperability*, even when the computers are manufactured by different vendors and owned by different organizations (Chapter 13).[34] The best analogy is banking's automated teller machine (ATM) system, in which interoperability allows customers to make transactions away from their own bank, almost anywhere in the world.

Recently, concerns have been raised about patient privacy and the unauthorized use of medical information, and these concerns have taken on additional force with the prospect of large, interoperable computer systems containing terabytes of sensitive patient data. These concerns, partly addressed in the United States by the *Health Insurance Portability and Accountability Act* (HIPAA), pose a real barrier to developing a national medical database, or even to moving patient information from clinic to hospital and back out again. While abuses are possible (and there have been several high-profile examples of them), policymakers will have to weigh the desirability of strict control over patient data (which sometimes means that important information is not shared reliably and that tests are repeated unnecessarily) against the value of linking healthcare systems in an increasingly mobile society.[35] Both individuals and organizations have experimented with having patients carry their own data (in the form of "smart cards" or even implantable chips) as a way of addressing these privacy concerns.[36] Because these systems seem a bit too unreliable and inflexible (one big challenge is that they will need to be updated after every clinical encounter), the more realistic hope will be for a single set of national, or even international, standards that would combine seamless interoperability with robust safeguards that ensure reasonable degrees of privacy.

BEST PRACTICES FOR SITE-TO-SITE HANDOFFS OTHER THAN HOSPITAL DISCHARGE

Before turning to the issues surrounding hospital discharge, it is worth reemphasizing that every transition carries the potential for harm, and all are worth scrutinizing for risk reduction opportunities. For example, transfers within the hospital itself—from the emergency department to the floor, the floor to the ICU, and the OR to the recovery room—are prone to error, as are interhospital transfers.[37] A systematic review of intrahospital transitions identified a number of key themes and evidence-based improvement strategies (Table 8-7).[38]

One particularly risky transition occurs when a patient leaves his or her hospital floor for a radiologic study or procedure. Unlike the patient transferring to the ICU or another service, where there are established nursing intake protocols and formalized physician handoffs, many of these intrahospital transports are done haphazardly, with an abrupt decrease in the level of

Table 8-7	KEY ISSUES IDENTIFIED BY A SYSTEMATIC REVIEW ON INTRAHOSPITAL TRANSFERS, ALONG WITH RECOMMENDED IMPROVEMENT STRATEGIES	
Setting	**Key Themes and Challenges**	**Improvement Strategies**
Transportation of critically ill patients	Failure to communicate arrival time and resources required results in delayed or inadequate care	Formalize pretransport coordination process
Discharge of patients from critical care to specialty ward	Ward nurses may lack expertise or confidence in handling critical care patients from the ICU Time constraints impede handoff communication during the discharge planning process Pretransfer communication is critical to ensure resource availability at the receiving ward	Introduce an ICU liaison nurse role to facilitate transfer, providing both coordination and clinical support Formalize handoff to allow for uninterrupted time to conduct handoff Early discharge planning
Transfer of surgical patients	Handoffs are informal and unstructured, leading to inadequate information transfer Surgical handoff is particularly poor Work pattern at recovery room is unpredictable; thus, timing of handoff is variable, and handoff takes place amidst other activities	Standardize handoff content and structure Involve all members of multidisciplinary team in handoff Formalize handoff to allow for uninterrupted time to conduct handoff
Transfers from ED	Content omission was common, in particular communication of the most recent set of vital signs Differing approaches to patient care between emergency department (ED) physicians and inpatient teams result in incomplete handoff and inter professional misunderstandings High workload, time constraint, and overcrowding at ED impede handoff communication Difficulty in assessing information and communicating with providers across units on different shifts	Standardize handoff content and structure Align physicians' view for referrals handoff communication across medical specialties through education and hospital-wide guidelines Increase staffing level Implement centralized information repository to ease access to patient information

Reproduced with permission from Ong MS, Coiera E. A systematic review of failures in handoff communication during intrahospital transfers. *Jt Comm J Qual Patient Saf* 2011;37:274–284.

nursing care and monitoring capability (e.g., telemetry), and substantial ambiguity regarding what actions to take in the event of deterioration.[39] One hospital uses a "Ticket to Ride" system, where the ticket—which includes patient identification, stability, and risk information—serves as the communication vehicle for the sending and receiving personnel. The transport personnel are responsible for ensuring the nurse completes the ticket, which stays with the patient until return to the home unit. Analysis of over 12,000 transports demonstrated improved transport documentation, higher patient satisfaction with transport, and fewer adverse events.[40] A well-designed checklist might serve the same function.

While the risks of intrahospital transfers are obvious, it is worth emphasizing that there are also major transition and handoff issues that occur in community practice. One study explored care coordination between hospitalists and primary care providers around hospitalizations and found that at times primary care providers did not even know that their patients were hospitalized and often could not find important information in discharge summaries.[41] This problem is magnified by the sheer volume of information that an outpatient provider needs to manage, and digitization has not completely solved this problem. In fact, there is evidence that computerization may even be contributing to information overload. One study of three large outpatient practices in Texas found that primary care providers received a mean of 76.9 electronic notifications per day (compared to 29.1 notifications per day for specialists). The authors estimated that it would take the physicians almost a minute to address each notification—likely on their own time.[42] In another study, only two-thirds of primary care physicians reported receiving consultation reports after referring patients to specialists, while over 80% of specialists reported that they sent such reports "always" or "most of the time." In addition, providers who did not receive timely clinical information were more likely to report that their ability to provide high-quality care was compromised.[43]

While the solutions here would seem to rest with better information technology, this is proving harder than it looks. In one study, the VA system created an electronic alert for abnormal imaging results—alerts went to both the receiving physician and the radiologist. Despite what appeared to be a foolproof system, flawed follow-up remained distressingly common.[44] Similarly, computerized order entry has been held out as the savior for many errors in transitions and medication reconciliation. Researchers examined 4000 computer-generated prescriptions and found a 12% error rate.[45] Clearly, our efforts to solve transitional problems with information technology will need to be accompanied by equal efforts to apply human factors thinking, be alert for unanticipated consequences, and remain attuned to the challenges of trying to change care patterns in complex systems (Chapters 2 and 7).

The issues surrounding one distinctive and risky handoff—the end-of-year transition that occurs when residents graduate and turn their practices over to new interns[46]—will be discussed in Chapter 16.

PREVENTING READMISSIONS: BEST PRACTICES FOR HOSPITAL DISCHARGE

As we've discussed, there is a body of evidence that the hospital discharge transition is one we manage exceptionally poorly. This was highlighted in the seminal study by Jencks et al., which found that 20% of Medicare patients are readmitted within a month of discharge and one-third return within 90 days.[14] The authors estimated the cost of preventable readmissions at $17 billion. A subsequent observational study combined physician surveys and chart review and found that about one quarter of all readmissions are preventable.[47]

Other studies have chronicled a litany of additional postdischarge disasters:

- Nearly 20% of patients experience adverse events within three weeks of discharge.[4]
- Forty percent of patients are discharged with tests pending, and many of these balls are dropped.[5]
- Fifteen percent of discharged patients have a discrepancy in their medication lists.[48]
- Astonishingly few discharge summaries reach the primary care physician by the time the patient returns for his or her first postdischarge visit.[49]

Despite powerful literature that shows that relatively simple interventions—such as *postdischarge phone calls* or the use of a *transitions coach*—can lead to striking improvements in postdischarge care and decreased readmission rates,[50,51] relatively few hospitals have implemented them. In addition, few hospitals that are not part of integrated delivery systems have become electronically linked to their referring physicians' offices.

Policy changes that have promoted value-based purchasing (Table 3-5) and financial penalties for excess readmissions[15] have turned improving the discharge transition into an imperative for hospitals, primary care doctors, and their respective systems. Luckily, a number of best practices have been identified, with proven beneficial effects on readmission rates and other meaningful outcomes.

In considering these best practices, several themes have emerged. First, hospitals will need to improve their discharge processes so that they can reliably: (a) get a meaningful discharge summary in the hands of the outpatient clinician on the day of discharge; (b) ensure that patients receive robust and understandable discharge instructions (not simply a check box on a form) (Figure 8-3 shows a discharge checklist, drawn from the Society of Hospital Medicine's Project BOOST[52]); and (c) keep in touch with patients via a follow-up phone call (or e-mail or video call or Tweet—whatever gets the job done!). Second, high-risk patients will require something more: a postdischarge clinic visit, perhaps, or a discharge or transitions coach or a high-risk case manager. This isn't rocket science—all these interventions make sense, have manageable costs, and are challenging but not impossible to implement. They simply take institutional will, strong teamwork, thoughtful integration of technology, and an appreciation of the principles of quality improvement and change management.

Of all of the discharge transition programs, perhaps the most creative has been *Project RED* ("Re-Engineered Discharge"), developed by a team at

Universal patient discharge checklist	Initials
1. GAP assessment (see below) completed with issues addressed................................YES ☐ NO ☐	_____
2. Medications reconciled with pre-admission list...YES ☐ NO ☐	_____
3. Medication use/side effects reviewed using Teach-Back with patient/caregiver(s)......................YES ☐ NO ☐	_____
4. Teach-Back used to confirm patient/caregiver understanding of disease, prognosis and self-care requirements..YES ☐ NO ☐	_____
5. Action plan for management of symptoms/side effects/complications requiring medical attention established and shared with patient/caregiver using Teach-Back..................YES ☐ NO ☐	_____
6. Discharge plan (including educational materials; medication list with reason for use and highlighted new/changed/discontinued drugs, follow-up plans) taught and provided to patient/caregiver at discharge..YES ☐ NO ☐	_____
7. Discharge communication provided to principal care provider(s)..................................YES ☐ NO ☐	_____
8. Documented receipt of discharge information from principal care provider(s)...............................YES ☐ NO ☐	_____
9. Arrangements made for outpatient follow-up with principal care provider(s)...................................YES ☐ NO ☐	_____
For increased risk patients, consider..Not applicable ☐	_____
1. Face-to-face multidisciplinary rounds pnor to discharge....................................YES ☐ NO ☐	_____
2. Direct communication with principal care provider *before* discharge..........................YES ☐ NO ☐	_____
3. Phone contact with patient/caregiver arranged within 72 hours postdischarge to assess condition, discharge plan comprehension and adherence, and to reinforce follow-up..................YES ☐ NO ☐	_____
4. Follow-up appointment with principal care provider within 7 days of discharge.........................YES ☐ NO ☐	_____
5. Direct contact information for hospital personnel familiar with patient's course provided to patient/caregiver to address questions/concerns *if unable to reach principal care provider* prior to first follow-up..................YES ☐ NO ☐	_____

Confirmed by: _____   _____   __/__/____
                          Signature   Print name   Date

Figure 8-3 ▪ An example of a discharge checklist, from Project BOOST®. (Copyright © Mark Williams et al. Project Boost Mentoring Program, Society of Hospital Medicine, 2010. Reproduced with permission.)

** Bring this Plan to ALL Appointments**

BOSTON MEDICAL CENTER

PROJECT RED

After Hospital Care Plan for:

John Doe

Discharge Date: October 20, 2006

Question or Problem about this Packet? Call your Discharge Advocate: (617) 444-1111

Serious health problem? Call Dr. Brian Jack: (617) 444-2222

PROJECT RED

EACH DAY follow this schedule:

MEDICINES

What time of day do I take this medicine?	Why am I taking this medicine?	Medication name Amount	How much do I take?	How do I take this medicine?
Morning	Blood pressure	PROCARDIA XL NIFEDIPINE 90 mg	1 pill	By mouth
	Blood pressure	HYDROCHLOROTHIAZIDE 25 mg	1 pill	By mouth
	Blood pressure	CLONIDINE HCl 0.1 mg	3 pills	By mouth
	cholesterol	LIPITOR ATORVASTATIN CALCIUM 20 mg	1 pill	By mouth
	stomach	PROTONIX PANTOPRAZOLE SODIUM 40 mg	1 pill	By mouth

Figure 8-4 ■ An example of a customized patient discharge care plan, from Project RED. (Courtesy of Boston University, Department of Family Medicine. Reproduced with permission.)

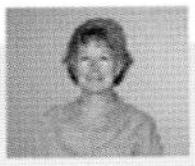

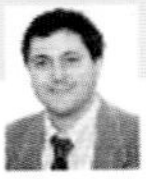

Boston University and supported by the U.S. Agency for Healthcare Research and Quality (AHRQ).[47] The RED protocol involves giving patients intensive predischarge counseling, a customized discharge document (Figure 8-4), an early postdischarge phone call, and a rapid follow-up appointment. The intervention resulted in a 30% decrease in readmissions and modest cost savings.

One of the most expensive parts of the intervention was the discharge counseling: an RN spent nearly 90 minutes with each patient and family, at significant cost. To address this issue, the BU investigators developed an animated conversational character, nicknamed "Louise." Louise is preprogrammed with individual patient information, which she combines with answers to disease-specific and general questions. She—a pleasant-looking middle-aged woman of purposely ambiguous race and ethnicity—appears on a computer screen wheeled to the patient's bedside (Figure 8-5). Speaking to the patient in a relatively fluent but unmistakable computer voice (with synchronized animation), she might say: *The doctors tell me that your primary condition is atrial fibrillation … it usually causes a rapid heartbeat. Do you have any questions about this condition?* Patients answer Louise's questions

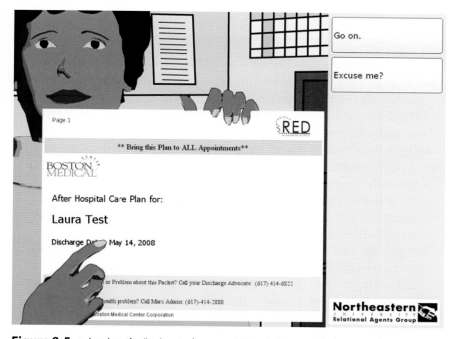

Figure 8-5 ■ Louise, the "animated conversational character" who provides discharge instructions to patients. From Project RED. (Courtesy of Boston University, Department of Family Medicine. Reproduced with permission.)

by picking choices off a touch-screen interface. She then responds according to her algorithm.

In a pilot study, Louise's performance was equivalent to that of the human discharge coach, while saving nearly $150 per encounter.[53] More interestingly, not only did most patients find Louise to be personable and responsive, but also three out of four preferred interacting with "her" to receiving discharge instructions from a live physician or nurse.

Let's be clear. While Louise can calmly walk a patient down an algorithmic path, answer simple questions, and test basic understanding, dealing with complex situations, managing ambiguity, and showing empathy are not her forte. Nevertheless, Louise's success indicates that certain job functions that we currently allocate to nurses or physicians can probably be accomplished by thoughtful use of other staff or technologies, at a lower cost. And, with rapid improvements in artificial intelligence technologies, Louise's successors are likely to be even more human-like. Ultimately, creatively combining technologies with human skills and empathy will be needed if we are to meet the challenges of providing high-quality, safe, reliable, and satisfying care at an affordable cost.

KEY POINTS

- Errors at the time of transitions (also known as handoff errors) are among the most common errors in healthcare.
- Handoffs can be site-to-site (e.g., hospital to skilled nursing faculty) or person-to-person (e.g., one physician signing out to another).
- Optimizing both types of handoffs requires improved information systems and standardized protocols.
- Handoffs should occur at designated times and without distraction, cover likely scenarios, include "if/then" statements, and utilize read backs and a phonetic alphabet. Implementation of the I-PASS mnemonic is increasingly widespread.
- It will be vital to have computer systems that "talk to each other" ("interoperability"); creating these systems will require that we address legitimate concerns about patient privacy.
- Increasing pressure to improve transitions is coming from a variety of policies (public reporting and financial penalties for high rates of readmissions). Luckily, several comprehensive programs have resulted in markedly decreased readmission rates, and practices have been identified that appear to improve other transitions and handoffs as well.

REFERENCES

1. Vidyarthi AR. Triple handoff [Spotlight] *AHRQ WebM&M* [serial online]; September 2006. Available at: https://psnet.ahrq.gov/webmm/case/134.

2. Patterson ES, Wears RL. Patient handoffs: standardized and reliable measurement tools remain elusive. *Jt Comm J Qual Patient Saf* 2010;36:52–61.

3. Cook RI, Render M, Woods DD. Gaps in the continuity of care and progress on patient safety. *BMJ* 2000;320:791–794.

4. Forster AJ, Murff HJ, Peterson JF, Gandhi TK, Bates DW. The incidence and severity of adverse events affecting patients after discharge from the hospital. *Ann Intern Med* 2003;138:161–167.

5. Roy CL, Poon EG, Karson AS, et al. Patient safety concerns arising from test results that return after hospital discharge. *Ann Intern Med* 2005;143:121–128.

6. Kitch BT, Cooper JB, Zapol WM, et al. Handoffs causing patient harm: a survey of medical and surgical house staff. *Jt Comm J Qual Patient Saf* 2008;34;563–570.

7. Starmer AJ, Spector ND, Srivastava R, et al. Changes in medical errors after implementation of a handoff program. *N Engl J Med* 2014;371:1803–1812.

8. Mueller SK, Yoon C, Schnipper JL. Association of a web-based handoff tool with rates of medical errors. *JAMA Intern Med* 2016;176:1400–1402.

9. Schoenfeld AJ, Wachter RM. The search for better patient handoff tools. *JAMA Intern Med* 2016;176:1402–1403.

10. Stimpfel AW, Aiken LH. Hospital staff nurses' shift length associated with safety and quality of care. *J Nurs Care Qual* 2013;28:122–129.

11. Landrigan CP, Rothschild JM, Cronin JW, et al. Effect of reducing interns' work hours on serious medical errors in intensive care units. *N Engl J Med* 2004;351:1838–1848.

12. Bilimoria KY, Chung JW, Hedges LV, et al. National cluster-randomized trial of duty-hour flexibility in surgical training. *N Engl J Med* 2016;374:713–727.

13. Wachter RM, Goldman L. The emerging role of "hospitalists" in American health care. *N Engl J Med* 2006;335:514–517.

14. Jencks SF, Williams MV, Coleman EA. Rehospitalizations among patients in the Medicare fee-for-service program. *N Engl J Med* 2009;360:1418–1428.

15. Epstein AM. Revisiting readmissions—changing the incentives for shared accountability. *N Engl J Med* 2009;360:1457–1459.

16. Naik G. A hospital races to learn lessons of Ferrari pit stop. *Wall Street Journal.* November 14, 2006:A1.

17. Catchpole KR, de Leval MR, McEwan A, et al. Patient handover from surgery to intensive care: using Formula 1 pit-stop and aviation models to improve safety and quality. *Paediatr Anaesth* 2007;17:470–478.

18. Catchpole K, Sellers R, Goldman A, McCulloch P, Hignett S. Patient handovers within the hospital: translating knowledge from motor racing to healthcare. *Qual Saf Health Care* 2010;19:318–322.

19. Horwitz LI, Moin T, Krumholz HM, Wang L, Bradley EH. What are covering doctors told about their patients? Analysis of sign-out among internal medicine house staff. *Qual Saf Health Care* 2009;18:248–255.

20. Wachter RM, Shojania KG. *Internal Bleeding: The Truth Behind America's Terrifying Epidemic of Medical Mistakes.* New York, NY: Rugged Land; 2004.

21. Boyd M, Cumin D, Lombard B, Torrie J, Civil N, Weller J. Read-back improved information transfer in simulated clinical crises. *BMJ Qual Saf* 2014;23:989–993.

22. Horwitz LI, Moin T, Krumholz HM, Wang L, Bradley EH. Consequences of inadequate sign-out for patient care. *Arch Intern Med* 2008;168:1755–1760.

23. Arora VM, Manjarrez E, Dressler DD, Basaviah P, Halasyamani L, Kripalani S. Hospitalist handoffs: a systematic review and task force recommendations. *J Hosp Med* 2009;4:433–440.

24. Starmer AJ, Spector ND, Srivastava R, et al. I-PASS, a mnemonic to standardize verbal handoffs. *Pediatrics* 2012;129:201–204.

25. Sheth S, McCarthy E, Kipps AK, et al. Changes in efficiency and safety culture after integration of an I-PASS-supported handoff process. *Pediatrics* 2016; 137:1–9.

26. Walia J, Qayumi Z, Khawar N, et al. Physician transition of care: benefits of I-PASS and an electronic handoff system in a community pediatric residency program. *Acad Pediatr* 2016;16:519–523.

27. Nabors C, Patel D, Khera S, et al. Improving resident morning sign-out by use of daily events reports. *J Patient Saf* 2015;11:36–41.

28. Seigel J, Whalen L, Burgess E, et al. Successful implementation of standardized multidisciplinary bedside rounds, including daily goals, in a pediatric ICU. *Jt Comm J Qual Patient Saf* 2014;40:83–90.

29. Sehgal NL, Green A, Vidyarthi AR, Blegen MA, Wachter RM. Patient whiteboards as a communication tool in the hospital setting: a survey of practices and recommendations. *J Hosp Med* 2010;5:234–239.

30. Committee on Quality of Healthcare in America, Institute of Medicine. *Crossing the Quality Chasm: A New Health System for the 21st Century*. Washington, DC: National Academies Press; 2001.

31. Struijs JN, Baan CA. Integrating care through bundled payments—lessons from the Netherlands. *N Engl J Med* 2011;364:990–991.

32. McClellan M, McKethan AN, Lewis JL, Roski J, Fisher ES. A national strategy to put accountable care into practice. *Health Aff (Millwood)* 2010;29:982–990.

33. Luft HS. Becoming accountable—opportunities and obstacles for ACOs. *N Engl J Med* 2010;363:1389–1391.

34. Blumenthal D, Tavenner M. The "meaningful use" regulation for electronic health records. *N Engl J Med* 2010;363:501–504.

35. Jacob J. On the road to interoperability, public and private organizations work to connect health care data. *JAMA* 2015;314:1213–1215.

36. Halamka J. Straight from the shoulder. *N Engl J Med* 2005;353:331–333.

37. Herrigel DJ, Carroll M, Fanning C, Steinberg MB, Parikh A, Usher M. Interhospital transfer handoff practices among US tertiary care centers: a descriptive survey. *J Hosp Med* 2016;11:413–417.

38. Ong MS, Coiera E. A systematic review of failures in handoff communication during intrahospital transfers. *Jt Comm J Qual Patient Saf* 2011;37:274–284.

39. Parmentier-Decrucq E, Poissy J, Favory R, et al. Adverse events during intrahospital transport of critically ill patients. *Ann Intensive Care* 2013;3:10.

40. Pesanka DA, Greenhouse PK, Rack LL, et al. Ticket to ride: reducing handoff risk during hospital patient transport. *J Nurs Care Qual* 2009;24:109–115.

41. Jones CD, Vu MB, O'Donnell CM, et al. A failure to communication: a qualitative exploration of care coordination between hospitalists and primary care providers around patient hospitalizations. *J Gen Intern Med* 2015;30:417–424.

42. Murphy DR, Meyer AN, Russo E, Sittig DF, Wei L, Singh H. The burden of inbox notifications in commercial electronic health records. *JAMA Intern Med* 2016;176:559–560.

43. O'Malley AS, Rescheovsky JD. Referral and consultation communication between primary care and specialist physicians: finding common ground. *Arch Intern Med* 2011;171:56–65.

44. Singh H, Thomas EJ, Mani S, et al. Timely follow-up of abnormal diagnostic imaging test results in an outpatient setting: are electronic medical records achieving their potential? *Arch Intern Med* 2009;169:1578–1586.

45. Nanji KC, Rothschild JM, Salzberg C, et al. Errors associated with outpatient computerized prescribing systems. *J Am Med Inform Assoc* 2011;18:767–773.

46. Garment AR, Lee WW, Harris C, Phillips-Caesar E. Development of a structured year-end sign-out program in an outpatient continuity practice. *J Gen Intern Med* 2013;28:114–120.

47. Auerbach AD, Kripalani S, Vasilevskis EE, et al. Preventability and causes of readmissions in a national cohort of general medicine patients. *JAMA Intern Med* 2016;176:484–493.

48. Coleman EA, Smith JD, Raha D, Min SJ. Posthospital medication discrepancies: prevalence and contributing factors. *Arch Intern Med* 2005;165:1842–1847.

49. Kripalani S, LeFevre F, Phillips CO, Williams MV, Basaviah P, Baker DW. Deficits in communication and information transfer between hospital-based and primary care physicians: implications for patient safety and continuity of care. *JAMA* 2007;297:831–841.

50. Schuller KA, Lin SH, Gamm LD, Edwardson N. Discharge phone calls: a technique to improve patient care during the transition from hospital to home. *J Healthc Qual* 2015;37:163–172.

51. Jack BW, Chetty VK, Anthony D, et al. A reengineered hospital discharge program to decrease rehospitalization: a randomized trial. *Ann Intern Med* 2009;150:178–187.

52. Society of Hospital Medicine. *BOOSTing Care Transitions Resource Room. Project BOOST (Better Outcomes for Older Adults Through Safe Transitions)*. Philadelphia, PA: Society of Hospital Medicine. Available at: http://www.hospitalmedicine.org/ResourceRoomRedesign/RR_CareTransitions/CT_Home.cfm.

53. Hendren R. Virtual discharge assistant cuts readmissions, costs. *HealthLeaders Media*. March 8, 2011. Available at: http://www.healthleadersmedia.com/page-1/NRS-263439/Virtual-Discharge-Assistant-Cuts-Readmissions-Costs.

ADDITIONAL READINGS

Care Transitions Program. Aurora, CO: The Division of Health Care Policy and Research, University of Colorado Health Sciences Center. Available at: http://www.caretransitions.org/.

Dalal AK, Poon EG, Karson AS, Gandhi TK, Roy CL. Lessons learned from implementation of a computerized application for pending tests at hospital discharge. *J Hosp Med* 2011;6:16–21.

Gandhi TK, Lee TH. Patient safety beyond the hospital. *N Engl J Med* 2010;363: 1001–1003.

Hansen LO, Young RS, Hinami K, Leung A, Williams MV. Interventions to reduce 30-day rehospitalization: a systematic review. *Ann Intern Med* 2011;155:520–528.

I-PASS Study Group. Boston, MA: Boston Children's Hospital. Available at: http://www.ipasshandoffstudy.com/home.

Project Red (Re-Engineered Discharge). Boston, MA: Boston University Medical Center. Available at: https://www.ahrq.gov/PROFESSIONALS/SYSTEMS/HOSPITAL/RED/TOOLKIT/INDEX.HTML.

Robertson ER, Morgan L, Bird S, Catchpole K, McCulloch P. Interventions employed to improve intrahospital handover: a systematic review. *BMJ Qual Saf* 2014;7:600–607.

Were MC, Li X, Kesterson J, et al. Adequacy of hospital discharge summaries in documenting tests with pending results and outpatient follow-up providers. *J Gen Intern Med* 2009;24:1002–1006.

Zakrison TL, Rosenbloom B, McFarlan A, et al. Lost information during the handover of critically injured trauma patients: a mixed-methods study. *BMJ Qual Saf* 2016;25:929–936.

TEAMWORK AND COMMUNICATION ERRORS | 9

A "Code Blue" is called when a hospitalized patient is discovered pulseless and not breathing. The code team rushes in and begins CPR. "Does anybody know this patient?" the code leader barks as the team continues its resuscitative efforts. A few moments later, a resident skids into the room, having pulled the patient's paper chart from the rack in the nurse's station. "This patient is a No Code!" he blurts, and all activity stops.

As the Code Blue team members collect their paraphernalia, the patient's young nurse wonders in silence. She received signout on this patient only a couple of hours ago, and was told that the patient was a "full code." She thinks briefly about questioning the physician, but reconsiders. One of the doctors must have changed the patient's code status to do not resuscitate (DNR) in the interim and forgotten to tell me, she decides. Happens all the time. So she keeps her concerns to herself.

Only later, after someone picks up the chart that the resident brought into the room, does it become clear that he had inadvertently pulled the wrong chart from the chart rack. The young nurse's suspicions were correct—the patient was a full code! A second Code Blue was called, but the patient could not be resuscitated.[1]

SOME BASIC CONCEPTS AND TERMS

All organizations need structure and hierarchies, lest there be chaos. Armies must have generals, large organizations must have CEOs, and children must have parents. This is not a bad thing, but taken to extremes, these hierarchies can become so rigid that frontline workers withhold critical information from leaders or reveal only the information they believe their leaders want to hear. This state can easily spiral out of control, leaving the leaders without the information they need to improve the system and the workers believing that the leaders are not listening, are not open to dissenting opinions, and are perhaps not even interested.

The psychological distance between a worker and a supervisor is sometimes called an *authority gradient*, and the overall steepness of this gradient is referred to as the *hierarchy* of an organization. Healthcare has traditionally been characterized by steep hierarchies and very large authority gradients, mostly between physicians and the rest of the staff. Errors like those in the wrong DNR case—in which the patient's nurse suspected that something was terribly wrong but did not feel comfortable raising her concerns in the face of a physician's forceful (but ultimately incorrect) proclamation—have alerted us to the safety consequences of this kind of a hierarchy.

THE ROLE OF TEAMWORK IN HEALTHCARE

Teamwork may have been less important in healthcare 50 years ago than it is today. The pace was slower, the technology less overwhelming, the medications less toxic (also less effective), and quality and safety appeared to be under the control of physicians; everyone else played a supporting role. But the last half century has brought a sea change in the provision of medical care, with massively increased complexity (think liver transplant or electrophysiology), huge numbers of new medications and procedures, and overwhelming evidence that the quality of teamwork often determines whether patients receive appropriate care, promptly and safely. For example, the outcomes of trauma care, obstetrical care, care of the patient with an acute myocardial infarction or stroke, and care of the immunocompromised patient are likely to hinge more on the quality of teamwork than the brilliance of the supervising physician.

After recognizing the importance of teamwork to safety and quality, healthcare looked to the field of aviation for lessons. In the late 1970s and early 1980s, a cluster of deadly airplane crashes occurred in which a steep authority gradient appeared to be an important culprit, as those lower in the hierarchy were reluctant to raise their concerns. Probably the best known of these tragedies was the 1977 collision of two 747s on the runway at Tenerife in the Canary Islands.

On March 27, 1977, Captain Jacob Van Zanten, a copilot, and a flight engineer sat in the cockpit of their KLM 747 awaiting clearance to take off on a foggy morning in Tenerife. Van Zanten was revered among KLM employees: as director of safety for KLM's fleet, he was known as a superb pilot. In fact, with tragic irony, in each of the KLM's 300 seatback pockets that morning there was an article about him, including his picture. The crew of the KLM had spotted a Pan Am 747 on the tarmac earlier that morning, but it was taxiing toward a spur off the lone main runway and it was logical to believe that it was out of the way. The fog now hung thick, and there was no ground radar to signal to the cockpit crew whether the runway was clear—the crew relied on its own eyes, and those of the air traffic controllers.

A transmission came from the tower to the KLM cockpit radio, but it was garbled—although the crew did hear enough of it to tell that it had something to do with the Pan Am 747. Months later, a report from the Spanish Secretary of Civil Aviation described what happened next:

> *On hearing this, the KLM flight engineer asked: "Is he not clear then?" The [KLM] captain didn't understand him and [the engineer] repeated, "Is he not clear, that Pan American?" The captain replied with an emphatic, "Yes" and, perhaps, influenced by his great prestige, making it difficult to imagine an error of this magnitude on the part of such an expert pilot, both the co-pilot and flight engineer made no further objections. [Italics added]*[2]

A few moments later, Van Zanten pulled the throttle and his KLM jumbo jet thundered down the runway. Emerging from the fog and accelerating for takeoff, the pilot and his crew now witnessed a horrifying sight: the Pam Am plane was sitting squarely in front of them on the main runway. Although Van Zanten managed to get the nose of the KLM over the Pan Am, doing so required such a steep angle of ascent that his tail first dragged along the ground, and then through the upper deck of the Pan Am's fuselage. Both planes exploded, causing the deaths of 583 people. Forty years later, the Tenerife accident remains the worst air traffic collision of all time.

Tenerife and similar accidents taught aviation leaders the risks associated with a hierarchical culture, one in which it was possible for individuals (such as the KLM flight engineer) to suspect that something was wrong yet not feel comfortable raising these concerns with the leader. Through many years of teamwork and communications training (called crew resource management [CRM], see Chapter 15), commercial airline crews have learned to speak up and raise concerns. Importantly, the programs have also taught pilots how to create an environment that makes it possible for those lower on the authority totem pole to raise issues. The result has been commercial aviation's remarkable safety record over the past 45 years (Figure 9-1), a record that many experts attribute largely to this "culture of safety"—particularly the dampening of the authority gradient.

How well do we do on this in healthcare? In a 2000 study, Sexton et al. asked members of operating room and aviation crews similar questions about culture, teamwork, and hierarchies.[3] While attending surgeons perceived that teamwork in their operating rooms was strong, the rest of the team members disagreed

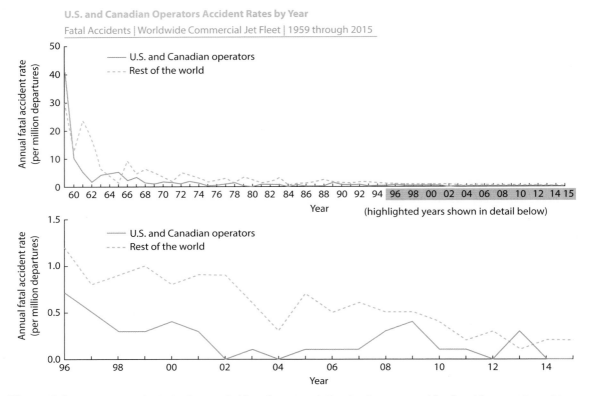

Figure 9-1 ■ Commercial aviation's remarkable safety record. Graphs shows annual fatal accident rate in accidents per million departures, broken out for U.S. and Canadian operators (solid line) and the rest of the world's commercial jet fleet (hatched line). (Source: http://www.boeing.com/news/techissues/pdf/statsum.pdf, Slide 18. Reproduced with permission from Boeing. © Boeing, 2016.)

(see Figure 15-3), proving that one should ask the followers, not the leader, about the quality of teamwork. Perhaps more germane to the patient safety question, while virtually all pilots would welcome being questioned by a coworker or subordinate, nearly 50% of surgeons would not (Figure 9-2). In subsequent studies, while these differences in perceptions among surgeons, anesthesiologists, and nurses had narrowed somewhat, they had not gone away.[4,5]

It is important to recognize that the attitudes still held by some surgeons were common among pilots in the past, until pilots recognized that these attitudes (and the culture they represented) made crashes far more likely. As we consider strategies to improve teamwork and dampen down hierarchies in healthcare, it is also worth noting that pilots did not immediately relish the prospect of teamwork training when it was first introduced in the early 1980s. (In fact, many pilots derisively referred to CRM training as "charm school.")

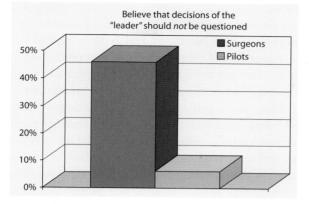

Believe that decisions of the
"leader" should *not* be questioned

■ Surgeons
□ Pilots

Figure 9-2 ■ Percent of pilots and surgeons who would not welcome being questioned by a subordinate. (Adapted from Sexton JB, Thomas EJ, Helmreich RL. Error, stress, and teamwork in medicine and aviation: cross sectional surveys. *BMJ* 2000;320:745–749.)

Yet today, it is difficult to find a pilot, or anyone else in commercial aviation, who questions the contribution of CRM training to airline safety. The adaptation of such training programs to medicine is further explored in Chapter 15, although it is worth foreshadowing that studies have demonstrated that they improve both culture and outcomes in healthcare.[6–8]

While enthusiasm for teamwork training in healthcare is warranted, it is important to appreciate the complexity of this undertaking and the limitations of the aviation analogy. Changing the cockpit environment to prevent the next Tenerife involved improving teamwork between two or three individuals—captain, first officer, and perhaps flight engineer—who share similar training, expertise, social status, income, and confidence. In a busy operating room, it may be the high school–educated clerk or young nursing assistant who harbors a crucial concern that needs to be transmitted to the senior surgeon, who as likely as not trained in an era when rigid hierarchy in the OR was the norm. Those interested in improving safety in healthcare need to recognize that transforming *this* culture is far more challenging than changing the culture of the cockpit.

FIXED VERSUS FLUID TEAMS

Some in healthcare point to our fluid teams—the fact that a surgeon is likely to work with multiple different sets of nurses, technicians, and perfusionists—as an additional obstacle to better teamwork. Many do not realize that commercial aviation has precisely the same problem: when you fly a commercial airliner, it is unlikely that your pilot and copilot have ever flown together before. Because fluid teams are so common, it is critical to develop strategies and protocols that do not rely on individuals having worked together to ensure safety. In fact, some observers of both healthcare and aviation believe that fixed teams (in which the same groups of people work together repetitively) may be *more* dangerous, because they are more likely to get sloppy, make incorrect assumptions, regenerate fixed hierarchies, and suffer from "groupthink."[9]

That said, there are significant logistical challenges in trying to promote teamwork when team members don't work together regularly, and the desire to be surrounded by familiar faces at stressful times is understandable. Some surgeons feel so strongly about this issue that they insist on working with "their team" in the operating room. Indeed, there are data that suggest that fixed OR teams may reduce turnover and preparation time[10] as well as procedure time, which may have implications for patient safety.[11]

On the medical ward, the concept of *geographic units* is increasingly popular—a unit in which the nurses and physicians are tied to a given locale. The hope is that this structure will lend itself to better team behaviors, both in the care of individual patients and in doing the hard work of improving systems of care. Recent studies have demonstrated that such units are generally associated with improved nurse–physician communication and—when combined with structured interdisciplinary rounds—fewer preventable adverse events, although not all studies support this conclusion.[12–14] The logistical and political complexity of guaranteeing fixed teams in the operating room and geographic units on the wards (particularly in hospitals that tend to run full) should not be underestimated.

TEAMWORK AND COMMUNICATION STRATEGIES

Data from the Joint Commission's sentinel event program have demonstrated that communication problems are among the most common root causes of serious medical errors (Table 9-1). Well-functioning teams employ a number of strategies (emphasized in CRM training programs, Chapter 15) to improve communication and teamwork. (In addition, many of the strategies to improve handoffs reviewed in Chapter 8 are relevant here as well.)

The first set of strategies focuses on ways to dampen authority gradients. These efforts can include very simple techniques, such as having the leader introduce him- or herself by name, learn the names of the other workers, admit his or her limitations, and explicitly welcome input from all the members of the team. These techniques can be incorporated into the surgical "time out" described in Chapter 5. But they shouldn't be limited to the presurgical or preprocedural pause: a medicine attending might employ them on the first day of a ward rotation, as might an obstetrician beginning a shift on the labor

Table 9-1	MOST FREQUENTLY IDENTIFIED ROOT CAUSES OF SENTINEL EVENTS REVIEWED BY THE JOINT COMMISSION BY YEAR*				
2013 (N=887)		**2014 (N=764)**		**2015 (N=936)**	
Human Factors	635	Human Factors	547	Human Factors	999
Communication	563	Leadership	517	Leadership	849
Leadership	547	Communication	489	Communication	744
Assessment	505	Assessment	392	Assessment	545
Information Management	155	Physical Environment	115	Physical Environment	202
Physical Environment	138	Information Management	72	Health Information Technology-related	125
Care Planning	103	Care Planning	72	Care Planning	75
Continuum of Care	97	Health Information Technology-related	59	Operative Care	62
Medication Care	77	Operative Care	58	Medication Use	60
Operative Care	76	Continuum of Care	57	Information Management	52

*Frequency of communication problems among Joint Commission sentinel events 2013, 2014, and 2015. (© The Joint Commission, 2017. Reprinted with permission.)

and delivery floor. For example, a surgeon might introduce himself (and have everyone else do the same) to all the members of his operating room crew, and then say, "You know, there will be times when I miss something, or when I'm going in the wrong direction in the middle of a complicated case. I really need all of you to be my eyes and ears. If you see anything that you're not comfortable with—anything—including things that I'm doing, I really want you to bring them up. As a team, we can be far safer than any of us can be individually." In *The Checklist Manifesto*, surgeon and safety expert Atul Gawande emphasizes the role of checklists in supporting such team behaviors—in contrast to the traditional view of checklists as tools to simply promote the completion of tasks (more on this in Chapter 15).[15]

There are also powerful opportunities to improve team performance after a procedure or a clinical encounter is over. Known in the military and aviation as a *debriefing*, all team members take a moment at the end of the procedure and explicitly, in a blame-free way, discuss what went wrong and right.[16,17] The lessons from these debriefings are often invaluable, and just as importantly, the sessions reinforce the value of team behaviors, the critical importance of speaking up, and the fact that everyone—even the leader—is fallible. Implementing standardized briefings and debriefings in the operating rooms of a regional medical center led to improved perceptions of teamwork and communication among the providers.[18]

It is one thing to tell nurses, clerks, or medical students to speak up, and another to give them the tools to do so productively. Many nurses recall having tried to raise concerns with physicians, only to be rebuffed. (Chapter 19 returns to the more serious issue of disruptive behaviors.) While most nurses are likely to speak up when they believe the patient is at risk, one study found that 12% of nurses would not do so even when they believed there was a high potential for patient harm.[19] To improve these odds and the quality of these exchanges, a number of techniques have been promoted, all designed to ensure that important messages are heard and acted upon. Two of these are *Situation, Background, Assessment, and Recommendations* (SBAR) and *CUS words*.

In most training programs, the focus of SBAR training is on nurses, for whom SBAR is a tool to structure their communication with physicians to capture the latter's attention and generate the appropriate action. There are data to suggest that SBAR improves nurse–physician communication.[20] The need for SBAR training grew from the recognition that many nurses have been trained to report in stories, while physicians have been taught to think and process information in bullet points. For example, a traditional nursing assessment of a postoperative patient with new chest pain might be:

> *Hi, doctor. Mr. Chow is having some chest pain. He was walking around the floor earlier, and he ate a good dinner. I don't really know what is going on, but I'm getting an electrocardiogram. He was a little sweaty when he had his pain, but I gave him the rest of his medicines, including his insulin and his antibiotic. He had surgery earlier today, and he's on a PCA pump right now.*

After SBAR training, the same nurse might call the physician and say:

> *This is Grace Jones. I'm a nurse on 7 North and I'm seeing your patient Edward Chow. He developed 8 out of 10 chest pain about five minutes ago, associated with shortness of breath, diaphoresis, and some palpitations (**Situation**). He is a 68-year-old man with no prior history of cardiac disease who had an uncomplicated abdominal-peritoneal resection yesterday (**Background**). I am obtaining an electrocardiogram, and my concern is that he might be having cardiac ischemia or a pulmonary embolism (**Assessment**). I'm giving him a nitroglycerin and would really appreciate it if you could be here in the next five minutes (**Recommendation**).*

Another technique to improve communication is the use of "CUS words." These involve escalating levels of concern, again usually on the part of a nurse, but they would be equally applicable to many other workers: medical students, respiratory therapists, pharmacists—anyone lower on a hierarchy who needs to get the attention of someone higher up. In escalating order, it begins with the use of the words, "I'm *concerned* about ...," then "I'm *uncomfortable* ...," and finally, "This is a *safety* issue!" It is important to teach those who might be receiving such messages (usually physicians) to appreciate their meaning and respond appropriately, and those who use CUS words to avoid overusing them to ensure that they have the intended impact.

Finally, strong teams depend on members—individually and collectively—responding appropriately to crises, particularly when the "fog of war" sets in. The concept of *situational awareness* refers to the degree to which one's perception of a situation matches reality.[21–23] Failure to maintain situational awareness during a crisis can result in various problems that compound the crisis. The classic examples come from certain airline crashes, where post-crash investigations revealed that the crew was focused, laser-like, on a trivial flashing light or gauge, as the plane ran out of fuel or crashed into a mountain.

We see similar problems in healthcare. For instance, during a resuscitation, an individual or entire team may focus on a particular task (such as a difficult central line insertion or administering a particular medication), while neglecting to address immediately life-threatening problems such as respiratory failure or a pulseless rhythm. In this context, maintaining situational awareness might be seen as equivalent to keeping the "big picture" in mind. Or, to cite one of the famous "Laws of the House of God" (the influential 1979 satire of the world of medical training), "at a cardiac arrest, the first procedure is to take your own pulse."[24]

KEY POINTS

- The provision of high-quality, safe healthcare is increasingly a team sport.
- Well-functioning teams are characterized by appropriate authority gradients and hierarchies that don't stifle the free flow of information.
- Healthcare has looked to the field of aviation for guidance regarding how best to dampen down hierarchies; the specific training model in aviation (which has been adapted to healthcare) is known as crew resource management (CRM).
- As long as effective teamwork and communication strategies are employed, the presence of fluid (rather than fixed) teams should not be a safety hazard.

- High-functioning teams use strategies such as effective introductions and debriefings.
- Strategies to improve communications, particularly up the authority gradient, include the use of SBAR and CUS words.
- Strong teams manage to maintain "situational awareness" (focusing on the big picture) even during crises.

REFERENCES

1. Wachter RM, Shojania KG. *Internal Bleeding: The Truth Behind America's Terrifying Epidemic of Medical Mistakes*. New York, NY: Rugged Land; 2004.
2. Secretary of Aviation (Spain) Report on Tenerife Crash. Aircraft Accident Digest (ICAO Circular 153-AN/56); 1978:22–68.
3. Sexton JB, Thomas EJ, Helmreich RL. Error, stress, and teamwork in medicine and aviation: cross sectional surveys. *BMJ* 2000;320:745–749.
4. Wauben LS, Dekker-van Doorn CM, van Wijngaarden JD, et al. Discrepant perceptions of communication, teamwork and situation awareness among surgical team members. *Int J Qual Health Care* 2011;23:159–166.
5. Bould MD, Sutherland S, Sydor DT, Naik V, Friedman Z. Residents' reluctance to challenge negative hierarchy in the operating room: a qualitative study. *Can J Anaesth* 2015;62:576–586.
6. Neily J, Mills PD, Young-Xu Y, et al. Association between implementation of a medical team training program and surgical mortality. *JAMA* 2010;304:1693–1700.
7. Weaver SJ, Dy SM, Rosen MA. Team-training in healthcare: a narrative synthesis of the literature. *BMJ Qual Saf* 2014;23:359–372.
8. Riley W, Davis S, Miller K, Hansen H, Sainfort F, Sweet R. Didactic and simulation nontechnical skills team training to improve perinatal patient outcomes in a community hospital. *J Qual Patient Saf* 2011;37:357–364.
9. In conversation with … Jack Barker. [Perspective]. *AHRQ PSNet* [serial online]; January 2006. Available at: https://psnet.ahrq.gov/perspectives/perspective/17.
10. Stepaniak PS, Vrijland WW, de Quelerij M, de Vries G, Heij C. Working with a fixed operating room team on consecutive similar cases and the effect on case duration and turnover time. *Arch Surg* 2010;145:1165–1170.
11. He W, Ni S, Chen G, Jiang X, Zheng B. The composition of surgical teams in the operating room and its impact on surgical team performance in China. *Surg Endosc* 2014;28:1473–1478.
12. Gordon MB, Melvin P, Graham D, et al. Unit-based care teams and the frequency and quality of physician–nurse communications. *Arch Pediatr Adolesc Med* 2011;165:424–428.
13. Seigel J, Whalen L, Burgess E, et al. Successful implementation of standardized multidisciplinary bedside rounds, including daily goals in a pediatric ICU. *Jt Comm J Qual Patient Saf* 2014;40:83–90.
14. Mueller SK, Schnipper JL, Giannelli K, Roy CL, Boxer R. Impact of regionalized care on concordance of plan and preventable adverse events on general medicine services. *J Hosp Med* 2016;11:620–627.

15. Gawande A. *The Checklist Manifesto: How to Get Things Right*. New York, NY: Metropolitan Books; 2009.

16. Bandari J, Schumacher K, Simon M, et al. Surfacing safety hazards using standardized operating room briefings and debriefings at a large regional medical center. *Jt Comm J Qual Patient Saf* 2012;38:154–160.

17. Wolfe H, Zebuhr C, Topjian AA, et al. Interdisciplinary ICU cardiac arrest debriefing improves survival outcomes. *Crit Care Med* 2014;42:1688–1695.

18. Berenholtz SM, Schumacher K, Hayanga AJ, et al. Implementing standardized operating room briefings and debriefings at a large regional medical center. *Jt Comm J Qual Patient Saf* 2009;35:391–397.

19. Lyndon A, Sexton JB, Simpson KR, Rosenstein A, Lee KA, Wachter RM. Predictors of likelihood of speaking up about safety concerns in labour and delivery. *BMJ Qual Saf* 2012;21:791–799.

20. De Meester K, Verspuy M, Monsieurs KG, Van Bogaert P. SBAR improves nurse-physician communication and reduces unexpected death: a pre and post intervention study. *Resuscitation* 2013;84:1192–1196.

21. Weick KE. The collapse of sensemaking in organizations: the Mann Gulch disaster. *Adm Sci Q* 1993;38:628–652.

22. Weick KE, Sutcliffe KM. *Managing the Unexpected: Assuring High Performance in an Age of Complexity*. 3rd ed. San Francisco, CA: Jossey-Bass; 2015.

23. Berwick DM. *Escape Fire: Lessons for the Future of Health Care*. New York, NY: The Commonwealth Fund; 2002.

24. Shem S. *The House of God*. New York, NY: Putnam; 1979.

ADDITIONAL READINGS

Berlinger N, Dietz E. Time-out: the professional and organizational ethics of speaking up in the OR. *AMA J Ethics* 2016;18:925–932.

Brown T. Healing the Hospital Hierarchy. *New York Times*. March 17, 2013.

Leape LL. Error in medicine. *JAMA* 1994;272:1851–1857.

Okuyama A, Wagner C, Binjen B. Speaking up for patient safety by hospital-based health care professionals: a literature review. *BMC Health Serv Res* 2014;14:61.

Raemer DB, Kolbe M, Minehart RD, Rudolph JW, Pian-Smith MC. Improving anesthesiologists' ability to speak up in the operating room: a randomized controlled experiment of a simulation-based intervention and a qualitative analysis of hurdles and enablers. *Acad Med* 2016;91:530–539.

Sachs BP. A 38-year-old woman with fetal loss and hysterectomy. *JAMA* 2005;294:833–840.

Srivastava R. Speaking up—when doctors navigate medical hierarchy. *N Engl J Med* 2013;368:302–305.

Sur MD, Schindler N, Singh P, Angelos P, Langerman A. Young surgeons on speaking up: when and how surgical trainees voice concerns about supervisors' clinical decisions. *Am J Surg* 2016;211:437–444.

Thomas EJ. Improving teamwork in healthcare: current approaches and the path forward. *BMJ Qual Saf* 2011;20:647–650.

Vincent C, Amalberti R. *Safer Healthcare: Strategies for the Real World*. New York, NY: SpringerOpen; 2016.

HEALTHCARE-ASSOCIATED INFECTIONS | 10

GENERAL CONCEPTS AND EPIDEMIOLOGY

Before the advent of the patient safety movement, the hospital epidemiology and other infection control staff were largely responsible for the prevention of hospital-acquired infections. Attempts to engage clinicians in prevention efforts were often unsuccessful. Branding healthcare-associated infections (HAIs) as a patient safety problem (which by extension rendered failure of clinicians to engage in appropriate infection control practices a form of medical error) has elevated the importance of preventing these infections in the minds of providers, leaders of healthcare organizations, and policymakers.

Gratifyingly, evidence is accumulating that healthcare organizations can markedly decrease the frequency of HAIs. Some hospitals, having religiously implemented a variety of prevention strategies, are reporting intervals of months, even years, between previously commonplace infections such as ventilator-associated pneumonias (VAP), methicillin-resistant *Staphylococcus aureus* (MRSA), and central line–associated bloodstream infections (CLABSI) (Figure 10-1).

If we consider HAIs resulting from failure to adhere to evidence-based practices preventable adverse events, then HAIs may well be the most common source of serious and preventable harm in healthcare. In the United States, HAIs are tracked and reported through the Center for Disease Control and Prevention's (CDC) National Healthcare Safety Network (NHSN). Based on the HAI Prevalence Survey, the CDC estimates that in 2011 there were about 722,000 HAIs in U.S. acute care hospitals, and that approximately 75,000 patients with HAIs died during their hospitalizations.[1] In addition, preventing HAIs is associated with significant cost savings. Indeed, it has been estimated that the federal government may have saved more than $1 billion in ICU-related costs alone from CLABSIs averted between 1990 and 2008.[2] Beginning in 2008, Medicare began withholding payments to hospitals for the care of certain HAIs (CLABSI, catheter-associated urinary tract infections

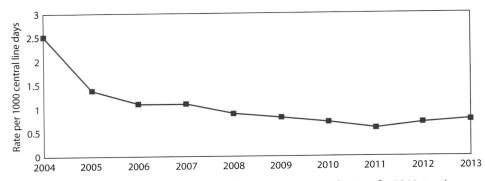

Figure 10-1 ■ Depicts mean rate of central line-associated bloodstream infections for 121 intensive care units from 73 hospitals from March 2004 through December 2013. (Reproduced with permission from Pronovost PJ, Watson SR, Goeschel CA, Hyzy RC, Berenholtz SM. Sustaining reductions in central line-associated bloodstream infections in Michigan intensive care units: a 10-year analysis. *Am J Med Qual* 2016;31:197–202.)

[CAUTIs], and *Clostridium difficile* infections) it considered largely preventable (Chapter 20 and Appendix VIII).[3]

For many HAIs (and other complications of healthcare, see Chapter 11), a variety of process or structural changes appear to be correlated with improvement. In the past, infection control experts and regulators underscored the need to increase adherence to individual prevention elements—for example, if there were five strategies thought to be effective in preventing a certain type of infection, a hospital might get "credit" for achieving 100% adherence on one of the five elements, 80% on another, and 50% on the other three. The Institute for Healthcare Improvement (IHI) has promoted a "*bundle*" approach, emphasizing that the chance of preventing complications seems to improve with complete adherence to a "bundle" of preventive strategies. There is evidence to suggest that this approach works.[4] Under this model, institutions receive credit for their quality and safety efforts only for above-threshold adherence (i.e., >80%) on *all* the preventive strategies, not just some. This approach rests on the theory that not only does better adherence to the individual elements increase the chances of prevention, but also that achieving high bundle adherence rates usually requires reengineering the entire clinical process. Changes born of this kind of reengineering may be more durable than those that result from short-term projects or cheerleading.

By this point in the book, you won't be surprised to learn that successfully eradicating HAIs is not as simple as creating and promoting the use of an evidence-based bundle of practices. In an insightful study, Saint et al. surveyed 86 people from a variety of disciplines (physicians, hospital executives, nurses, infection control preventionists, and others) to determine barriers to successful implementation of evidence-based HAI prevention strategies.[5]

They identified two kinds of personnel—active resistors and "organizational constipators"—who impeded these efforts. To illustrate the resistor category, the authors quote one hospital chief of staff, who gave the following advice to those charged with getting surgeons to follow HAI guidelines:

> *Surgeons are very tribal so if you … have something that you think is a best practice at your hospital … you need to get…either the chair of surgery or some reasonable surgeon … If you come in and you're an internist … into a group of surgeons … the first thing we're going to do is we're going to say, "Look, you're not one of us" … the way to get buy-in from surgeons is you got to have a surgeon on your team.*

Table 10-1 chronicles some of the major themes from this study and best practices for overcoming both sources of resistance.

It is beyond the scope of this book to cover all aspects of HAIs in great detail; the interested reader is referred to other resources.[6–8] Instead, this chapter will highlight some of the patient safety principles involved in preventing the most common HAIs, ending with a discussion of what the patient safety movement can learn from the more established field of infection prevention. Table 10-2 summarizes some of the key evidence-based practices for the prevention of surgical site infections, VAP, CLABSI, and CAUTI.[6,9] (Note that hand hygiene is an essential practice for the prevention of *all* HAIs.)

SURGICAL SITE INFECTIONS

Surgical site infections represent a serious form of postoperative complications, occur in about 2% of all surgical procedures, and comprise about a fifth of HAIs.[10] They cause substantial increases in mortality, readmission rates, and costs. Approximately 1 in 30 "clean" surgeries (surgeries characterized by an uninfected wound, a respiratory, gastrointestinal, or genitourinary tract that has not been entered, and primary closure; examples include mastectomy, neck dissection, and thyroid surgery) will be complicated by a surgical site infection. The rate is significantly higher for "dirty" (surgeries involving trauma or existing infection, e.g., abscess incision and drainage or perforated bowel) emergency, or prolonged surgeries, and for patients with medical comorbidities.

The following strategies[6] are recommended to prevent surgical site infections: appropriate use of prophylactic antibiotics (giving guideline-endorsed antibiotics within an hour or two of the incision, depending on the half-life, and stopping it/them within 24 hours after surgery), avoiding hair removal

Table 10-1   MAJOR UNIFYING AND RECURRENT THEMES SURROUNDING THE ROLES OF HOSPITAL PERSONNEL IN THWARTING HEALTHCARE-ASSOCIATED INFECTION PREVENTION EFFORTS, WITH IDEAS FOR OVERCOMING THESE BARRIERS

1. *Active resistance* to a change in practice is pervasive, whether by attending physicians, resident physicians, or nurses. Successful efforts to overcome active resistance included the following:
   (a) Data feedback comparing local infection rates to national rates
   (b) Data feedback comparing rates of compliance with the practices to rates of others in the same area
   (c) Effective championing by an engaged and respected change agent who can speak the language of the staff he or she is guiding (e.g., a surgeon to motivate other surgeons)
   (d) Participation in collaborative efforts that generally align hospital leadership and clinicians in the goal of reducing healthcare-associated infection

2. *Organizational constipators*: mid- to high-level executives who act as insidious barriers to change—they present added challenges to change in practice. Once leadership recognizes the problem and the negative effect on other staff, various techniques were used to overcome this barrier:
   (a) Include the organizational constipator early in group discussions in order to improve communication and obtain buy-in
   (b) Work around the individual, realizing that this is likely a shorter-term solution
   (c) Terminate the constipator's employment
   (d) Take advantage of turnover opportunities when the constipator leaves the organization by hiring a person who has a very high likelihood of being effective

Reproduced with permission from Saint S, Kowalski CP, Banaszak-Holl J, Forman J, Damschroder L, Krein SL. How active resisters and organizational constipators affect health care–acquired infection prevention efforts. *Jt Comm J Qual Patient Saf* 2009;35:239–246.

unless necessary and if removal is required, use of clippers (rather than razors) for hair removal, maintenance of postoperative normothermia, and maintain blood glucose levels less than 180 mg/dL.[11]

The last recommendation has an interesting history, one that illustrates the importance of following new evidence and adjusting guidelines over time as such evidence emerges. Based on an influential 2001 study,[12] early bundles recommended far tighter glucose control. However, subsequent research[6] found that tight control did not reduce the incidence of surgical site infections and was associated with other adverse outcomes such as stroke and death.[13] Today's recommendation to aim for glucoses less than 180 mg/dL reflects these newer studies.[6]

Table 10-2	SPECIFIC MEASURES FOR PREVENTION OF FOUR MAJOR HEALTHCARE-ASSOCIATED INFECTIONS*	
Healthcare-Associated Infection	**Preventive Measure**	**Definition or Comment**
All healthcare-associated infections	Hand hygiene	Cleaning hands before and after each patient contact
Surgical site infection	Appropriate use of perioperative antibiotics	Administration of appropriate prophylactic antibiotic, generally begun within 1 hour of skin incision and discontinued within 24 hours
	Avoidance of shaving the operative site	Use clippers or other methods for hair removal in the area of incision(s)
	Perioperative normothermia	Maintain normothermia during the perioperative period
	Glucose control	Aim for less than 180 mg/dL
Ventilator-associated pneumonia	Semirecumbent positioning	Elevation of the head of the bed to more than 30° for all mechanically ventilated patients
	Daily assessment of readiness for weaning	Minimize duration of mechanical ventilation by limiting sedative administration and/or using protocolized weaning
	Regular antiseptic oral care	*Recommended by some guidelines but data is mixed*
	Use of endotracheal tubes with subglottic secretion drainage ports for patients expected to require mechanical ventilation for more than 48 or 72 hours	Minimize pooling of secretions above the endotracheal tube cuff
Central line–associated bloodstream infection	Maximum barrier precautions	Use aseptic technique, including cap, mask, sterile gown, sterile gloves, and a large sterile sheet for the insertion of all central venous catheters
	Chlorhexidine skin antisepsis	Use 2% chlorhexidine gluconate solution for skin sterilization at the insertion site
	Appropriate insertion site selection	Subclavian vein is preferred site for nontunneled catheters; avoid femoral site for nonemergency insertions; consider risk benefit of different insertion sites with regard to infectious and noninfectious complications; use ultrasound guidance for internal jugular catheter insertion
	Prompt removal of unnecessary catheters	Remove when no longer essential for care

(continued)

Table 10-2 SPECIFIC MEASURES FOR PREVENTION OF FOUR MAJOR HEALTHCARE-ASSOCIATED INFECTIONS* *(continued)*		
Healthcare-Associated Infection	Preventive Measure	Definition or Comment
Catheter-associated urinary tract infection	Aseptic insertion and catheter care	Use of skin antisepsis at insertion and proper technique for maintenance of catheter and drainage bag; use of closed drainage system
	Prompt removal of unnecessary catheters	Remove catheter when no longer essential for care
Methicillin-resistant *S. aureus* infection	Conduct MRSA risk assessment	Assess patients' risk for contracting MRSA
	Use contact precautions for MRSA-colonized and MRSA infected patients	*Wear appropriate personal protective equipment when entering rooms of patients on contact precautions*
	Ensure cleaning and disinfection of equipment and environment	Equipment and environment must be disinfected appropriately
C. difficile infection	Antibiotic stewardship	Use antibiotics only when needed and narrow from broad spectrum when pathogen identified
	Use contact precautions for infected patients, single-patient room preferred	Wear appropriate personal protective equipment when entering infected patients' rooms and wash hands with soap and water to minimize spore transmission
	Ensure cleaning and disinfection of equipment and environment	Equipment and environment must be disinfected appropriately to prevent transmission via spores

*Drawn from References 6, 9, 27, 35. Controversial or no longer recommended items in italics.

VENTILATOR-ASSOCIATED PNEUMONIA

Of all HAIs, VAP is the most deadly, with an attributable mortality of about 10%. About 10% to 20% of patients receiving mechanical ventilation, particularly for long periods, will develop VAP, which in turn results in prolonged mechanical ventilation, longer hospital stays, and increased mortality.[14]

Many cases of VAP can be prevented by strict adherence to several preventive strategies. The first is elevation of the head of the bed to semirecumbent (at least 30°) position, which in one trial resulted in an 18% decrease in VAP cases.[15] Head-of-bed (HOB) elevation decreases the risk of microaspiration of gastrointestinal tract and upper respiratory tract secretions into the lungs, which can serve as a nidus for infection. Although this intervention might seem like a relatively simple undertaking, experience has demonstrated that it can be a challenge, usually because of changes in patient position.[16] Several tactics have been recommended to increase adherence with HOB elevation, including enlisting the support of respiratory therapists and family members and placing a visual cue (such as a line on the wall) to help identify whether the bed is in the correct position. Some modern ICU beds come with a built-in tool to provide continuous monitoring of the angle of incline.[6]

A second effective strategy is minimizing sedation for ventilated patients.[17] Under one popular protocol, patients' sedative infusions are stopped each day, allowing patients to "lighten" to the point that they can answer simple questions. This strategy, when coupled with a program of systematic assessment (usually by trained respiratory therapists) regarding readiness for weaning, results in shorter duration of mechanical ventilation, presumably lowering the risk of VAP.[18,19]

Several other strategies have been included in various "VAP bundles." Studies regarding the effectiveness of regular antiseptic oral care have produced mixed results,[19,20] with some demonstrating decreased VAPs and others showing increased mortality.[21] The use of endotracheal tubes with subglottic secretion drainage ports for patients expected to require mechanical ventilation for more than 48 or 72 hours is also recommended.[14,22] Finally, while there is evidence to support the use of silver-coated endotracheal tubes to prevent biofilm generation and ultimately VAP,[23] recent guidelines generally do not recommend their use, citing insufficient data to support a decrease in length of stay, duration of mechanical ventilation, and mortality.[14]

VAP, like the other HAIs, has been considered for inclusion in a variety of public reporting and payment policies. One challenge, though, is that there are several VAP definitions, which means that the determination of whether an individual patient has VAP may be subject to interpretation. This, of course, opens the door to the possibility that hospitals may apply definitions differently, making rates of VAP difficult to interpret.[24,25]

The broader topic of hospital-acquired pneumonia[26,27] will not be covered here, nor will additional categories of ventilator complications. Together, this group of complications is now referred to as *ventilator-associated events* (VAEs). The increasing popularity of this term owes to the CDC's introduction of a new surveillance paradigm in 2013. It uses objective criteria to identify four types of VAEs: ventilator-associated conditions (VACs), infection-related ventilator-associated conditions (IVACs), possible VAPs, and probable VAPs.[28,29]

| CENTRAL LINE–ASSOCIATED BLOODSTREAM INFECTIONS

As catheter access to the central circulation has become ubiquitous (to provide long-term antibiotics, nutrition, and vasoactive medications, as well as to permit central blood sampling), so too have infectious complications of these lines. The vast majority of CLABSI cases are associated with central venous catheters (CVCs). Patients in ICUs, nearly half of whom have CVCs, are particularly vulnerable. While the past decade has witnessed a significant decline in the incidence of CLABSI (from 3.64 to 1.65 infections per 1000 central line days in ICU patients, between 2001 and 2009),[30,31] estimates from 2009 suggest that there were still approximately 23,000 CLABSIs among hospitalized patients in the United States.[32] A meta-analysis found that a CLABSI led to a nearly threefold increase in the odds of in-hospital death.[33] In addition, CLABSI is associated with longer lengths of hospital stay and increased costs—the annual national cost associated with these infections has been estimated to be as much as $2.7 billion.[34] Recommended practices to prevent central line infections are outlined in Table 10-2.[35]

The prevention of CLABSI has been one of the great success stories of the patient safety movement. Analyzing the history of this success is instructive, as it is built on a series of small-scale, then increasingly ambitious, interventions—interventions that blended tools and recommended practices with change and measurement strategies.

First, of course, came the science: identifying a series of evidence-based practices that each reduced the incidence of CLABSI, and had an even more powerful effect when bundled together. Next, Berenholtz et al. demonstrated that high rates of adherence to these practices (Table 10-2) led to a near-zero rate of CLABSI in the ICUs at Johns Hopkins Hospital.[36] This was followed by the *Keystone Project*, in which widespread implementation of this bundle of practices in more than 100 ICUs in Michigan resulted in a breathtaking 66% reduction in CLABSIs over 18 months, a result sustained over 18 additional months.[37,38] A recent 10-year analysis demonstrated sustained reductions in CLABSIs in 121 ICUs across 73 hospitals in Michigan, with a decrease in mean rate of CLABSI from 2.5 infections/1000 catheter days in 2004 to 0.76 in 2013 (Figure 10-1).[39]

While the results in Michigan have famously been attributed to the use of a checklist that prompted the providers to adhere to the recommended practices,[40] the Hopkins-based investigators and colleagues have taken pains to highlight the importance of co-interventions aimed at improving teamwork, leadership, and culture (Chapter 15).[41,42] An analysis of the Michigan experience led by the British sociologist Mary Dixon-Woods is a masterful guide to understanding the pathophysiology of change in complex organizations.[42] Dixon-Woods and her coworkers proposed a

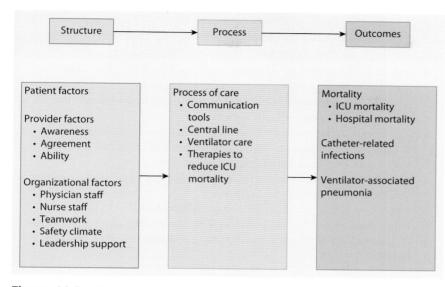

Figure 10-2 ▪ The conceptual model for the Michigan study. (Reproduced with permission from Dixon-Woods M, Bosk CL, Aveling EL, Goeschel CA, Pronovost PJ. Explaining Michigan: developing an ex post theory of a quality improvement program. *Milbank Q* 2011;89:167–205.)

conceptual model (Figure 10-2) and six macrolevel key success factors to "explain Michigan" (Table 10-3). Anyone interested in promoting large-scale change in complex systems of care would do well to read this analysis, as well as the lessons from a subsequent, and unsuccessful, UK-based effort to "match Michigan."[43]

Moving from the macro/sociopolitical to the bedside, the Michigan investigators did a number of things right here as well. Institutions that have made major gains in hand hygiene often empower nurses (and patients or families; Chapter 21) to question those entering patient rooms about whether they've cleaned their hands, and the Michigan team encouraged this kind of culture change.[44] The use of maximal sterile barrier precautions prior to line insertion, which has been strongly associated with lower infection rates,[45] was facilitated by the availability of a dedicated cart containing all the necessary equipment (a human factors intervention; Chapter 7). Importantly, although removal of central lines at the earliest possible date is a key preventive strategy (and should be encouraged by a daily team discussion of the risks and benefits of continued central access), routine line replacement (either by a new line at a fresh site or by a line placed over a guidewire at the same site) does not result in fewer catheter-related infections, and was not part of the intervention.[46]

Table 10-3   **PROPOSED MECHANISMS BY WHICH THE MICHIGAN KEYSTONE PROJECT ACHIEVED ITS SUCCESSES**

1. It generated isomorphic pressures (the desire to conform to a group norm) for ICUs to join the program and conform to its requirements
2. It created a densely networked community with strong horizontal links that exerted normative pressure on its members
3. It reframed catheter-associated bloodstream infections as a social problem and addressed it through a professional movement that combined "grassroots" features and a vertically integrating program structure
4. It used several interventions that functioned in different ways to shape a culture of commitment to doing better in practice
5. It harnessed data on infection rates as a disciplinary force
6. It used "hard edges" (i.e., the leaders were not afraid to be tough at times, using "activist tactics," and threatening sanctions against laggards) when they were needed

Adapted from Dixon-Woods M, Bosk CL, Aveling EL, Goeschel CA, Pronovost PJ. Explaining Michigan: developing an ex post theory of a quality improvement program. *Milbank Q* 2011;89:167–205.

The Keystone Project is an important model for successfully implementing patient safety practices on a broad scale, accompanied by rigorous measures of effectiveness. One of the key questions for the safety field going forward is whether the factors that led to Michigan's success can be replicated in other venues, under different circumstances, and for other safety targets. We offer our assessment of this provocative issue in Table 10-4.

CATHETER-ASSOCIATED URINARY TRACT INFECTIONS

Urinary tract infections are the most common HAIs, accounting for about 40% of HAIs in the United States. The vast majority are associated with indwelling urinary catheters, and the duration of catheterization is the biggest risk factor for infection.[47] Although more common than VAP and CLABSI, catheter-associated urinary tract infections (CAUTIs) are less often fatal, and thus have received less attention in the patient safety and infection control literatures. But they have received more notice in the past decade, particularly after they were included on Medicare's "no pay" list in 2008 (Appendix VIII) and, in 2012, became the subject of a Joint Commission National Patient Safety Goal (Appendix IV).

The strategies for preventing healthcare-associated urinary tract infections are similar to those used to prevent central line infections. Specifically,

Table 10-4 SUCCESS FACTORS IN MICHIGAN, AND QUESTIONS REGARDING THEIR GENERALIZABILITY*	
Factor at Play in Michigan	**Questions Regarding Generalizability**
The target (CLABSI) was one in which a relatively small number of evidence-based practices resulted in near 100% preventability	For many other safety targets, the interventions are more complex and preventability is lower (often 30–50%). Seeing clear evidence that one's interventions are paying off creates momentum, which may be harder to achieve with less preventable targets, such as falls or medication errors
The target (CLABSI) was unambiguously measurable, leaving little debate about rates or opportunity for gaming	Many other targets (falls with harm, VAP) have more ambiguous definitions, leading to the possibility that different measurement strategies will influence the results. Some potential targets, such as diagnostic errors, are not measurable without very expensive chart review (and even then, not very accurately)
A medium-sized state with a strong hospital association and some history of cross-hospital collaborations	Many states or networks lack this tradition and leadership
A team of investigators from another state	Many projects will be run by local personnel, who may have the advantage of insider's insight but lack the cachet of the outside expert
In particular, the outside group was from a prestigious academic medical center, and its leader was an accomplished and well-known figure nationally	All of this gave the study considerable luster, which helped with participation and adherence. Most projects will not have these advantages
Grant funding, from local and national funders	Many projects will lack sufficient financial resources to carry out all the necessary tasks, including training, data gathering and feedback, meetings, and more

*Authors' own analysis.

in patients with indwelling catheters, maintaining a closed drainage system, using aseptic technique during insertion and maintenance, providing appropriate catheter care, and removing the catheter as quickly as possible are all beneficial.[47,48] Saint et al. have demonstrated that historically, nearly one-third of hospital doctors were unaware that their patient even had a Foley catheter.[49] In a systematic review, Saint and colleagues describe evidence supporting the use of automatic stop orders and reminders to ensure that catheters are removed when they are no longer needed.[50] Studies regarding the use of both silver alloy- and antibacterial-coated urinary catheters have produced conflicting results,[51–53] and they are not recommended for routine use.[6] In men, condom catheters are safer than indwelling catheters.[54]

In the last few years, significant progress has been made in CAUTI prevention. A 2016 study demonstrated that implementation of a multicomponent intervention in 603 hospitals across 32 states achieved marked success in decreased urinary catheter usage and CAUTI rates in non-ICU patients.[55] In another article, authors describe in greater detail the implementation efforts, include multistakeholder collaborations, associated with a large national program to reduce CAUTIs.[56]

METHICILLIN-RESISTANT *S. AUREUS* INFECTION

The four infections reviewed so far—surgical site infections, CLABSI, VAP, and CAUTI—were considered the main infectious targets of the patient safety field until recently. The four comprise the majority of HAIs, tend to strike very sick patients, and are, to varying degrees, preventable. In the past decade, MRSA and *C. difficile* (Table 10-2) have been added to this list, since many of the prevention strategies are similar and these infections are becoming subject to the same kinds of policy maneuvers—public reporting of rates, inclusion among accreditation standards, and, in some cases, financial penalties—as the other HAIs.

MRSA is the most common multidrug-resistant organism in U.S. hospitals and, according to recent estimates, is responsible for over 50% of CLABSIs, almost 60% of CAUTIs, almost 50% of VAPs, and just over 40% of surgical site infections.[57] Infections with MRSA carry a significantly higher mortality rate than infections with methicillin-sensitive *S. aureus*.[58] While there is a general consensus regarding several of the prevention strategies for MRSA (hand hygiene, contact precautions, recognizing and isolating previously colonized patients, selective surveillance and rapid reporting of MRSA lab results, and engaging caregivers in prevention efforts), there is considerable controversy surrounding the role of screening newly admitted hospital patients for nasal carriage of MRSA ("active surveillance").[59–61] Notwithstanding the controversy within the scientific community, multiple U.S. states have mandated active screening at hospital admission, a dangerous intrusion of the political process into a clinical area in which the evidence remains unsettled.

Probably the most impressive MRSA prevention effort to date was reported by the Veterans Affairs (VA) system in 2011.[62] The VA implemented an MRSA bundle, consisting of universal nasal surveillance for MRSA, contact precautions for patients found to be infected or colonized, promotion of hand hygiene, and efforts to create a culture in which all staff members took responsibility for infection control. Fourteen percent of patients were found to be colonized or infected at the time of admission. (Importantly, there were no recommendations to try to decolonize patients who tested positive with either topical mupirocin or chlorhexidine baths; there is no good evidence that either strategy improves outcomes.[63,64]) Over two years, the VA's ICU MRSA infection rate fell by 62% (from 1.64 infections per 1000 patient-days to 0.62), and the non-ICU rate fell by 45% (0.47 per 1000 patient-days to 0.26).

Before we get too excited about having identified the magic bullet—or bundle—it is worth noting, with frustration, that another large MRSA prevention trial, reported in the same issue of the *New England Journal of Medicine*, found no impact on infection rates[65] despite employing a similar array of activities. For now, the optimal approach to surveillance remains up in the air, pending additional research.[66] Many institutions follow a strategy of selective active surveillance (sometime required by state law), focusing on high-risk patients such as those admitted to the ICU or receiving chronic hemodialysis.

C. DIFFICILE INFECTION

C. difficile is the most common cause of infectious diarrhea in hospitalized patients, and both its incidence and severity have increased in recent years.[67] It is associated with substantial morbidity and mortality; a 2014 study found that the incidence of *C. difficile* in hospitalized patients nearly doubled from 2001 to 2010, and the mortality rate increased from 6.6% to 7.2% during that same period,[68] perhaps as the result of a true increase as well as increasingly sensitive diagnostics (which may contribute to overdiagnosis). It is well established that *C. difficile* is associated with increased length of stay and healthcare costs.[69]

The mainstays of prevention are strict contact precautions, hand hygiene (most authorities recommend the use of traditional hand washing with soap and water, rather than alcohol hand gels, which do not kill the organism), cleaning and disinfecting rooms and equipment, and *antibiotic stewardship*.[70] The latter is vital since the main risk factor for *C. difficile* is prior antibiotic use, and decreasing unnecessary use will not only prevent this infection but also decrease antibiotic resistance. The mainstays of antibiotic stewardship are: avoid prolonged use of empiric antibiotics, narrow the spectrum of antibiotics whenever possible, and discontinue antibiotics promptly when appropriate.[71] Boston's Brigham and Women's Hospital combined an educational campaign, a prevention bundle (including newly designed "Contact Precautions Plus" signs for the doors of patients with *C. difficile*, Figure 10-3), and a treatment bundle (which guides the use of metronidazole or oral vancomycin, as well as the need for abdominal imaging and consultation), and saw a 40% decrease in the incidence of *C. difficile*.[72]

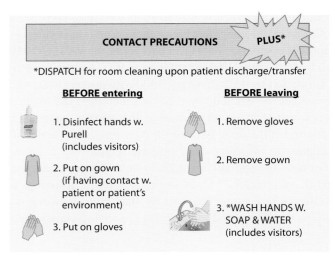

Figure 10-3 ■ The Contact Precautions Plus sign, developed by Brigham and Women's Hospital, to be displayed outside the room of patients with *C. difficile* infection. (Reproduced with permission from Abbett SK, Yokoe DS, Lipsitz SR, et al. Proposed checklist of hospital interventions to decrease the incidence of healthcare-associated *Clostridium difficile* infection. *Infect Control Hosp Epidemiol* 2009;30:1062–1069.)

WHAT CAN PATIENT SAFETY LEARN FROM THE APPROACH TO HOSPITAL-ASSOCIATED INFECTIONS?

As a relatively nascent field, patient safety has looked outside of healthcare—to fields such as commercial aviation, clinical psychology, informatics, and engineering—for many of its lessons and guiding principles (Chapter 1). However, the patient safety movement can also learn from the much older fields of infection control and hospital epidemiology. Former CDC director Julie Gerberding made this important point in 2002, in the early years of the patient safety movement:

> *Precise and valid definitions of infection-related adverse events, standardized methods for detecting and reporting events, confidentiality protections, appropriate rate adjustments for institutional and case-mix differences, and evidence-based intervention programs come to mind. Perhaps most important, reliance on skilled professionals to promote ongoing improvements in care has contributed to the 30-year track record of success in infection prevention and control.*
>
> *Analogously, in approaching patient safety, standard definitions should be used as much as possible when discussing adverse events and preventability. Healthcare organizations should be encouraged to*

pool data on adverse events in a central repository to permit bench-marking, and such data should be appropriately adjusted and reported. Finally, institutions should consider hiring dedicated, trained patient safety officers (comparable to infection control practitioners) ....[73]

KEY POINTS

- Since the start of the patient safety movement, infection control activities have been considered a subset of patient safety, implying that many HAIs are best seen as preventable adverse events caused by medical errors (failure to adhere to evidence-based prevention strategies).
- Many surgical site infections can be prevented by appropriate use of prophylactic antibiotics, clipping rather than shaving the surgical site, maintaining perioperative normothermia and reasonable postoperative glucose control.
- Many cases of VAP can be prevented by elevating the head of the bed and by strategies designed to minimize the duration of mechanical ventilation (particularly daily interruption of sedation).
- Many cases of CLABSIs and CAUTIs can be prevented by rigorous hand hygiene, strict infection control procedures at the time of insertion, and removal of the foreign bodies at the earliest possible time. The Keystone Project, which demonstrated major reductions in CLABSI rates across Michigan ICUs, is one of the striking successes of the field of patient safety.
- MRSA and *C. difficile* infection are considered largely preventable HAIs, and thus fair game for the kinds of policy pressures that we've seen with the other HAIs.
- The still-young field of patient safety can learn much from the older fields of hospital epidemiology and infection control, particularly the use of standardized definitions, the importance of data collection and analysis, and the key role of professionals to monitor safety problems and implement safe practices.

REFERENCES

1. Centers for Disease Control and Prevention. *HAIs at a Glance; Centers for Disease Control and Prevention*. Available at: http://www.cdc.gov/hai/surveillance/.
2. Scott RD II, Sinkowitz-Cochran R, Wide ME, et al. CDC central-line bloodstream infection prevention efforts produced net benefits of at least $640 million during 1990-2008. *Health Aff (Millwood)* 2014;33:1040–1047.
3. Wachter RM, Foster NE, Dudley RA. Medicare's decision to withhold payment for hospital errors: the devil is in the details. *Jt Comm J Qual Patient Saf* 2008;34:116–123.

4. Sacks GD, Diggs BS, Hadjizacharia P, Green D, Salim A, Malinoski DJ. Reducing the rate of catheter-associated bloodstream infections in a surgical intensive care unit using the Institute for Healthcare Improvement Central Line Bundle. *Am J Surg* 2014;207:817–823.

5. Saint S, Kowalski CP, Banaszak-Holl J, Forman J, Damschroder L, Krein SL. How active resisters and organizational constipators affect health care–acquired infection prevention efforts. *Jt Comm J Qual Patient Saf* 2009;35:239–246.

6. Yokoe DS, Anderson DJ, Berenholtz SM, et al. A compendium of strategies to prevent healthcare-associated infections in acute care hospitals: 2014 updates. *Infect Control Hosp Epidemiol* 2014;35(Supple 2):S21–S31.

7. Lautenbach E, Woeltje KF, Malani PN. *Practical Healthcare Epidemiology*. 3rd ed. Chicago, IL: University of Chicago Press; 2010.

8. Jarvis WR. *Bennett & Brachman's Hospital Infections*. 6th ed. Philadelphia, PA: Lippincott Williams & Wilkins; 2014.

9. Mauger Rothenberg B, Marella A, Pines E, Chopra R, Black ER, Aronson N. Closing the quality gap: revisiting the state of the science (vol. 6: prevention of healthcare-associated infections). Evidence Report/Technology Assessment 208. Rockville, MD: Agency for Healthcare Research and Quality; 2012. AHRQ Publication No. 12(13)-E012-EF.

10. de Lissovoy G, Fraeman K, Hutchins V, Murphy D, Song D, Vaughn BB. Surgical site infection: incidence and impact on hospital utilization and treatment costs. *Am J Infect Control* 2009;37:387–397.

11. Anderson DJ, Podgomy K, Berrios-Torres SI, et al. Strategies to prevent surgical site infections in acute care hospitals: 2014 update. *Infect Control Hosp Epidemiol* 2014;35(Suppl 2):S66–S88.

12. Van den Berghe G, Wouters P, Weekers F, et al. Intensive insulin therapy in the critically ill patients. *N Engl J Med* 2001;345:1359–1367.

13. Gandhi GY, Nuttall GA, Abel MD, et al. Intensive intraoperative insulin therapy versus conventional glucose management during cardiac surgery: a randomized trial. *Ann Intern Med* 2007;146(4):233–243.

14. Klompas M, Branson R, Eichenwald EC, et al. Strategies to prevent ventilator-associated pneumonia in acute care hospitals: 2014 update. *Infect Control Hosp Epidemiol* 2014;35(Suppl 2):S133–S154.

15. Keeley L. Reducing the risk of ventilator-acquired pneumonia through head of bed elevation. *Nurs Crit Care* 2007;12:287–294.

16. van Nieuwenhoven CA, Vandenbroucke-Grauls C, van Tiel FH, et al. Feasibility and effects of the semirecumbent position to prevent ventilator-associated pneumonia: a randomized study. *Crit Care Med* 2006;34:396–402.

17. Klompas M. Potential strategies to prevent ventilator-associated events. *Am J Respir Crit Care Med* 2015;192:1420–1430.

18. Girard TD, Kress JP, Fuchs BD, et al. Efficacy and safety of a paired sedation and ventilator weaning protocol for mechanically ventilated patients in intensive care (Awakening and Breathing controlled trial): a randomised controlled trial. *Lancet*. 2008;371:126–134.

19. Klompas M, Li L, Kleinman K, Szumita PM, Massaro AF. Associations between ventilator bundle components and outcomes. *JAMA Intern Med* 2016;176:1277–1283.

20. Labeau SO, Vyver VD, Brusselaers N, Vogelaers D, Blot SI. Prevention of ventilator-associated pneumonia with oral antiseptics: a systematic review and meta-analysis. *Lancet Infect Dis* 2011;11:845–854.

21. Klompas M, Speck K, Howell MD, Greene LR, Berenholtz SM. Reappraisal of routine oral care with chlorhexidine gluconate for patients receiving mechanical ventilation: systematic review and meta-analysis. *JAMA Intern Med* 2014;174(5):751–761.

22. Muscedere J, Rewa O, McKechnie K, Jiang X, Laporta D, Heyland DK. Subglottic secretion drainage for the prevention of ventilator-associated pneumonia: a systematic review and meta-analysis. *Crit Care Med* 2011;39:1985–1991.

23. Afessa B, Shorr AF, Anzueto A, Craven DE, Schinner R, Kollef MH. Association between a silver-coated endotracheal tube and reduced mortality in patients with ventilator-associated pneumonia. *Chest* 2010;137:1015–1021.

24. Magill SS, Fridkin SK. Improving surveillance definitions for ventilator-associated pneumonia in an era of public reporting and performance measurement. *Clin Infect Dis* 2012;54:378–380.

25. Metersky ML, Wang Y, Klompas M, Eckenrode S, Bakullari A, Eldridge N. Trend in ventilator-associated pneumonia rates between 2005 and 2013. *JAMA* 2016;316:2427–2429.

26. Amin A, Kollef MH. Health care-associated pneumonia. *Hosp Pract (Minneap)* 2010;38:63–74.

27. Kalil AC, Metersky ML, Klompas M, et al. Executive summary: management of adults with hospital-acquired and ventilator-associated pneumonia: 2016 clinical practice guideline by the Infectious Disease Society of America and the American Thoracic Society. *Clin Infect Dis* 2016;63:575–582.

28. Klompas M, Anderson D, Trick W, et al. The preventability of ventilator-associated events. The CDC prevention epicenters wake up and breathe collaborative. *Am J Respir Crit Care Med* 2015;191:292–301.

29. Magill SS, Klompas M, Balk R, et al. Developing a new, national approach to surveillance for ventilator-associated events. *Crit Care Med* 2013;41:2467–2475.

30. Centers for Disease Control and Prevention. Vital signs: central line-associated blood stream infections—United States 2001, 2008, and 2009. *MMWR Morb Mortal Wkly Rep* 2011;60:243–248.

31. Fagan RP, Edwards JR, Park BJ, Fridkin SK, Magill SS. Incidence trends in pathogen-specific central line-associated bloodstream infections in US intensive care units, 1990-2010. *Infect Control Hosp Epidemiol* 2013;34:893–899.

32. Centers for Disease Control and Prevention. Vital signs: central line-associated blood stream infections—United States 2001, 2008, and 2009. *MMWR Morb Mortal Wkly Rep* 2011;60:243–248.

33. Ziegler MJ, Pellegrini DC, Safdar N. Attributable mortality of central line associated bloodstream infection: systematic review and meta-analysis. *Infection* 2015;43: 29–36.

34. Chopra V, Krein SL, Olmsted RN, et al. Prevention of Central Line-Associated Bloodstream Infections: Brief Update Review. In: *Making Health Care Safer II: An Updated Critical Analysis of the Evidence for Patient Safety Practices*. Shekelle PG, Wachter RM, Pronovost PJ, eds. Rockville, MD: Agency for Healthcare Research and Quality; March 2013. (Evidence Reports/Technology Assessments, No. 211) Chapter 10. Available at: http://www.ncbi.nlm.nih.gov/books/NBK133364/.

35. Marschall J, Mermel LA, Fakih M, et al. Strategies to prevent central line-associated bloodstream infections in acute care hospitals: 2014 update. *Infect Control Hosp Epidemiol* 2014;35(Suppl 2):S89–S107.

36. Berenholtz SM, Pronovost PJ, Lipsett PA, et al. Eliminating catheter-related bloodstream infections in the intensive care unit. *Crit Care Med* 2004;32:2014–2020.

37. Pronovost P, Needham D, Berenholtz S, et al. An intervention to decrease catheter-related bloodstream infections in the ICU. *N Engl J Med* 2006;355:2725–2732.

38. Pronovost PJ, Goeschel CA, Colantuoni E, et al. Sustaining reductions in catheter related bloodstream infections in Michigan intensive care units: observational study. *BMJ* 2010;340:c309.

39. Pronovost PJ, Watson SR, Goeschel CA, Hyzy RC, Berenholtz SM. Sustaining reductions in central line-associated bloodstream infections in Michigan intensive care units: a 10-year analysis. *Am J Med Qual* 2016;31:197–202.

40. Gawande A. *The Checklist Manifesto: How to Get Things Right.* New York, NY: Metropolitan Books; 2009.

41. Bosk CL, Dixon-Woods M, Goeschel CA, Pronovost PJ. Reality check for checklists. *Lancet* 2009;374:444–445.

42. Dixon-Woods M, Bosk CL, Aveling EL, Goeschel CA, Pronovost PJ. Explaining Michigan: developing an ex post theory of a quality improvement program. *Milbank Q* 2011;89:167–205.

43. Dixon-Woods M, Leslie M, Tarrant C, Bion J. Explaining matching Michigan: an ethnographic study of a patient safety program. *J Implement Sci* 2013;8:70.

44. Gawande A. *Better: A Surgeon's Notes on Performance.* New York, NY: Metropolitan Books; 2007.

45. Hu KK, Lipsky BA, Veenstra DL, Saint S. Using maximal sterile barriers to prevent central venous catheter-related infection: a systematic evidence-based review. *Am J Infect Control* 2004;32:142–146.

46. Cook D, Randolph A, Kernerman P, et al. Central venous catheter replacement strategies: a systematic review of the literature. *Crit Care Med* 1997;25:1417–1424.

47. Lo E, Nicolle LE, Coffin SE, et al. Strategies to prevent catheter-associated urinary tract infections in acute care hospitals: 2014 update. *Infect Control Hosp Epidemiol* 2014;35(Suppl 2):S32–S47.

48. Rebmann T, Greene LR. Preventing catheter-associated urinary tract infections: an executive summary of the Association for Professionals in Infection Control and Epidemiology, Inc, Elimination Guide. *Am J Infect Control* 2010;38:644–646.

49. Saint S, Wiese J, Amory JK, et al. Are physicians aware of which of their patients have indwelling urinary catheters? *Am J Med* 2000;109:476–480.

50. Meddings J, Rogers MA, Krein SL, Fakih MG, Olmstead RN, Saint S. Reducing unnecessary urinary catheter use and other strategies to prevent catheter-associated urinary tract infection: an integrative review. *BMJ Qual Saf* 2014;23:277–289.

51. Saint S, Veenstra DL, Sullivan SD, Chenoweth C, Fendrick AM. The potential clinical and economic benefits of silver alloy urinary catheters in preventing urinary tract infection. *Arch Intern Med* 2000;160:2670–2675.

52. Johnson JR, Kuskowski MA, Wilt TJ. Systematic review: antimicrobial urinary catheters to prevent catheter-associated urinary tract infection in hospitalized patients. *Ann Intern Med* 2006;144:116–126.

53. Pickard R, Lam T, MacLennan G, et al. Antimicrobial catheters for reduction of symptomatic urinary tract infections in adults requiring short-term catheterization in hospital: a multicenter randomized controlled trial. *Lancet* 2012;380:1927–1935.

54. Saint S, Kaufman SR, Rogers MA, Baker PD, Ossenkop K, Lipsky BA. Condom versus indwelling urinary catheters: a randomized trial. *J Am Geriatr Soc* 2006;54:1055–1061.

55. Saint S, Greene MT, Krein SL, et al. A program to prevent catheter-associated urinary track infection in acute care. *N Engl J Med* 2016;374:2111–2119.

56. Fakih MG, George C, Edson BS, Goeschel CA, Saint S. Implementing a national program to reduce catheter-associated urinary tract infection: a quality improvement collaboration of state hospital associations, academic medical centers, professional societies and governmental agencies. *Infect Control Hosp Epidemiol* 2013;34:1048–1054.

57. Calfee DP, Salgado CD, Milstone AM, et al. Strategies to prevent methicillin-resistant Staphylococcus aureus transmission and infection in acute care hospitals: 2014 update. *Infect Control Hosp Epidemiol* 2014;35(Suppl 2):S108–S132.

58. Cosgrove SE, Sakoulas G, Perencevich EN, Schwaber MJ, Karchmer AW, Carmeli Y. Comparison of mortality associated with methicillin-resistant and methicillin-susceptible Staphylococcus aureus bacteremia: a meta-analysis. *Clin Infect Dis* 2003;36:53–59.

59. Harbarth S, Fankhauser C, Screnzel J, et al. Universal screening for methicillin-resistant Staphylococcus aureus at hospital admission and nosocomial infection in surgical patients. *JAMA* 2008;229:1149–1157.

60. Robicsek A, Beaumont JL, Paule SM, et al. Universal surveillance for methicillin-resistant Staphylococcus aureus in 3 affiliated hospitals. *Ann Intern Med* 2008;148:409–418.

61. Cohen Al, Calfee D, Fridkin SK, et al. Recommendations for metrics for multidrug-resistant organisms in healthcare settings: SHEA/HICPAC position paper. *Infect Control Hosp Epidemiol* 2008;29:901–913.

62. Jain R, Kralovic SM, Evans ME, et al. Veterans Affairs initiative to prevent methicillin-resistant Staphylococcus aureus infections. *N Engl J Med* 2011;364:1419–1430.

63. Hebert C, Robicsek A. Decolonization therapy in infection control. *Curr Opin Infect Dis* 2010;23:340–345.

64. Robicsek A, Beaumont JL, Thomson RB Jr, Govindarajan G, Peterson LR. Topical therapy for methicillin-resistant Staphylococcus aureus colonization: impact on infection risk. *Infect Control Hosp Epidemiol* 2009;30:623–632.

65. Huskins WC, Huckabee CM, O'Grady NP, et al. STAR*ICU Trial Investigators. Intervention to reduce transmission of resistant bacteria in intensive care. *N Engl J Med* 2011;364:1407–1418.

66. Platt R. Time for a culture change? *N Engl J Med* 2011;364:1464–1465.

67. Zilberberg MD, Shorr AF, Kollef MH. Increase in adult Clostridium difficile related hospitalizations and case-fatality rate, United States, 2000–2005. *Emerg Infect Dis* 2008;14:929–931.

68. Reveles KR, Lee GC, Boyd NK, Frei CR. The rise in *Clostridium difficile* infection incidence among hospitalized adults in the United States: 2001-2010. *Am J Infect Control* 2014;42:1028–1032.

69. Dubberke ER, Olsen MA. Burden of Clostridium difficile on the healthcare system. *Clin Infect Dis* 2012;55:S88–S92.

70. Dubberke ER, Carling P, Carrico R, et al. Strategies to prevent Clostridium difficile infections in acute care hospitals: 2014 update. *Infect Control Hosp Epidemiol* 2014;35(Suppl 2):S48–S65.

71. Rebmann T, Carrico RM. Association for Professionals in Infection Control and Epidemiology. Preventing Clostridium difficile infections: an executive summary of the Association for Professionals in Infection Control and Epidemiology's elimination guide. *Am J Infect Control* 2011;39:239–242.

72. Abbett SK, Yokoe DS, Lipsitz SR, et al. Proposed checklist of hospital interventions to decrease the incidence of healthcare-associated Clostridium difficile infection. *Infect Control Hosp Epidemiol* 2009;30:1062–1069.

73. Gerberding JL. Hospital-onset infections: a patient safety issue. *Ann Intern Med* 2002;137:665–670.

ADDITIONAL READINGS

Allegranzi B, Bischoff P, de Jonge S, et al. New WHO recommendations on preoperative measures for surgical site infection prevention: an evidence-based global perspective. *Lancet Infect Dis* 2016;16:e276–e287.

Allegranzi B, Zayed B, Bischoff P, et al. New WHO recommendations on intraoperative and postoperative measures for surgical site infection prevention: an evidence-based global perspective. *Lancet Infect Dis* 2016;16:e288–e303.

Fan CJ, Pawlik TM, Daniels T, et al. Association of safety culture with surgical site infection outcomes. *J Am Coll Surg* 2016;222:122–128.

Hugonnet S, Chevrolet JC, Pittet D. The effect of workload on infection risk in critically ill patients. *Crit Care Med* 2007;35:76–81.

Jeeva RR, Wright D. Healthcare-associated infections: a national patient safety problem and coordinated response. *Med Care* 2014;52:S4–S8.

Lee GM, Kleinman K, Soumerai SB, et al. Effect of nonpayment for preventable infections in U.S. hospitals. *N Engl J Med* 2012;367:1428–1437.

Lin MY, Hota B, Khan YM, et al.; CDC Prevention Epicenter Program. Quality of traditional surveillance for public reporting of nosocomial bloodstream infection rates. *JAMA* 2010;304:2035–2041.

Magill SS, Edwards JR, Bamberg W, et al.; Emerging Infections Program Healthcare-Associated Infections and Antimicrobial Use Prevalence Survey Team. Multistate point-prevalence survey of health care-associated infections. *N Engl J Med* 2014; 370:1198–1208.

Stelfox HT, Bates DW, Redelmeier DA. Safety of patients isolated for infection control. *JAMA* 2003;290:1899–1905.

Stulberg JJ, Delaney CP, Neuhauser DV, Aron DC, Fu P, Korukian SM. Adherence to Surgical Care Improvement Project measures and the association with postoperative infections. *JAMA* 2010;303:2479–2485.

Umscheid CA, Mitchell MD, Doshi JA, Agarwal R, Williams K, Brennan PJ. Estimating the proportion of healthcare-associated infections that are reasonably preventable and the related mortality and costs. *Infect Control Hosp Epidemiol* 2011;32:101–114.

Waters HR, Korn R Jr, Colantuoni E, et al. The business case for quality: economic analysis of the Michigan Keystone Patient Safety Program in ICUs. *Am J Med Qual* 2011;26:333–339.

Zimlichman E, Henderson D, Tamir O, et al. Health care-associated infections: a meta-analysis of costs and financial impact on the US health care system. *JAMA Intern Med* 2013;173:2039–2046.

OTHER COMPLICATIONS OF HEALTHCARE

11

GENERAL CONCEPTS

As with healthcare-associated infections (Chapter 10), the patient safety movement has broadened the concept of "adverse event" to include outcomes such as patient falls, delirium, pressure ulcers, and venous thromboembolism (VTE) occurring in healthcare facilities. The rationale for this inclusion is that the strategies to prevent these complications of medical care are similar to those used to prevent other harms. Such strategies include education, culture change, audit and feedback, improved teamwork, and the use of checklists and bundles.

Moreover, as a practical matter, inclusion of these complications under the broad umbrella of patient safety has increased their visibility, making available more resources to combat them. It has also facilitated their inclusion within policy initiatives being used to promote safety. For example, postoperative VTE is on the Agency for Healthcare Research and Quality (AHRQ) Patient Safety Indicators list (Appendix V), and is included among the preventable adverse events that are no longer reimbursed by Medicare (Appendix VIII).[1]

This chapter will highlight a few key complications of healthcare and the strategies that can help prevent them. Strategies to prevent readmissions and other handoff-related adverse events are covered in Chapter 8.

PREVENTING VENOUS THROMBOEMBOLISM

Hospitalized or institutionalized patients often have conditions that place them at high risk for VTE, including inactivity, comorbid diseases and conditions that increase the risk of clotting (e.g., cancer, nephrotic syndrome, heart failure, recent surgery), and indwelling catheters. Moreover, because such patients often have limited cardiopulmonary reserve, a pulmonary embolism (PE) can be quite consequential, even fatal. In fact, autopsy studies have shown that among patients dying in the hospital, PE remains among the most frequently missed diagnoses.[2,3]

The risk of VTE in a hospitalized patient is hard to determine with certainty, because it varies widely depending on the ascertainment method. Studies relying on clinical diagnosis have found rates of 20% for deep venous thrombosis and 1% to 2% for PE after major surgical procedures in the absence of prophylaxis. Rates after certain orthopedic procedures are even higher. Studies using more aggressive observational methods (i.e., Doppler ultrasounds on every postoperative patient) have found much higher rates. It is not known how many of these asymptomatic clots would have caused clinical problems, but surely some would have.

A detailed review of strategies to prevent VTE is beyond the scope of this chapter; the interested reader is referred to a number of excellent reviews, particularly the regularly updated guidelines published by the American College of Chest Physicians (ACCP).[4,5] Instead, in keeping with the patient safety focus on systems, our emphasis will be on creating systems that ensure that every eligible patient receives appropriate, evidence-based prophylaxis.

Given the complexity of the VTE prophylaxis decision (which varies by patient group and clinical situation, and changes rapidly with new research and pharmacologic agents), it seems unlikely that physician education, the traditional approach, is the best strategy to ensure that research is translated into practice. Rather, the emphasis should be on developing standardized protocols, through order sets and similar mechanisms and, when possible, building these protocols into clinical decision support systems (Chapter 13). In fact, ACCP guidelines strongly recommend that "every hospital develop a formal strategy that addresses the prevention of VTE."[4,5]

In a study of 2500 hospitalized patients, half the patients received standard care, while the other half's physicians received a computerized notice of their patient's risk of thromboembolism. The latter group was required to acknowledge the notice and then explicitly choose to withhold prophylaxis or order it (graduated compression stockings, pneumatic boots, unfractionated or low-molecular-weight heparin, or warfarin). Physicians receiving the alerts were far more likely to order appropriate prophylaxis, and the rates of clinically diagnosed deep venous thrombosis or PE fell by 41% in their patients.[6] Two ICU-based studies reported on the adoption of a series of tools that promoted team communication, prompted clinicians with evidence-based recommendations for ICU prophylaxis (for VTE and other targets including ventilator-associated pneumonia and stress ulcers), and gave clinicians real-time feedback on their performance. Both studies found significant improvements in the use of evidence-based prophylaxis.[7,8] A recent review concluded that while many interventions are effective in preventing VTE to varying degrees, active tools, such as computerized VTE prophylaxis alerts, are more likely to succeed than passive ones. Of course, for alerts to work well, they must be thoughtfully integrated into provider workflow.[9] Another analysis found that many patients diagnosed with VTE while hospitalized had been prescribed prophylaxis appropriately but did not receive all doses.[10] This study highlights the importance of measuring what matters – in this case, the actual receipt of prophylaxis, rather than just the prescription.

As with many patient safety targets, moving from local improvement strategies to national reporting and payment changes involves some complexity. Many national programs determine the presence of VTE based on hospital administrative records, largely created for billing purposes. Several studies have shown that such data lack specificity for hospital-acquired VTE, because either the thrombosis was present on admission or the coding was inaccurate, and that diagnosing VTE may be subject to significant surveillance bias.[11–13]

In addition to accuracy of coding, the issue of preventability arises when hospitals are no longer reimbursed for certain cases of VTE.[1] In one study, almost 50% of the hospitalized patients found to have VTE received what is considered to be optimal prophylaxis, suggesting that not all VTEs are preventable adverse events.[10] This is of greater concern now that diagnosis of VTE carries financial implications for hospitals. In 2014, the Centers for Medicare and Medicaid Services (CMS) began using AHRQ's Patient Safety for Selected Indicators (PSI-90) in both the Hospital-Acquired Condition (HAC) Reduction program and the Hospital Value-Based Purchasing (VBP) program—programs in which hospitals that perform poorly on the metric are financially penalized. One component of PSI-90 is PSI-12, the measure for postoperative PE or deep vein thrombosis. PSI-90 has been heavily criticized for surveillance bias associated with some of its component measures (including postoperative VTE), for inadequate risk adjustment, and for the challenges associated with accurate identification of adverse events.[14]

Streiff and Haut have argued for a reimbursement strategy in which the presence of the adverse event—VTE in this case—would lead to a chart review to determine whether the evidence-based processes were carried out; reimbursement would be withheld only if they were not.[12] Although unwieldy and expensive, such a strategy seems fairer than penalizing hospitals when they did everything right. A similar argument, of course, can be made for the other events on Medicare's "no pay" list that are only partly preventable (Appendix VIII). Of course, one must keep in mind that some adverse events initially thought to be unavoidable, such as central line-associated bloodstream infections (CLABSIs), were later proven to be completely preventable through implementation of appropriate prevention strategies. This is unlikely to be the case with VTEs.

PREVENTING PRESSURE ULCERS

Pressure ulcers—damage to skin or underlying structures caused by unrelieved pressure—cause pain, delay functional recovery, and predispose patients to local and systemic infections. It is estimated that about one in seven hospitalized patients in the United States has or develops a pressure ulcer, that 2.5 million patients are treated for pressure ulcers each year, that more than 60,000 patients die each year from complications, and that the incidence of pressure ulcers is increasing.[15]

Similar to patient falls (see Section "Preventing Falls"), the first step in preventing pressure ulcers is identifying at-risk patients with a validated risk assessment tool. A variety of such tools are available; most assess nutritional status, mobility, incontinence, and sensory deficiencies. In the United States, the most commonly used tool is the Braden Scale.[16,17] Risk should be assessed on admission (to the hospital or skilled nursing facility), then subsequently (daily, in the case of hospitalized patients). The goals of risk assessment are both overall prevention and preventing early stage pressure ulcers from becoming more severe (i.e., Stages III and IV) with deep tissue injury (Table 11-1).

These risk assessments are followed by a variety of preventive activities focused on at-risk patients. The Institute for Healthcare Improvement's (IHI) bundle includes the following strategies: daily inspection of skin from head to toe (with a special focus on high-risk locations such as sacrum, buttocks, and heels), keeping the patient dry while treating overly dry skin with moisturizers, optimizing nutrition and hydration, and minimizing pressure through frequent repositioning and the use of pressure relieving surfaces such as special beds. To date, no large-scale, methodologically strong clinical trial has defined evidence-based best practices or the degree to which pressure ulcers are truly preventable. Systematic reviews suggest that implementation of multicomponent interventions is the most appropriate prevention strategy.[15,18]

PREVENTING FALLS

Patient falls are common—each year, more than one-third of community-dwelling elders fall—and frequently morbid. As older patients are hospitalized or institutionalized, placed on multiple medications, and often immobilized, the risk of falls grows, with a fall rate in acute care hospitals ranging from about 1 to 9 per 1000 bed-days.[19] When hospitalized patients do fall, 30% to 50% of falls result in injuries, and a substantial fraction of these injuries are serious.[19] Interestingly, when asked about what they fear during a hospitalization, adult patients rate "falling and getting hurt" as a greater concern than

Table 11-1	PRESSURE ULCER STAGING SYSTEM

Suspected deep tissue injury

Purple or maroon localized area of discolored intact skin or blood-filled blister due to damage of underlying soft tissue from pressure and/or shear. The area may be preceded by tissue that is painful, firm, mushy, boggy, warmer, or cooler as compared to adjacent tissue

Stage I

Intact skin with nonblanchable redness of a localized area usually over a bony prominence. Darkly pigmented skin may not have visible blanching; its color may differ from the surrounding area

Stage II

Partial thickness loss of dermis presenting as a shallow open ulcer with a red pink wound bed, without slough. May also present as an intact or open/ruptured serum-filled blister

Stage III

Full thickness tissue loss. Subcutaneous fat may be visible but bone, tendon, or muscle is not exposed. Slough may be present but does not obscure the depth of tissue loss. May include undermining and tunneling

Stage IV

Full thickness tissue loss with exposed bone, tendon, or muscle. Slough or eschar may be present on some parts of the wound bed. Often includes undermining and tunneling

Unstageable

Full thickness tissue loss in which the base of the ulcer is covered by slough (yellow, tan, gray, green, or brown) and/or eschar (tan, brown, or black) in the wound bed.

Reproduced with permission from National Pressure Ulcer Advisory Panel and European Pressure Ulcer Advisory Panel. *Pressure Ulcer Prevention and Treatment: Clinical Practice Guideline*. Washington, DC: National Pressure Ulcer Advisory Panel; 2014. Available at: http://www.npuap.org/resources/educational-and-clinical-resources/npuap-pressure-injury-stages/.

"being misdiagnosed," "having the wrong test or procedure done," or "being mistaken for another patient," and only a bit below "errors with your medications" and "mistakes by nurses."[20] Patients who suffer serious fall-related injuries while hospitalized cost $14,000 more and stay seven days longer than age- and disease-matched controls.[21] This cost includes only the hospital stay, not the cost of rehabilitation or of any liability payments.[22]

All institutionalized patients should formally be assessed for fall risk in a manner that incorporates both clinical judgment (usually during nurses' admission assessment) and results from a validated screening tool. It is important to note that multiple studies have produced conflicting results as to which screening tool is best. A systematic review and meta-analysis examined 51 distinct evaluations of fall risk screening tools and found that while the Morse Falls Scale and the St. Thomas Risk Assessment Tool In Falling elderlY inpatients (*STRATIFY*) tool[23] may be useful in some situations, it's not clear that either is better than nurses' clinical judgment.[24] In addition to the patient-centered risk factors captured in these tools, environmental (such as room clutter, the lack of a clear path to the door and bathroom, and having necessary items beyond the patient's reach) and extrinsic (such as polypharmacy) risk factors need to be considered.[19] A systematic review found that the best predictors of future falls were a history of falls in the past year and the presence of active gait or balance problems.[25]

Particularly in patients found to be at risk for falls, active prevention efforts should be instituted. Although the use of restraints (such as vests, bed rails, and wrist restraints) might appear to be a fall prevention strategy, evidence suggests just the opposite.[26] For this reason (as well as on ethical grounds), restraints should be used as a fall prevention strategy only as a last resort. Other important strategies include early mobilization and efforts to preserve patient strength. Using hip protectors to prevent hip fractures in high-risk patients who do fall has shown benefit in some studies but not others; their use remains controversial.[27,28] A number of other commonsensical practices have not been convincingly demonstrated to help, including the use of bed alarms to signal patient egress[29] and the use of specially padded floors (which appear to decrease harm from falls but may increase fall risk from tripping).

Camera monitoring is sometimes used for patient deemed to be high risk for falls. One study found that the use of webcams and virtual bed rail alarms was associated with fewer patient falls.[30] In some hospitals, a staff member, sometimes referred to as a "sitter," may be individually assigned to watch patients at increased risk for falls, but this intervention is expensive. A recent review of the literature on sitters suggests that their effectiveness in reducing falls is mixed at best.[31] There are some data to suggest that centralized video monitoring (patients' rooms are outfitted with a camera and an individual monitors multiple patients simultaneously from a centralized location, alerting the bedside nurse if the patient is demonstrating concerning behavior) may effectively prevent falls and cost less than one-on-one observation.[32]

In order to prevent inpatient falls, hospitals should develop and implement a program that consists of three general components: (1) screening for patient risk, (2) creating an individualized fall prevention plan for patients at risk, and (3) implementing the individualized plan, along with universal fall precautions for all patients.[19] Best practices for preventing falls in hospitalized patients are summarized in Table 11-2.

Two rigorous studies have demonstrated that fall prevention strategies truly work. In one, conducted at two Australian hospitals, patients received a comprehensive educational program, which included both written and video-based materials and follow-up by a physical therapist.[33] Falls were reduced by approximately 50% among cognitively intact patients. Importantly, simply providing the educational materials without the physical therapist follow-up carried no benefit.

Table 11-2	FALL PREVENTION BEST PRACTICES FOR HOSPITALIZED PATIENTS

Universal fall precautions for all patients:

- Evaluation of the condition of the patient's feet can identify anatomic abnormalities that can impair ability to walk securely and may also reveal need for corrective footwear
- Ensure a safe environment with room free of clutter and a clear path to the door and bathroom
- Place all necessary items (such as call light, telephone, and water) within patient's reach
- Maintain bed in proper position with wheels locked

Interventions to reduce anticipated physiological falls (*tailored to patient-specific areas of risk*):

- Previous fall: safety precautions, communicate risk status via plan of care, change of shift report, and signage, document circumstances of previous fall
- Medication adverse effects: review medications with pharmacist and physician, consider adverse effects of medications used to treat comorbidities, consider toileting schedule
- Need for assisted toileting: implement toileting/rounding schedule (assist to bathroom, assist to commode, or provide bedpan)
- Urinary incontinence/frequency: implement toileting/rounding schedule (assist to bathroom, assist to commode, or provide bedpan), ambulatory aid at bedside if appropriate, consider PT consult
- Gait instability: assist with out of bed (one or two person(s)), consider PT consult
- Lower limb weakness: assist with out of bed (one or two person(s)), consider PT consult
- Agitation, confusion, impaired judgment: turn on bed alarm/chair alarm, place patient in visible location, encourage family presence, frequent rounding

Reprinted with permission from AHRQ Patient Safety Network: Dykes PC, Leung WY, Vacca V. Falling through the crack (in the bedrails) [Spotlight]. *AHRQ WebM&M* [serial online]; May 2016. Available at: https://psnet.ahrq.gov/webmm/case/374.

The second study tested the value of a fall prevention tool kit in four teaching hospitals.[34] The tool kit, which was implemented through a sophisticated hospital information technology system, included a risk assessment, tailored fall prevention interventions aimed at both patients and different providers (Figure 11-1), and a tailored educational intervention. The results were impressive: falls in older patients were reduced by about half. The study was not sufficiently powered to detect a change in fall-related injuries. Together, these studies suggest that fall rates can be cut through thoughtful implementation of programs that include risk assessment, comprehensive multidisciplinary prevention strategies, patient education, and use of information technology.

While these successes suggest that some falls are preventable, it's important to note that the evidence around fall prevention remains controversial. A 2016 cluster randomized controlled trial across six Australian hospitals examined the impact of a bundled intervention on the rate of falls on adult inpatients and found no difference in the fall rate between control and intervention groups, even though the bundle was successfully implemented.[35]

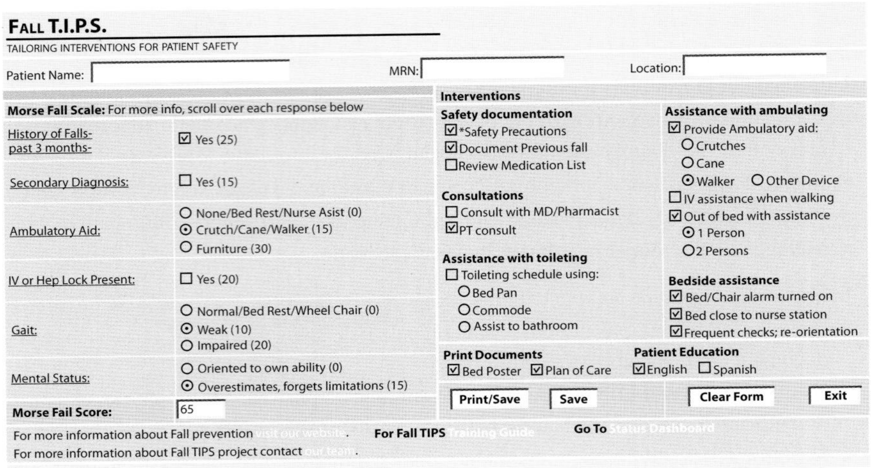

Figure 11-1 ▪ Fall prevention tool kit user interface (Reproduced with permission from Partners HealthCare System and Dykes PC, Carroll DL, Hurley A, et al. Fall prevention in acute care hospitals. A randomized trial. *JAMA* 2010;304:1912–1918. Copyright © 2010 American Medical Association. All rights reserved.)

PREVENTING DELIRIUM

Healthcare-acquired delirium is increasingly recognized as an important patient safety issue. Its attributes largely follow those of the other noninfectious topics covered earlier: there are clear risk factors for its occurrence, many cases relate to errors in management and/or can be prevented with evidence-based interventions, and policymakers are increasingly scrutinizing these adverse events for possible public reporting requirements and payment changes.

One difference from VTE, falls, and even pressure ulcers, though, is that the diagnosis of delirium is often challenging to make, since there are many underlying causes and not all changes in mental status in hospitalized patients represent delirium. That said, because delirium is so common and morbid in institutionalized patients, one should *assume that altered mental status in a patient in the hospital or long-term care facility is delirium* until proven otherwise.[36] The *Confusion Assessment Method* (CAM), a diagnostic algorithm based on this history and physical examination, is the most useful tool in diagnosing delirium (Figure 11-2).[37] It is noteworthy that published guidelines preclude making the diagnosis of dementia in the inpatient setting; many such diagnoses prove incorrect, the true cause being delirium.[36]

Delirium is common, affecting approximately half of all hospitalized elderly patients, and leads to increased costs.[38] Certain patients, especially

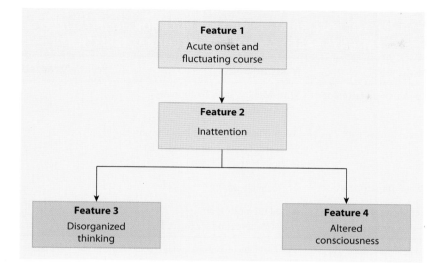

Figure 11-2 ▪ The Confusion Assessment Method (CAM) for the diagnosis of delirium. The diagnosis of delirium using the CAM requires the presence of both features 1 and 2, and either feature 3 or 4. (Reprinted with permission from AHRQ Patient Safety Network: Rudolph JL. Delirium or dementia? [Spotlight]. *AHRQ WebM&M* [serial online]; May 2009. Available at: https://psnet.ahrq.gov/webmm/case/200/delirium-or-dementia? q=delirium+or+dementia.)

those with underlying dementia, are at higher risk for delirium than others, and as a result may experience adverse outcomes including increased mortality and length of stay, discharge to a nursing home, and irreversible cognitive decline.[39,40] While treating delirium is challenging, it is important to make the diagnosis early. A risk assessment using a validated tool should be performed at the time of admission to a hospital, ICU, or long-term care facility. One such tool, for use in medical patients, is shown in Table 11-3.[41]

Delirium carries several risks that go beyond the diagnosis itself. Making the correct diagnosis of the delirious patient's primary illness is often delayed, both because patients are unable to provide accurate histories and because providers become consumed with managing the delirium itself. Patients, particularly those who are agitated, are at risk for adverse events from the medications or restraints that are often administered. The general risks of hospitalization in older patients, including malnutrition, loss of muscle mass, aspiration, and line infections, are also magnified.

A detailed description of delirium diagnosis and management is beyond our scope; interested readers would do well to read Rudolph's discussion of a misdiagnosed case of delirium,[36] as well as Merrilees and Lee's discussion of a case involving the mismanagement of delirium in *AHRQ WebM&M*.[42] For our purposes, suffice it to say that many cases of delirium can be prevented

Table 11-3 **DELIRIUM PREDICTION RULE FOR HOSPITALIZED PATIENTS BASED ON ADMISSION CHARACTERISTICS***		
Feature	**Measurement**	**Points Awarded**
Cognitive impairment	Mini-Mental State Examination (MMSE) score <24	1
Acute illness	Acute Physiology Age and Chronic Health Evaluation (APACHE) score >16	1
Visual impairment	Corrected >20/70	1
Evidence of dehydration	Blood urea nitrogen (BUN):creatinine ratio ≥18	1

*The points are added. The incidence of delirium in patients scoring 0 points is 3% to 9%, 1 to 2 points is 16% to 23%, and ≥3 points is 32% to 83%.

Adapted from Inouye SK, Viscoli CM, Horwitz RI, Hurst LD, Tinetti ME. A predictive model for delirium in hospitalized elderly medical patients based on admission characteristics. *Ann Intern Med* 1993;119:474–481.

through a program that includes risk assessment, careful medication management,[43] attention to psychosocial aspects of care (reorientation by caregivers and family, appropriate cognitive stimulation, preventing sleep deprivation), and rapid diagnosis and management of underlying precipitants, which are often infections, electrolyte disorders, medication effects, and even constipation. Studies in hospitalized older patients and in patients after hip fracture have demonstrated that these types of multicomponent interventions can prevent many cases of this highly morbid and, until recently, underemphasized adverse event.[44,45]

KEY POINTS

- Like healthcare-associated infections, several other complications of healthcare have been included under the patient safety umbrella. These include venous thromboembolism (VTE), pressure ulcers, patient falls, and delirium.
- VTE guidelines are complex and rapidly changing. Improving adherence to appropriate prophylactic strategies depends on building systems (including checklists and computerized decision support) to prompt their use.

- Many cases of pressure ulcers can be prevented with systematic risk assessment using validated tools, followed (particularly in at-risk patients) by extra attention to skin hygiene, nutrition and hydration, and avoiding undue pressure.
- Similarly, the approach to preventing falls begins with risk assessment, developing multicomponent interventions tailored to individual patients, and implementing fall prevention plans with universal fall precautions.
- Delirium is a common complication of healthcare and is associated with considerable morbidity and mortality. All hospitalized patients with altered mental status should be assumed to have delirium until proven otherwise. Multimodal prevention efforts, targeted to high-risk patients, can decrease the frequency of this adverse event.

REFERENCES

1. Wachter RM, Foster NE, Dudley RA. Medicare's decision to withhold payment for hospital errors: the devil is in the details. *Jt Comm J Qual Patient Saf* 2008;34:116–123.
2. Tejerina E, Esteban A, Fernandez-Segoviano P, et al. Clinical diagnoses and autopsy findings: discrepancies in critically ill patients. *Crit Care Med* 2012;40:842–846.
3. Winters B, Custer J, Galvagno SM Jr, et al. Diagnostic errors in the intensive care unit: a systematic review of autopsy studies. *BMJ Qual Saf* 2012;21:894–902.
4. Gould MK, Garcia DA, Wren SM, et al. Prevention of VTE in nonorthopedic surgical patients: antithrombotic therapy and prevention of thrombosis. 9th ed. American College of Chest Physicians evidence-based clinical practice guidelines. *Chest* 2012;141:e227S–e277S.
5. Kearon C, Akl EA, Ornelas J, et al. Antithrombotic therapy for VTE disease: Chest guideline and expert panel report. *Chest* 2016;149:315–352.
6. Kucher N, Koo S, Quiroz R, et al. Electronic alerts to prevent venous thromboembolism among hospitalized patients. *N Engl J Med* 2005;352:969–977.
7. Byrnes MC, Scheurer DJ, Schallom ME, et al. Implementation of a mandatory checklist of protocols and objectives improves compliance with a wide range of evidence-based intensive care unit practices. *Crit Care Med* 2009;37:2775–2781.
8. Krimsky WS, Mroz IB, McIlwaine JK, et al. A model for increasing patient safety in the intensive care unit: increasing the implementation rates of proven safety measures. *Qual Saf Health Care* 2009;18:74–80.
9. Lau BD, Haut ER. Practices to prevent venous thromboembolism: a brief review. *BMJ Qual Saf* 2014;23:187–195.
10. Haut ER, Lau BD, Kraus PS, et al. Preventability of hospital-acquired venous thromboembolism. *JAMA Surg* 2015;150:912–915.
11. Bahl V, Thompson MA, Kau T-Y, Hu HM, Campbell DA Jr. Do the AHRQ Patient Safety Indicators flag conditions that are present at the time of hospital admission? *Med Care* 2008;46:516–522.

12. Streiff MB, Haut ER. The CMS ruling on venous thromboembolism after total knee or hip arthroplasty: weighing risks and benefits. *JAMA* 2009;301:1063–1065.

13. Bilimoria KY, Chung J, Ju MH, et al. Evaluation of surveillance bias and the validity of the venous thromboembolism quality measure. *JAMA* 2013;310:1482–1489.

14. Rajaram R, Barnard C, Bilimoria KY. Concerns about using the patient safety indicator-90 composite in pay-for-performance programs. *JAMA* 2015;313:897–898.

15. Sullivan N, Schoelles KM. Preventing in-facility pressure ulcers as a patient safety strategy: a systematic review. *Ann Intern Med* 2013;158:410–416.

16. Comfort EH. Reducing pressure ulcer incidence through Braden Scale risk assessment and support surface use. *Adv Skin Wound Care* 2008;21:330–334.

17. Prevention Plus. Home of the Braden Scale. Available at: http://www.bradenscale.com/.

18. Soban LM, Hempel S, Munjas BA, Miles J, Rubenstein LV. Preventing pressure ulcers in hospitals: a systematic review of nurse-focused quality improvement interventions. *Jt Comm J Qual Patient Saf* 2011;37:245–252.

19. Dykes PC, Leung WY, Vacca V. Falling through the crack (in the bedrails) [Spotlight]. *AHRQ WebM&M* [serial online]; May 2016. Available at: https://psnet.ahrq.gov/webmm/case/374.

20. Burroughs TE, Waterman BM, Gallagher TH, et al. Patients' concerns about medical errors during hospitalization. *Jt Comm J Qual Improv* 2007;33:5–14.

21. Wong CA, Recktenwald AJ, Jones ML, Waterman BM, Bollini ML, Dunagan WC. The cost of serious fall-related injuries at three midwestern hospitals. *Jt Comm J Qual Patient Saf* 2011;37:81–87.

22. Oliver D, Killick S, Even T, Willmott M. Do falls and falls-injuries in hospital indicate negligent care—and how big is the risk? A retrospective analysis of the NHS Litigation Authority Database of clinical negligence claims, resulting from falls in hospitals in England 1995 to 2006. *Qual Saf Health Care* 2008;17:431–436.

23. Oliver D, Britton M, Seed P, Martin FC, Hopper AH. Development and evaluation of evidence based risk assessment tool (STRATIFY) to predict which elderly inpatients will fall: case–control and cohort studies. *BMJ* 1997;315:1049–1053.

24. Haines TP, Hill K, Walsh W, Osborne R. Design-related bias in hospital fall risk screening tool predictive accuracy evaluations: systematic review and meta-analysis. *J Gerontol A Biol Sci Med Sci* 2007;62:664–672.

25. Ganz DA, Bao Y, Shekelle PG, Rubenstein LZ. Will my patient fall? *JAMA* 2007;297:77–86.

26. Castle NG, Engberg J. The health consequences of using physical restraints in nursing homes. *Med Care* 2009;47:1164–1173.

27. Parker MJ, Gillespie WJ, Gillespie LD. Effectiveness of hip protectors for preventing hip fractures in elderly people: systematic review. *BMJ* 2006;332:571–574.

28. Kiel DP, Magaziner J, Zimmerman S, et al. Efficacy of a hip protector to prevent hip fracture in nursing home residents: the HIP PRO randomized controlled trial. *JAMA* 2007;298:413–422.

29. Shorr RI, Chandler AM, Mion LC, et al. Effects of an intervention to increase bed alarm use to prevent falls in hospitalized patients: a cluster randomized trial. *Ann Intern Med* 2012;157:692–699.

30. Hardin SR, Dienemann J, Rudisill P, Mills KK. Inpatient fall prevention: use of in-room Webcams. *J Patient Saf* 2013;9:29–35.

31. Lang CE. Do sitters prevent falls? A review of the literature. *J Gerontol Nurs* 2014;40:24–33.

32. Sand-Jecklin K, Johnson JR, Tylka S. Protecting patient safety: can video monitoring prevent falls in high-risk patient populations? *J Nurs Care Qual* 2016;31:131–138.

33. Haines TP, Hill AM, Hill KD, et al. Patient education to prevent falls among older hospital inpatients: a randomized controlled trial. *Arch Intern Med* 2011;171: 516–524.

34. Dykes PC, Carroll DL, Hurley A, et al. Fall prevention in acute care hospitals. A randomized trial. *JAMA* 2010;304:1912–1918.

35. Barker AL, Morello RT, Wolfe R, et al. 6-PACK programme to decrease fall injuries in acute hospitals: cluster randomised controlled trial. *BMJ* 2016;352:h6781.

36. Rudolph JL. Delirium or dementia? [Spotlight]. *AHRQ WebM&M* [serial online]; May 2009. Available at: https://psnet.ahrq.gov/webmm/case/200/delirium-or-dementia?q=delirium+or+dementia.

37. Inouye SK, van Dyck CH, Alessi CA, Balkin S, Siegal AP, Horwitz RI. Clarifying confusion: the confusion assessment method. A new method for detection of delirium. *Ann Intern Med* 1990;113:941–948.

38. Leslie DL, Marcantonio ER, Zhang Y, Leo-Summers L, Inouye SK. One-year health care costs associated with delirium in the elderly population. *Arch Intern Med* 2008;168:27–32.

39. Fick DM, Steis MR, Waller JL, Inouye SK. Delirium superimposed on dementia is associated with prolonged length of stay and poor outcomes in hospitalized older adults. *J Hosp Med* 2013;8:500–505.

40. Tropea J, LoGiudice D, Liew D, Gorelik A, Brand C. Poorer outcomes and greater healthcare costs for hospitalized older people with dementia and delirium: a retrospective cohort study. *Int J Geratr Psychiatry* 2017;32:539–547.

41. Inouye SK, Viscoli CM, Horwitz RI, Hurst LD, Tinetti ME. A predictive model for delirium in hospitalized elderly medical patients based on admission characteristics. *Ann Intern Med* 1993;119:474–481.

42. Merrilees J, Lee K. Mismanagement of delirium. *AHRQ WebM&M* [serial online]; May 2016. Available at: https://psnet.ahrq.gov/webmm/case/375/mismanagement-of-delirium.

43. Hamilton H, Gallagher P, Ryan C, Byrne S, O'Mahony D. Potentially inappropriate medications defined by STOPP criteria and the risk of adverse drug events in older hospitalized patients. *Arch Intern Med* 2011;171:1013–1019.

44. Brodaty H, Arasaratnam C. Meta-analysis of nonpharmacological interventions for neuropsychiatric symptoms of dementia. *Am J Psychiatry* 2012;169:946–953.

45. Reston JT, Schoelles KM. In-facility delirium prevention programs as a patient safety strategy: a systematic review. *Ann Intern Med* 2013;158:375–380.

ADDITIONAL READINGS

Clegg A, Siddiqi N, Heaven A, Young J, Holt R. Interventions for preventing delirium in older people in institutional long-term care. *Cochrane Database Syst Rev* 2014;1:CD009537.

Inouye SK, Westendorp RG, Saczynski JS. Delirium in elderly people. *Lancet* 2014; 383:911–922.

Hill AM, McPhail SM, Waldron N, et al. Fall rates in hospital rehabilitation units after individualized patient and staff education programs: a pragmatic, stepped-wedge, cluster-randomized controlled trial. *Lancet* 2015;385:2592–2599.

Lederle FA, Zylla D, Macdonald R, Wilt TJ. Venous thromboembolism prophylaxis in hospitalized medical patients and those with stroke: a background review for an American College of Physicians clinical practice guideline. *Ann Intern Med* 2011;155:602–615.

Michael YL, Whitlock EP, Lin JS, Fu R, O'Connor EA, Gold R; US Preventive Services Task Force. Primary care-relevant interventions to prevent falling in older adults: a systematic evidence review for the US Preventive Services Task Force. *Ann Intern Med* 2010;153:815–825.

Moore ZEH, Webster J, Samuriwo R. Wound-care teams for preventing and treating pressure ulcers. *Cochrane Database Syst Rev* 2015;9:CD011011.

Qaseem A, Mir TP, Starkey M, Denberg TD; Clinical Guidelines Committee of the American College of Physicians. Risk assessment and prevention of pressure ulcers: a clinical practice guideline from the American College of Physicians. *Ann Intern Med* 2015;162:359–369.

Reade MC, Finfer S. Sedation and delirium in the intensive care unit. *N Engl J Med* 2014;370:444–454.

PATIENT SAFETY IN THE AMBULATORY SETTING | 12

GENERAL CONCEPTS AND EPIDEMIOLOGY

The point has been well made that while most of the patient safety literature focuses on the inpatient setting, the majority of healthcare encounters occur in the clinic. Consider this: for each inpatient hospitalization, approximately 28 outpatient medical visits take place each year—a ratio that has remained relatively stable over the last 20 years.[1] Indeed, ambulatory visits now account for over one-third of all healthcare spending in the United States.[2] Nevertheless, early emphasis on patient safety in the hospital was a natural first step. Inpatients are sicker, making the stakes higher. Hospital errors are often more visible. Additionally, when compared to most community-based physician practices, hospitals have greater resources to research and address safety challenges.

The landscape is shifting. With the passage of the Affordable Care Act, millions of Americans previously uninsured are now covered and able to access outpatient care more easily. According to the Agency for Healthcare Research and Quality, 30% of previously uninsured adults under 65 became insured between 2013 and 2014.[3] Moreover, new payment models – including readmission penalties, bundled payments, and Accountable Care Organizations—place greater emphasis on maintaining the health of patients across the continuum, and patient safety is an important component of population health. All of these factors are prompting increased focus on ambulatory safety, and healthcare delivery organizations and researchers (and research funders) are responding accordingly.

While some of the key principles of safety are the same regardless of setting, ambulatory safety does present some new challenges and opportunities. The scope of potential errors may be larger in the hospital. For example, major hospital safety targets, including healthcare-associated infections, pressure ulcers, and blood clots, are less relevant in the clinic. But both settings are plagued by medication and laboratory errors as well as transitions of care and communication problems. And although the ambulatory setting has histori-cally seen fewer surgical errors, the rapid growth in outpatient surgery makes this an increasingly significant problem.

Recent research has helped to better characterize the frequency and types of safety issues associated with outpatient medicine, as well as potential solu-tions for them. One study estimated that approximately 75,000 hospitalizations per year in the United States are due to preventable adverse events that occur in the ambulatory setting.[4] In the clinic, adverse drug events and diagnostic errors are particularly common, with some estimates suggesting that about 5% of all U.S. adults experience a diagnostic error in outpatient medicine every year.[5–7] Prescribing errors occur at a particularly high rate: one study found that nearly one in four prescriptions contained at least one mistake involving dosing, patient instructions, or legibility.[8] Adverse events occurring soon after hospital discharge are especially common,[9,10] and may result from communi-cation breakdown between inpatient and outpatient providers,[11] pending test results at the time of hospital discharge,[12] incorrect medication reconcilia-tion,[13] and increased stress on patients and families coping with illness.

Efforts to advance ambulatory safety are being directed toward improving care coordination and transitions, establishing reliable medication prescribing practices and test result management systems, providing adequate resources to support ambulatory safety efforts, and engaging patients and families in their care. The growing implementation of ambulatory electronic health records and computerized prescribing[14,15] has the potential to help reduce medication-prescribing errors and improve test result follow-up. While care coordination between inpatient and outpatient providers as well as between physicians from different health systems remains challenging, improving interoperability of electronic health records and targeted post-discharge inter-ventions, such as follow-up phone calls and timely outpatient follow-up, may help mitigate this problem.

Sarkar et al. proposed a model for ambulatory safety[16] modified from Wagner's Chronic Care Model.[17] It encompasses the three interrelated roles and relationships that influence outpatient safety:

- The role of the community and health system
- The relationship between patients and providers
- The role of patient and caregiver behaviors

The model emphasizes that errors and adverse events in the ambulatory setting may stem from problems in each of these areas and particularly high-lights the patient's role. More often than in the hospital, patients in the ambu-latory setting may become unwitting participants in the genesis of errors, while others may assume some degree of responsibility for catching mistakes (Chapter 21).

This chapter highlights some of the emerging literature on ambulatory safety and the differences between the inpatient and outpatient settings that may impact improvement efforts.[18]

HOSPITAL VERSUS AMBULATORY ENVIRONMENTS

In the ambulatory world, the pace is slower and the patient flow is generally more predictable than in the hospital. While the average error in the office may be less consequential—because patients are less fragile and their medications and procedures are less potent—the cumulative impact of errors may be surprisingly large given the high volume. In the hospital, most care delivery centers around the patient's room. When the patient does travel for a procedure or to the operating room, the distances are relatively short, the patient remains within the same system, and all involved caregivers are able to communicate with one another and view the same clinical information in real time. In the ambulatory environment, on the other hand, the patient may travel many miles to obtain a test or see a specialist, often traversing practices that use different information systems and have vastly different clinical and operational cultures and policies (Chapter 8).

The structural and organizational differences may have even more important implications for improving ambulatory safety than the clinical ones. In all but the tiniest hospital, it is possible to have individuals on staff who specialize in safety-related tasks, addressing problems as they arise (Chapter 22). For example, even a modest-sized hospital is likely to have a quality officer, a compliance officer, a risk manager, and several IT experts. A larger hospital will have armies of people in these departments, and may even employ a human factors specialist and a patient safety officer. In the average small office practice, on the other hand, a physician (or nurse or practice administrator) will wear all of these hats. Moreover, because none of these specialized staff members generate patient care revenue, the ability of a small practice to support them is far more limited than in the hospital, which can cross-subsidize patient safety efforts with other profit-generating activities.

There are other important policy and cultural differences that influence ambulatory safety. Office practice is less highly regulated, and, because most of the care takes place behind closed doors (with just doctor and patient in the room), it is easier for errors to avoid the light of day. Even the cultural issues (Chapters 9 and 15) have a very different flavor. For example, consider programs that aim to improve physician–nurse relationships and flatten the steep authority gradients that are often present in healthcare settings. In American hospitals (where the physician is usually self-employed while the nurse works for the hospital), the shape of such programs is likely to be very different from the office, where the doctor is frequently the nurse's employer.

Many of these differences would appear to favor the hospital as an environment to establish a flourishing patient safety enterprise. However, the ambulatory setting also has unique advantages. First, simplification, standardization, and the implementation of IT may yield more palpable efficiency advantages. When a single clerk or nurse is working with three physicians in an office practice, the impact of implementing a standard procedure for following up lab results is often profound. And the office space freed up by converting to a paperless medical record system can yield major economic advantages for a practice. Second, efforts to engage patients in helping to ensure their own safety are more likely to be productive (Chapter 21) in the outpatient setting. Ambulatory patients are less apt to be physically and mentally impaired and, therefore, are in a better position to intervene when they see something amiss.

The previously mentioned organizational structure of most American outpatient practices can become another advantage. In many hospitals, the doctors are not particularly invested in the safety enterprise (because, in most settings, they use the hospital to provide care but don't own the organization), whereas most office practices in the United States are owned by the physicians themselves. The old saying "nobody ever washes a rented car" helps explain the challenge faced by those who try to engage nonemployed physicians in hospital safety efforts (Chapter 22).

IMPROVING AMBULATORY SAFETY

The implications of these ambulatory versus hospital differences are important as we turn our attention to outpatient safety. Most clinics will be able to identify areas in which adverse events are common and target their efforts accordingly. These likely include improving medication prescribing, test result follow-up, communication with referring physicians and hospital providers, and patient engagement and education. In a far-reaching discussion of a delayed diagnosis of a renal mass, safety expert Gordon Schiff highlights a number of Swiss cheese–related (Chapter 2) problems, along with the many opportunities for improvement in ambulatory test follow-up (Table 12-1).[19]

While the advent of computerized provider order carries potential to decrease outpatient prescribing errors,[20] and the growing adoption of IT systems has the potential to improve the safety of ambulatory medicine more generally, a robust electronic backbone is only one component of a safer system. Indeed, a recent study of EHR-related malpractice claims (in which most of the cases came from ambulatory settings) concluded that unintended consequences of healthcare IT are real and associated with adverse events that can cause significant harm.[21]

Table 12-1	**BUILDING A SYSTEM FOR MORE RELIABLE TEST FOLLOW-UP IN THE AMBULATORY ENVIRONMENT***	
Redesign Recommendation	**Logic**	**Specifications**
Tests need to be tracked from order to completion, receipt, and action.	Failures need to be visible, rather than invisibly falling through cracks.	Each step needs to be acknowledged and documented. Critical tests ordered but not performed and results lacking acknowledgment or expected action need to be tracked.
Develop standardized approach for every test and test-generating area to define and flag clinically significant abnormal results.	"Panic values" were a major advance in the 1970s, but nonurgent, action-requiring abnormal results are now the biggest problem. Lack of standardized, coded system is difficult for clinicians and for systematic tracking.	Each testing area should delineate criteria for abnormal results using three levels of urgency—immediate/ life threatening, urgent, and nonurgent but critical to follow up—defining time frames for receipt and action for each level of urgency and tagging results meeting criteria.
Eliminate ambiguities regarding whom to contact for critical abnormal results, and delineate their responsibilities.	Confusion leads to errors, particularly related to responsibilities of ordering specialists and cross-covering physicians versus primary caregivers. Redesign is needed to overcome fragmented outpatient services and increasing inpatient "shift work."	Emerging consensus that initial responsibility belongs to the *ordering* clinician to receive, act on, and/or relay critical results, backed up by the *covering* clinician when ordering clinician is unavailable, for more urgent results.
Outpatients should be informed about all test results, even normal results.	Creating expectation that they will hear about all results allows patients to serve as reliability backstop for unreported results.	Multiple ways to communicate with patients depending on the result, the patient, and available technology. Web-based secure patient "portals" are increasingly useful as ways to post results.
Tracking and system oversight monitoring	Just as someone needs to "own" each critical result, someone needs to be responsible for tracking outstanding results and identifying problems and system improvement opportunities.	Create test result quality office/ person to track abnormal results unaddressed after predefined intervals, to troubleshoot/investigate when clinicians are not reachable or results are sent to wrong physician, and to monitor and improve performance based on incidents and aggregated data.

(*continued*)

Table 12-1 **BUILDING A SYSTEM FOR MORE RELIABLE TEST FOLLOW-UP IN THE AMBULATORY ENVIRONMENT* (*continued*)**		
Redesign Recommendation	**Logic**	**Specifications**
Advanced systems to support clinicians in test results management	Further overloading busy clinicians with more tests to follow up without supporting ability to do so is not effective system redesign. Need automation, delegation, and cognitive support tools.	Results management system redesign and tools featuring interoperability with all testing areas (e.g., cardiology, endoscopy), linking to contextual information (past results, problems, drugs), and electronic decision support to identify and streamline carrying out next actions.

*Adapted from multiple consensus guidelines and recommendations, including the Massachusetts Coalition for the Prevention of Medical Errors Communicating Critical Test Results Collaborative; the Partners Communicating Clinically Significant Test Results Task Force; the Alert Notification of Critical Radiology Results collaboration project of the Brigham and Women's Hospital, Beth Israel Deaconess Medical Center, and the University of Chicago; and the CRICO Risk Management Foundation's Office Practice: What Works.

As with IT in all healthcare settings, it is relatively easy—natural, even—to think of IT as the Holy Grail: "if we just had a good IT system" is a common refrain. And there is no question that the need for such systems exists—just consider these sobering statistics:

- In a typical week, the average primary care physician is responsible for following up on 800 chemistry/hematology tests, 40 radiographs, and 12 pathology specimens.[22]
- A recent survey study suggests that follow-up of test results remains a major concern for primary care providers.[23]
- Fewer than half of primary care physicians are satisfied with their system for managing test results, more than four in five reports having had at least one test result "they wished they had known about earlier" in the prior two months.[24]
- More often than not, some crucial piece of information (lab and radiology results, consultant and pathology reports, procedure notes, and more) is missing in primary care visits.[25] Another study showed that information from one outpatient visit was available at the next visit less than one-quarter of the time.[26]

Unfortunately, early evidence from ambulatory IT implementations demonstrates that IT is not a panacea. One primary care group nearly broke up over the challenges that accompanied implementing a new system (after the dust settled, none of the physicians could imagine going back to paper, though).[27] More sobering, several recent studies have found persistently high rates of errors in both medication and radiology information flow even after IT implementations,[28–30] and early evidence that the presence of an ambulatory health record was associated with improved quality was limited.[31]

At the same time, it is inconceivable that we can achieve highly reliable ambulatory care without effective IT. These sobering results illustrate, as always, that building and implementing IT is harder than it looks, that systems need to evolve based on provider and patient feedback, and that human factors need to be considered in the development and implementation of these systems (Chapters 7 and 13). Addressing these challenges is increasingly crucial, as adoption in the ambulatory setting has grown rapidly over the last decade. According to data from the Office of the National Coordinator for Health Information Technology, 83% of outpatient physicians had implemented some type of EHR by 2014, about twice as many as in 2008.[32] And while the flaws of healthcare IT continue to be well recognized, findings from a 2015 national survey of primary care providers suggest that physicians recognize the potential for health IT to improve quality and safety, with 50% of physicians and 64% of nurse practitioners and physician assistants responding that implementation has had a favorable impact.[33] In addition, more recent studies have shown a positive impact of health IT adoption on ambulatory care.[34–36] As healthcare IT adoption continues to grow rapidly, some commonsensical steps that can be taken to improve ambulatory medication safety are worth reviewing (Table 12-2).[37]

Table 12-2 PRACTICES THAT MAY LEAD TO IMPROVED AMBULATORY MEDICATION SAFETY

Use an electronic prescribing system, if available. An electronic prescribing system, especially when interfaced with an electronic health record, has the potential to decrease errors from illegibility and interactions. Direct electronic transmission to pharmacies may decrease errors even further.

If using a paper system, write understandable, legible prescriptions, and include the indication on the prescription. Use English instead of Latin abbreviations (i.e., writing "four times daily" or "once daily" instead of "qid" and "qd," respectively), and write the indication on the prescription (e.g., "for high blood pressure").

Use sample medications with care, if at all. Pharmacists serve as an important safety check when prescribing medications, often catching interactions and allergies that physicians miss.

Maintain accurate and usable medication lists and reconcile medications regularly. Use the "brown bag checkup" (i.e., ask patients to bring all the medicines in their medicine cabinet to a visit). Physicians and their staff need to confirm the medications at every visit. When discrepancies are found, it is the physician's task to resolve these.

Empower patients to serve as safety double checkers. Most patients can assume significant responsibility for discovering—and preventing—many medical errors from becoming harmful events.

Reprinted with permission from AHRQ Patient Safety Network: Elder NC. Patient safety in the physician office setting [Perspective]. *AHRQ PSNet* [serial online]; May 2006. Available at: https://psnet.ahrq.gov/perspectives/perspective/24.

The role of the patient is crucial in ambulatory safety, particularly since patients spend so little time with their providers and far more at home managing their health. Strong emphasis should be placed on patient education (using proven methods such as the "teach back"[38]) and empowerment, with particular attention paid to the issues of health literacy and cultural differences. We will discuss these in more detail in Chapter 21.

Overall, improving safety in the ambulatory setting will not necessarily be harder or easier than in the hospital, just different.[18] As with much of the patient safety field, which often involves extrapolating experiences (Table P-1) from other settings (i.e., *Will crew resource management, which worked so well in commercial aviation, work in the labor and delivery suite? Will bar coding, which works so well in the supermarket, actually decrease medication errors?*), it will be important to remain sensitive to the differences in structure and culture as we try to translate what we know about safety from the hospital to the office setting.

Moving forward, experts suggest that research in ambulatory safety should focus on several areas. These include: broadening the data on the epidemiology of ambulatory safety, focusing on areas where tangible improvements to prevent harm can be made, improving patient and family engagement around safety in outpatient care, tying ambulatory safety to "high-profile" issues like care transitions and readmissions, and improving the infrastructure around ambulatory research.[39]

While ambulatory safety was all but ignored during the first few years of the safety movement, research funders, accreditors, regulators, and specialty societies have come to appreciate its importance, as have patients and their advocates. All these stakeholders are now exerting their influence, so the next decade is likely to see far more activity in the ambulatory safety arena, and far more pressure to improve.

KEY POINTS

- Until recently, the patient safety field's focus has been on hospital safety. Attention is now shifting to the ambulatory setting. In the United States, some of the change is being driven by the Affordable Care Act and payment models that increasingly emphasize care across the continuum.
- Efforts to improve ambulatory safety should focus on decreasing medication errors, improving the management of test results, improving communication between outpatient and inpatient providers, and engaging patients in their care.

■ In approaching ambulatory safety, it will be important to appreciate major clinical, structural, and organizational differences between the hospital and the office. These include the inability to support specialized experts in many safety-related areas, and the employer–employee relationship between physicians and many nurses and other staff found in most U.S. office practices.

■ The development and implementation of effective IT tools is essential to improving ambulatory safety, particularly in the areas of medication management and test results handling. Early experience with ambulatory IT has been sobering, with unexpectedly high rates of errors and significant numbers of unanticipated consequences. Effective systems will need to integrate provider and patient feedback and take better account of human factors.

REFERENCES

1. Johansen ME, Kircher SM, Huerta TR. Reexamining the ecology of medical care. *N Engl J Med* 2016;374:495–496.
2. Chang JE, Brundage SC, Chokshi DA. Convenient ambulatory care—promise, pitfalls, and policy. *N Engl J of Med* 2016;372:382–388.
3. Vistnes J, Cohen S. Statistical brief #467—transitions in health insurance coverage over time, 2012–2014 (selected intervals): estimates for U.S. civilian non-institutionalized adult population under age 65. *Agency for Healthcare Research and Quality* 2015. Available at: http://meps.ahrq.gov/mepsweb/data_files/publications/st467/stat467.shtml.
4. Woods DM, Thomas EJ, Holl JL, Weiss KB, Brennan TA. Ambulatory care adverse events and preventable adverse events leading to a hospital admission. *Qual Saf Health Care* 2007;16:127–131.
5. Sarkar U, López A, Maselli JH, Gonzales R. Adverse drug events in U.S. adult ambulatory medical care. *Health Services Research* 2011;46:1517–1533.
6. Singh H, Giardina TD, Meyer AN, Forjuoh SN, Reis MD, Thomas EJ. Types and origins of diagnostic errors in primary care settings. *JAMA Intern Med* 2013;173:418–425.
7. Singh H, Meyer AD, Thomas EJ. The frequency of diagnostic errors in outpatient care: estimations from three large observational studies involving U.S. adult populations. *BMJ Qual Saf* 2014;23:727–731.
8. Abramson EL, Bates DW, Jenter C, et al. Ambulatory prescribing errors among community-based providers in two states. *J Am Med Inform Assoc* 2012;19:644–648.
9. Forster AJ, Murff HJ, Peterson JF, et al. The incidence and severity of adverse events affecting patients after discharge from the hospital. *Ann Intern Med* 2003;138:161–167.
10. Tsilimingras D, Schnipper J, Duke A, et al. Post-discharge adverse events among urban and rural patients of an urban community hospital: a prospective cohort study. *J Gen Intern Med* 2015;30:1164–1171.

11. Kripalani S, LeFevre F, Phillips CO, Williams MV, Basaviah P, Baker DW. Deficits in communication and information transfer between hospital-based and primary care physicians: implications for patient safety and continuity of care. *JAMA* 2007; 297:831–841.

12. Ong MS, Magrabi F, Jones G, Coiera E. Last order: follow-up of tests ordered on the day of hospital discharge. *Arch Intern Med* 2012;172:1347–1349.

13. Belda-Rustarazo S, Cantero-Hinojosa J, Salmeron-García A, González-García L, Cabeza-Barrera J, Galvez J. Medication reconciliation at admission and discharge: an analysis of prevalence and associated risk factors. *Int J Clin Pract* 2015;69:1268–1274.

14. DesRoches CM, Campbell EG, Rao SR, et al. Electronic health records in ambulatory care—a national survey of physicians. *N Engl J Med* 2008;359:50–60.

15. Bruen BK, Ku L, Burke MF, Buntin MB. More than four in five office-based physicians could qualify for federal electronic health record incentives. *Health Aff (Millwood)* 2011;30:472–480.

16. Sarkar U, Wachter RM, Schroeder SA, Schillinger D. Refocusing the lens: patient safety in ambulatory chronic disease care. *Jt Comm J Qual Patient Saf* 2009;35:377–383.

17. Wagner EH, Austin BT, Von Korff M. Organizing care for patients with chronic illness. *Milbank Q* 1996;74:511–544.

18. Wachter RM. Is ambulatory patient safety just like hospital safety, only without the "stat?" *Ann Intern Med* 2006;145:547–549.

19. Schiff GD. A 60-year-old man with delayed care for a renal mass. *JAMA* 2011; 305:1890–1898.

20. Kaushal R, Kern LM, Barrón Y, Quaresimo J, Abramson EL. Electronic prescribing improves medication safety in community-based office practices. *J Gen Intern Med* 2010;25:530–536.

21. Graber ML, Siegal D, Riah H, Johnston D, Kenyon K. Electronic health record-related events in medical malpractice claims. *J Patient Safety* November 6, 2015. [Epub ahead of print].

22. Poon EG, Wang SJ, Gandhi TK, Bates DW, Kuperman GJ. Design and implementation of a comprehensive outpatient results manager. *J Biomed Inform* 2003; 36:80–91.

23. Litchfield I, Bentham L, Lilford R, McManus RJ, Hill A, Greenfield S. Test results communication in primary care: a survey of current practice. *BMJ Qual Saf* 2015; 24:691–699.

24. Poon EG, Gandhi TK, Sequist TD, Murff HJ, Karson AS, Bates DW. "I wish I had seen this test result earlier!": dissatisfaction with test result management systems in primary care. *Arch Intern Med* 2004;164:2223–2228.

25. Smith PC, Araya-Guerra R, Bublitz C, et al. Missing clinical information during primary care visits. *JAMA* 2005;293:565–571.

26. van Walraven C, Taljaard M, Bell CM, et al. Information exchange among physicians caring for the same patient in the community. *CMAJ* 2008;179:1013–1018.

27. Baron RJ, Fabens EL, Schiffman M, Wolf E. Electronic health records: just around the corner? Or over the cliff? *Ann Intern Med* 2005;143:222–226.

28. Singh H, Thomas EJ, Mani S, et al. Timely follow-up of abnormal diagnostic imaging test results in an outpatient setting: are electronic medical records achieving their potential? *Arch Intern Med* 2009;169:1578–1586.

29. Dhavle AA, Yang Y, Rupp MT, Singh H, Ward-Charlerie S, Ruiz J. Analysis of prescribers' notes in electronic prescriptions in ambulatory practice. *JAMA Intern Med* 2016;176:463–470.

30. Overhage JM, Gandhi TK, Hope C, et al. Ambulatory computerized prescribing and preventable adverse drug events. *J Patient Saf* 2016;12:69–74.

31. Romano MJ, Stafford RS. Electronic health records and clinical decision support systems: impact on national ambulatory care quality. *Arch Intern Med* 2011;171:897–903.

32. Office of the National Coordinator for Health Information Technology. Office-based Physician Electronic Health Record Adoption: 2004–2014, Health IT Quick-Stat #50. Available at: http://dashboard.healthit.gov/quickstats/pages/physician-ehr-adoption-trends.php.

33. The Commonwealth Fund and The Kaiser Family Foundation. *Primary Care Providers' Views of Recent Trends in Health Care Delivery and Payment*, August 2015. Available at: http://www.commonwealthfund.org/publications/issue-briefs/2015/aug/primary-care-providers-views-delivery-payment.

34. Kern LM, Barrón Y, Dhopeshwarkar RV, Edwards A, Kaushal R; HITEC Investigators. Electronic health records and ambulatory quality of care. *J Gen Intern Med* 2013; 28:496–503.

35. Ancker JS, Kern LM, Edwards A, et al.; HITEC Investigators. Associations between healthcare quality and use of electronic health record functions in ambulatory care. *J Am Med Inform Assoc* 2015;22:864–871.

36. Lammers EJ, McLaughlin CG, Barna M. Physician EHR adoption and potentially preventable hospital admissions among Medicare beneficiaries: panel data evidence, 2010–2013. *Health Serv Res* 2016;51:2056–2075.

37. Elder NC. Patient safety in the physician office setting [Perspective]. *AHRQ PSNet* [serial online]; May 2006. Available at: https://psnet.ahrq.gov/perspectives/perspective/24.

38. Bertakis KD. The communication of information from physician to patient: a method for increasing patient retention and satisfaction. *J Fam Pract* 1977;5:217–222.

39. Wynia MK, Classen DC. Improving ambulatory patient safety. *JAMA* 2011; 306:2504–2505.

ADDITIONAL READINGS

Bowie P, Price J, Hepworth N, Dinwoodie M, McKay J. System hazards in managing laboratory tests requests and results in primary care: medical protection database analysis and conceptual model. *BMJ Open* 2015;5:e008968.

Elder NC. Laboratory testing in general practice: a patient safety blind spot. *BMJ Qual Saf* 2015;24:667–670.

Gandhi TK, Lee TH. Patient safety beyond the hospital. *N Engl J Med* 2010;363:1001–1003.

Gandhi TK, Weingart SN, Seger AC, et al. Outpatient prescribing errors and the impact of computerized prescribing. *J Gen Intern Med* 2005;20:837–841.

Hatoun J, Chan JA, Yaksic E, et al. A systematic review of patient safety measures in adult primary care. *Am J Med Qual* 2017;32:237–245.

Hickner J, Smith SA, Yount N, Sorra J. Differing perceptions of safety culture across job roles in the ambulatory setting: analysis of the AHRQ medical office survey on patient safety culture. *BMJ Qual Saf* 2016;25:588–594.

Kravet SJ, Bailey J, Demski R, Pronovost P. Establishing an ambulatory medicine quality and safety oversight structure: leveraging the fractal model. *Acad Med* 2016; 91:962–966.

Modak I, Sexton JB, Lux TR, Helmreich RL, Thomas EJ. Measuring safety culture in the ambulatory setting: the Safety Attitudes Questionnaire—ambulatory version. *J Gen Intern Med* 2007;22:1–5.

Nassaralla CL, Naessens JM, Chaudhry R, Hansen MA, Scheitel SM. Implementation of a medication reconciliation process in an ambulatory internal medicine clinic. *Qual Saf Health Care* 2007;16:90–94.

Panesar SS, deSilva D, Carson-Stevens A, et al. How safe is primary care? A systematic review. *BMJ Qual Saf* 2016;25:544–553.

Roy CL, Rothschild JM, Dighe AS, et al. An initiative to improve the management of clinically significant test results in a large health care network. *Jt Comm J Qual Patient Saf* 2013;39:517–527.

Schiff GD, Reyes Nieva H, Griswold P, et al. Addressing ambulatory safety and malpractice: the Massachusetts PROMISES project. *Health Serv Res* 2016;51:2634–2641.

Shekelle PG, Sarkar U, Shojania K, et al. Patient Safety in Ambulatory Settings. Technical Brief No. 27. Agency for Healthcare Research and Quality; October 2016. AHRQ Publication No. 16-EHC033-EF.

Singh H, Schiff GD, Graber ML, Onakpoya I, Thompson MJ. The global burden of diagnostic errors in primary care. *BMJ Qual Saf* 2017;26:484–494.

Taché SV, Sönnichsen A, Ashcroft DM. Prevalence of adverse drug events in ambulatory care: a systematic review. *Ann Pharmacother* 2011;45:977–989.

SOLUTIONS

INFORMATION TECHNOLOGY | 13

HEALTHCARE'S INFORMATION PROBLEM

The provision of healthcare is remarkably information intensive. A large integrated healthcare system processes tens of millions of information exchanges per day, through multiple pathways, including its electronic health record, as well as via beepers, text messages, and e-mails.

But high volume is just the beginning. Consider the task of tracking a single patient's current diseases, past medical history, medications, allergies, test results, risk factors, and personal preferences (such as for cardiopulmonary resuscitation). Tricky? Sure, but now do it over months or years, and then add in the fact that the patient is seen by many different providers, scattered across a region, often using different medical record systems that generally do not communicate with one another.

Want more? To make payment decisions, the insurer needs access to some of this information, as does the source of the insurance, which in the United States is often the patient's employer. But, because of privacy concerns, both should receive only essential information; to tell them of the patient's HIV status, or her psychiatric or sexual history, would be highly inappropriate, damaging, and possibly illegal.

Now let's make it really hard. Assume that the patient is in a car accident and taken to an emergency department (ED) in a nearby state, where she is stabilized and admitted to the hospital. Ideally, the doctors and nurses would see the relevant clinical details of her past history, preferably in a format that highlighted the information they needed without overwhelming them with extraneous data. Orders must be processed instantaneously (none of "the system is down for planned maintenance" or "orders are processed on the next business day" so familiar from commercial transactions). During the patient's hospital stay, not only would there be seamless links among all of the new observations (the neurosurgeon can easily view the ED doctor's notes; the resident can quickly find the patient's vital signs and laboratory studies), but also the various components would weave together seamlessly. For example:

- The system would prompt the doctor with information regarding the appropriate therapy or test for a given condition (along with links to the evidence supporting any recommendations).
- The system would warn the nurse that the patient is allergic to a medicine before she administers it.
- The system would tell the doctor or pharmacist which medications are on the formulary and steer them to the preferred ones.

Meanwhile, the vast trove of data being created through this patient's case—and millions of others like it—would be chronicled and analyzed ("mined"), searching for new patterns of disease, evidence of preferred strategies, and more. All of this would be iterative—as new information emerged from this and other research about disease risk factors or best practices, it would seamlessly flow into the system, spurring the next patient's care to be even better.

Contrast this vision of information nirvana with the prevailing state of most doctors' offices and hospitals.[1,2] Although federal policies have spurred rapid digitization of health information in recent years—almost 87% of outpatient physicians and over 96% of nonfederal acute care hospitals in the United States were recorded as using an electronic health record (EHR) as of 2015[3,4]—in some places vital patient information is still stored on paper charts, and thus unavailable to anyone who lacks physical possession of the relevant piece of paper (in some cases, the notes are sufficiently illegible that even physical custody of the paper does not insure information access). Notes are often entered as free text, not in a format that facilitates analysis or productive interaction with other pieces of system data. When the patient moves across silos—from outpatient to inpatient, from state to state, from hospital to hospice—crucial information rarely moves with her, although work is ongoing to change this. Communication of facts (e.g., medication lists, allergies, past medical history), which should be streamed through the system, instead is at the mercy of person-to-person interactions or a haphazard pinball game of photocopies bouncing from place to place.

Even at the level of the individual practitioner, the impact of this data chaos is profoundly demoralizing, wasteful, and most importantly, dangerous. Just watch a nurse take a patient's vital signs on a typical hospital ward. The nurse looks at the numbers on the screen of an automated blood pressure cuff: **165/92**. Even in digitally advanced hospitals, as often as not she records them on an index card (or, sometimes, on a paper towel, her forearm, or the cuff of her scrub suit), hopefully next to the correct patient's name.

Later, she returns to the nurses' station and types these numbers (again, hopefully belonging to the correct patient) into the appropriate place in the chart (hopefully the right chart). Then, in a teaching hospital, an intern transcribes these vital signs onto another index card (or maybe an iPad) during morning rounds. He presents these data to his resident and later to his attending, who each do the same thing. Eventually, each of these practitioners writes, or dictates, separate notes for the medical record. Any wonder that this information (which, you'll recall, began life in digital form!) is frequently wrong? Or that busy healthcare professionals find that huge chunks of their valuable time are squandered? Or that the patient has the sense (particularly after she has been asked the same question by 10 different people) that the right hand has no idea what the left hand is doing?

Why has healthcare, the most information intensive of industries, entered our remarkable age of computers so sluggishly, reluctantly, and haphazardly? Part of the reason is that, until recently, the business or clinical case for healthcare information technology (HIT) was far from ironclad. Such justification was needed because HIT is extraordinarily expensive (about $50,000 per doctor in an ambulatory office, up to $200 million to wire a 600-bed teaching hospital, and over $1 billion in some cases for large, multihospital health systems), unreimbursed, and extremely challenging to implement. Moreover, healthcare computer systems have traditionally been relatively clunky and user unfriendly, in part because the market for them was too weak to fund vigorous research and development, and to generate the user feedback and refinement cycles needed for complex systems to mature.

We are now at a turning point for HIT. The patient safety movement has catalyzed the widespread recognition that robust digital scaffolding is absolutely essential to efforts to improve quality, safety, efficiency, and coordination of care. There are striking examples of successes, such as that enjoyed by the huge Veterans Affairs (VA) system, whose early adoption of EHRs and computerized provider order entry (CPOE) sparked a substantially improved quality of care.[5] A large and convincing literature demonstrates that well-designed and implemented electronic systems can lead to significant benefits for systems and patients.[6–10]

Yet there is a more troubling, though not entirely surprising, side of the story. Over a decade ago, safety experts expressed concern that the early glowing evidence about HIT's benefits had come from a handful of institutions that lovingly built their own systems, possessed highly committed leaders, and invested heavily in computerization.[11] As Wachter and Shojania wrote in their 2004 book *Internal Bleeding*:

> *But the average hospital will not share these conditions, any more than your local Gilbert and Sullivan troupe resembles the Metropolitan*

Opera ... More than one CIO has tried to airlift a commercial system into her hospital, then stood scratching her head at how slick the system seemed to be during the vendor's demo, and how poorly it performed in real life.[12]

As you've already seen, our suspicions—that the implementation of commercial IT systems at thousands of hospitals and hundreds of thousands of ambulatory offices might not go quite so smoothly—have, sadly, been proven correct. A growing literature tells stories of HIT implementation failures, unanticipated consequences, and even harm.[13–18] Indeed, in *The Digital Doctor*, Wachter describes a serious medication error that occurred at our own hospital, an error that vividly illustrates how the unintended consequences of HIT implementation can lead to significant harm. In the case, a 16-year-old boy with a chronic genetic immunodeficiency was supposed to receive one antibiotic tablet (trimethoprim-sulfamethoxazole, or Septra) twice a day, but instead was given 38 ½ of them.[19] The overdose, which led to a near-fatal grand mal seizure, stemmed from a combination of poorly designed user interfaces, alert fatigue, undue trust in the technology, and failure to speak up (Table 13-1).

This case is a sobering but useful tale, one that highlights the immense challenges of fundamental change in complex adaptive systems (Chapter 2), the critical need to use human factors design principles (Chapter 7), the overwhelming complexity underlying tasks that might initially seem routine (ordering and administering medications), and the tremendous impact that errors can have on both patients as well as on the providers and nurses who care for them (Chapter 16). It is also a classic illustration of the Swiss cheese model of error (Chapter 2).

This chapter will describe the main types of HIT systems, some of their safety advantages, and some of the problems—including new kinds of errors—they can create. Because HIT addresses so many safety targets and is a component of so many solutions, considerable information about HIT's role in specific areas can also be found throughout the book.

ELECTRONIC HEALTH RECORDS

Because most medical errors represent failures in communication and data transmission, computerization of the medical record would seem like a safety lynchpin. (While the old term was "electronic medical record" [EMR], today the term "electronic health record" [EHR] is generally preferred, since it emphasizes the role of the patient in viewing and even contributing to the record and the fact that the EHR may chronicle and even influence health

Table 13-1	KEY ERRORS IN THE SEPTRA OVERDOSE CASE
Error	**Comment**
After being prompted by pharmacist's text message to clarify an order, a physician mistakenly orders 160 mg/kg of the antibiotic Septra, rather than intended 160 mg. This means that the order is for 38 ½ pills, rather than the intended single pill.	EHR provides no visual or other cues about whether the MD is in "mg" mode or "mg/kg" mode (weight-based dosing).
An overdose alert fires, but the physician clicks out of it.	Classic problem with alert fatigue.
Pharmacist now sees the physician's order, but doesn't catch the overdose. He too clicks out of the alert.	In addition to alert fatigue, the pharmacists are working in a busy, cramped space and are constantly multitasking.
The order for 38 ½ pills goes to a pharmacy robot, which fills it accurately.	The robot has replaced the pharmacy tech since it is faster and more accurate. But it is not programmed to question a nonsensical order.
A young nurse, working on an unfamiliar floor ("floating") sees the order for 38 ½ pills, finds it odd, but checks it with her bar code scanner. Bar code confirms that 38 ½ pills is correct, which reassures the nurse.	Classic Swiss cheese model, with an inexperienced nurse working on an unfamiliar floor (on top of all the other problems). In addition, a cultural issue, in that the nurse didn't want to call the doctor or pharmacist for fear of looking dumb. Finally, overtrust in the technology: the bar code's confirmation was enough to convince the nurse that the order was correct (at that phase of the medication safety process, the bar code's job is to ensure that the nurse gives the medication as it is written).

Excerpted with permission from Wachter RM. *The Digital Doctor: Hope, Hype, and Harm at the Dawn of Medicine's Computer Age.* New York, NY: McGraw-Hill; 2015.

status, not just a patient's medications and diagnoses.) But to realize this benefit, attention must be paid to a variety of system and user factors. System factors include the ease of use, the speed with which data can be entered and retrieved, the quality of the user interface, and the presence of value-added features such as order entry, decision support, sign-out and scheduling systems, links to all the necessary data (e.g., imaging and electrocardiograms), and automatic reports. User factors primarily relate to the training and readiness of the provider and nonprovider workforce (Chapters 7 and 16). Both system and user factors played a role in the case of the Septra overdose described above.

User efficiency is particularly important. Despite the hope that computerization would save time for providers, evidence indicates that the opposite is often true, particularly for physicians. Many doctors now complain that they have become "glorified data entry clerks," while also struggling to manage an overabundance of data[20] and a large volume of electronic communication with both patients and other providers. All of this has been associated with a troubling increase in rates of physician burnout.[21,22]

Some of this cost in time may be repaid in more efficient information retrieval, but increasing attention will need to be focused on workflow. (Remember that digital blood pressure reading?—in the "wired" hospital, it will magically leap from the blood pressure machine into the EHR, where it can be seamlessly imported into each provider's note and trigger useful decision support.) Effective systems will, of course, provide huge efficiency benefits to administrators, researchers, and insurers by capturing data in standardized formats and allowing electronic transmission.

Unfortunately, this facilitated movement of bits and bytes has a dark side, in the form of the *copy-and-paste phenomenon*.[23] One tongue-in-cheek essayist captured the problem beautifully:

> *The copy-and-paste command allows one day's note to be copied and used as a template for the next day's note. Ideally, old information and diagnostic impressions are deleted and new ones added. In reality, however, there is no deletion, only addition. Daily progress notes become progressively longer and contain senescent information. The admitting diagnostic impression, long since discarded, is dutifully noted day after day. Last month's echocardiogram report takes up permanent residence in the daily results section. Complicated patients are on "post-op day 2" for weeks. One wonders how utilization review interprets such statements.[24]*

A cohort study performed in the ICU of an academic medical center found copying and pasting of notes to be prevalent among both trainees and attendings. In fact, in almost 75% of the notes examined, more than one-fifth of the content of the daily progress note was copied from the prior day's note.[25] Some IT systems can disable the copy-and-paste function, although this may be unacceptable to providers[26] (some information really *does* remain static from day to day, and having to retype or redictate it is wasteful and annoying), and resourceful providers can usually find a way to bypass such restrictions anyway.[27] In the end, copy-and-paste resembles many elements of patient safety, in that introducing structural changes without ensuring that caregivers possess the requisite education and professionalism is likely to lead to new types of mischief, or even harm.

One important choice for EHR developers is the use of *structured versus unstructured data*. Physicians, in particular, have always preferred entering data as unstructured prose (captured through typing, transcription services, or increasingly, speech recognition software), which has the advantages of ease of use and familiarity, and is consistent with the long tradition of "telling the patient's story."[28,29] On the other hand, unstructured data are difficult to analyze for patterns, to use to support quality improvement and public reporting activities, and to link to computerized decision support.[30] Structured, or coded, data (captured via templates or automatically fed into the EHR after being recorded by electronic devices) can support these functions, but they clash with clinicians' mental model for data acquisition and analysis. Ongoing research is attempting to identify the best mix of structured and unstructured EHR inputs, and to develop new ways (through computerized "natural language processing") to mine narrative prose for key data elements. One study performed in the Veterans Affairs Health System demonstrated that natural language processing algorithms could accurately identify postoperative complications by screening providers' notes.[31] This finding is supported by additional research.[32] It is likely that advanced EHRs of the future will combine the best of both types of data capture and analysis, thereby decreasing today's documentation and information retrieval burdens.

Another important advance in EHRs is the ability to promote *patient engagement* (Chapter 21). At the very least, allowing patients access to their laboratory data and giving them the ability to schedule their own appointments represents real progress.[33] As of this writing, some 10 million patients in the United States have full access to their entire health record, including physician notes ("OpenNotes"). While many clinicians worried that such access would lead to confused or anxious patients,[34] evidence from several studies has allayed these concerns.[35]

Patients, who are increasingly accustomed to managing their own affairs (financial, travel, dating) with the support of digital systems, are likely to demand new kinds of tools to help with their medical care and overall health.[36] Many patients now keep *personal health records* (PHRs), and these are increasingly electronic.[37] Future developments in this area are likely to weave patient- and provider-facing electronic systems together (including information gleaned from apps and sensors), facilitate new kinds of information flow and communications (e-mails, text messaging, video consultations, and more), and raise a host of issues surrounding reimbursement, liability, privacy, data integrity (what happens when the provider and patient disagree about what should be in a jointly created record?), and more.[38,39] Obviously, PHRs hold important implications for patient safety,[40] with the capacity both for great leaps forward and some new hazards.

EHRs raise yet another profound challenge. As the physician-author Abraham Verghese has observed, clinicians' focus is increasingly centered on the data in the computer, sometimes at the cost of the human connections so fundamental to the practice of medicine and the art of healing. After discussing the traditional approach to patients, in which "the [patient's] body is the text," Verghese writes of a new, more expedient approach that he sees in today's trainees:

> *The patient is still at the center, but more as an icon for another entity clothed in binary garments: the "iPatient." Often, emergency room personnel have already scanned, tested, and diagnosed, so that interns meet a fully formed iPatient long before seeing the real patient. The iPatient's blood counts and emanations are tracked and trended like a Dow Jones Index, and pop-up flags remind caregivers to feed or bleed. iPatients are handily discussed (or "card-flipped") in the bunker [the conference room where the team does its work], while the real patients keep the beds warm and ensure that the folders bearing their names stay alive on the computer.*[41]

Taking full advantage of the remarkable potential for EHRs to improve safety and quality while heeding Verghese's cautionary tale may be one of the most subtle yet important challenges facing caregivers in the modern age.

COMPUTERIZED PROVIDER ORDER ENTRY

Because the prescribing process is one of the Achilles' heels of medication safety (Figure 4-3), efforts to computerize this process have long been a focus of safety efforts. In 1998, Bates et al. demonstrated that a CPOE system with decision support reduced serious medication errors by 55%, mediated by improved communication, better availability of information, constraints to prevent the use of inappropriate drugs, doses, and frequencies, and assistance with monitoring.[42] Another early study of more sophisticated decision support found an 83% reduction in medication errors.[43] A subsequent meta-analysis demonstrated that the risk of inpatient prescribing errors was reduced by almost half when CPOE replaced paper orders.[44] Studies in the outpatient setting have shown similar effectiveness.[45] The advantages of CPOE over paper-based systems are many; in addition to those listed in Table 13-2, the installation of CPOE systems inevitably leads organizations to standardize chaotic processes (the equivalent of cleaning out your closet before moving), which has its own safety benefits.[46]

Although CPOE initially centered around medication ordering, the use of the technology has grown rapidly in both inpatient and outpatient settings and now facilitates the ordering of much more than medications: procedures,

Table 13-2	ADVANTAGES OF CPOE SYSTEMS OVER PAPER-BASED SYSTEMS

- Free of handwriting identification problems
- Faster to reach the pharmacy
- Less subject to error associated with similar drug names
- More easily integrated into medical records and decision support systems
- Less subject to errors caused by use of apothecary measures
- Easily linked to drug–drug interaction warnings
- More likely to identify the prescribing physician
- Able to link to ADE reporting systems
- Able to avoid specification errors, such as trailing zeros
- Available and appropriate for training and education
- Available for immediate data analysis, including postmarketing reporting
- Claimed to generate significant economic savings
- With online prompts, CPOE systems can:
  Link to algorithms to emphasize cost-effective medications
  Reduce underprescribing and overprescribing
  Reduce incorrect drug choices

Abbreviation: ADE, adverse drug event.

Reproduced with permission from Koppel R, Metlay JP, Cohen A, et al. Role of computerized physician order entry systems in facilitating medication errors. *JAMA* 2005;293:1197–1203. Copyright © 2005 American Medical Association. All rights reserved.

tests, labs, consults and more. In the case of medication safety, much of CPOE's value comes from identifying out-of-range results or potentially unsafe medication interactions, and rapidly alerting providers so that they can decide whether their plan is correct.[47] For example, a CPOE system can alert a provider to a potentially fatal medication–allergy interaction (Figure 13-1) or a potentially dangerous laboratory result. These systems can also be used at the healthcare system level to identify and track errors via trigger tools (Chapters 2 and 14).

In addition to helping clinicians avoid mistakes, CPOE systems can suggest actions that should always accompany certain orders. In an ideal world, these "if A, then do B" should be second nature, but our memories are fallible and we sometimes forget to check a creatinine and potassium after starting an angiotensin-converting enzyme (ACE) inhibitor, a PTT after starting heparin, or a glucose level after starting insulin. We'll say more about these functions—which go under the general name of clinical decision support systems (CDSS)—later in this chapter.

Despite the great appeal of CPOE, issues with workflow and implementation continue to raise concerns about patient safety. Patient harm from adverse

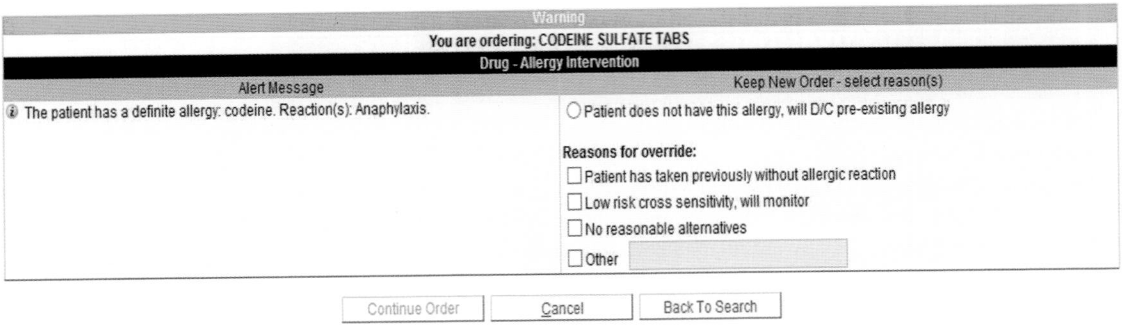

Figure 13-1 ▪ Example of a CPOE system's warning of a potentially fatal medication–allergy interaction in the outpatient setting. (Reproduced with permission from Slight SP, Beeler PE, Seger DL, et al. A cross-sectional observational study of high override rates of drug allergy alerts in inpatient and outpatient settings, and opportunities for improvement. *BMJ Qual Saf* 2017;26:217–225.)

drug events still occurs frequently in some institutions where CPOE has been implemented.[48] While one would think that combining decision support with CPOE would solve this problem, research has demonstrated that, even in systems with decision support, unsafe medication orders are still processed,[49] suggesting that there is opportunity to improve the usability of decision support alerts.[50] In one study, researchers developed 21 examples of concerning medication orders and tested them in a variety of commercially available CPOE systems. Most of these orders were entered fairly easily or required the use of minimal workarounds such as overriding an alert,[51] a finding consistent with prior research.[52]

Table 13-3 describes eight themes identified as contributing to CPOE-related prescribing errors and offers recommendations for improvement.[53]

We can expect that, as the market for CPOE grows and commercial products experience many user-feedback-generated improvement cycles, the systems will become better, errors associated with them will become less common, and the full safety benefits of the technology will begin to be realized. Table 13-4 highlights the many categories of IT-related errors that have been identified and suggests several mitigating strategies.[17]

IT SAFETY SOLUTIONS TO IMPROVE MEDICATION SAFETY

Bar coding and radio-frequency identification systems

Even when rigorous safety checks are embedded into the prescribing process, errors at the time of medication administration can still lead to great harm, in both hospital and ambulatory settings (Chapter 4). To prevent these errors on

Table 13-3   KEY THEMES CONTRIBUTING TO PRESCRIBING ERRORS ASSOCIATED WITH COMPUTERIZED PROVIDER ORDER ENTRY AND RECOMMENDATIONS FOR IMPROVEMENT

Main Error Facilitator	Key Themes	Specific Issues	Recommendations
System-related	Computer screen display	Incomplete display Navigation between multiple sources Confusing data labels	All medications (oral, intravenous, etc.) and all statuses (active and discontinued, etc.) should be clearly displayed in one area if possible The naming of data labels should be unambiguous Post-implementation testing is crucial to identify any issues Consistent use of color and design throughout the system
System-related	Drop-down menus and auto-population	Mis-selection errors: Similar named medications or patients located next to each other Orders listed above or below the intended order Delays in the system response time and the consequent use of "multiple clicks" Scrolling onto the wrong order Erroneous suggestions of medications, doses, or patients	Avoid overly long lists of patient's names or medications Distinction between "look-alike-sound-alike" medications using tall man lettering, color or bold font Indication based CDS alerts Improved sensitivity and specificity of CDS functions
System-related	Wording	Confusion between the system's wording and user's interpretation of that meaning Unnecessary "trailing zeros" i.e., 20.000 mg instead of 20 mg	Pre- and post-evaluation of user's normal workflow and practice to ensure user-informed design Enable local customization according to local practice and terminology
System-related and user-related	Default settings	User-related: Failure to change suggested default settings Lack of knowledge about default settings System-related: Orders hidden within predefined order sentences and order sets	User education and training about complex prescribing functions and challenges that may be encountered with using the system Development of more sophisticated, patient specific predefined order sentences and order sets

(continued)

Main Error Facilitator	Key Themes	Specific Issues	Recommendations
System-related	Nonintuitive ordering or information transmission	Lack of standardized terminology Interoperability issues	Facilitate local customization to incorporate local terminology Consistent use of key terms between systems Addressing interoperability issues between standalone systems, particularly at the transmission of information stage
System-related	Repeat prescriptions and automated processes	Repetition of previously corrected errors Reduced visibility of computerized errors	Introduce additional checks into the prescribing process User training and education about the risks of using workarounds
User-related	User's work processes	Batch order entry Users working under another colleague's log-in	User education and training about the risks of using workarounds
System-related and user-related	CDS systems	User-related: Lack of knowledge about the CDS checks that are being performed System-related: Inconsistent and insufficient use of CDS to safeguard against errors Poor CDS design Erroneous suggestions due to issues with, CDS sensitivity, specificity, and accuracy of information	Education and training about the systems functions (and lack of) Use of CDS, where a clinical need has been identified Refining the sensitivity and specificity of CDS

Abbreviations: CDS, Clinical Decision Support.
Reprinted with permission from Brown CL, Mulcaster HL, Triffitt KL, et al. A systematic review of the types and causes of prescribing errors generated from using computerized provider order entry systems in primary and secondary care. *J Am Med Inform Assoc* 2017;24:432–440.

the inpatient side, many institutions are implementing bar coding or radiofrequency identification (RFID) solutions. In bar code medication administration (BCMA), a nurse must swipe a bar code on the medication, the patient's wristband, and her own badge to confirm a three-way match before a medication can be administered.[54] In RFID systems, the medication package has an

Sociotechnical Model Dimension	Examples of Types of Possible Errors	Examples of Potential Ways to Reduce Likelihood of These Errors
Hardware and software: required to run the healthcare applications	Computer or network is not functioning Input data truncated (i.e., buffer overflow): some entered data lost	Provide redundant hardware for all essential patient care activities Warn users when data entered exceed amount that can be stored
Clinical content: data, information, and knowledge entered, displayed, or transmitted	Allowable item cannot be ordered (e.g., no amoxicillin in the antibiotic pick list) Incorrect default dose for given medication	Conduct extensive prerelease testing on all system–system data interfaces and human–computer interfaces to ensure that new features are working as planned and that existing features are working as before
Human–computer interface: aspects of the system that users can see, touch, or hear	Data entry or review screen does not show complete data (e.g., missing patient name, medical record number, birthdate) Two buttons with same label but different functionality Wrong decision about KCl administration based on poor data presentation on the computer screen	Encourage and provide methods for clinicians to report when patient-specific screens do not contain key patient demographics so that the software can be fixed Prerelease inspection of all screens for duplicate button names Improve data displays and train users to routinely review and cross-validate all data values for appropriateness before making critical decisions
People: the humans involved in the design, development, implementation, and use of HIT	Two patients with same name: data entered for wrong patient Incorrect merge of two patients' data Nurses scan duplicate patient bar code taped to their clipboard rather than bar code on patient to save time	Alert providers to potential duplicate patient names and require reconfirmation of patient identity before saving data (e.g., display patient photo before signing) Develop tools to compare key demographic data and calculate a probability estimate of similarity Improve user training, user interfaces, work processes, and organizational policies to reduce need for workarounds
Workflow and communication: the steps needed to ensure that each patient receives the care he or she needs at the time he or she needs it	Computer discontinues a medication order without notifying a human Critical abnormal test result alerts not followed up	Implement fail-safe communication (e.g., resend message to another hospital designee if no response from physician or nurse) for all computer-generated actions Implement robust quality assurance systems to monitor critical alert follow-up rates; use dual notification for alerts judiciously

Table 13-4 **EXAMPLES OF INFORMATION TECHNOLOGY–RELATED ERRORS AND CORRESPONDING SUGGESTED MITIGATING PROCEDURES**

(continued)

Table 13-4   EXAMPLES OF INFORMATION TECHNOLOGY–RELATED ERRORS AND CORRESPONDING SUGGESTED MITIGATING PROCEDURES (*continued*)

Sociotechnical Model Dimension	Examples of Types of Possible Errors	Examples of Potential Ways to Reduce Likelihood of These Errors
Organizational policies and procedures: internal culture, structures, policies, and procedures that affect all aspects of HIT management and healthcare	Policy contradicts physical reality (e.g., required bar code medicine administration readers not available in all patient locations) Policy contradicts personnel capability (e.g., one pharmacist to verify all orders entered via CPOE in large hospital) Incorrect policy allows "hard stops" on clinical alerts, causing delays in needed therapy	Before and after implementation, conduct inspections and interviews and monitor feedback from users in all physical locations Before and after implementation, conduct interviews with all affected users to better gauge workload Disallow "hard stops" on almost all alerts; users should be able to override the computer in all but the most egregious cases (e.g., ordering promethazine as intravenous push by peripheral vein)
External rules, regulations, and pressures: external forces that facilitate or place constraints on the design, development, implementation, use, and evaluation of HIT in the clinical setting	Billing requirements lead to inaccurate documentation in EHR (e.g., inappropriate copy and paste) Joint Commission-required medication reconciliation processes causing rushed development of new medication reconciliation applications that were difficult to use and caused errors: safety goal rescinded only to be reinstated July 1, 2011	Highlight all "pasted" material and include reference to source of material Carefully consider potential adverse unintended consequences before making new rules or regulations: conduct interviews and observations of users to gauge effects of rules and regulations on patient safety, quality of care, and clinician work life
System measurement and monitoring: evaluation of system availability, use, effectiveness, and unintended consequences of system use	Incomplete or inappropriate (e.g., combining disparate data) data aggregation leads to erroneous reporting Incorrect interpretation of quality measurement data	Increase measurement and monitoring transparency by providing involved stakeholders with access to raw data, analytical methods, and reports

Abbreviations: CPOE, computerized provider order entry; EHR, electronic health record; HIT, health information technology; KCl, potassium chloride.

implanted chip that transmits a signal, allowing for passive identification (like driving through an automated toll booth) rather than requiring a scan. Despite its intuitive appeal, RFID remains more expensive, and—because patients are taking multiple medications and nurses often have the medications for several patients on their carts—somewhat trickier to implement. For now, most hospitals seeking to improve their medication administration process have favored BCMA.

Like all HIT systems, BCMA has its challenges. Nurses worry that it will take too much time (although one study demonstrated that it did not[55])—and workarounds (such as when a nurse takes a handful of patient wristbands and scans them outside the patient's room to save time) that bypass the systems' safety features remain possible.[56] Moreover, BCMA must be rooted in an environment of robust safety processes. We documented one case in which two patients (one a poorly controlled diabetic) were mistakenly given each other's bar-coded wristbands, nearly leading to a fatal insulin overdose in the nondiabetic whose computerized record erroneously indicated that he had a stratospheric blood sugar.[57]

Like all IT systems, BCMA can become a very efficient error propagator if the inputted data are incorrect. For example, in the case of the Septra overdose, although the nurse thought to question the extraordinarily high number of pills (38 ½ of them), she placed implicit trust in our hospital's bar-coding system, which was mistakenly programmed (per the order placed by the provider and approved by the pharmacist) to prompt the administration of 38 ½ pills, rather than the correct dose of one.[19]

Concerns notwithstanding, effective use of BCMA technology can substantially reduce medication dispensing errors. After a long period during which bar coding was supported more by face validity than hard evidence, two studies by Poon et al. have demonstrated that bar coding really does work. The first focused on a process invisible to most doctors and nurses: the drug dispensing system in the pharmacy. There, a bar code scanning system reduced both errors and potential adverse drug events.[58] The other, of a bedside bar coding system, is probably the more important one for the field of patient safety.[9] In it, a "closed-loop" system that combined CPOE, BCMA, and an electronic medication administration record (eMAR) led to an approximately 50% decrease in drug administration errors and potential adverse drug events. More recent research continues to support the role of BCMA in reducing adverse drug events.[59–61]

Although the system is not foolproof, it is comforting that BCMA is now supported by robust evidence. In the end, of course, hospitals will need both BCMA *and* CPOE. The studies of Poon et al.[9,58] demonstrate the synergistic value of blending these technologies together in a "closed loop."

Smart intravenous pumps

Progress in medication safety through BCMA still leaves a large gap: the safety of medications infused intravenously. Approximately 90% of hospitalized patients receive at least one intravenous medication. Because many of these medications are far more dangerous than pills, and their doses are more variable (often calculated by the hour, or through complex weight- and size-based formulae), the opportunity for harm is significant. As with BCMA, the problem is that there is no downstream opportunity to catch errors at the administration phase. Because of this, there has been considerable interest in so-called "smart intravenous pumps."

Smart pumps are engineered to have built-in danger alerts, clinical calculators, and drug libraries that include information on the standard concentrations of frequently used drugs. They also can record every infusion, creating a database that can identify risky situations and medications for future interventions. Studies have shown that these pumps can prevent many infusion errors,[62–64] but that attention must be paid to seamlessly interfacing these systems with other computerized medication systems such as CPOE and BCMA.[65] Studies also find that workarounds continue to pose a problem.[63]

One group of researchers compared three types of pumps—traditional pumps, smart pumps, and smart pumps with bar coding technology—and found that the smart pumps were most effective either when they had bar coding (to ensure that the pharmacy-prepared bag was the correct one for a given patient) or when "hard" (i.e., unchangeable by the bedside nurse) dosing limits were used.[66] When one considers the increasing number and complexity of intravenous infusions in hospitalized (Figure 7-1), and now even homebound, patients, perfecting this technology and working through the complex machine–person interaction issues should be high priorities.

Automated drug dispensing systems and robots

When people think of information technology and patient safety, they generally think of EHRs, CPOE, and perhaps BCMA and smart pumps. It is worth adding several others to the list of IT tools that can help improve medication safety, such as automated drug dispensing systems and robots.[67]

Automated drug dispensing systems or cabinets are computerized pharmaceutical storage devices that facilitate the storing and dispensing of medications as well as tracking of user access. They are often located near the site of care on the inpatient floors. Use of such systems has been shown to decrease both medication errors and costs.[68,69]

In addition, there are a variety of robot dispensing systems, which take over many of the tasks previously performed by clinical pharmacists and pharmacy technicians. The goal of these systems is to reduce the potential for human error. Yet even these technologies can cause errors. In *The Digital Doctor*, Wachter describes the role of UCSF's $7 million Swiss-made pharmacy robot, which, ironically, contributed to the massive Septra overdose by following its orders precisely.[19] After the physician ordered, and the pharmacist approved, the errant order, it was sent electronically to the robot. At that point, recounts Wachter,

> [the] robot dutifully collected 38 ½ Septra tablets—with perfect accuracy—placed them on a half-dozen rings, and sent them to Pablo's floor, where they came to rest in a small bin waiting for the nurse to administer them at the appointed time…. there is no final pharmacist check of the robot's handiwork, the way there is for the medications prepared by the technicians in the seventh-floor pharmacy. "If the order goes to the robot, the techs just sort it by location and put it in a bin, and that's it," [said the pharmacist]. "They eliminated the step of the pharmacist checking on the robot, because the idea is you're paying so much money because it's so accurate."[19]

This case again highlights the need to carefully consider workflow, human factors, and the inevitability of unanticipated consequences when implementing HIT. Once the bugs are worked out of all of these different HIT systems, hospitals' challenges will be to find the money to purchase, maintain, and train people on all of them, and then to weave them together into a seamless whole (Chapter 7).

IT SOLUTIONS FOR IMPROVING COMMUNICATION AND ACCESS

It is worth pointing out that a wide range of other IT-based solutions can help improve patient safety outside the sphere of medication safety. The rise of social media platforms, widespread adoption of smartphones, and the advent of highly effective communication technologies hold the potential to improve both the ways in which care team members connect with each another and with their patients. This may have powerful implications for patient safety.

Social media platforms

Patients are increasingly using social media platforms, such as Facebook and Yelp, to highlight quality and safety issues they perceive in healthcare, often discussing events in real-time.[70] In addition, the stories that patients publicly communicate about their care online may prove valuable to efforts dedicated to improving the patient experience, a growing area of focus for hospitals.[71,72] While the role of social media in identifying safety issues and improving hospital quality is not yet clear,[73] healthcare institutions will need to think about how to integrate this information with safety data from more traditional sources such as the incident reporting system (Chapter 14).

Provider communication technologies

In many hospitals, new systems modeled on social media platforms like Facebook and Twitter are being used to facilitate instant communication among caregivers[74,75] (Figure 13-2). While healthcare providers have historically used paging as the main form of communication, app-based or text-based

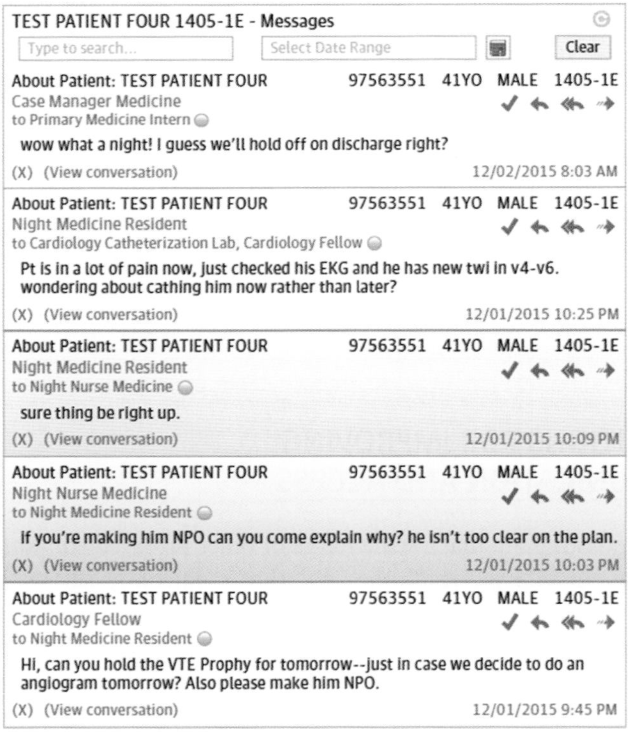

Figure 13-2 ▪ This provides a fictitious example viewed from the perspective of "Night Nurse Medicine" and demonstrates how clinicians communicate about a patient's plan of care. The blue rectangle represents a message sent by the viewing provider and the gray color indicates a received message. The white boxes are messages about the same patient but between other clinicians. (Reproduced with permission from Khanna RR, Wachter RM, Blum M. Reimagining electronic clinical communication in the post-pager, smartphone era. *JAMA* 2016;315:21–22.)

communication is becoming increasingly common and may improve the quality of provider-to-provider communication by improving efficiency and the accuracy of information transfer.[76]

One concern is security. Texting patients' protected health information on a nonsecure site may be a privacy violation. The development of secure apps and platforms may mitigate these concerns. Smartphone-enabled communication systems may also improve handover processes,[77] particularly when used in conjunction with some of the IT-based sign-out systems discussed in Chapter 8.

Telemedicine

In addition to improving provider communication to better facilitate patient care within a single hospital or health system, technologies have evolved to diagnose, monitor, manage, treat, and support patients remotely—a practice referred to as *telemedicine* or *telehealth*. Research demonstrates that remote monitoring or telemonitoring can reduce mortality rates and hospitalizations for heart failure,[78] and decrease the frequency of medication errors.[79,80] Telemonitoring has also been used successfully to mitigate adverse events in diabetic outpatients[81] and reduce inappropriate shocks in patients with implantable defibrillators.[82] Finally, telemedicine consults also seem to improve access to specialty expertise not readily available at all hospitals and may obviate the need for some patients to transfer to hospitals with a higher level of care.[83]

While the impact of telemedicine has been generally favorable, challenges and safety concerns persist.[84] Critics argue that providers may miss crucial details, leading to inaccurate diagnosis or mismanagement of a medical condition.

This likely suggests that, just as with other forms of HIT, thoughtful implementation of telemedicine is required. Table 13-5 outlines suggestions to improve patient safety with regard to telemedicine.

In addition, we shouldn't forget the importance of other forms of clinically-oriented HIT, such as the picture archiving and communication systems (PACS) that allow digital radiographs to be reviewed from a few miles, or a few thousand miles, away from the hospital or clinic.[85] In addition to their convenience, PACS can decrease x-ray interpretation errors by facilitating double reads, computerized enhancements of images, and access to prior radiographs.[86]

Mobile applications

The use of direct-to-consumer technology in healthcare is growing, especially with regard to mobile applications (or apps, as they are commonly referred to), often used by patients for assistance in monitoring or managing

Table 13-5	SUGGESTIONS FOR IMPROVING SAFETY IN TELEMEDICINE

- Patient safety awareness should permeate all phases of the telemedicine project life cycle
- Integrate safety testing as part of usability and efficacy trials, such evaluations should not be limited to academic medical settings
- Use the latest data security and encryption systems to protect patient privacy
- Increase regulatory, professional, and healthcare organizations' involvement in creating consensus-driven guidelines, operational protocols, and standards, all of which should be updated regularly
- Full disclosure of possible risks prior to patient enrollment in telemedicine interventions
- Create systems for clinicians to document telemedicine services and integrate them as part of regular workflow
- Increase efforts to lessen social risks by creating more solutions for patients with low health literacy, along with solutions for non-English speakers

Reprinted with permission from AHRQ Patient Safety Network: Agboola S, Kvedar J. Telemedicine and patient safety [Perspective]. *AHRQ PSNet* [serial online]; September 2016. Available at: https://psnet. ahrq.gov/perspectives/perspective/206/telemedicine-and-patient-safety?q=telemedicine.

certain health concerns and increasingly, by providers for a variety of reasons. Although mobile apps hold the potential to assist with diagnosis and management of disease, especially in the case of chronic medical conditions,[87] concerns persist regarding the regulation and vetting of the thousands of available apps. Indeed, a recent review of mobile applications designed to improve diagnostic accuracy found that consumers and providers should use these apps cautiously.[88] One study found that one app misdiagnosed almost 90% of melanomas that had been confirmed by biopsy.[89] Experts have also raised concerns that consumers' privacy may be compromised by the use of apps.[90]

COMPUTERIZED CLINICAL DECISION SUPPORT SYSTEMS

Although much of HIT's emphasis has been on replacing the paper chart and moving information around, its ultimate value may lie more in computerized clinical decision support systems (CDSS) that can provide guidance to clinicians at the point of care. For example, some systems offer simple alerts such as drug–drug, drug–allergy, or drug–lab interactions (Figure 13-1),[91] or links to evidence-based guidelines (the clinician types in a diagnosis of "pneumonia" and a link to a recent pneumonia management guideline pops up).

But that is just the start. More advanced decision support systems can "hard wire" certain kinds of care. For example, order sets for common

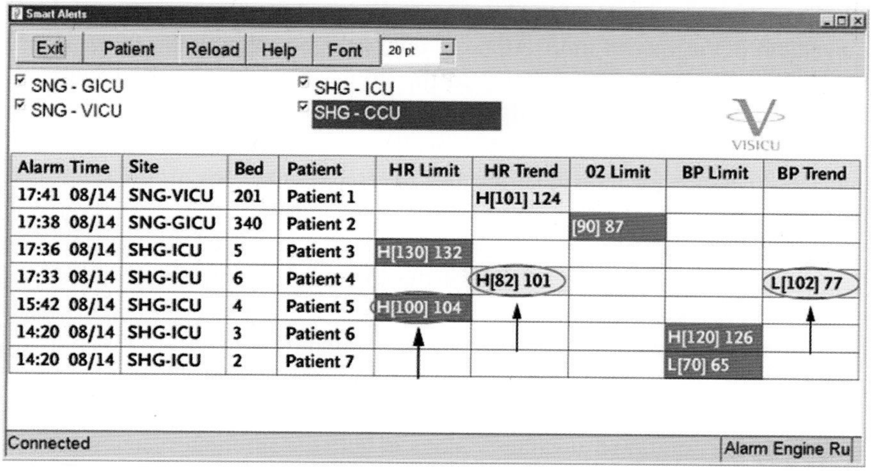

Alarm Time	Site	Bed	Patient	HR Limit	HR Trend	02 Limit	BP Limit	BP Trend
17:41 08/14	SNG-VICU	201	Patient 1		H[101] 124			
17:38 08/14	SNG-GICU	340	Patient 2			[90] 87		
17:36 08/14	SHG-ICU	5	Patient 3	H[130] 132				
17:33 08/14	SHG-ICU	6	Patient 4		H[82] 101			L[102] 77
15:42 08/14	SHG-ICU	4	Patient 5	H[100] 104				
14:20 08/14	SHG-ICU	3	Patient 6				H[120] 126	
14:20 08/14	SHG-ICU	2	Patient 7				L[70] 65	

Figure 13-3 ■ "Smart" monitoring system in an ICU. This screen highlights physiologic changes that are occurring (in this case, a rapid pulse and a trend toward increasing pulse and decreasing blood pressure [BP]); such monitoring can help clinicians detect and respond to such changes before an adverse event occurs. The heart-rate (HR) limit alert is triggered when the heart rate crosses a high (H) or low (L) limit, which are determined according to the patient's active medical conditions. Patient 5 (thick arrow) has had surgery and is at risk for perioperative coronary events. The limit value is given in brackets, followed by the patient's current value. The heart-rate or blood-pressure trend alert is triggered if the heart rate or blood pressure changes substantially over a period of several hours. Patient 4 (thin arrows) has an increasing heart rate and a decreasing blood pressure; on evaluation, this patient was found to have hypovolemia. The baseline value is given in brackets, followed by the current value. (Reproduced with permission from Bates DW, Gawande AA. Improving safety with information technology. *N Engl J Med* 2003;348:2526–2534.)

diagnoses can be loaded into a CPOE system, making it easy to do the right thing by simply clicking a few boxes.[92] Or an intensive care unit (ICU) system can alert the physician or nurse when a patient's vital signs veer outside preset parameters (Figure 13-3). Note that these prescriptive systems usually permit clinicians to deviate from recommended protocols, but this takes more time, because the doctor needs to type out the orders instead of accepting an order set, and may even be asked to document the reason for deviation. Even more prescriptively, the computer could all but force a given practice, making the clinician jump through several hoops (such as "call a specialist for approval") before being allowed to bypass a recommendation.

Of course, this is tricky stuff, as humans worry both about machines taking over their lives and that guidelines embedded in computer systems may not completely apply to the situation and patient at hand. Many healthcare experts and providers are also troubled by the possibility that prescriptive guidelines may stand in the way of innovation or "out of the box thinking." These issues are real and will need to be worked through over time, but for healthcare systems, which are increasingly being judged both on their adherence to evidence-based processes of care as well as clinical outcomes (Chapters 3 and 19), tolerance for individual practice differences that vary from established best practices is diminishing rapidly.

More pragmatically, one of the great challenges of CDSS systems has been *alert fatigue*.[93] This was one of the root causes in the Septra case, as both the busy resident and pharmacist clicked out of alerts designed to warm them of the impending overdose.[19] One study of approximately 5000 computerized alerts showed that clinicians overrode "critical drug interaction" and "allergy–drug interaction" alerts approximately 75% of the time.[94] Another looked at over 150,000 drug allergy alerts in both the ambulatory and inpatient settings of one healthcare system and found that close to 80% of these warnings were overridden and 96% of the overrides were thought to be appropriate when evaluated by clinician reviewers.[95] Finally, another study found that, in one large teaching hospital, the ICU monitors threw off more than 2.5 million alerts each month, the vast majority of which were false positives.[96] As systems become more prescriptive, clinicians may also bristle at hardwired care protocols that appear to lack flexibility (*cookbook medicine*).

All of this creates a daunting calibration challenge for designers of CDSS: making sure clinicians are alerted when appropriate but not so much that they simply learn to ignore or click out of every alert (especially the important ones). Because the experience of virtually every HIT implementation has been that the vast majority of alerts are ignored, most modern installations begin with a "less is more" philosophy: retaining the truly life-threatening, mission-critical alerts while jettisoning the "nice to know" ones. This philosophy, which has been taken to high art by Google (think about how uncluttered your Google search page is) and Apple (ditto your iPhone), is deeply rooted in human factors thinking and also has implications for alarm systems in ICUs and hospital wards (Chapter 7).

Increasingly sophisticated solutions are in the works. One version involves better integration between different data sources. Taking the example of ICU alarms, a smarter system would weave together the heart rate and blood pressure data streams, such that an alarm wouldn't fire if the heart rate abruptly increased from 70 to 180 if the blood pressure didn't budge (since this would be physiologically impossible).[19] Another type of solution, which comes more from the realm of "big data" and artificial intelligence, would mine clinician responses to millions of alerts, so as to say, "it looks like this particular alarm or alert, when fired on this unit with this type of patient, is always ignored. So I won't fire the next one." We are also starting to see the blending together of computerized systems and multidisciplinary patient safety and quality improvement programs. In Chapter 11, we discussed a fall prevention protocol that was embedded in a computerized environment: the IT system calculated the patient's risk of falling and created a customized educational program for the patient and family, while also targeting actions for the various providers (Figure 11-1).[97] We can expect to see more of this type of integration—an exciting development.

Just as exciting, a new philosophy of "*measure-vention*" is emerging, in which real-time computerized measurement of performance is fed back to providers not one or two weeks (or one or two years) later, but immediately, allowing for "just in time" improvements. For example, one program improved adherence to a variety of quality and safety measures in a pediatric ICU by using an electronic dashboard to display real-time data on informed consent, urinary catheters, use of restraints, deep venous thrombosis prophylaxis, pressure ulcer risk, and medication reconciliation status to frontline providers (Figure 13-4).[98] In another application of the same principle,

Pediatric ICU (PICU) Dashboard

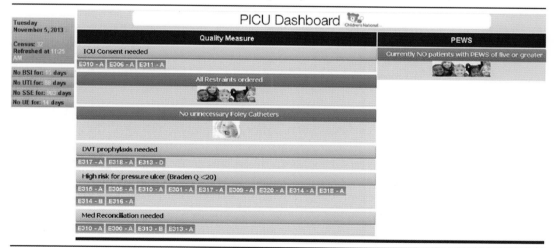

Figure 13-4 ▪ The measure-vention strategy depicted in this figure is a real-time dashboard as it is displayed in the PICU at Children's National Health System and shows each patient's status with regard to six elements of care including documentation of caregiver consent to treatment, the use of restraints without an accompanying order, duration of urinary catheter placement >96 hours, pharmacologic or mechanical DVT prophylaxis use, risk for pressure ulcer development, and completion of medication reconciliation. Each patient not in compliance with a recommended practice remains on the dashboard until the appropriate action is taken in the electronic record. (Reproduced with permission from Shaw SJ, Jacobs B, Stockwell DC, Futterman C, Spaeder MC. Effect of a real-time pediatric ICU safety bundle dashboard on quality improvement measures. *Jt Comm J Qual Patient Saf* 2015;41:414–420.)

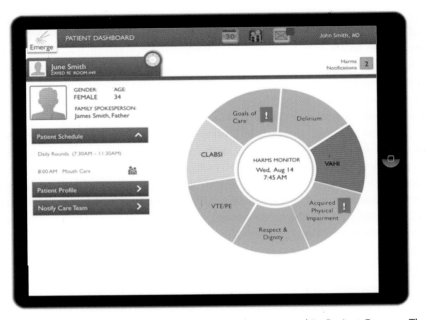

Figure 13-5 ▪ Screenshot from the tablet application used in Project Emerge. The application integrates data from monitoring equipment and information systems so that clinicians can view the data easily. The application displays a "harms monitor" that tracks tasks performed for patients and alerts providers when patients may be at risk. (Reproduced with permission from Dr. Peter Pronovost, Johns Hopkins Armstrong Institute for Patient Safety and Quality.)

a real-time electronic surveillance dashboard allows pharmacists to intercept and prevent medication errors and optimize therapy.[99] In an effort known as Project Emerge, researchers from Johns Hopkins are seeking to improve the safety and experience of patients in the ICU using a tablet dashboard that captures real-time patient data and displays it to clinicians.[100] The tablet application viewed by clinicians integrates data from many sources and updates a "harms monitor" that alerts providers to which patients may be at risk (Figure 13-5). These innovative strategies hold real promise for improving safety.

IT SOLUTIONS FOR IMPROVING DIAGNOSTIC ACCURACY

Finally, another type of decision support focuses on improving diagnostic accuracy (Chapter 6). Early clinical artificial intelligence programs—in which clinicians entered key elements from the history, physical examination, and laboratory studies and the computer fashioned a list of diagnoses—were disappointing, because the computer-generated diagnostic lists mixed plausible possibilities with nonsensical ones, and the data entry time (which came over and above clinical charting time) was prohibitive.[101]

Recent advances have generated new interest in diagnostic decision support. Some programs now pull data directly from the EHR, bypassing the need for redundant data entry. Others mine textbooks and journal articles to find diagnoses most frequently associated with citations of certain symptoms and signs.[102] Most modern programs not only suggest possible diagnoses but also link to helpful resources and references. The accuracy of today's top programs, such as Isabel (Figure 13-6) and DxPlain, far surpasses that of earlier models,[103,104] although none can yet compete with seasoned human diagnosticians.[105]

Diagnostic decision support systems are likely to be judged on the seamlessness of the inputting process and the helpfulness of the diagnostic

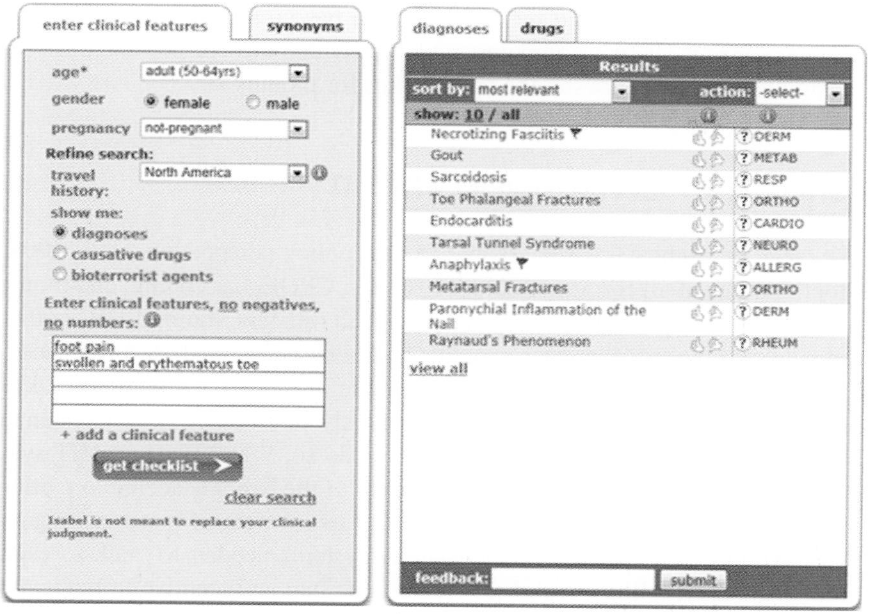

Figure 13-6 ▪ Screenshot from the Isabel diagnostic system. Signs, symptoms, and laboratory abnormalities are entered on the list on the left, and a differential diagnosis is generated. Clicking on any of the diagnoses takes the user to textbook chapters and online literature with additional information. (Available at: http://isabelhealthcare.files. wordpress.com/2011/07/isabelblog-pic.png.)

possibilities they offer. As of yet, no studies convincingly prove that these systems improve patient outcomes, but this may more reflect the challenges of measuring the frequency and impact of diagnostic errors (Chapter 6) rather than the quality or usefulness of the tools.

One can envision future computerized decision aids that draw their information directly from the EHR (facilitated as either data are entered in more structured formats or as computerized deep learning improves so that key information can more easily be extracted from narrative notes), produce possible diagnoses that are automatically updated with new information, and actually "learn" by integrating prior experiences from the system itself, making them ever more accurate over time. In a world in which Netflix helpfully suggests, "People who liked this movie also liked that one," how about a decision support system that says, "Patients at our hospital with this constellation of findings often turned out to have diagnoses X or Y"? While this might have seemed like fantasy a decade ago, anyone who observed the IBM computer "Watson" defeat the world's top *Jeopardy!* contestants or has seen a driverless car rolling down the street has become convinced that it may be just a matter of time before this kind of computerized firepower transforms the diagnostic process. Oh, and by the way, IBM has created a medical version of its *Jeopardy!*-playing computer: which provided the correct diagnosis in 10 minutes in a case that stumped physicians for months.[106]

THE POLICY ENVIRONMENT FOR HIT

The story of health IT is remarkable from a policy perspective. Until 2008, adoption rates of all forms of health IT (EHRs, CPOE, bar coding, and more) were low; fewer than 10% of U.S. hospitals had full-functioning EHRs at that time, despite the fact that such systems had been on the market for decades. This represented a market failure, in that none of the players who needed to make the large investment in health IT (mostly physicians, health systems, and hospitals) were sufficiently motivated to do so. Why? Because HIT systems are so complex and expensive and many of the benefits accrue to parties other than those shelling out the money (such as insurers). Moreover, to gain the maximum benefit from HIT, disparate systems needed to "talk to each other" (interoperability), and, here too, no one had an incentive to make the investment to weave the systems together.

Federal investment was needed to overcome this market failure, and it came in late 2008, as the American economy tumbled into crisis and Congress passed a $700 billion stimulus package to rescue it. In that package was tucked a provision known as HITECH (Health Information Technology for Economic and Clinical Health), which allocated $30 billion for doctors'

Table 13-6 THE CORE OBJECTIVES OF THE "MEANINGFUL USE" STANDARDS*,†

- Use computerized physician order entry (CPOE) for medication orders
- Implement drug–drug and drug–allergy checks
- Generate and transmit permissible prescriptions electronically
- Maintain an up-to-date problem list, active medication list, and allergy list
- Record demographics, vital signs, and smoking status
- Implement at least one clinical decision rule
- Report ambulatory clinical quality measures to CMS or to states
- Provide patients with an electronic copy of their health information, including: diagnostic test results, problem list, medication lists, and medication allergies
- Provide clinical summaries of each office visit (or, for hospitals, a summary of the hospitalization)
- Have the capability to exchange key clinical information among providers of care and patient-authorized entities electronically
- Protect electronic protected health information (ePHI) created or maintained by the EHR through implementation of appropriate technical capabilities

*Specific features of an EHR that providers were required to use to qualify for incentive payments under the HITECH Act.[107,108]

†In 2016, CMS announced the end of Meaningful Use, with new standards, known as Advancing Care Information, to be folded into the broader set of quality measurements under the Medicare Access and CHIP Reauthorization Act (MACRA).

Abbreviations: CMS, Centers for Medicare & Medicaid Services.

offices and hospitals that purchased and installed EHRs that met certain criteria ("Meaningful Use" see Table 13-6).[107,108] While Meaningful Use was criticized for creating a large regulatory burden and for failing to ensure widespread interoperability, there is little doubt that HITECH achieved its primary goal: to digitize the American healthcare system. Implementation is also being driven by changes in the payment system, emphasizing value over volume. These changes add to the motivation of health systems to capture clinical and financial data, and to build tools to analyze individual patient and population health outcomes.

Driven by all of these forces, HIT adoption rates rose from 20.8% in 2008 to 86.9% in 2015 in physician offices,[109] and from 9% in 2008 to 96.9% in 2015 in hospitals[110] (Figures 13-7 and 13-8). Given the importance of digitization to patient safety, this represents a seminal development for the field. However, as we have described, the results of health IT have been somewhat disappointing. This should have been predictable, since the trajectory has followed a couple of well-known principles that relate to technology adoption more generally: the "*Technology Hype Cycle*" and the "*Productivity Paradox*."

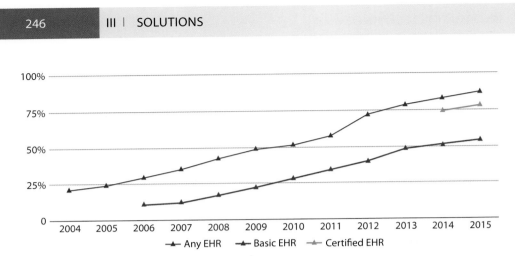

Figure 13-7 ■ Graph depicting increased office-based physician electronic health record adoption over time. (From the Office of the National Coordinator for Health Information Technology. 'Office-based Physician Electronic Health Record Adoption,' Health IT Quick-Stat #50. December 2016. Available at: https://dashboard.healthit.gov/quickstats/pages/physician-ehr-adoption-trends.php.)

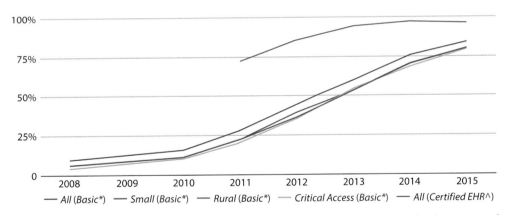

Figure 13-8 ■ Graph depicting increased electronic health record adoption by nonfederal acute care hospitals over time. (From the Office of the National Coordinator for Health Information Technology. 'Non-federal Acute Care Hospital Electronic Health Record Adoption,' Health IT Quick-Stat #47. May 2016. Available at: https://dashboard.healthit.gov/quickstats/pages/FIG-Hospital-EHR-Adoption.php.)

The "Technology Hype Cycle" (Figure 13-9),[111] originally described by the consulting firm Gartner, is made up of a predictable series of phases that technologies tend to traverse after their introduction:

- "Technology Trigger": after its initial launch, the technology reaches the attention of the public and industry.
- "Peak of Inflated Expectations": A few successful applications of the technology (often by highly selected individuals or organizations—sound familiar?) catalyze unrealistic expectations, often pushed along

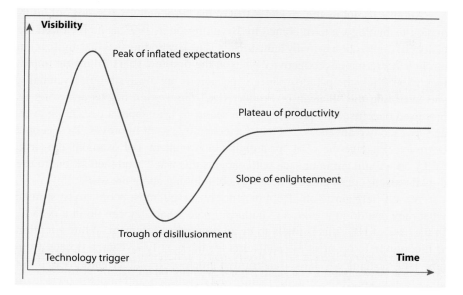

Figure 13-9 ■ The Technology Hype Cycle. (Reproduced with permission from Gartner. Gartner Hype Cycle. Available at: http://www.gartner.com/technology/research/methodologies/hype-cycle.jsp.)

by word of mouth, the blogosphere, or the marketing prowess of the vendor.

- "Trough of Disillusionment": Virtually no technology can live up to its initial hype. As negative experience grows, the balloon is pricked and air rushes out. The media move on to cover another "hotter" technology, and the cycle repeats.
- "Slope of Enlightenment": A few hardy individuals and organizations, seeing the technology's true potential, begin experimenting with it, no longer burdened by inflated expectations. Assuming that the technology is worthwhile, they begin to see and demonstrate its value.
- "Plateau of Productivity": As more organizations ascend the "Slope of Enlightenment," the benefits of the technology (which has improved from its initial clunky phase based on user feedback and the self-preserving instincts of the developers) become widely demonstrated and accepted. The height of the plateau, of course, depends on the quality of the technology and the size of its market.

This cycle perfectly describes the history of CPOE (over the last 20 years) and diagnostic artificial intelligence tools (over the past 40 years). The hope is that these technologies—all HIT, really—are now somewhere on either the Slope of Enlightenment or the Plateau of Productivity.

Another useful mental model is that of the "Productivity Paradox" of information technology, a term coined by Brynjolfsson in 1993 as he reviewed the history of digitization in many industries.[112] The key finding was that digitization rarely leads to major productivity gains in the first few years following implementation (thus, the paradox, since expectations are always high). Eventually, and mirroring the "Plateau of Productivity," digitization begins achieving its promised benefits. This process, which seems to take about a decade on average, owes to two advances.[113] One, the technology itself improves. Two, people begin to reimagine the work for a digital environment. For example, they ask, "Why do we still communicate with patients this way?" and then set out to use digital tools to create entirely new ways of thinking about the work.

As self-help guru Tony Robbins once observed, most people overestimate what they can do in a year, and underestimate what they can do in a decade. In the case of HIT, this is likely to be an accurate assessment. While adoption will continue to occur in fits and starts for the next few years, a decade from now HIT systems will have transformed much of the safety enterprise, if not all of healthcare. If the systems mature and developers and implementers learn from past mistakes, this will be decidedly for the better.

KEY POINTS

- The implementation of HIT had been remarkably slow until about a decade ago, when a combination of federal policy changes (including $30 billion in incentive payments in the United States) and a growing business case have led to a marked uptick in adoption rates.
- Many healthcare activities require multiple providers (and others) to view patient-level information simultaneously, a powerful argument for EHRs.
- CPOE can ensure that physicians' orders are legible and respect preset parameters.
- Bar coding or other similar systems can help decrease the frequency of medication administration (and other patient identification–related) errors.
- Ultimately, much of the benefit of HIT will come through the thoughtful implementation of computerized decision support, which ranges from simply providing information to clinicians at the point of care to more prescriptive systems that "hardwire" certain care processes.
- While HIT has tremendous appeal, its history to date has been characterized by a surprising number of failures and unanticipated consequences, illustrating the importance of human factors and the ongoing challenge of implementing major changes in complex organizations.

REFERENCES

1. Jha AK, Desroches CM, Campbell EG, et al. Use of electronic health records in US hospitals. *N Engl J Med* 2009;360:1628–1638.

2. DesRoches CM, Campbell EG, Rao SR, et al. Electronic health records in ambulatory care—a national survey of physicians. *N Engl J Med* 2008;359:50–60.

3. Office of the National Coordinator for Health Information Technology. 'Office-based physician electronic health record adoption. Health IT Quick-Stat #50; December 2016. Available at: https://dashboard.healthit.gov/quickstats/pages/physician-ehr-adoption-trends.php.

4. Henry J, Pylypchuk Y, Searcy T, et al. *Adoption of Electronic Health Record Systems among U.S. Non-Federal Acute Care Hospitals: 2008-2015*. ONC Data Brief, no.35. Office of the National Coordinator for Health Information Technology: Washington, DC; May 2016. Available at: https://dashboard.healthit.gov/evaluations/data-briefs/non-federal-acute-care-hospital-ehr-adoption-2008-2015.php.

5. Jha AK, Perlin JB, Kizer KW, Dudley RA. Effect of the transformation of the Veterans Affairs Health Care System on the quality of care. *N Engl J Med* 2003;348:2218–2227.

6. Furukawa MF, Eldridge N, Wang Y, Metersky M. Electronic health records adoption and rates of in-hospital adverse events. *J Patient Saf* February 6, 2016. [Epub ahead of print].

7. Radley DC, Wasserman MR, Olsho LE, Shoemaker SJ, Spranca MD, Bradshaw B. Reduction in medication errors in hospitals due to adoption of computerized provider order entry systems. *J Am Med Inform Assoc* 2013;20:470–476.

8. Kaushal R, Kern LM, Barrón Y, Quaresimo J, Abramson EL. Electronic prescribing improves medication safety in community-based office practices. *J Gen Intern Med* 2010;25:530–536.

9. Poon EG, Keohane CA, Yoon CS, et al. Effect of bar-code technology on the safety of medication administration. *N Engl J Med* 2010;362:1698–1707.

10. Buntin MB, Burke MF, Hoaglin MC, Blumenthal D. The benefits of health information technology: a review of the recent literatures shows predominantly positive results. *Health Aff (Millwood)* 2011;30:464–471.

11. Shojania KG, Duncan BW, McDonald KM, Wachter RM. Safe but sound: patient safety meets evidence-based medicine. *JAMA* 2002;288:508–513.

12. Wachter RM, Shojania KG. *Internal Bleeding: The Truth Behind America's Terrifying Epidemic of Medical Mistakes*. New York, NY: Rugged Land; 2004.

13. Harrington L, Kennerly D, Johnson C. Safety issues related to the electronic medical record (EMR): synthesis of the literature from the last decade, 2000–2009. *J Healthc Manag* 2011;56:31–43.

14. Meeks DW, Smith MW, Taylor L, Sittig DF, Scott JM, Singh H. An analysis of electronic health record-related patient safety concerns. *J Am Med Inform Assoc* 2014;21:1053–1059.

15. Wachter RM. Expected and unanticipated consequences of the quality and information technology revolutions. *JAMA* 2006;295:2780–2783.

16. Wright A, Hickman TT, McEvoy D, et al. Analysis of clinical decision support system malfunctions: a case series and survey. *J Am Med Inform Assoc* 2016;23:1068–1076.

17. Sittig DF, Singh H. Defining health information technology–related errors: new developments since 'to err is human'. *Arch Intern Med* 2011;171:1281–1284.

18. Cheung KC, van der Veen W, Bouvy ML, Wensing M, van den Bemt PM, de Smet PA. Classification of medication incidents associated with information technology. *J Am Med Inform Assoc* 2014;21:e63–e70.

19. Wachter RM. *The Digital Doctor: Hope, Hype, and Harm at the Dawn of Medicine's Computer Age*. New York, NY: McGraw-Hill; 2015.

20. Singh H, Spitzmueller C, Petersen NJ, et al. Primary care practitioners' views on test result management in EHR-enabled health systems: a national survey. *J Am Med Inform Assoc* 2013;20:727–735.

21. Babbott S, Manwell LB, Brown R, et al. Electronic medical records and physician stress in primary care: results from the MEMO Study. *J Am Med Inform Assoc* 2014;21(e1):e100–e106.

22. Shanafelt TD, Hasan O, Dyrbye LN, et al. Changes in burnout and satisfaction with work-life balance in physicians and the general US working population between 2011 and 2014. *Mayo Clin Proc* 2015;90:1600–1613.

23. Weis JM, Levy PC. Copy, paste, and cloned notes in electronic health records: prevalence, benefits, risks, and best practice recommendations. *Chest* 2014;145:632–638.

24. Hirschtick RE. A piece of my mind. Copy-and-paste. *JAMA* 2006;295:2335–2336.

25. Thornton JD, Schold JD, Venkateshaiah L, Lander B. Prevalence of copied information by attendings and residents in critical care progress notes. *Crit Care Med* 2013;41:382–388.

26. O'Donnell HC, Kaushal R, Barrón Y, Callahan MA, Adelman RD, Siegler EL. Physicians' attitudes towards copy and pasting in electronic note writing. *J Gen Intern Med* 2009;24:63–68.

27. Siegler EL, Adelman R. Copy and paste: a remediable hazard of electronic health records. *Am J Med* 2009;122:495–496.

28. Rosenbloom ST, Denny JC, Xu H, Lorenzi N, Stead WW, Johnson KB. Data from clinical notes: a perspective on the tension between structure and flexible documentation. *J Am Med Inform Assoc* 2011;18:181–186.

29. Johnson SB, Bakken S, Dine D, et al. An electronic health record based on structured narrative. *J Am Med Inform Assoc* 2008;15:54–64.

30. Polnaszek B, Gilmore-Bykovskyi A, Hovanes M, et al. Overcoming the challenges of unstructured data in multisite, electronic medical record-based abstraction. *Med Care* 2016;54:e65–e72.

31. Murff HJ, FitzHenry F, Matheny ME, et al. Automated identification of postoperative complications within an electronic medical record using natural language processing. *JAMA* 2011;306:848–855.

32. Alemzadeh H, Raman J, Leveson N, Kalbarczyk Z, Iyer RK. Adverse events in robotic surgery: a retrospective study of 14 years of FDA data. *PLoS One* 2016;11:e0151470.

33. de Lusignan S, Mold F, Sheikh A, et al. Patients' online access to their electronic health records and linked online services: a systematic interpretative review. *BMJ Open* 2014;4:e006021.

34. Delbanco T, Walker J, Bell SK, et al. Inviting patients to read their doctors' notes: a quasi-experimental study and a look ahead. *Ann Intern Med* 2012;157:461–470.

35. Bell SK, Mejilla R, Anselmo M, et al. When doctors share visit notes with patients: a study of patient and doctor perceptions of documentation errors, safety opportunities and the patient-doctor relationship. *BMJ Qual Saf* 2017;26:262–270.

36. Tang PC, Lee TH. Your doctor's office or the Internet? Two paths to personal health records. *N Engl J Med* 2009;360:1276–1278.

37. Roehrs A, da Costa CA, Righi RD, de Oliveira KS. Personal health records: a systematic literature review. *J Med Internet Res* 2017; 19:e13.

38. Archer N, Fevrier-Thomas U, Lokker C, McKibbon KA, Straus SE. Personal health records: a scoping review. *J Am Med Inform Assoc* 2011;18:515–522.

39. Halamka JD, Mandl KD, Tang PC. Early experiences with personal health records. *J Am Med Inform Assoc* 2008;15:1–7.

40. Schnipper JL, Gandhi TK, Wald JS, et al. Effects of an online personal health record on medication accuracy and safety: a cluster-randomized trial. *J Am Med Inform Assoc* 2012;19:728–734.

41. Verghese A. Culture shock—patient as icon, icon as patient. *N Engl J Med* 2008;359:2748–2751.

42. Bates DW, Leape LL, Cullen DJ, et al. Effect of computerized physician order entry and a team intervention on prevention of serious medication errors. *JAMA* 1998;280:1311–1316.

43. Bates DW, Teich JM, Lee J, et al. The impact of computerized physician order entry on medication error prevention. *J Am Med Inform Assoc* 1999;6:313–321.

44. Radley DC, Wasserman MR, Olsho LE, Shoemaker SJ, Spranca MD, Bradshaw B. Reduction in medication errors in hospital due to adoption of computerized provider order entry systems. *J Am Med Inform Assoc* 2013;20:470–476.

45. Kaushal R, Kern LM, Barrón Y, Quaresimo J, Abramson EL. Electronic prescribing improves medication safety in community-based office practices. *J Gen Intern Med* 2010;25:530–536.

46. Bates DW, Gawande AA. Improving safety with information technology. *N Engl J Med* 2003;348:2526–2534.

47. Boling B, McKibben M, Hingl J, Worth P, Jacobs BR, the Clinical Informatics Outcomes Research Group. Effectiveness of computerized provider order entry with dose range checking on prescribing errors. *J Patient Saf* 2005;1:190–194.

48. Ranji SR, Rennke S, Wachter RM, et al. Computerized provider order entry combined with clinical decision support systems to improve medication safety: a narrative review. *BMJ Qual Saf* 2014;23:773–780.

49. Amato MG, Salazar A, Hickman TT, et al. Computerized prescriber order entry-related patient safety reports: analysis of 2522 medication errors. *J Am Med Inform Assoc* 2017;24:316–322.

50. Payne TH, Hines LE, Chan RC, et al. Recommendations to improve the usability of drug-drug interaction clinical decision support alerts. *J Am Med Inform Assoc* 2015;22:1243–1250.

51. Schiff GD, Amato MG, Eguale T, et al. Computerized physician order entry-related medication errors: analysis of reported errors and vulnerability testing of current systems. *BMJ Qual Saf* 2015;24:264–271.

52. Metzger J, Welebob E, Bates DW, Lipsitz S, Classen DC. Mixed results in the safety performance of computerized physician order entry. *Health Aff (Millwod)* 2010; 29:655–663.

53. Brown CL, Mulcaster HL, Triffitt KL, et al. A systematic review of the types and causes of prescribing errors generated from using computerized provider order entry systems in primary and secondary care. *J Am Med Inform Assoc* 2017;24:432–442.

54. Wright AA, Katz IT. Bar coding for patient safety. *N Engl J Med* 2005;454:329–331.

55. Poon EG, Keohane CA, Bane A, et al. Impact of barcode medication administration technology on how nurses spend their time providing patient care. *J Nurs Adm* 2008;38:541–549.

56. Voshall B, Piscotty R, Lawrence J, Targosz M. Barcode medication administration workarounds: a systematic review and implications for nurse executives. *J Nurs Am* 2013;43:530–535.

57. McDonald CJ. Computerization can create safety hazards: a bar-coding near miss. *Ann Intern Med* 2006;144:510–516.

58. Poon EG, Cina JL, Churchill W, et al. Medication dispensing errors and potential adverse drug events before and after implementing bar code technology in the pharmacy. *Ann Intern Med* 2006;145:426–434.

59. Truitt E, Thompson R, Blazey-Martin D, NiSai D, Salem D. Effect of the implementation of barcode technology and an electronic medication administration record on adverse drug events. *Hosp Pharm* 2016;51:474–483.

60. Bonkowski J, Carnes C, Melucci J, et al. Effect of barcode-assisted medication administration on emergency department medication errors. *Acad Emerg Med* 2013;20:801–806.

61. Leung AA, Denham CR, Gandhi TK, et al. A safe practice standard for barcode technology. *J Patient Saf* 2015;11:89–99.

62. Keohane CA, Hayes J, Saniuk C, Rothschild JM, Bates DW. Intravenous medication safety and smart infusion systems: lessons learned and future opportunities. *J Infus Nurs* 2005;28:321–328.

63. Ohashi K, Dalleur O, Dykes PC, Bates DW. Benefits and risks of using smart pumps to reduce medication error rates: a systematic review. *Drug Saf* 2014;37:1011–1020.

64. Williams CK, Maddox RR, Heape E, et al. Application of the IV Medication Harm Index to assess the nature of harm averted by "smart" infusion safety systems. *J Patient Saf* 2006;2:132–139.

65. Husch M, Sullivan C, Rooney D, et al. Insights from the sharp end of intravenous medication errors: implications for infusion pump technology. *Qual Saf Health Care* 2005;14:80–86.

66. Trbovich PL, Pinkney S, Cafazzo JA, Easty AC. The impact of traditional and smart pump infusion technology on nurse medication administration performance in a simulated inpatient unit. *Qual Saf Health Care* 2010;19:430–434.

67. Chapuis C, Roustit M, Bal G, et al. Automated drug dispensing system reduces medication errors in an intensive care setting. *Crit Care Med* 2010;38:2275–2281.

68. Cousein E, Mareville J, Lerooy A, et al. Effect of automated drug distribution systems on medication error rates in a short-stay geriatric unit. *J Eval Clin Pract* 2014;20:678–684.

69. Chapuis C, Bedouch P, Detavernier M, et al. Automated drug dispensing systems in the intensive care unit: a financial analysis. *Crit Care* 2015;19:318.

70. Golder S, Norman G, Loke YK. Systematic review on the prevalence, frequency and comparative value of adverse events data in social media. *Br J Clin Pharmacol* 2015;80:878–888.

71. Lee V. Transparency and trust—online patient reviews of physicians. *N Engl J Med* 2017;376:197–199.

72. Greaves F, Ramirez-Cano D, Millett C, Darzi A, Donaldson L. Harnessing the cloud of patient experience: using social media to detect poor quality healthcare. *BMJ Qual Saf* 2013;22:251–255.

73. Lagu T, Goff SL, Craft B, et al. Can social media be used as a hospital quality improvement tool? *J Hosp Med* 2016;11:52–55.

74. Khanna RR, Wachter RM, Blum M. Reimagining electronic clinical communication in the post-pager, smartphone era. *JAMA* 2016;315:21–22.

75. Frizzell JD, Ahmed B. Text messaging versus paging: new technology for the next generation. *J Am Coll Cardiol* 2014;64:2703–2705.

76. Bhavesh P, Johnston M, Cookson N, King D, Arora S, Darzi A. Interprofessional communication of clinicians using a mobile phone app: a randomized crossover trial using simulated patient. *J Med Internet Res* 2016;18:e79.

77. Wu R, Lo V, Morra D, et al. A smartphone-enabled communication system to improve hospital communication: usage and perceptions of medical trainees and nurses on general internal medicine wards. *J Hosp Med* 2015;10:83–89.

78. Kitsou S, Paré G, Jaana M. Effects of home telemonitoring interventions on patients with chronic heart failure: an overview of systematic review. *J Med Internet Res* 2015;17:e63.

79. Dharmar M, Kupperman N, Romano PS, et al. Telemedicine consultations and medication errors in rural emergency departments. *Pediatrics* 2013;132:1090–1097.

80. Scott DM, Friesner DL, Rathke AM, Doherty-Johnsen S. Medication error reporting in rural critical access hospitals in the North Dakota Telepharmacy Project. *Am J Health Syst Pharm* 2014;71:58–67.

81. Sarkar U, Handley MA, Gupta R, et al. Use of an interactive, telephone-based self-management support program to identify ambulatory diabetes patients. *J Gen Intern Med* 2008;23:459–465.

82. Bifulco P, Argenziano L, Romano M, et al. Frequent home monitoring of ICD is effective to prevent inappropriate defibrillator shock delivery. *Case Rep Med* 2014;2014:579526.

83. Fang JL, Collura CA, Johnson RV, et al. Emergency video telemedicine consultation for newborn resuscitations: the Mayo Clinic experience. *Mayo Clin Proc* 2016;91:1735–1743.

84. Kahn JM. Virtual visits—confronting the challenges of telemedicine. *N Engl J Med* 2015;372:1684–1685.

85. Wachter RM. International teleradiology. *N Engl J Med* 2006;354:662–663.

86. Bryan S, Weatherburn G, Buxton M, Watkins J, Keen J, Muris N. Evaluation of a hospital picture archiving and communication system. *J Health Serv Res Policy* 1999;4:204–209.

87. Steinhubl SR, Muse ED, Topol EJ. Can mobile health technologies transform health care? *JAMA* 2013;310:2395–2396.

88. Jutel A, Lupton D. Digitizing diagnosis: a review of mobile applications in the diagnostic process. *Diagnosis* 2015;2:89–96.

89. Ferrero NA, Morrell DS, Burkhart CN. Skin scan: a demonstration of the need for FDA regulation of medical apps on iPhone. *J Am Acad Dermatol* 2013;68:515–516.

90. Wicks P, Chiauzzi E. 'Trust but verify'—five approaches to ensure safe medical apps. *BMC Med* 2015;13:205.

91. Classen DC, Phansalkar S, Bates DW. Critical drug–drug interactions for use in electronic health records systems with computerized physician order entry: review of leading approaches. *J Patient Saf* 2011;7:61–65.

92. Bright TJ, Wong A, Dhurjati R, et al. Effect of clinical decision-support systems: a systematic review. *Ann Intern Med* 2012;157:29–43.

93. Nanji KC, Slight SP, Seger DL, et al. Overrides of medication-related clinical decision support alerts in outpatients. *J Am Med Inform Assoc* 2014;21:487–491.

94. Payne TH, Nichol WP, Hoey P, Savarino J. Characteristics and override rates of order checks in a practitioner order entry system. *Proc AMIA Symp* 2002:602–606.

95. Slight SP, Beeler PE, Seger DL, et al. A cross-sectional observational study of high override rates of drug allergy alerts in inpatient and outpatient settings, and opportunities for improvement. *BMJ Qual Saf* 2017;26:217–225.

96. Drew BJ, Harris P, Zégre-Hemsey JK, et al. Insights into the problem of alarm fatigue with physiologic monitor devices: a comprehensive observational study of consecutive intensive care unit patients. *PLoS One* 2014;9:e110274.

97. Dykes PC, Carroll DL, Hurley A, et al. Fall prevention in acute care hospitals. A randomized trial. *JAMA* 2010;304:1912–1918.

98. Shaw SJ, Jacobs B, Stockwell DC, Futterman C, Spaeder MC. Effect of a real-time pediatric ICU safety bundle dashboard on quality improvement measures. *Jt Comm J Qual Patient Saf* 2015;41:414–420.

99. Waitman LR, Phillips IE, McCoy AB, et al. Adopting real-time surveillance dashboards as a component of an enterprise-wide medication safety strategy. *Jt Comm J Qual Patient Saf* 2011;37:326–332.

100. Rice S. Ambitious checklist app comes as hospitals struggle with basic checklists. *Modern Healthcare.* June 21, 2014. Available at: http://www.modernhealthcare.com/article/20140621/MAGAZINE/306219979.

101. Berner ES, Webster GD, Shuerman AA, et al. Performance of four computer-based diagnostic systems. *N Engl J Med* 1994;330:1792–1796.

102. Ramnarayan P, Winrow A, Coren M, et al. Diagnostic omission errors in acute paediatric practice: impact of a reminder system on decision-making. *BMC Med Inform Decis Mak* 2006;6:37.

103. Bond WF, Schwartz LM, Weaver KR, Levick D, Giuliano M, Graber ML. Differential diagnosis generators: an evaluation of currently available computer programs. *J Gen Intern Med* 2012;27(2):213–219.

104. Graber ML, Mathew A. Performance of a web-based clinical diagnosis support system for internists. *J Gen Intern Med* 2008;23:37–40.

105. Semigran HL, Levine DM, Nundy S, Mehrotra A. Comparison of Physician and Computer Diagnostic Accuracy. *JAMA Intern Med* 2016;176:1860–1861.

106. Ng Alfred. IBM's Watson gives proper diagnosis for Japanese leukemia patient after doctors were stumped for months. *New York Daily News.* August 7, 2016. Available at: http://www.nydailynews.com/news/world/ibm-watson-proper-diagnosis-doctors-stumped-article-1.2741857.

107. Blumenthal D. Launching HITECH. *N Engl J Med* 2010;362:382–385.

108. Blumenthal D, Tavenner M. The "meaningful use" regulations for electronic health records. *N Engl J Med* 2010;363:501–504.

109. Office of the National Coordinator for Health Information Technology. 'Office-based Physician Electronic Health Record Adoption', Health IT Quick-Stat #50. December 2016. Available at: dashboard.healthit.gov/quickstats/pages/physician-ehr-adoption-trends.php.

110. Office of the National Coordinator for Health Information Technology. 'Non-federal Acute Care Hospital Electronic Health Record Adoption', Health IT Quick-Stat #47. May 2016. Available at: dashboard.healthit.gov/quickstats/pages/FIG-Hospital-EHR-Adoption.php.

111. Gartner Hype Cycle. Available at: http://www.gartner.com/technology/research/methodologies/hype-cycle.jsp.

112. Brynjolfsson E. The productivity paradox of information technology: review and assessment. *Communications of the ACM* 1993;36:12.

113. Brynjolfsson E, Hitt L. Is information systems spending productive? New evidence and new results. *ICIS 1993 Proceedings* 1993; Paper 43. Available at: http://aisel.aisnet.org/icis1993/43/?utm_source=aisel.aisnet.org%2Ficis1993%2F43&utm_medium=PDF&utm_campaign=PDFCoverPages.

ADDITIONAL READINGS

Aspden P, Wolcott J, Bootman JL, et al., eds. *Preventing Medication Errors: Quality Chasm Series*. Committee on Identifying and Preventing Medication Errors. Washington, DC: National Academies Press; 2007.

Black AD, Car J, Pagliari C, et al. The impact of eHealth on the quality and safety of health care: a systematic overview. *PLoS Med* 2011;8:e1000387.

Classen DC, Bates DW. Finding the meaning in meaningful use. *N Engl J Med* 2011;365:855–858.

Committee on Patient Safety and Health Information Technology, Board on Health Care Services, Institute of Medicine. *Health IT and Patient Safety: Building Safer Systems for Better Care*. Washington, DC: National Academies Press; 2011.

Dorsey ER, Topol EJ. State of telehealth. *N Engl J Med* 2016;375:154–161.

Jha AK. The promise of electronic records. Around the corner or down the road? *JAMA* 2011;306:880–881.

Mahajan AP. Health information exchange—obvious choice or pipe dream? *JAMA Intern Med* 2016;176:429–430.

Obermeyer Z, Emanuel E. Predicting the future—big data, machine learning, and clinical medicine. *N Engl J Med* 2016;375:1216–1219.

Rudin RS, Bates DW, MacRae C. Accelerating innovation in health IT. *N Engl J Med* 2016;375:815–817.

Singh H, Thomas EJ, Mani S, et al. Timely follow-up of abnormal diagnostic imaging test results in an outpatient setting: are electronic medical records achieving their potential? *Arch Intern Med* 2009;169:1578–1586.

Topol E. *The Creative Destruction of Medicine: How the Digital Revolution Will Create Better Health Care*. New York, NY: Basic Books; 2012.

Topol E. *The Patient Will See You Now: The Future of Medicine is in Your Hands*. New York, NY: Basic Books; 2015.

REPORTING SYSTEMS, ROOT CAUSE ANALYSIS, AND OTHER METHODS OF UNDERSTANDING SAFETY ISSUES | 14

OVERVIEW

In the late 1990s, as patients, reporters, and legislators began to appreciate the scope of the medical errors problem, the response was nearly Pavlovian: we need more reporting! This commonsensical appeal had roots in several places, including the knowledge that transparency often drives change, the positive experiences with reporting in the commercial aviation industry,[1] the desire by many interested parties (patients, legislators, the media, healthcare leaders) to understand the dimensions of the safety problem, and the need of individual healthcare organizations to know which problems to work on.

We will begin this chapter by focusing on reporting within the walls of a healthcare delivery organization such as a hospital or clinic, and then widen the lens to consider extra-institutional reporting systems. Further discussion on these issues, from somewhat different perspectives, can be found in Chapters 3, 20, and 22.

The systems designed to capture safety issues within a healthcare organization are generally known as *incident reporting* (IR) *systems.* Incident reports come from frontline personnel (e.g., the nurse, pharmacist, or physician caring for a patient when a medication error occurred) rather than, say, from supervisors. From the perspective of those receiving the data, IR systems are *passive* forms of surveillance, relying on involved parties to choose to report. More *active* methods of surveillance, such as retrospective chart review, direct observation, and trigger tools, have already been discussed in Chapter 1, though we'll have more to say about them later in this chapter.

Although IR systems capture only a fraction of incidents, they have the advantages of relatively low cost and the involvement of caregivers in the process of identifying important problems. Yet the experience with them has been disappointing[2]—while well-organized IR systems can yield important insights, they can also waste substantial resources, drain provider goodwill, and divert attention from more important problems.

One should understand the following realities when evaluating the role of reporting in patient safety:

- Errors occur one at a time, to individual patients—often already quite ill—scattered around hospitals, nursing homes, and doctors' offices. This generates tremendous opportunity to cover up errors, and requires that providers be engaged in efforts to promote transparency.
- Because reporting errors takes time and can lead to shame and (particularly in the United States) legal liability, providers who choose to report need to be protected from unfair blame, public embarrassment, and legal risk.
- Reporting systems need to be easy to access and use, and reporting must yield palpable improvements. Busy caregivers are not likely to report if systems are burdensome to use or reports seem to disappear into the dark corners of a bureaucracy.
- Many different stakeholders need to hear about and learn from errors. However, these stakeholders— doctors, nurses, hospital administrators, educators, researchers, regulators, legislators, the media, and patients— all have different levels of understanding and may need to see very different types of reports. This diversity makes error reporting particularly challenging.
- Although most errors do reflect systems problems, some *can* be attributed to bad providers. The public—and those charged with defending the public's interest, such as licensing and credentialing boards—have a legitimate need to learn of these cases and take appropriate (including, at times, disciplinary) action (Chapter 19).
- Similarly, even when the problem is systemic and not one of "bad apples," the public has a right to know about systems that are sufficiently unsafe that a reasonable person would hesitate before receiving care from them.
- Medical errors are so breathtakingly common that the admonition to "report everything" is silly. Estimates suggest that preventable medication errors affect around 7 million patients annually across healthcare settings.[3] A system that captured every error and near miss would quickly accumulate unmanageable mountains of data, require armies of analysts, and result in caregivers spending much of their time reporting and digesting the results instead of caring for patients.

Taken together, these "facts on the ground" mean that error reporting, while conceptually attractive, must be approached thoughtfully. IR systems need to be easy to use, nonpunitive, and manned by people skilled at analyzing the data and putting them to use. The energy and resources invested in designing action plans that respond to IRs should match the level of energy and resources invested in the IR system itself. After all, the goal of an IR system is not data collection but meaningful improvements in safety and quality.

There is yet another cautionary note to be sounded regarding IR systems: voluntary reporting systems cannot be used to derive rates—of errors, or harm, or anything, really.[4] If the reports at a particular hospital have gone up by, let's say, 20% in the past year, those in charge of patient safety might invariably exclaim, "Look at these numbers. You see, we've established a culture of reporting, and people are confident that reports lead to action. We're getting safer!"

That all sounds great until those in charge of patient safety at a comparable institution, whose IR volume has fallen, say "This is great, we've had fewer errors!" The problem is obvious: there is no way to know which explanation is correct.

Given the limitations of IR systems,[5] healthcare organizations need to employ other techniques to capture errors and identify risky situations.[6,7] This chapter will cover a few of them, including *failure mode and effects analysis* and *trigger tools*. Errors and adverse events that *are* reported must be put to good use, such as by turning them into stories that are shared within organizations, in forums such as *Morbidity and Mortality (M&M) conferences,* and perhaps by shifting the focus from number of reports to system-level changes resulting from reports. Finally, errors that are of particular concern—often called *sentinel events*—must be analyzed in a way that rapidly generates the maximum amount of institutional learning and catalyzes the appropriate changes. The method of doing this is known as *root cause analysis* (RCA). The following sections discuss each of these issues and techniques.

GENERAL CHARACTERISTICS OF REPORTING SYSTEMS

Error reports, whether filed on paper or through the Web, and whether routed to the hospital's safety officer or to a federal regulator, can be divided into three main categories: anonymous, confidential, and open. *Anonymous reports* are ones in which there is no identifying information asked of the reporter. Although they have the advantage of encouraging reporting, anonymous systems have the disadvantage of preventing necessary follow-up questions from being answered. In a *confidential reporting system*, the identity of the reporter is known but shielded from authorities such as regulators and representatives of the legal system (except in cases of clear professional misconduct or criminal acts). Such systems tend to capture more useful data than anonymous systems, because follow-up questions can be asked. The key to these systems, of course, is that reporters must trust that they are truly confidential. Finally, in *open reporting systems* all people and places are publicly identified. These systems have a relatively poor track record in healthcare, because the potential for unwanted publicity and blame is very strong, and it is often easy for individuals to cover up errors (even with "mandatory" reporting).

Another distinguishing feature of reporting systems is the organizational entity that receives the reports. With that in mind, let's first consider the local system managed by a healthcare delivery organization—the IR system—before expanding the discussion to systems that move reports to other entities beyond the clinical organization's walls.

HOSPITAL INCIDENT REPORTING SYSTEMS

Hospitals[*] have long had IR systems, but prior to the patient safety movement these systems received little attention. Traditional IR systems relied on providers—nearly always nurses (most studies show that nurse reports outnumber physician reports by at least five to one[8])—to fill out paper reports. The reports generally went to the hospital's risk manager, whose main concern was often to limit his or her institution's potential legal liability (Chapter 18). There was little emphasis on systems improvement, and dissemination of incidents to others in the system (other managers, caregivers, educators) was unusual. Most clinicians felt that reporting was a waste of time, and so few did it.

Despite the growing emphasis on patient safety reporting, until recently, reporting systems have been studied insufficiently. Based on a 2008 survey of 1600 U.S. hospitals' error reporting systems, Farley et al. described four key components of effective systems (Table 14-1). Unfortunately, they found that only a minority of hospitals met these criteria.[9] Specifically, only a small fraction of hospitals showed evidence of a safety culture that encouraged reporting, properly analyzed error reports, and effectively disseminated the results of these analyses.

These failures are not for lack of effort or, in many hospitals, lack of investment. In fact, many hospitals have invested heavily in their IR systems, mostly in the form of new computerized infrastructure. However, the resources and focus needed to change the culture around incident reporting and management, to properly analyze reports, and to create useful and durable action plans have been less forthcoming.[2]

---

*We'll use the term "hospital" in this chapter while recognizing that the same issues hold true for healthcare systems that include ambulatory and hospital sites.

Table 14-1	**CHARACTERISTICS OF AN EFFECTIVE REPORTING SYSTEM**

- Institution must have a supportive environment for event reporting that protects the privacy of staff who report occurrences.
- Reports should be received from a broad range of personnel.
- Summaries of reported events must be disseminated in a timely fashion.
- A structured mechanism must be in place for reviewing reports and developing action plans.

Reproduced with permission from Farley DO, Haviland A, Champagne S, et al. Adverse-event-reporting practices by US hospitals: results of a national survey. *Qual Saf Health Care* 2008;17:416–423.

That said, the computerized systems do have their advantages. For example, most systems now allow any provider to submit an incident and categorize it by error type (e.g., medication error, patient fall; Table 14-2) and level of harm (e.g., no harm, minimal harm, serious harm, death). In confidential systems, the reporter can be contacted electronically to provide additional detail if needed. Computerized systems also make it easy to create aggregate statistics about reports, although it is important to reemphasize that voluntary systems are incapable of providing accurate error rates.[5] As with other aspects of digital data (see Chapter 13), increasingly sophisticated analytics and artificial intelligence systems may soon be able to mine IR data to identify meaningful trends and to suggest, or even implement, solutions.[10]

Probably most importantly, incident reports can be routed to the managers positioned to take action or spot trends (unfortunately, not all computerized IR systems have this functionality). For example, when an error pertaining to the medical service is reported through a hospital's computerized IR system, the system might automatically send an e-mail to the chief of the service, as well as the service's head nurse, the hospital's risk manager, the "category manager" (an appropriate individual is often assigned to each item in Table 14-2), and the hospital's director of patient safety. Each individual can review the error, have a discussion about it (verbally over the phone or in person, or within the IR system's computerized environment), and document the action taken in response.

Although this represents great progress, it is important to appreciate the amount of time, skill, and energy all of these functions require. Many hospitals have built or purchased fancy IR systems, exhorted their staff to "report everything—errors, near misses, everything," and found themselves overwhelmed by thousands of reports. A system that generated fewer reports but was able to act on those reports promptly and effectively would likely be more effective than one with far more reports that end up in the black hole of the

Table 14-2	TYPICAL MAJOR CATEGORIES IN A HOSPITAL IR SYSTEM

- Anesthesia issues
- Behavior management (including restraint use/seclusion)
- Cardiac and respiratory arrest
- Confidentiality and consent issues
- Controlled substance issues
- Diagnosis/treatment issues
- Dietary services
- Environmental safety
- Falls/injuries (involving patients)
- Home care issues
- Infection control (including blood-borne pathogens, isolation issues)
- IVs, tubes, catheter, and drain issues (including broken, infiltrated catheters)
- Laboratory results (including result errors, tests not performed, wrong specimens)
- Medical devices (including device malfunction, improper use)
- Medication-related events (including errors, delays, and adverse drug reactions)
- Patient flow issues
- Patient property loss
- Radiology issues
- Security issues
- Skin issues (including pressure ulcers)
- Surgical issues (including death in operating room, retained objects, unplanned return to OR)
- Sterile processing issues
- Skin issues
- Transfusion issues
- Unprofessional staff behavior

hospital's hard drive. In addition, using informatics technology to screen incident reports for high-risk events may be helpful.[11] As you can see, developing thoughtful ways to manage data overload—whether the goal is to prevent alert fatigue in a CPOE system (Chapter 13) or to handle thousands of error reports—is an overarching theme in the field of patient safety.

In an increasingly computerized environment and with the advent of trigger tools and other new methods of identifying cases of error and harm, some patient safety experts are starting to question the role of voluntary error reporting by frontline personnel. For example, some wonder whether every medication error and every fall really need to be reported through an IR system. We don't think so. Perhaps we should be sampling common error categories in depth for short periods of time. Consider, for example, a system in which January is Falls Month, February is Pressure Ulcer Month, and so on.

Table 14-3   WAYS TO IMPROVE THE CURRENT STATE OF IR SYSTEMS
■ Make reporting easier so that it is self-explanatory and requires minimal training
■ Make reporting meaningful to the reporter by developing feedback mechanisms
■ Focus on system changes as the real measure of success as opposed to number of events reported
■ Prioritize which events should be reported and investigated
■ For those countries with national IR systems, consider meeting with healthcare provider organizations and other stakeholders to reduce preventable harm

Adapted from: Pham JC, Girard T, Pronovost PJ. What to do with healthcare incident reporting systems. *J Public Health Res* 2013;2(3):e27.

A hospital employing this strategy would likely learn everything it needed to know about its latent errors (Chapter 1) in these areas after such a sampling.

On the other hand, organizations *do* need ways to disseminate the lessons they have learned from serious errors and to understand their error patterns in order to plan strategically (Chapter 22), to meet regulatory reporting requirements (Chapter 20), and to pursue their risk management and error disclosure responsibilities (Chapter 18). Given these realities, experts agree that IR systems must be improved, not abolished.[12] Suggested mechanisms for improving the current states of IR systems are outlined in Table 14-3.

THE AVIATION SAFETY REPORTING SYSTEM

Turning to reports that "leave the building," the pressure to build statewide or federal reporting systems grew in part (like so much of the patient safety field) from the experience of commercial aviation.[1,13] As we consider extra-institutional reporting systems, it is worth reflecting on whether this particular aviation analogy is apt.

On December 1, 1974, a Trans World Airlines (TWA) flight crashed into the side of a small mountain in Virginia, killing all 92 passengers and crew. As tragic as the crash was, the subsequent investigation added to the tragedy, because the problems leading to the crash (poorly defined minimum altitudes on the Dulles Airport approach) were well known to many pilots but not widely disseminated. A year later, the Federal Aviation Administration (FAA) launched the *Aviation Safety Reporting System* (ASRS). Importantly, recognizing that airline personnel might be hesitant to report errors and near misses to their primary regulator, FAA contracted with a third party (NASA) to run the system and broadcast its lessons to the industry.

There is general agreement that the ASRS is a primary reason for aviation's remarkable safety record (a 10-fold decrease in fatalities over the past generation; Figure 9-1). Five attributes of the ASRS have helped create these successes: ease of reporting, confidentiality, third-party administration, timely analysis and feedback, and the possibility of regulatory action. The ASRS rules are straightforward: if anyone witnesses a near miss (note an important difference from healthcare: non-near misses in aviation—that is, crashes— don't need a reporting system, because they appear on the news within minutes), that person *must* report it to ASRS within 10 days. The reporter is initially identified so that he or she can be contacted, if needed, by ASRS personnel; the identifying information is subsequently destroyed. In 40 years of operation, there have been no reported confidentiality breaches of the system. Trained ASRS personnel analyze the reports for patterns, and they have several pathways to disseminate key information or trigger actions (including grounding airplanes or shutting down airports, if necessary).

Even as healthcare tries to emulate these successes, it is worth highlighting some key differences between its problems and those of commercial aviation. The biggest is the scale of the two enterprises and their errors. The ASRS receives about 8000 reports per month, across the entire U.S. commercial aviation system—a fivefold increase from 1988 to 2015.[14] If all errors and near misses were being reported in American healthcare, this would almost certainly amount to millions of reports per month! Our own 800-bed hospital system generates 12,000 yearly reports, and (a) we certainly don't report everything, (b) we are one of the 6000 hospitals in the country, and (c) you would need to add in the errors and adverse events from nonhospital facilities and ambulatory practices to come up with an overall estimate. There are simply many more things that go wrong in the healthcare system than in the aviation system. This makes prioritizing and managing error reports a much knottier problem for us than it is in aviation.

REPORTS TO ENTITIES OUTSIDE THE HEALTHCARE ORGANIZATION

As the patient safety field gained momentum, the pressure to report errors or harm beyond the walls of provider institutions grew rapidly, driven in part by the inspiring example of the ASRS. As of 2015, there were 28 state reporting programs in the United States (including the District of Columbia). All of these state programs include hospital adverse event reporting; some also collect reports from a broader array of institutions including outpatient surgery centers, long-term care facilities, outpatient clinics and home health providers. Most programs have moved from manual, paper-based systems to electronic ones.[15]

The best approach to reporting outside the walls of the provider institution—to states, federal authorities, or other regulators and accreditors—remains unsettled and controversial. Further complicating the issue is a lack of standardization among states regarding what is reported. In 2014, of the states that did require reporting, 8 had adopted the National Quality Forum's (NQF) list of serious reportable events (sometimes called the "Never Events" list; Appendix VI and Chapter 20), 7 were using a revised version of the NQF list, and the remaining 12 were using a state-specific list.[15]

Other regulators have taken a broader approach to reporting. For example, Pennsylvania requires hospitals to report all "serious events," "incidents," and hospital-acquired infections. In 2013, it received hundreds of thousands of submissions, compared to 51 reports received by New Hampshire.[15] Similarly, the UK's National Patient Safety Agency (NPSA) launched a national reporting system for "patient safety incidents" in England and Wales in the early 2000s. The NPSA (which was absorbed into the National Health Service Commissioning Board Special Health Authority in 2012) received one million reports *in the year 2007 alone!* Sixteen states release periodic reports to the public with aggregation of state data while only three states include both aggregate data and more specific information about particular facilities; some states do share data across facilities to a varying degree of transparency.[15] The Pennsylvania system produces a newsletter describing key trends and suggested solutions.[16]

But we remain skeptical that broad-scale, "report everything"–type state or federal systems will be worth the substantial resources they require. We are more enthusiastic about the limited approach to reporting pioneered by Minnesota, which in 2005 began to require hospitals (and later ambulatory surgical centers) to report only those cases of error or harm that rose to the level of the "Never Events" list (Appendix VI). During the 2014–2015 reporting period, Minnesota received 316 such reports, a much more manageable number than Pennsylvania's hundreds of thousands. In our view, Minnesota's analyses of its database, and the programs it has developed in response to these reports,[17] are as useful as Pennsylvania's, with a savings of many thousands of person-hours of both reporting and analysis time.

Before leaving the subject of outside reporting systems, it is worth highlighting several specialized reporting systems that have made important contributions to patient safety. The MEDMARX voluntary error reporting system and the system maintained by the Institute for Safe Medication Practices (ISMP) have led to valuable insights about medication errors (Chapter 4).[18–20] Useful research and analysis has also come out of specialty reporting systems such as the ICU Safety Reporting System developed by Johns Hopkins and an online surgical reporting system at Northwestern University.[21,22] Finally, we are part of a UCSF-based team that produces a Web site, *AHRQ WebM&M*,[23]

which is, at its core, a reporting and learning system.[24] We receive confidential anonymous reports of cases of medical errors or adverse events, and choose three interesting ones to post each month, accompanied by an expert commentary (Figure 14-1). The site (along with its sister site, AHRQ Patient Safety Network) receives approximately 1.3 million unique visits yearly. Further illustrating the point that the question is not how many reports you receive but what you do with them, over the 14 year history of *WebM&M* we have received only about 800 case report submissions, not a huge number but easily enough to cull three useful cases each month.

The lessons are clear: as with hospital IR systems, reporting is not a numbers game where the person or system with the most reports "wins." Rather, the goal is the most efficient system that produces the greatest amount of learning and productive change. We believe that external reporting works best when the reports are confidential and cover only a limited number of serious events (i.e., events on the NQF list). This too is an area that is begging for innovative approaches and rigorous research.

PATIENT SAFETY ORGANIZATIONS

In 2005, the U.S. Congress passed the Patient Safety and Quality Improvement Act, which authorized the creation of *patient safety organizations* (PSOs) to encourage "voluntary, provider-driven initiatives to improve the safety and quality of patient care." The U.S. Agency for Healthcare Research and Quality (AHRQ) was charged with overseeing the development of PSOs, private or public entities that agree to adhere to common reporting standards and are granted federal protection for shared data.[25]

AHRQ has published its criteria for becoming a PSO: they include a signed commitment to collect and analyze patient safety data for the purposes of improving healthcare and the presence of robust confidentiality and privacy protections.[26] As of October 2016, 81 organizations, including state hospital associations, large healthcare provider networks, and information technology and data management companies, had been certified as a federal PSO (Table 14-4).[27] In addition, AHRQ has developed a set of common definitions and reporting formats (the "Common Format") to facilitate the collection and analysis of safety events.

PSOs receive robust legal protections for their patient safety and quality data. This is particularly important in some states, which—in a misguided effort to promote public accountability—have stripped away all prior protections for peer review and quality improvement data. In one (Florida), the passage of such legislation reportedly led most hospitals, fearful of liability, to discontinue error analysis and learning sessions such as M&M conferences.[28]

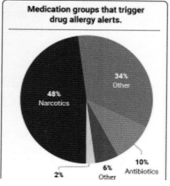

Figure 14-1 ■ Screenshot of the home page of the January 11, 2017 edition of *AHRQ PSNet*. (Available at: https://psnet.ahrq.gov/. Reproduced with permission.)

Table 14-4	EXAMPLES OF PATIENT SAFETY ORGANIZATIONS (PSOs) CERTIFIED BY AHRQ*	
Type of Organization	**Representative Examples**
State hospital associations or state safety organizations	Texas Hospital Association PSO, Virginia PSO
Large healthcare delivery systems	Baptist Health Patient Safety Partnership, Ascension Health PSO
Malpractice carriers	MCIC Vermont, Academic Medical Center PSO (an entity of the Risk Management Foundation of Harvard Medical Institutions)
Medical specialty societies	Society of NeuroInterventional Surgery PSO, Society for Vascular Surgery PSO
Private provider networks	Emergency Consultants PSO
Private vendors	Quantros Patient Safety Center (computerized incident reporting system vendor)

*As of October 2016, 81 organizations had been officially listed as federal PSOs by the Agency for Healthcare Research and Quality. The full list is available at: https://www.pso.ahrq.gov/listed.

While PSOs are a welcome option (particularly in light of these legal issues), their impact on safety remains unclear. Given how difficult it is for even a single hospital to effectively manage its own incident reports and disseminate the lessons from them without being overwhelmed by an avalanche of data, a healthy skepticism about the ability of 5 hospitals—or 50—to do this successfully is warranted.

ROOT CAUSE ANALYSIS AND OTHER INCIDENT INVESTIGATION METHODS

After we learn of a significant error, what should we do? The technique of *root cause analysis* (RCA) involves a deliberate, comprehensive dissection of an error, laying bare all of the relevant facts and searching assiduously for underlying ("root") causes rather than being satisfied by facile explanations (such as "the doctor pulled the wrong chart" or "the pharmacist stocked the wrong medicine"). Some U.S. states now require RCAs after serious events[15] (and require that reports from them be submitted along with error notifications), and the Joint Commission mandates an RCA after every "sentinel event."

To ensure that RCAs are maximally productive, certain elements appear to be important:

1. *Strong leadership and facilitation*: it is easy for an RCA to drift away from the search for root causes and toward the assignment of blame. The leader must be skilled at steering the conversation toward key systems defects, including complex and potentially charged issues involving culture and communication. The use of a structured tool to prompt participants to consider the full range of potential contributing factors can be helpful (Table 2-1).[29–31]

2. *An interdisciplinary approach*: the RCA committee should include representatives of all of the relevant disciplines (at a minimum, physicians, nurses, pharmacists, and administrators). In addition, a risk manager is often present and generally helpful, although the discussion should focus on what can be learned from the error rather than on how to reduce the institution's liability. In larger organizations, content experts (such as in information technology and human factors) can add their insights. Some experts favor including a patient representative unrelated to the event being discussed.

3. *Individuals who participated in the case should be invited to "tell their stories."* These discussions can be highly emotional, and the RCA leader needs to skillfully manage the presentation of facts to ensure maximum benefit, paying particular attention to avoiding finger-pointing and the defensiveness it invariably provokes. It is often useful for someone (usually the patient safety officer or risk manager) to have gathered many of the key facts and timelines and present them to the RCA committee to streamline the discussion. However, even when this has been done, it is important to confirm the facts with the participants early in the meeting and offer them the opportunity to share their perspectives. In most cases, all the involved caregivers should be present at the same meeting to share their views; in rare instances, this will be too emotionally charged and sequential presentations may be preferable.

4. *Some institutions routinely invite other frontline workers (such as an uninvolved nurse or physician) to RCAs to help educate them in the process and demystify the ritual.* The hope is that they can serve as ambassadors for the process with their colleagues. Other organizations have found that the participation of lay individuals adds an important perspective.

5. *Focus on identifying corrective actions that will prevent future harm.* Essential to the RCA process is the identification of strong corrective actions that will mitigate the root cause(s) down the road to prevent the same harm or near miss from happening again.[32]

6. *Ensure that corrective actions are implemented and sustained, that feedback is provided to those involved, and that learnings from the RCA are shared across the institution.*[32] Implementing and sustaining the corrective action items can be challenging. It is critical that those participating in the process understand the outcome and that there is a mechanism for sharing lessons learned with the institution at large.

Ultimately, the goal of the RCA is to identify systems factors that led to the error, and to suggest solutions that can prevent similar errors from causing harm in the future.[33–37] Some have suggested that the term "root cause analysis" is misleading since—as we learned from the discussion of the Swiss cheese model (Chapter 1)—most adverse events and errors have multiple "holes in the cheese." In fact, it is nearly unheard of for an effective RCA to identify a single root cause of an error, particularly if the committee has deeply considered all the potential systems issues.

In its zeal to emphasize contributory systems factors, an RCA committee should not shy away from identifying human error, nor from taking appropriate steps to ensure accountability (such as when there is evidence of repetitive errors by a single individual or failure to adhere to sensible safety rules) (Chapter 19). But, for individuals to truly trust the RCA process, this part of the discussion should be moved to a different venue, such as a medical staff credentialing or a peer review committee. As with many aspects of trying to improve patient safety, finding the appropriate balance between a systems approach and individual accountability is the most challenging aspect of the RCA process.

At UCSF Medical Center, we transformed our RCA process several years ago, and this may be one of the most important things we have done to improve safety. These changes are described in Table 14-5. Recently, we have audited the sustainability of the action items coming out of prior RCAs to help understand the effectiveness of our process. Although measuring sustainability is time intensive, preliminary data suggests that stronger corrective action items are often sustained (particularly those that led to system changes, such as eliminating certain equipment and devices from use or changing the processes for specimen labeling and collection to minimize opportunity for human error) but that weaker action items like reminders and education may not be. There are few studies in the literature comparing different ways of conducting, and following up on, RCAs.

Although RCA remains a valuable process for understanding adverse events and near misses, there are clearly opportunities for improvement. Indeed, some experts argue that many institutions have not optimally adapted the RCA process to healthcare, that flaws with the investigative process persist, that organizations often settle for "weak" corrective actions such as

Table 14-5	THE UCSF MEDICAL CENTER ROOT CAUSE ANALYSIS PROCESS	
Prior Structure	**New Model**	**Comment or Rationale**
RCAs were scheduled in a haphazard way following a safety-related event	A weekly, scheduled 2-hour meeting, with the first hour devoted to performing an RCA of a recent event	New structure ensures same committee members (including senior administrators) present, and permits rapid RCA (within days of event)
Frontline caregivers invited to participate in RCA	Clear directive from hospital leadership to attend any RCA that discusses a case provider was involved in	E-mail to involved caregivers (after initial fact-finding by staff member) directing them to attend next meeting; substantial pressure to do so
Lots of time spent fact-finding before RCA meeting	Less time on fact-finding; first segment of RCA meeting relatively free-form discussion by involved personnel about "what happened"	Prior requirement for detailed fact-finding often delayed RCA by weeks. We have found it better to get the right people to the table and let them tell their story
Action plan often fuzzy as to next steps and who was responsible for carrying them out	No meeting ends without clear action plan and assigned responsibilities	Often requires additional meetings of assigned personnel, but clarity regarding what is to be done (or needs to be learned) and who is responsible for doing it is crucial
No discussion of disclosure to patient/family	No meeting ends without discussion about how/whether disclosure was accomplished, whether more needs to be done, and whether payment was (or should be) waived	Important to make this issue visible and demonstrate support for full disclosure and payment waiver policies
Follow-up reports not expected, haphazard process	Second hour of RCA meeting reserved for 15-minute follow-up reports from previously charged groups	Standing committee members become better at learning what did and didn't work; follow-up requirement forces accountability for those charged with carrying out action plan and allows senior administrators to intervene if implementation stalled by need for resources or political pressure

education or reminders, that findings/results are not fed back to those involved, and that learning is not disseminated beyond the walls of the organization[38] (Table 14-6). The formation of PSOs may help us test whether, in fact, aggregating RCAs across many institutions improves efficiency, or, by removing so much of the local context and including fewer directly involved participants, strips away some of its effectiveness.

Table 14-6	**PROBLEMS WITH ROOT CAUSE ANALYSIS**
The name "root cause analysis"	Promotes linear thinking toward a single root cause when most adverse events are complex and have multiple interacting parts and potential intervention points. Tools also tend to focus on a linear or temporal view of event, rather than a systems view of events.
Investigations of questionable quality	Teams may not have in-depth training in accident investigation and human factors; clinicians may be unwilling or unable to provide relevant data to the investigation; patients and families often are not included in the investigative process.
"Political hijack"	Investigations are usually conducted under significant time pressure, lack independence from the organization where the events occurred, and are subject to hindsight bias. These factors may significantly limit the scope of the investigation, the recommendations, and the report.
Poor design and implementation of risk controls	Tendency to focus on weak solutions such as reminders, education, and training over stronger solutions addressing flawed technology or flawed systems design; lack of evidence for effectiveness of solutions; lack of follow-up on implementation of solutions.
Feedback does not support learning	Learning is supported when outcomes of investigation are shared and the recommended solutions are "salient and actionable." This type of feedback is often missing in healthcare settings.
Focus on single incidents and institutions	Incidents tend to be investigated in isolation—single events within single institutions. This limits opportunity for understanding recurrence vulnerability and may lead to focusing resources on preventing very rare events over solving broader systems issues that have greater potential to prevent harm. Systematic ways of aggregating root causes are lacking.
Confusion about blame	The balance between individual and organizational responsibility is complex. While most accidents are the result of systems defects, serious individual transgressions also occur and need to be addressed. Taking an overly algorithmic approach to just culture can obscure complicated relationships between individual action and organizational defects.
Problem of many hands	Many actors, both within and outside the healthcare organization, may be implicated. RCA-derived risk controls tend to focus on solutions that are within the internal control of the organization or team, and not assign responsibility to broader problems outside of their control (e.g., equipment design or medication labeling).

Adapted from Peerally MF, Carr S, Waring J, Dixon-Woods M. The problem with root cause analysis. *BMJ Qual Saf* 2017;26:417–422.

In 2015, the National Patient Safety Foundation (NPSF) released a report entitled, "RCA^2: Improving Root Cause Analyses and Actions to Prevent Harm." The report suggests many ways to improve the RCA process, addressing many of the oft-cited criticisms.[32] NPSF recommends renaming the process to emphasize both the *analyses* and the resulting *actions*, hence the name RCA^2. The report's nine recommendations are outlined in Table 14-7.

Table 14-7 RCA^2 IMPROVING ROOT CAUSE ANALYSES AND ACTIONS TO PREVENT HARM: NINE RECOMMENDATIONS FROM NPSF	
Leadership	Leadership (e.g., CEO, board of directors) should be actively involved in the root cause analysis and action (RCA^2) process. This should be accomplished by supporting the process, approving and periodically reviewing the status of actions, understanding what a thorough RCA^2 report should include, and acting when reviews do not meet minimum requirements.
Re-evaluate the process regularly	Leadership should review the RCA^2 process at least annually for effectiveness.
Determine which events should not go through RCA	Blameworthy events that are not appropriate for RCA^2 review should be defined.
Prioritize which events to review	Facilities should use a transparent, formal, and explicit risk-based prioritization system to identify adverse events, close calls, and system vulnerabilities requiring RCA^2 review.
Expedite the RCA process	An RCA^2 review should be started within 72 hours of recognizing that a review is needed.
Train a designated team	RCA^2 teams should be composed of 4 to 6 people. The team should include process experts as well as other individuals drawn from all levels of the organization, and inclusion of a patient representative unrelated to the event should be considered. Teams should not include individuals who were involved in the event or close call being reviewed, but those individuals should be interviewed for information.
Provide time to conduct the investigation	Time should be provided during the normal work shift for staff to serve on an RCA^2 team, including attending meetings, researching, and conducting interviews.
Use appropriate tools and identify viable corrective actions	RCA^2 tools (e.g., interviewing techniques, Flow Diagramming, Cause and Effect Diagramming, Five Rules of Causation, Action Hierarchy, Process/Outcome Measures) should be used by teams to assist in the investigation process and the identification of strong and intermediate strength corrective actions.
Provide feedback	Feedback should be provided to staff involved in the event as well as to patients and/or their family members regarding the findings of the RCA^2 process.

Adapted from *RCA^2: Improving Root Cause Analyses and Actions to Prevent Harm.* Boston, MA: National Patient Safety Foundation; 2015. Available at: http://www.npsf.org/?page=RCA2.

MORBIDITY AND MORTALITY CONFERENCES

While the RCA process is confidential, many institutions have recognized the value of presenting cases of medical errors to diverse groups of providers, usually in an *M&M conference*. Cases of medical errors are often quite interesting and dramatic, and a well-constructed "M&M" can quickly become one of the premier educational sessions in an institution. As with RCAs, it is vital that the leader be a skilled facilitator—striving to protect the presenter (if he or she participated in the care of the patient) from public humiliation, and working to elucidate system factors that bear improvement or general lessons for the audience.

Traditionally, most M&M conferences have involved physicians only, focused on a single discipline (i.e., surgery or medicine), and not comported with modern patient safety thinking. One UCSF study demonstrated that internal medicine M&M conferences rarely classify errors as errors (tending instead to divert into academic discussions of pathophysiology or more traditional aspects of diagnosis and therapy), while surgical conferences often focus on individual fault at the cost of insufficient discussion of system issues.[39] In another study, the leaders of 12 clinical departments at Johns Hopkins Hospital were interviewed about their M&Ms. Patient safety and quality improvement were an explicit goal in only 42%. Only one department (8%) used a structured tool to elicit systems issues, and only seven (58%) had a plan for assigning individuals to follow up on recommendations.[40]

Some innovative approaches have recently been brought to this time-honored exercise, including interdisciplinary M&M conferences (e.g., with both physicians and nurses), cross-specialty M&M conferences (e.g., surgeons and internists), integrating a focus on patient safety and systems thinking, and conferences that involve institutional administrators and catalyze action and follow-up.[41–45] In the latter model, after systems issues are uncovered in the M&M, a group is charged with returning later to present what was learned about them and how they were fixed. One teaching hospital applied a systems audit framework (Table 14-8) to its M&M conferences, and found that this change led to an improved safety culture and enhanced resident awareness of systems issues.[46]

Unfortunately, many hospitals (particularly nonacademic ones) and departments lack M&M conferences, and they are rare in outpatient settings. Reasons cited include fear of medicolegal risk (the content of M&M conferences and peer review processes is protected from legal exposure in most U.S. states if they are performed under the hospital's quality assurance umbrella[47]) and the absence of time or expertise. Luckily, there are now several academic series—both print and on-line—that provide M&M-type analyses of errors.[23,35,48–50]

Table 14-8	**SIX STEPS OF THE SYSTEMS AUDIT USED IN AN INNOVATIVE M&M CONFERENCE FORMAT**

1. Review all documentation related to the case and identify all involved providers.
2. Interview stakeholders, including those who directly provided care and those involved in the system.
3. Use a quality improvement tool (such as a fishbone diagram or mind map*) to conduct a root cause analysis.
4. Determine overall cost of care and the cost of the adverse outcome.
5. Identify a systems issue that contributed to the outcome.
6. Propose systems-level interventions and prioritize based on effort–yield projections.

*__Fishbone diagram__: a cause-and-effect diagram where the "head" of the fish represents the adverse outcome or systems problem and the "bones" represent contributing factors. **Mind map**: A diagram representing the relationships between a systems problem and its root causes. The adverse outcome or problem is typically depicted in the center with contributing factors branching outward to multiple levels. Reproduced with permission from Baker S, Darin M, Lateef O. Multidisciplinary morbidity and mortality conferences: improving patient safety by modifying a medical tradition. *Jt Comm Perspect Patient Saf* 2010;10:8–10.

OTHER METHODS OF CAPTURING SAFETY PROBLEMS

It is important to recognize that IR systems are only one of several methods to capture safety problems. Increasingly, methods to identify "system safety" through certain measurable structures, processes, and outcomes (Donabedian's Triad, Chapter 3) have been developed that do not depend on voluntary reporting. Over time, more and more (though certainly not all) of these measures will be captured via an institution's information technology system (Chapter 13). A detailed discussion of these methods, including the increasingly popular *Global Trigger Tool* (GTT) to identify adverse events, can be found in Chapters 1 and 3. Table 1-3 shows the test characteristics (sensitivity and specificity) of voluntary incident reports, the AHRQ Patient Safety Indicators, and the GTT, illustrating that the GTT is by far the most sensitive.[51] Table 1-4 highlights some of the advantages and disadvantages of the most common methods of measuring errors and harm. The take-away message is that there are various ways of measuring the safety of an organization, and a well-constructed safety program will use several of them to get a robust picture of its challenges and opportunities.[6,7,52]

Just as IRs are not the only way to identify safety problems, RCAs are not the sole means of analyzing such problems and developing fixes. For example, the technique of *failure mode and effects analysis* (FMEA), borrowed from engineering, is being used by many healthcare institutions to identify active and latent threats to safety.[53] In an FMEA, the likelihood that a particular process will fail is combined with an estimate of the relative impact of that failure to produce a "criticality index." This index allows one to assign priorities to specific processes as improvement targets.

As one illustration, an FMEA of the medication dispensing process on a hospital ward might break down all the steps, from receipt of orders in the central pharmacy to filling automated dispensing machines by pharmacy technicians (Chapter 4). Each step would be assigned a probability of failure and an impact score, allowing it to be ranked according to the product of these two numbers. Steps ranked at the top would be prioritized for error-proofing. The strength of the FMEA technique is that it taps into the insights of both experts and frontline workers to prioritize hazards and create an agenda for improvement. Anecdotally, some institutions have reported that FMEAs led to useful insights not obtainable from other methods,[54–56] and a recent review examining 117 FMEAs from three hospitals found that the resulting action items were implemented in over 75% of cases within a few years.[57]

KEY POINTS

- Although it is natural to see error reporting as an important component of improving patient safety, several factors (including the ubiquity of errors, the difficulty capturing errors without voluntary reporting, and the multiple perspectives and stakeholders) make reporting quite challenging.
- The most common reporting systems are institutionally-based voluntary incident reporting (IR) systems. Increasingly, hospitals and other healthcare organizations are required to submit certain reports to extra-institutional entities such as states, the federal government, and regulators, with mixed results.
- Significant errors should be thoroughly investigated by a root cause analysis (RCA), seeking system problems that merit improvement. A prominent safety organization has suggested the term RCA^2, signifying the importance of both analysis and action.
- Sharing stories of errors is an important part of improving safety. This is usually done through an institutional M&M conference, though there are now outside resources that carry out similar functions. Recent innovations in the M&M format are bringing the conference in line with modern patient safety thinking.
- Other methods of capturing safety problems include identifying the lack of evidence-based safety structures, processes, and outcomes, and using trigger tools and FMEA. A robust institutional safety program will integrate multiple methods to get a broad view of its safety challenges and opportunities.

REFERENCES

1. Helmreich RL. On error management: lessons from aviation. *BMJ* 2000;320:781–785.
2. Macrae C. The problem with incident reporting. *BMJ Qual Saf* 2016;25:71–75.
3. da Silva BA, Krishnamurthy M. The alarming reality of medication error: a patient case review of Pennsylvania and national data. *J Community Hosp Intern Med Perspect* 2016;6:31758.
4. Pronovost PJ, Miller MR, Wachter RM. Tracking progress in patient safety: an elusive target. *JAMA* 2006;296:696–699.
5. Pham JC, Girard T, Pronovost PJ. What to do with healthcare incident reporting systems. *J Public Health Res* 2013;2:e27.
6. Levtzion-Korach O, Frankel A, Alcalai H, et al. Integrating incident data from five reporting systems to assess patient safety: making sense of the elephant. *Jt Comm J Qual Patient Saf* 2010;36:402–410.
7. Shojania KG. The elephant of patient safety: what you see depends on how you look. *Jt Comm J Qual Patient Saf* 2010;36:399–401, AP1–AP3.
8. Rowin EJ, Lucier D, Pauker SG. Does error and adverse event reporting by physicians and nurses differ. *Jt Comm J Qual Patient Saf* 2008;34:537–545.
9. Farley DO, Haviland A, Champagne S, et al. Adverse-event-reporting practices by US hospitals: results of a national survey. *Qual Saf Health Care* 2008;17:416–423.
10. Benin AL, Fodeh SJ, Lee K, Koss M, Miller P, Brandt C. Electronic approaches to making sense of the text in the adverse event reporting system. *J Healthc Risk Manag* 2016;36:10–20.
11. Ong MS, Magrabi F, Coiera E. Automated identification of extreme-risk events in clinical incident reports. *J Am Med Inform Assoc* 2012;10:e110–e118.
12. Mitchell I, Schuster A, Smith K, Pronovost P, Wu A. Patient safety incident reporting: a qualitative study of thoughts and perceptions of experts 15 years after 'To Err is Human.' *BMJ Qual Saf* 2016;25:92–99.
13. Ross J. Aviation tools to improve patient safety. *J Perianesth Nurs* 2014;29:508–510.
14. Aviation Safety Reporting System. ASRS Program Briefing. Available at: https://asrs.arc.nasa.gov/docs/ASRS_ProgramBriefing2015.pdf.
15. Hanlon C, Sheedy K, Kniffin T, et al. *2014 Guide to State Adverse Event Reporting Systems*. National Academy for State Health Policy; 2015. Available at: http://www.nashp.org/sites/default/files/2014_Guide_to_State_Adverse_Event_Reporting_Systems.pdf.
16. Commonwealth of Pennsylvania Patient Safety Authority. *Pennsylvania Patient Safety Advisory*. Available at: http://patientsafetyauthority.org/ADVISORIES/Advisory Library/2016/dec;13(4)/Pages/home.aspx.
17. Minnesota Department of Health. *Adverse Health Events in Minnesota, Twelfth Annual Public Report*. St. Paul, MN: Minnesota Department of Health; February 2016. Available at: http://www.health.state.mn.us/patientsafety/ae/2016ahereport.pdf.
18. Latif A, Rawat N, Pustavoitau A, Pronovost PJ, Pham JC. National study on the distribution, causes, and consequences of voluntarily reported medication errors between the ICU and non-ICU settings. *Crit Care Med* 2013;41:389–398.
19. Schiff GD, Amato MG, Eguale T, et al. Computerised physician order entry-related medication errors: analysis of reported errors and vulnerability testing of current systems. *BMJ Qual Saf* 2015;24:264–271.

20. Institute for Safe Medication Practices. *ISMP Medication Errors Reporting Program.* Available at: https://www.ismp.org.

21. Wu AW, Holzmueller CG, Lubomski LH, et al. Development of the ICU safety reporting system. *J Patient Saf* 2005;1:23–32.

22. Bilimoria KY, Kmiecik TE, DaRosa DA, et al. Development of an online morbidity, mortality, and near-miss reporting system to identify patterns of adverse events in surgical patients. *Arch Surg* 2009;144:305–311.

23. *AHRQ WebM&M: Morbidity and Mortality Rounds on the Web.* Available at: https://psnet.ahrq.gov/webmm.

24. Wachter RM, Shojania KG, Minichiello T, et al. AHRQ WebM&M, online medical error reporting and analysis. In: Henriksen K, Battles JB, Marks ES, Lewin DI, eds. *Advances in Patient Safety: From Research to Implementation (Volume 4: Programs, Tools, and Products).* Rockville, MD: Agency for Healthcare Research and Quality; February 2005.

25. In conversation with William B. Munier, MD, MBA [Perspective]. *AHRQ PSNet* (serial online); July 2011. Available at: https://psnet.ahrq.gov/perspectives/perspective/105/in-conversation-with-william-b-munier-md-mba?q=munier.

26. Jaffe R. Becoming a patient safety organization [Perspective]. *AHRQ PSNet* (serial online); July 2011. Available at: https://psnet.ahrq.gov/perspectives/perspective/106.

27. Agency for Healthcare Research and Quality. *Listed Patient Safety Organizations.* Available at: https://www.pso.ahrq.gov/listed.

28. Barach P. The unintended consequences of Florida medical liability legislation [Perspective]. *AHRQ PSNet* (serial online); December 2005. Available at: https://psnet.ahrq.gov/perspectives/perspective/14.

29. Vincent C. Understanding and responding to adverse events. *N Engl J Med* 2003;348:1051–1056.

30. Vincent C, Taylor-Adams S, Stanhope N. Framework for analyzing risk and safety in clinical medicine. *BMJ* 1998;316:1154–1157.

31. Nicolini D, Waring J, Mengis J. Policy and practice in the use of root cause analysis to investigate clinical adverse events: mind the gap. *Soc Sci Med* 2011;73:217–225.

32. National Patient Safety Foundation. *RCA^2: Improving Root Cause Analysis and Actions to Prevent Harm.* Boston, MA: National Patient Safety Foundation; 2015.

33. Bagian JP, Gosbee J, Lee CZ, Williams L, McKnight SD, Mannos DM. The Veterans Affairs root cause analysis system in action. *Jt Comm J Qual Improv* 2002;28:531–545.

34. Rex JH, Turnbull JE, Allen SJ, Vande Voorde K, Luther K. Systematic root cause analysis of adverse drug events in a tertiary referral hospital. *Jt Comm J Qual Improv* 2000;26:563–575.

35. Chassin MR, Becher EC. The wrong patient. *Ann Intern Med* 2002;136:826–833.

36. Flanders SA, Saint S. Getting to the root of the matter [Spotlight]. *AHRQ WebM&M* (serial online); July 2005. Available at: http://webmm.ahrq.gov/case.aspx?caseid=98.

37. Charles R, Hood B, Derosier JM, et al. How to perform a root cause analysis for workup and future prevention of medical errors: a review. *Patient Saf Surg* 2016;10:20.

38. Peerally MF, Carr S, Waring J, Dixon-Woods M. The problem with root cause analysis. *BMJ Qual Saf* 2017;26:417–422.

39. Pierluissi E, Fischer MA, Campbell AR, Landefeld CS. Discussion of medical errors in morbidity and mortality conferences. *JAMA* 2003;290:2838–2842.

40. Aboumatar HJ, Blackledge CG Jr, Dickson C, Heitmiller E, Freischlag J, Pronovost PJ. A descriptive study of morbidity and mortality conferences and their conformity to medical incident analysis models: results of the morbidity and mortality conference improvement study, phase 1. *Am J Med Qual* 2007;22:232–238.

41. Berenholtz SM, Hartsell TL, Pronovost PJ. Learning from defects to enhance morbidity and mortality conferences. *Am J Med Qual* 2009;24:192–195.

42. Ksouri H, Balanant PY, Tadié JM, et al. Impact of morbidity and mortality conferences on analysis of mortality and critical events in intensive care practice. *Am J Crit Care* 2010;19:135–145.

43. Baker S, Darin M, Lateef O. Multidisciplinary morbidity and mortality conferences: improving patient safety by modifying a medical tradition. *Jt Comm Perspect Patient Saf* 2010;10:8–10.

44. Mitchell EL, Lee DY, Arora S, et al. Improving the quality of the surgical morbidity and mortality conference: a prospective intervention study. *Acad Med* 2013;88:824–830.

45. Singh HP, Durani P, Dias JJ. Enhanced mobidity and mortality meeting and patient safety education for specialty trainees. *J Patient Saf.* 2015 Jun 22; [Epub ahead of print].

46. Szostek JH, Wieland ML, Loertscher LL, et al. A systems approach to morbidity and mortality conference. *Am J Med* 2010;123:663–668.

47. Stewart RM, Corneille MG, Johnston J, et al. Transparent and open discussion of errors does not increase malpractice risk in trauma patients. *Ann Surg* 2006;243:645–651.

48. Wachter RM, Shojania KG, Markowitz AJ, Smith M, Saint S. Quality grand rounds: the case for patient safety. *Ann Intern Med* 2006;145:629–630.

49. Wachter RM, Shojania KG. *Internal Bleeding: The Truth Behind America's Terrifying Epidemic of Medical Mistakes*. New York, NY: Rugged Land; 2004.

50. Wachter RM, Shojania KG. The faces of errors: a case-based approach to educating providers, policy makers, and the public about patient safety. *Jt Comm J Qual Saf* 2004;31:665–670.

51. Classen DC, Resar R, Griffin F, et al. 'Global Trigger Tool' shows that adverse events in hospitals may be ten times greater than previously measured. *Health Aff (Millwood)* 2011;30:581–589.

52. Lipczak H, Knudsen JL, Nissen A. Safety hazards in cancer care: findings using three different methods. *BMJ Qual Saf* 2011;20:1052–1056.

53. McDermott RE, Mikulak RJ, Beauregard MR. *The Basics of FMEA*. Portland, OR: Resources Engineering, Inc; 1996.

54. Singh R, Hickner J, Mold J, Singh G. "Chance favors only the prepared mind": preparing minds to systematically reduce haards in the testing process in primary care. *J Patient Saf* 2014;10:20–28.

55. Manrique-Rodríguez S, Sánchez-Galindo AC, López-Herce J, et al. Risks in the implementation and use of smart pumps in a pediatric intensive care unit: application of the failure mode and effects analysis. *Int J Technol Assess Health Care* 2014;30: 210–217.

56. Alamry A, Al Owais SM, Marini AM, Al-Dorzi H, Alsolamy S, Arabi Y. Application of failure mode effect analysis to improve the care of septic patients admitted through the emergency department. *J Patient Saf* 2017;13:76–81.

57. Öhrn A, Ericsson C, Andersson C, Elfström J. High rate of implementation of pro-
    posed actions for improvement with the healthcare failure mode effect analysis
    method: evaluation of 117 analyses. *J Patient Saf* 2015 Feb 24; [Epub ahead of print].

ADDITIONAL READINGS

Classen DC, Lloyd RC, Provost L, Griffin FA, Resar R. Development and evaluation of the
    Institute for Healthcare Improvement global trigger tool. *J Patient Saf* 2008;4:169–177.

Franklin BD, Shebl NA, Barber N. Failure mode and effects analysis: too little for too
    much? *BMJ Qual Saf* 2012;21:607–611.

Howell AM, Burns EM, Bouras G, Donaldson LJ, Athanasiou T, Darzi A. Can patient
    safety incident reports be used to compare hospital safety? Results from a quantita-
    tive analysis of the English National Reporting and Learning System data. *PLoS One*
    2015;10:e0144107.

Milch CE, Salem DN, Pauker SG, Lundquist TG, Kumar S, Chen J. Voluntary electronic
    reporting of medical errors and adverse events. *J Gen Intern Med* 2006;21:165–170.

Perez B, Knych SA, Weaver SJ, et al. Understanding the barriers to physician error
    reporting and disclosure: a systemic approach to a systemic problem. *J Patient Saf*
    2014;10:45–51.

Pronovost PJ, Holzmueller CG, Young J, et al. Using incident reporting to improve patient
    safety: a conceptual model. *J Patient Saf* 2007;3:27–33.

Vincent C, Amalberti R. *Safer Healthcare: Strategies for the Real World.* New York, NY:
    SpringerOpen; 2016.

CREATING A CULTURE OF SAFETY | 15

OVERVIEW

In Chapter 9, we discussed the tragic collision of two 747s on a foggy morning in Tenerife, the crash that vividly illustrated to everyone in the field of commercial aviation the risks associated with steep and unyielding *authority gradients*. In response to Tenerife and similar accidents, aviation began a series of training programs, generally called "crew resource management" or "cockpit resource management" (CRM) programs, designed to train diverse crews in communication and teamwork. Some of these programs also incorporate communication skills, such as training in Situation, Background, Assessment, and Recommendations (SBAR) and briefing/debriefing techniques (Chapter 9). There is widespread agreement that these programs helped transform the culture of aviation, a transformation that was largely responsible for the remarkable safety record of commercial airlines over the past generation (Figure 9-1).

As the healthcare field began to tackle patient safety, it naturally looked to other organizations that seemed to have addressed their error problems effectively.[1] The concept of *high reliability organizations* (HROs) became shorthand for the relatively mistake-free state enjoyed by airlines, computer chip manufacturers, nuclear power plants, and naval aircraft carriers—but certainly not healthcare organizations.[2,3] According to Weick and Sutcliffe, HROs share the following characteristics:[2]

- *Preoccupation with failure*: the acknowledgment of the high-risk, error-prone nature of an organization's activities and the determination to achieve consistently safe operations.
- *Commitment to resilience*: the development of capacities to detect unexpected threats and contain them before they cause harm, or to recover from them when they do occur.
- *Sensitivity to operations*: attentiveness to the issues facing workers at the frontline, both when analyzing mistakes and in making decisions about how to do the work. Management units at the frontline are given

some autonomy in identifying and responding to threats, rather than being forced to work under a rigid top-down approach.

■ *A culture of safety*: in which individuals feel comfortable drawing attention to potential hazards or actual failures without fear of censure from management.

Over the past decade, the patient safety world has embraced the concept of HROs. While conceptually attractive, one wonders whether organizations that commit themselves to become a HRO (as many do) are embracing a vague, albeit laudatory, goal without committing themselves to any actionable or measurable targets. As British safety expert Charles Vincent wrote, "Put simply, reading the HRO literature offers a great deal of inspiration, but little idea of what to do in practice to enhance safety."[4,5]

This hints at an overarching challenge we face as we enter the crucial but hazy world of safety culture, which can sometimes feel like the weather—*everybody talks about it but nobody does anything about it*. When it comes to safety culture, everyone seems to have an opinion. As with many complex matters in life, the truth lies somewhere between the commonly polarized viewpoints. Is a safe culture top down or bottom up? Both. Is it "no blame" or dependent on a strong framework for accountability? Both. Is it a local phenomenon ("microculture") or an attribute of an entire organization? Both. Is it enhanced by following a set of rules and standards or by creating a nimble frontline staff, able to innovate, think on its feet, and even break a rule or two when that's required for safe care? Well, both.

The gossamer nature of safety culture—sometimes defined as "the way we do things around here"—can be frustrating to those entering the field, whether their goal is to improve the safety of their own practice or that of an entire hospital. It seems to be nowhere and everywhere. Yet the past decade has seen real progress in the area of safety culture: our understanding of what it means is growing richer and more nuanced, and we are discovering robust ways of measuring it and, to a degree, improving it. This, thankfully, provides something for even the pragmatist to grab on to.

▌ AN ILLUSTRATIVE CASE

In a large teaching hospital, an elderly woman ("Joan Morris"*) is waiting to be discharged after a successful neurosurgical procedure. A floor away, another woman with a similar last name ("Jane Morrison") is scheduled to receive the day's first cardiac electrophysiology study (EPS), a procedure in which a catheter is threaded

---

* Joan Morris and Jane Morrison are fictitious names, but are designed to illustrate the fact that the two patients' real last names were similar to each other, but not identical.

into the heart to start and stop the heart repetitively to find the cause of a potentially fatal rhythm disturbance. The EPS laboratory calls the floor to send "Morrison" down, but the clerk hears "Morris" and tells that patient's nurse that the EP lab is ready for her patient. That's funny, she thinks, my patient was here for a neurosurgical procedure. Well, she assumes, one of the docs must have ordered the test and not told me. So she sends the patient down.

Later that morning, the neurosurgery resident enters Joan Morris's room to discharge his patient, and is shocked to learn that his patient is in the EPS laboratory. He sprints there, only to be told by the cardiologists that they are in the middle of a difficult part of the procedure and can't listen to his concerns. Assuming that his attending physician ordered the test without telling him, he returns to his work.

Luckily, the procedure, which was finally aborted when the neurosurgery attending came to discharge his patient and learned she was in the EPS laboratory, caused no lasting harm (in fact, the patient later remarked, "I'm glad my heart checked out OK").[6]

The case illustrates several process problems, and it would be easy, even natural, to focus on them. Many hospitals would respond to such a case by mandating that procedural units use complete patient names, hospital numbers, and birthdays when calling for a patient; by requiring a written (or electronic) order from the physician before allowing his or her patient to leave a floor for a procedure; by directing that important information be read back to ensure accuracy; or by implementing a bar coding system that matches a patient's identity with the name in the computerized scheduling system. These would all be good things to do.

But these changes would leave an important layer of Swiss cheese (Chapter 1)—perhaps the most crucial one of all—unaddressed, the one related to the cultural issues that influence, perhaps even determine, the actions of many of the participants. A closer look at the case, now through a safety culture lens, reveals issues surrounding hierarchies, the "culture of low expectations," production pressures, and rules.[6] After a brief discussion about measuring safety culture, we will address each of these topics in turn, and then consider solutions such as teamwork training and checklists. Rapid Response Teams and dealing with disruptive behavior are covered in Chapters 16 and 19, respectively.

MEASURING SAFETY CULTURE

While one could try to assess safety culture by directly observing provider behavior (and some studies do just that[7,8]), the usual method is through self-reports of caregivers and managers, collected via a survey instrument.

The two most popular instruments are the *AHRQ Patient Safety Culture Survey* and the *Safety Attitudes Questionnaire* (SAQ).[9–11] A core benefit of using one of these validated instruments is that they have been administered to tens of thousands of healthcare workers and leaders, which means that benchmarks (for various types of clinical units and healthcare organizations) have been established. There has also been considerable research performed using these instruments, with results that have been surprising, sometimes even eye-popping. They include:

- Safety culture is mostly *a local phenomenon*.[12] Pronovost and Sexton administered the SAQ to clinicians at 100 hospitals.[13] While they found considerable variation in safety culture *across* hospitals (with positive scores ranging from 40% to 80%, Figure 15-1), there was even more variation when they looked at 49 individual units *within* a single hospital (positive scores ranging from 0% to 100%, Figure 15-2). It is not an oversimplification to say that your *hospital* doesn't have a safety culture—rather, your fourth floor ICU has one, your step-down unit 50 ft away has a different one, and your emergency department has still another one. This is liberating in a way, since one need not look far

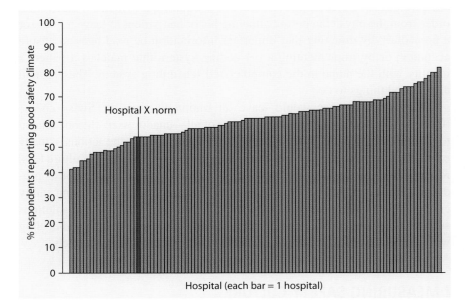

Figure 15-1 ■ Safety climate scores across 100 different hospitals. (Reproduced with permission from Pronovost PJ, Sexton B. Assessing safety culture: guidelines and recommendations. *Qual Saf Health Care* 2005;14:231–233. © 2005 by BMJ Publishing Group Ltd.)

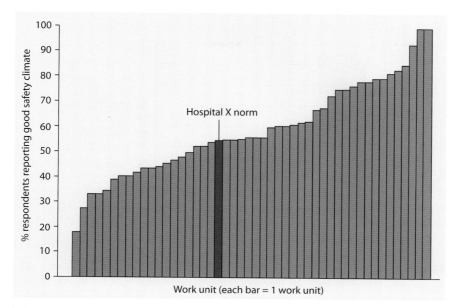

Figure 15-2 ▪ Safety climate scores across 49 different work units within a single hospital. (Reproduced with permission from Pronovost PJ, Sexton B. Assessing safety culture: guidelines and recommendations. *Qual Saf Health Care* 2005;14:231–233. © 2005 by BMJ Publishing Group Ltd.)

afield for the secrets of a strong safety culture—it's likely that some unit in your organization has already figured them out.

- Safety culture *varies markedly among different providers*, and it is important to query all of them to paint a complete picture of a unit's culture. In a seminal 2000 study, Sexton et al. administered the SAQ to members of operating room teams (Figure 15-3).[14] Whereas nearly 80% of the surgeons felt that teamwork was strong in their OR, only one in four nurses and 10% of the residents felt the same way. More recent studies, including one in the ambulatory setting, have found that these differences persist.[15–17]

- Safety culture is *perceived differently by caregivers and administrators*. Singer et al. found that problematic views of culture were much more common among frontline providers than hospital managers working in the same facilities.[18] They argue that this difference may be an important determinant of an organization's safety: if frontline workers perceive poor safety culture but the leaders remain blissfully unaware, the two groups are unlikely to be able to make appropriate decisions regarding how to prioritize safety concerns. Interestingly, another study by the

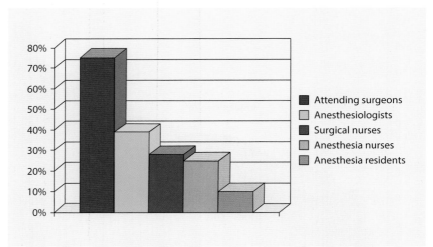

Figure 15-3 ■ Members of different groups of operating room personnel who rated teamwork as "high" in their OR. (Reproduced with permission from Sexton JB, Thomas EJ, Helmreich RL. Error, stress, and teamwork in medicine and aviation: cross-sectional surveys. *BMJ* 2000;320:745–749.)

same group found that there were differences even *among* managers, with senior managers having rosier views of culture than lower-level administrators.[19]

There is increasingly powerful evidence that safety culture scores correlate with clinical outcomes, including infection and readmission rates.[10,20–24] The Joint Commission now requires that accredited organizations administer and analyze safety culture surveys each year, and doing so is one of the National Quality Forum's "safe practices" (Appendix VII). Some have argued that, since safety culture survey results correlate with many safety outcomes, they should be publicly reported,[25] although this suggestion has not received much support. Of course, simply measuring safety culture without a strategy to improve it will be of limited value.

HIERARCHIES, SPEAKING UP, AND THE CULTURE OF LOW EXPECTATIONS

In Chapter 9, we introduced the topic of *authority gradients*—the psychological distance between a worker and his or her supervisor. These gradients are often referred to in terms of hierarchies; an organization is said to have *steep hierarchies* if these gradients tend to be large. In the wrong patient case described at the start of this chapter, the nurse's reluctance to raise concerns when told that her patient was being called for a procedure she didn't know about, or the neurosurgery resident's decision to acquiesce after getting pushback from the cardiology staff, can be attributed at least partly to steep authority gradients. So too can the tragic events that doomed the KLM 747 in Tenerife (Chapter 9). You may also recall the case that begins Chapter 9, in which a Code Blue is aborted when a physician finds a "no code" order in the wrong patient's chart. There too, a young nurse was reluctant to question the resident's confident proclamation, even though she had received sign-out an hour earlier that portrayed the patient's status as "full code."

Authority gradients are natural and, to a degree, useful. But when they prevent caregivers with important knowledge or concerns from sharing them with superiors for fear of being wrong or angering the boss, they become dangerous. This issue pertains not only to direct clinical care but also to whether the ward clerk, pharmacist, or intern will point out hazardous conditions to his or her floor manager, pharmacy director, or department chair. Safe organizations find ways to tamp down hierarchies at all levels, encouraging individuals (including patients, Chapter 21) to speak up when they see unsafe conditions or suspect that something might be awry.

In their masterful discussion of the wrong patient case in our *Quality Grand Rounds* series in the *Annals of Internal Medicine* (Appendix I), Chassin and Becher introduced the concept of "the culture of low expectations."[6] In reflecting on the actions—or inactions—of the nurse and the resident, they wrote:

> *We suspect that these physicians and nurses had become accustomed to poor communication and teamwork. A 'culture of low expectations' developed in which participants came to expect a norm of faulty and incomplete exchange of information [which led them to conclude] that these red flags signified not unusual, worrisome harbingers but rather mundane repetitions of the poor communication to which they had become inured.*[6]

Fighting the culture of low expectations is a crucial step in creating a safety culture. Doing this requires a change in default setting of all the providers, from:

A. If you're not sure it is wrong, assume it is right (*it's probably just another glitch, we have them all the time around here*) **to**
B. If you're not sure it is right, assume that it is wrong—and do whatever it takes to become sure, even at the cost of delaying the first case in the operating room or making someone important a little irritated.

There is no shortcut to fighting the culture of low expectations. Yes, it is important to clean up communications with tools such as SBAR (Chapter 9) and information technology (Chapter 13)—making the instinct to think, "another glitch, but it must be right," less automatic. (We sometimes tell healthcare leaders that they can improve their organization's safety immediately by simply purging the four words—*it must be right*—from their staff's vocabulary.)

But healthcare organizations will always have examples of faulty, ambiguous communication or rapid changes that cannot be communicated to everyone. Therefore, changing the dominant mindset from "A" to "B" requires a powerful and consistent message from senior leadership (Chapter 22). As importantly, when a worker *does* take the time to perform a double check after noticing something that seems amiss—and it turns out that everything was okay—it is vital for senior leaders to vocally and publicly support that person.[26] If praise is reserved for the "great save" but withheld for the clerk who voiced a concern when nothing later proved to be wrong, staff are unlikely to adopt mindset "B," because they will still fret about the repercussions of being mistaken.

PRODUCTION PRESSURES

Another, perhaps more subtle, culprit in the EPS wrong patient case—and in safety culture more generally—is *production pressure*.[27,28] In a nutshell, every industry, whether it produces hip replacements or cappuccinos, has to deal with the tension between safety and throughput. The issue is not whether they experience this tension—that would be like asking if they experience the Laws of Gravity. Rather, it is how they balance these twin demands.

Next time you find yourself in a low- or mid-price eating establishment, take a moment to notice the impact of production pressures. Customers are seated promptly, their orders are taken rapidly, and someone asks "is there anything else I can get you today?" when the diner appears to be nearly done with his or her food. The reason for this pace is obvious: in the fast food business, with large boluses of customers arriving en masse and relatively low profit margins per customer, corporate survival depends on throughput. The food may not be great, and there may be periodic errors (of the two-forks, no-knife type). But that's what happens when production trumps safety and reliability.

Now consider a large airport, such as San Francisco International (SFO). The tension between production and safety is particularly acute at SFO, since its two main runways are merely 738 ft apart.

The Federal Aviation Administration (FAA) enforces inviolable rules about throughput at SFO and every other airport. For example, when the cloud cover falls below 3000 ft (which, in foggy San Francisco, happens often), one of the two runways is closed, gumming up the entire U.S. air traffic control system. And whatever the weather, planes cannot land more often than one each minute. The explanation for these rules is as simple as the explanation for the restaurant's speed: when the aviation industry has to choose between production and safety, safety wins. The result: despite 400,000 takeoffs and landings each year, there has been only one fatal crash at SFO in over 50 years (Asiana 214, which killed three people in 2013). The question for healthcare organizations is this: as they balance production and safety, do they look more like the fast food restaurant or the airport? Although things in healthcare have improved a bit in the last few years, most still act more like the restaurant.

Addressing production pressures sometimes involves creating more efficient processes that free up time to do the work safely (just recall the description in Chapter 13 of the maddening waste of time and effort that often occurs when a nurse has to chart a blood pressure measurement). But it also involves choices, such as slowing down the operating rooms or the rate of inbound transfers when things reach a state of chaos. This is expensive and disruptive, but so is closing a runway. In aviation, our society willingly pays this price to ensure safety, but we have not done so in healthcare.

As always, it is vital to appreciate the limits of analogies between healthcare and other industries. When SFO closes Runway 10R, planes sit on the ground (or circle overhead) and passengers are inconvenienced. But if we close our emergency department to new ambulances ("go on divert") because of safety concerns, patients, some quite ill, need to be taken to other facilities. This carries its own safety cost, one that needs to be weighed as we address this challenging balance.

Charles Vincent quotes an oil industry executive who captured the tension beautifully. The executive said:

> *Safety is not our top priority. Our top priority is getting oil out of the ground. However, when safety and productivity conflict, then safety takes priority.*[4]

The sign in Figure 15-4 is from the gate outside a construction site in London. Can you imagine a similar sign in the entrance to your hospital's operating room or emergency department? Until you can, we need to reflect more on the nexus between production pressures and patient safety.

TEAMWORK TRAINING

It should be clear from the above discussion that safety culture involves far more than what happens in the operating room, in the labor and delivery suite, or on the wards. It is influenced, and sometimes determined, by

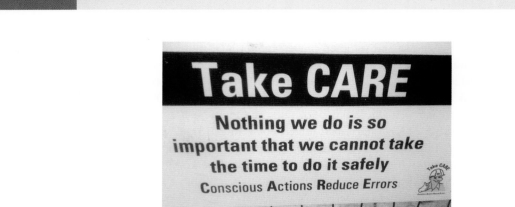

Figure 15-4 ▪ A sign outside a roadway construction site in London. Can you imagine a similar sign outside a clinical unit in a hospital?

the organizational culture, leadership, context, incentives, and more. For this reason, there has been increasing emphasis on the engagement of healthcare boards and other leaders.[29,30] We will return to their crucial role at the end of this section and again in Chapter 22.

But much of the discussion around safety culture *does* center on the world of caregivers. You have already heard a fair amount about this in our discussions of handoffs and teamwork (Chapters 8 and 9). But let's now turn to efforts to improve culture, most specifically through team training, checklists, and the thoughtful use of rules.

One of the key ways that the commercial aviation industry transformed its culture in the 1980s was through team training (CRM) programs.[1] Healthcare was relatively slow to embrace this kind of training for several reasons: it was not required by regulators or accreditors (Chapter 20), it was often challenging to get clinicians (particularly physicians) to participate, many people found the concept unattractive (some dismissively wondering whether they will be required to sing "Kumbaya" during the training), and the evidence for its effectiveness was relatively weak.

The last objection has been largely answered by the experience of the U.S. Veterans Affairs (VA) healthcare system. Neily et al. compared surgical outcomes at 74 VA hospitals in which surgical teams had undergone team training with those of 34 facilities that had not yet implemented such training.[31] They found that the risk-adjusted mortality rate had fallen 50% more in team training hospitals than in controls. Moreover, there was evidence of a dose–response curve, with additional training yielding even further cuts in mortality. The particular training program used by the VA emphasized four core areas of competency: team leadership, situation monitoring, mutual support, and communication.[32] Several other studies have also demonstrated the benefits of team training,[33–37] but there have also been negative trials[38] and the impact of team training in the context of other interventions, such as checklists, is less clear.[39] Still, after a period of high hopes but substantial uncertainty, the weight of the evidence now supports the premise that teamwork training improves both safety culture and clinical outcomes.[40]

Healthcare CRM programs come in a variety of shapes and sizes, though all focus on improving communication skills, forging a more cohesive environment, encouraging caregivers to speak up when they have concerns, addressing errors in a nonjudgmental fashion, and implementing tools such as time outs and briefs/debriefs (Chapter 5). The general experience is that, even when using an "off the shelf" program, it is best to allow for some local customization. In Table 15-1, Mayer et al. outline a number of implementation factors that help determine success[33] and, in Table 15-2, Weaver et al. enumerate 12 best practices for evaluating team training programs.[41]

From the literature and our personal experience in implementing team training[42] (the outline of the UCSF program is shown in Table 15-3), we'd emphasize the following practices and strategies:

1. *Employ strong leadership and "champions"*: Changing culture is hard, and one person's "empowerment" might be another's loss of power and status. The case for culture change has to be clearly articulated, and buy-in—particularly from the physicians, nurses, and hospital executives at the top of the authority ladder—is vital. Luckily, thoughtful leaders now appreciate the safety risks associated with poor teamwork and steep authority gradients, and many are welcoming CRM-type programs.

2. *Use aviation and other relevant nonhealthcare analogies, but don't overdo them*: At UCSF, we used actual airline pilots in some of our training, and this was helpful. Pilots can confess to medical audiences that their culture was previously similar to that of physicians, and that they participated in team training programs reluctantly at first, but that they now have come to believe that such training is essential to improving culture and decreasing errors. The Tenerife story and others like it are powerful ways to energize a healthcare audience, and—particularly for physicians—the pilots' experiences are quite relevant.

   However, healthcare providers will be quick to highlight differences between an operating room and a cockpit. The biggest difference: a cockpit "team" is made up of two or three individuals with similar training, expertise, income, and social status—operating in quiet behind a hermetically sealed door. Dampening this hierarchy is easy compared with doing so in a busy operating or delivery room, where the authority ladder might span from the chief of neurosurgery

Table 15-1	**IMPLEMENTATION FACTORS FOR SUCCESSFUL TEAM TRAINING**
Success Factor	**Implementation Strategy**
1. Align team training objectives and safety aims with organizational goals	Communication to organizational leaders and unit staff linked potential impact of teamwork on meeting organizational goals for employee satisfaction, patient satisfaction, and quality of care.
2. Provide organizational support for the team training initiative	The patient safety officer and a program manager each dedicated 40% effort to this project. Physician, nurse, and respiratory therapy senior leaders approved change team members' time on the project. Continuing education units for nurses, physicians, and respiratory therapists was approved and provided.
3. Get frontline care leaders on board	Both formal and informal unit leaders were recruited for active involvement in the project, either through inclusion in change team or by determining best approach and timing for training. Individuals were recognized for involvement by wearing TeamSTEPPS badges that identified them as TeamSTEPPS Master Trainers (Coach badge) or participants (Ready badge).
4. Prepare the environment and trainees for team training	Before training and during regular staff meetings, we provided trainees with information about why the unit was selected, what training would be provided, and expected outcomes. In addition, TeamSTEPPS was framed as a way to standardize and increase consistency of already good team performance as opposed to implementation for remediation purposes.
5. Determine required resources and time commitment and ensure their availability	Training sessions were scheduled at times that would minimize schedule disruptions for staff and were offered on all shifts and days of the week. If needed, overtime training hours were budgeted and approved.
6. Facilitate application of trained teamwork skills on the job	Staff were trained together in interdisciplinary groups to remove hierarchy barriers. The training included an opportunity to practice, and, following training, unit-based change team leaders modeled and encouraged use of TeamSTEPPS skills. Multiple reinforcement aids were developed and used (e.g., chocolates with TeamSTEPPS labels were handed out after good teamwork events and TeamSTEPPS note cards were printed to provide a handwritten note of recognition for good teamwork).
7. Measure the effectiveness of the team training program	Metrics of success were identified early and periodically reported back to staff. Training effectiveness was measured on multiple levels.

Reproduced with permission from Mayer CM, Cluff L, Lin WT, et al. Evaluating efforts to optimize TeamSTEPPS implementation in surgical and pediatric intensive care units. *Jt Comm J Qual Patient Saf* 2011;37:365–374.

Table 15-2	**BEST PRACTICES FOR EVALUATING TEAM TRAINING PROGRAMS**

Planning

- **Best Practice 1.** Before designing training, start backwards: think about traditional frameworks for evaluation in reverse.
- **Best Practice 2.** Strive for robust, experimental design in your evaluation: it is worth the headache.
- **Best Practice 3.** When designing evaluation plans and metrics, ask the experts—your frontline staff.
- **Best Practice 4.** Do not reinvent the wheel; leverage existing data relevant to training objectives.
- **Best Practice 5.** When developing measures, consider multiple aspects of performance.
- **Best Practice 6.** When developing measures, design for variance.
- **Best Practice 7.** Evaluation is affected by more than just training itself. Consider organizational, team, or other factors that may help (or hinder) the effects of training (and thus evaluation outcomes).

Implementation

- **Best Practice 8.** Engage socially powerful players early. Physician, nursing, and executive engagement is crucial to evaluation success.
- **Best Practice 9.** Ensure evaluation continuity: have a plan for employee turnover at both the participant and evaluation administration team levels.
- **Best Practice 10.** Environmental signals before, during, and after training must indicate that the trained knowledge, skills, and attitudes and the evaluation itself are valued by the organization.

Follow-up

- **Best Practice 11.** Get in the game, coach! Feed evaluation results back to frontline providers and facilitate continual improvement through constructive coaching.
- **Best Practice 12.** Report evaluation results in a meaningful way, both internally and externally.

Reproduced with permission from Weaver SJ, Salas E, King HB. Twelve best practices for team training evaluation in health care. *Jt Comm J Qual Patient Saf* 2011;37:341–349.

or obstetrics to a ward clerk who is a recent immigrant with a high school degree (Chapter 9). Moreover, the process of flying is now so automated that, like control room workers at nuclear power plants, pilots are mostly in the cockpit to react to emergencies. Medicine is a long way from being that routinized. These differences mean that aviation examples should rapidly give way to medical ones.

Table 15-3	ELEMENTS OF THE UCSF CREW RESOURCE MANAGEMENT ("TRIAD FOR OPTIMAL PATIENT SAFETY," TOPS) CURRICULUM*	
Topic	Description	Time (Minutes)
Welcome	From a system leader (i.e., chief medical officer)	10
"Laying the foundation"	Brief overview, goals of the day	15
First, Do No Harm	Video shown, followed by facilitated discussion to serve as icebreaker	40
Lecture on healthcare team behaviors and communication skills	Delivered by a commercial airline pilot. Introduces key principles of safety culture, communication, including SBAR, CUS words (Chapter 9)	60
Small-group facilitated "scenarios"	Two case scenarios, groups of ~8 people (must be interdisciplinary) to teach and practice standardized communication, team behaviors	80

*The TOPS project was funded by the Gordon and Betty Moore Foundation. Reproduced with permission from Sehgal NL, Fox M, Vidyarthi AR, et al.; TOPS Project. A multidisciplinary teamwork training program: the Triad for Optimal Patient Safety (TOPS) experience. *J Gen Intern Med* 2008;23: 2053–2057.

3. *Consider whether to use simulation*: Experts debate the utility of adding simulation to culture and communication training programs (there is less debate on the utility of simulation for improving technical skills; Chapters 5 and 17).[43,44] Proponents of simulation in CRM training argue that it "raises the stakes," allows participants to suspend disbelief more readily, and makes lessons more memorable.[45] Others feel that simulation (particularly high-fidelity, realistic simulation, as opposed to role-playing case scenarios) is not worth the added cost and complexity, and might even distract providers from the lessons regarding communication and collaboration.[46] Whether simulation is or is not used, it is critical to "get everybody in the room" to work through case-based scenarios, and to provide an opportunity for skillful debriefing and interdisciplinary cross-talk. Didactics can go only so far in transforming deep-seated attitudes and beliefs.

4. *Programs must live on beyond the initial training*: Although a brief (e.g., 4–6 hours) CRM program can sensitize workers to some of the key cultural and communication issues, effective programs outlive their initial training phase. Whether the programs live on in the

form of "unit-based safety teams" or other vehicles, the new emphasis on teamwork and collaboration must be supported by structures that endure (see also Chapter 22).[47,48]

Before leaving the topic of teamwork training, we'd like to loop back to where we began this section. Team training may seem like a convenient solution to poor safety culture, and the evidence now confirms that it generally does help. But, as Salas et al. point out, such training likely accounts for a small fraction of a team's effectiveness; the rest is determined by the culture and actions of the organization.[49] They continue:

> *The organizational system matters. What the top leadership does, matters. What policies and procedures are in place to support teamwork, matters. The formal and informal signs and symbols of what is important in the organization—as conveyed through the norms, conditions, policies, procedures, metrics in place, and the messages that top leadership sends—make or break transformational culture change. One cannot forget that organizations tend to obtain the behaviors, cognitions, and attitudes that they measure and reinforce. We need to shift from thinking about a "team training intervention" to creating and sustaining an organizational system that supports teamwork. The best team training in the world will not yield the desired outcomes unless the organization is aligned to support it.*

CHECKLISTS AND CULTURE

We've mentioned checklists several times throughout this book, mostly as a method to ensure adherence to key care processes. It may seem strange to now see a section on checklists in a chapter on safety culture. Yet in his book, *The Checklist Manifesto*, surgeon and author Atul Gawande reminds us that checklists can address a number of safety targets.[50] In leading the multicenter study that established the value of the World Health Organization's surgical checklist (Figure 5-2),[51] Gawande came to appreciate that the value of "the lowly checklist" was not simply in ensuring that the team gave the right preoperative antibiotics at the correct time, but in prompting team members in the operating room to introduce themselves to each other before a procedure begins. In other words, it was as much a culture-changing intervention as a cookbook.

Of course, concerns about "cookbook medicine" explain much of the resistance to the use of checklists, particularly among physicians. Gawande writes:

> *... we have the means to make some of the most complex and dangerous work we do ... more effective than we ever thought possible.*

But the prospect pushes against the traditional culture of medicine, with its central belief that in situations of high risk and complexity what you want is a kind of expert audacity.... Checklists and standard operating procedures feel like exactly the opposite, and that's what rankles many people.[50]

Reflecting further on the intersection between checklists and physician culture, Gawande writes; "All learned occupations have a definition of professionalism, a code of conduct ... [with] at least three common elements": selflessness, an expectation of skill, and an expectation of trustworthiness. He continues:

Aviators, however, add a fourth expectation, discipline; discipline in following prudent procedure and in functioning with others. This is a concept almost entirely outside the lexicon of most professions, including my own. In medicine, we hold up 'autonomy' as a professional lodestar, a principle that stands in direct opposition to discipline .... The closest our professional codes come to articulating the goal [of discipline] is an occasional plea for 'collegiality.' What is needed, however, isn't just that people working together be nice to each other. It is discipline.[50]

Gawande would doubtlessly agree that checklists can't solve all our problems, but they—and other safety-oriented activities such as standardization, simplification, forcing functions, and double checks—*can* help us deliver healthcare that is safer and more reliable. In applying these solutions, though, we need to grapple with the fact that checklists challenge some of physicians' most deeply held beliefs about what it means to be an excellent doctor.

The relationship between checklists and culture is a two-way street: checklists can influence culture, but their success can also be determined by an organization's ambient culture. While today's enthusiasm for checklists is well grounded, it is worth reading descriptions by Bosk et al.[52] and Dixon-Woods et al.[53] of the co-interventions crucial to the remarkable success of the Michigan central line–associated bloodstream infection study (which is often characterized—too simplistically—as a "checklist intervention"; Chapter 10).[54] We are already beginning to see failures of interventions that were organized around the naive assumption that simply embedding a checklist into a complex clinical process, without addressing matters of culture and barriers to implementation, will enhance safety.[55,56]

One other point about checklists has emerged from recent research. After participating in the WHO surgical safety intervention, 21% of clinicians disagreed with or gave neutral responses to the statement, "The checklist prevents errors in the operating room." Yet 93% of the same respondents stated that they would want the checklist to be used *if they themselves were having an operation.*[57] This is Lake Wobegon Meets Patient Safety: humans naturally believe they are above average in their carefulness.[58] Accordingly, tools such as checklists might seem useful for "the other guy"—you know, the one who isn't quite as careful as I am. But life doesn't work that way. Inserting checklists—to be used by everyone—into error-prone processes as part of a comprehensive strategy to improve culture represents one of the major recent advances in patient safety.[59]

Developing a great checklist is not a trivial undertaking. Like many good checklists, the WHO surgical checklist went through scores of iterations before the final version was produced.[50] Experiences like this and collaboration with other industries that have been using checklists for decades have allowed us to begin to understand some of the design principles for effective healthcare checklists. Figure 15-5, from McLaughlin, depicts a poor and an improved surgical checklist, illustrating some of these tenets.[60]

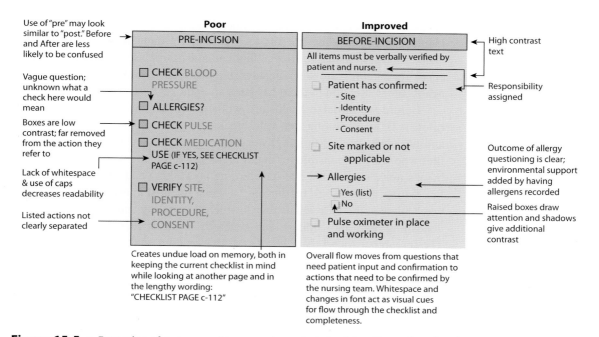

Figure 15-5 ▪ Examples of a poor and improved surgical checklist. (Reproduced with permission from AHRQ Patient Safety Network: McLaughlin AC. What makes a good checklist [Perspective]. *AHRQ PSNet* [serial online]; October 2010. Original image available at: https://psnet.ahrq.gov/media/perspectives/images/persp92_f01.gif.)

▌RULES, RULE VIOLATIONS, AND WORKAROUNDS

Gawande's comments on discipline naturally lead us into a discussion of rules and standard procedures. Healthcare providers are, of course, familiar with clinical rules: treat hypovolemia with fluids, don't give gadolinium to patients in renal failure, abscesses need to be drained. Although such rules were developed informally in the past and handed down by experts to trainees, our modern paradigm is to base clinical guidelines on firm scientific evidence (Chapter 3).

The field of patient safety is not agnostic about such clinical guidance. Providing high-quality, safe care requires that we pay attention to evidence-based rules and guidelines while allowing clinicians the flexibility to deviate when their patients do not fit the template (such as in patients with multiple and overlapping diseases).[61] In Chapter 13, we discussed the role of computerized clinical decision support systems, which should make it easier for clinicians to follow such rules by providing up-to-date guidance at the point of care.

But these clinical rules fall largely in the domain of quality of care (Chapter 3). In the safety field, we are more concerned with rules and policies enacted to prevent patient harm. Examples might include: perform a "time out" prior to the first incision (Chapter 5), read back a critical lab value, use a checklist before inserting a central line (Chapter 10), and check the patient's identity before sending her off to a potentially dangerous procedure (this chapter's case). Such rules (e.g., "flight attendants, please arm doors and cross check for takeoff") are the mainstays of many industries' safety programs, but healthcare's attention to them has been sporadic, at best.

Before we criticize healthcare workers too harshly for breaking safety rules, it is worth noting that rule breaking is part of the human condition, and not always a bad thing. History, of course, is filled with stories of gadflies who were responsible for major breakthroughs. And who among us never breaks rules, such as the ones concerning jaywalking and speed limits?[62] In a fascinating study quoted by Vincent,[4] a social scientist interviewed British railway shunters, the individuals responsible for coupling and uncoupling trains, depositing them into sidings, and generally ensuring their safe movement.[63] The researcher found that, despite the risky nature of the work, the shunters frequently violated established safety procedures, sometimes for reasons of inexperience, sometimes because they felt a rule was unnecessary or silly, and sometimes because they believed their action did not pose any serious risk (Table 15-4). James Reason calls the last category a *routine rule violation*, and most times they are harmless enough.[64]

The problem is that an unblinking acceptance of rule violations has diffused throughout medicine, particularly among physicians, whose status atop the hierarchy and, at least in the United States, as independent entrepreneurs (rather than employees of the hospital or healthcare system, although this is

Table 15-4 RAILWAY SHUNTERS' REASONS FOR VIOLATING RULES	
Reason for Violation	**Percent**
This is a quicker way of working	39
Inexperienced shunter	38
Time pressure	37
High workload	30
The shunter is lazy	19
A skilled shunter can work safely this way	17
The rule can be impossible to work to	16
Design of the sidings makes the violation necessary	16
Management turns a blind eye	12
Physical exhaustion	7
No one understands the rule	6
It is a more exciting way of working	6
It is a macho way to work	5
The rule is outdated	5

Reproduced with permission from Lawton R. Not working to rule: understanding procedural violations at work. *Saf Sci* 2004;28:199–211.

changing) has traditionally given them license to ignore rules. But, just as with the broken windows theory of policing (which holds that letting people get away with minor violations, such as breaking windows in abandoned houses, tacitly encourages them to try their hand at larger crimes),[65] it can be argued that our permissiveness toward healthcare rule violators is responsible for the high rate of violations of some very important rules, such as hand hygiene. As Henry Kissinger famously said, "History teaches that weakness is provocative …."[66]

Yet before we embrace a more punitive approach to rule-breakers (which we discuss more fully in Chapter 19), it is worth recognizing the extraordinary complexity swirling around this area. Vincent[4] highlights the contributions of Diana Vaughan (whose study of the Challenger shuttle disaster introduced the concept of *normalization of deviance*) and Rene Amalberti (whose studies have illuminated the frequent migration of workers from the "legal" to the "illegal-normal," sometimes driven by differences in risk perception by individuals).[67,68] Vincent and coworkers also describe a fascinating study by French anesthesiologists documenting the brief lifespan of many safety rules.[69] "They are born," Vincent writes, "they have a vigorous youth where most people take note of them, they begin to get old and less notice is taken of them, and finally they die."[4]

As our quest to improve safety drives us to pay more attention to rules and procedures, we need to be sure that the rules we promulgate are important enough to be worth paying attention to, that we distinguish "must follow" from "nice to follow" rules (some organizations call the inviolable ones "*Red Rules*"),[70] and that we enlist teams and peers to help enforce crucial rules. One aspect of high functioning teams is that they reach consensus that deviations from certain rules will not be tolerated, and then enforce such decisions with everything from gentle reminders to outright sanctions. You'll know you've achieved a safe culture when you see someone low in the hierarchy—say, a new nurse—reminding a senior physician to wash his or her hands, and the physician responds by simply saying, "thank you," then turns to the sink or gel dispenser.

SOME FINAL THOUGHTS ON SAFETY CULTURE

We end the chapter with a few general reflections on the remarkably rich and challenging issue of safety culture. Rather than emphasizing the issues above (promoting teamwork and collaboration, dampening down authority gradients, fighting the culture of low expectations, staying attuned to production pressures, mandating adherence to key rules and policies), some institutions define a safety culture in terms of the following questions:

- Do workers report errors?
- Is there a "no blame" culture?
- Is "improving patient safety" listed in the strategic plan?

Let's consider these points one by one.

As we discussed in Chapter 14, pushing workers to report, report, and report some more (particularly to an institutional or governmental reporting system) is not likely to generate a stronger safety culture. That said, local reporting (especially when there is a supportive unit leader who listens to problems and helps fix them, and when reports fuel engaging M&M conferences and unit-based problem solving) is important. Moreover, reporting can be a useful part of a broader effort to discover problems and engage frontline workers.

The issue of "no blame" is one of the most complex in the safety field. Throughout the book, we have discussed the importance of a systems approach, fighting the instinct to blame and replacing it with a focus on identifying system flaws that allow our inevitable human errors to cause harm. This mental model has been responsible for much of the progress we have made in the first 15 years of the patient safety movement.

That said, the "no blame" mantra has been taken by some to absurd levels. Blame *is* appropriate for individuals who make frequent, careless errors, who fail to keep up with their specialty, who come to work intoxicated, or who choose to ignore reasonable safety rules. David Marx and others have promoted the concept of a "*Just Culture*" (rather than a "no blame" culture) as a way to reconcile an appropriate focus on "no blame" when caring, competent workers make errors with the need to hold individuals (and institutions) accountable for blameworthy errors or conditions.[71] This concept is explored more fully in Chapter 19.

Finally, placing patient safety in, or even atop, an institution's strategic plan is no guarantee of a safe culture (Chapter 22). Senior leadership and hospital boards make an important statement when they prioritize patient safety among their values and missions, but too many organizations and leaders offer lip service without promoting the effort and allocating the resources to make this commitment real.[29,30] Creating a safe culture is hard work. But once it is created, it is easy to identify its presence, as well as its absence.

KEY POINTS

- Safe cultures are ones in which people willingly speak up when they see risky situations and behaviors, there are relatively flat hierarchies, workers follow critical safety rules, and the need for throughput is balanced against the need for safety.
- Some institutions are employing teamwork training programs, usually modeled on aviation's crew resource management (CRM) programs, and emerging research on the results of well-implemented programs is promising.
- Validated survey instruments are available to measure safety culture and to benchmark against like clinical units or organizations.
- One aspect of a safe culture is fighting "the culture of low expectations," in which workers assume faulty communication and therefore fail to perform double checks despite clear warning signs.
- Checklists can not only encourage compliance with safe processes of care but also facilitate culture change by improving teamwork and communication. Their success, in turn, can also be influenced by the ambient culture and implementation process.
- The concept of a "Just Culture" has been advanced to emphasize the importance of blending a systems focus with appropriate individual and institutional accountability.

REFERENCES

1. Helmreich RL. On error management: lessons from aviation. *BMJ* 2000;320:781–785.
2. Weick KE, Sutcliffe KM. *Managing the Unexpected: Assuring High Performance in an Age of Complexity*. 2nd ed. San Francisco, CA: John Wiley & Sons; 2007.
3. Pronovost PJ, Berenholtz SM, Goeschel CA, et al. Creating high reliability in health care organizations. *Health Serv Res* 2006;41:1599–1617.
4. Vincent C. *Patient Safety*. 2nd ed. West Sussex, UK: Wiley-Blackwell; 2010:282.
5. Vincent C, Benn J, Hanna GB. High reliability in healthcare. *BMJ* 2010;340:c84.
6. Chassin MR, Becher EC. The wrong patient. *Ann Intern Med* 2002;136:826–833.
7. Berridge EJ, Mackintosh NJ, Freeth DS. Supporting patient safety: examining communication within delivery suite teams through contrasting approaches to research observation. *Midwifery* 2010;26:512–519.
8. Knight LJ, Gabhart JM, Earnest KS, Leong KM, Anglemyer A, Franzon D. Improving code team performance and survival outcomes: implementation of pediatric resuscitation team training. *Crit Care Med* 2014;42:243–251.
9. Agency for Healthcare Research and Quality. *Surveys on Patient Safety Culture*. Rockville, MD: Agency for Healthcare Research and Quality; October 2016. Available at: http://www.ahrq.gov/professionals/quality-patient-safety/patientsafety culture/index.html.
10. Sexton JB, Helmreich RL, Neilands TB, et al. The Safety Attitudes Questionnaire: psychometric properties, benchmarking data, and emerging research. *BMC Health Serv Res* 2006;6:44.
11. Etchegaray JM, Thomas EJ. Comparing two safety culture surveys: Safety Attitudes Questionnaire and Hospital Survey on Patient Safety. *BMJ Qual Saf* 2012;490–498.
12. Campbell EG, Singer S, Kitch BT, Iezzoni LI, Meyer GS. Patient safety climate in hospitals: act locally on variation across units. *Jt Comm J Qual Patient Saf* 2010;36:319–326.
13. Pronovost PJ, Sexton B. Assessing safety culture: guidelines and recommendations. *Qual Saf Health Care* 2005;14:231–233.
14. Sexton JB, Thomas EJ, Helmreich RL. Error, stress, and teamwork in medicine and aviation: cross sectional surveys. *BMJ* 2000;320:745–749.
15. Listyowardojo TA, Nap RE, Johnson A. Variations in hospital worker perceptions of safety culture. *Int J Qual Health Care* 2012;24:9–15.
16. Bump GM, Coots N, Liberi CA, et al. Comparing trainee and staff perceptions of patient safety culture. *Acad Med* 2017;92:116–122.
17. Hickner J, Smith SA, Yount N, Sorra J. Differing perceptions of safety culture across job roles in the ambulatory setting: analysis of the AHRQ Medical Office Survey on Patient Safety Culture. *BMJ Qual Saf* 2016;25:588–594.
18. Singer SJ, Gaba DM, Geppert JJ, Sinaiko AD, Howard SK, Park KC. The culture of safety: results of an organization-wide survey in 15 California hospitals. *Qual Saf Health Care* 2003;12:112–118.
19. Singer SJ, Falwell A, Gaba DM, Baker LC. Patient safety climate in US hospitals: variation by management level. *Med Care* 2008;46:1149–1156.
20. Huang DT, Clermont G, Kong L, et al. Intensive care unit safety culture and outcomes: a US multicenter study. *Int J Qual Health Care* 2010;22:151–161.

21. Singer S, Lin S, Falwell A, Gaba D, Baker L. Relationship of safety climate and safety performance in hospitals. *Health Serv Rev* 2009;44:399–421.

22. Mardon RE, Khanna K, Sorra J, Dyer N, Famolaro T. Exploring relationships between hospital patient safety culture and adverse events. *J Patient Saf* 2010;6:226–232.

23. Hansen LO, Williams MV, Singer SJ. Perceptions of hospital safety climate and incidence of readmission. *Health Serv Res* 2011;46:596–616.

24. DiCuccio MH. The relationship between patient safety culture and patient outcomes: a systematic review. *J Patient Saf* 2015;11:135–142.

25. Makary M. *Unaccountable: What Hospitals Won't Tell You and How Transparency Can Revolutionize Health Care*. New York, NY: Bloomsbury Press; 2012.

26. Okuyama A, Wagner C, Bijnen B. Speaking up for patient safety by hospital-based health care professionals: a literature review. *BMC Health Serv Res* 2014;14:61.

27. Carayon P. Production pressures. *AHRQ WebM&M* (serial online); May 2007. Available at: https://psnet.ahrq.gov/webmm/case/150.

28. Gaba DM, Howard SK, Jump B. Production pressure in the work environment. California anesthesiologists' attitudes and experiences. *Anesthesiology* 1994;81:488–500.

29. Millar R, Mannion R, Freeman T, Davies HTO. Hospital board oversight of quality and patient safety: a narrative review and synthesis of recent empirical research. *Milbank Q* 2013;91:738–770.

30. Goeschel CA, Wachter RM, Pronovost PJ. Responsibility for quality improvement and patient safety: hospital board and medical staff leadership challenges. *Chest* 2010;138:171–178.

31. Neily J, Mills PD, Young-Xu Y, et al. Association between implementation of a medical team training program and surgical mortality. *JAMA* 2010;304:1693–1700.

32. Dunn EJ, Mills PD, Neily J, Crittenden MD, Carmack AL, Bagian JP. Medical team training: applying crew resource management in the Veterans Health Administration. *Jt Comm J Qual Patient Saf* 2007;33:317–325.

33. Mayer CM, Cluff L, Lin WT, et al. Evaluating efforts to optimize TeamSTEPPS implementation in surgical and pediatric intensive care units. *Jt Comm J Qual Patient Saf* 2011;37:365–374.

34. Weaver SJ, Dy SM, Rosen MA. Team-training in healthcare: a narrative synthesis of the literature. *BMJ Qual Saf* 2014;23:359–372.

35. Wolf FA, Way LW, Stewart L. The efficacy of medical team training: improved team performance and decreased operating room delays: a detailed analysis of 4863 cases. *Ann Surg* 2010;252:477–485.

36. Morey JC, Simon R, Jay GD, et al. Error reduction and performance improvement in the emergency department through formal teamwork training: evaluation results of the MedTeams project. *Health Serv Res* 2002;37:1553–1581.

37. Riley W, Davis S, Miller K, Hansen H, Sainfort F, Sweet R. Didactic and simulation nontechnical skills team training to improve perinatal patient outcomes in a community hospital. *Jt Comm J Qual Patient Saf* 2011;37:357–364.

38. Fransen AF, van de Ven J, Schuit E, et al. Simulation-based team training for multiprofessional obstetric care teams to improve patient outcome: a multicenter, cluster randomized controlled trial. *BJOG* 2017;124:641–650.

39. Duclos A, Peix JL, Piriou V, et al. Cluster randomized trial to evaluate the impact of team training on surgical outcomes. IDILIC Study Group. *Br J Surg* 2016;103(13): 1804–1814.

40. Hughes AM, Gregory ME, Joseph DL, et al. Saving lives: a meta-analysis of team training in healthcare. *J Appl Psychol* 2016;101:1266–1304.

41. Weaver SJ, Salas E, King HB. Twelve best practices for team training evaluation in health care. *Jt Comm J Qual Patient Saf* 2011;37:341–349.

42. Sehgal NL, Fox M, Vidyarthi AR, et al.; TOPS Project. A multidisciplinary teamwork training program: the Triad for Optimal Patient Safety (TOPS) experience. *J Gen Intern Med* 2008;23:2053–2057.

43. Schmidt E, Goldhaber-Fiebert SN, Ho LA, McDonald KM. Simulation exercises as a patient safety strategy: a systematic review. *Ann Intern Med* 2013;158:426–432.

44. Cook DA, Hatala R, Brydges R, et al. Technology-enhanced simulation for health professions education. *JAMA* 2011;306:978–988.

45. Gaba DM. What does simulation add to teamwork training? [Perspective]. *AHRQ PSNet* (serial online); March 2006. Available at: https://psnet.ahrq.gov/perspectives/perspective/20.

46. Pratt SD, Sachs BP. Team training: classroom training vs. high-fidelity simulation [Perspective]. *AHRQ PSNet* (serial online); March 2006. Available at: http://www.webmm.ahrq.gov/perspective.aspx?perspectiveID=21.

47. Timmel J, Kent PS, Holzmueller CG, Paine L, Schulick RD, Pronovost PJ. Impact of the Comprehensive Unit-Based Safety Program (CUSP) on safety culture in a surgical inpatient unit. *Jt Comm J Qual Patient Saf* 2010;36;252–260.

48. Pronovost P, King J, Holzmueller CG, et al. A web-based tool for the Comprehensive Unit-based Safety Program (CUSP). *J Comm J Qual Patient Saf* 2006;32:119–129.

49. Salas E, Gregory ME, King HB. Team training can enhance patient safety—the data, the challenge ahead. *J Comm J Qual Patient Saf* 2011;37:339–340.

50. Gawande A. *The Checklist Manifesto: How to Get Things Right.* New York, NY: Metropolitan Books; 2009.

51. Haynes AB, Weiser TG, Berry WR, et al.; for the Safe Surgery Saves Lives Study Group. A surgical safety checklist to reduce morbidity and mortality in a global population. *N Engl J Med* 2009;360:491–499.

52. Bosk CL, Dixon-Woods M, Goeschel CA, Pronovost PJ. Reality check for checklists. *Lancet* 2009;374:444–445.

53. Dixon-Woods M, Bosk CL, Aveling EL, Goeschel CA, Pronovost PJ. Explaining Michigan: developing an ex post theory of a quality improvement program. *Milbank Q* 2011;89:167–205.

54. Pronovost P, Needham D, Berenholtz S, et al. An intervention to decrease catheter-related bloodstream infections in the ICU. *N Engl J Med* 2006;355:2725–2732.

55. Urbach DR, Govindarajan A, Saskin R, Wilton AS, Baxter NN. Introduction of surgical safety checklists in Ontario, Canada. *N Engl J Med* 2014;370:1029–1038.

56. Catchpole K, Russ S. The problem with checklists. *BMJ Qual Saf* 2015;24: 545–549.

57. Haynes AB, Weiser TG, Berry WR, et al.; Safe Surgery Saves Lives Study Group. Changes in safety attitude and relationship to decreased postoperative morbidity and

mortality following implementation of a checklist-based surgical safety intervention. *BMJ Qual Saf* 2011;20:102–107.

58. Kruger J. Lake Wobegon be gone! The "below-average effect" and the egocentric nature of comparative ability judgments. *J Pers Soc Psychol* 1999;77:221–232.

59. Treadwell JR, Lucas S, Tsou AY. Surgical checklists: a systematic review of impacts and implementation. *BMJ Qual Saf* 2014;23:299–318.

60. McLaughlin AC. What makes a good checklist? [Perspective]. *AHRQ PSNet* (serial online); October 2010. Available at: https://psnet.ahrq.gov/perspectives/perspective/92.

61. Boyd CM, Darer J, Boult C, Fried LP, Boult L, Wu AW. Clinical practice guidelines and quality of care for older patients with multiple comorbid diseases. Implications for pay for performance. *JAMA* 2005;294:716–724.

62. McKenna FP, Horswill MS. Risk taking from the participant's perspective: the case of driving and accident risk. *Health Psychol* 2006;25:163–170.

63. Lawton R. Not working to rule: understanding procedural violations at work. *Saf Sci* 1998;28:77–95.

64. Reason JT. *Human Error.* New York, NY: Cambridge University Press; 1990.

65. Wilson JQ, Kelling GL. Broken windows: the police and neighborhood safety. *The Atlantic Monthly*. March 1982.

66. Nuclear Age Peace Foundation. *Statement of the Honorable Henry A. Kissinger Before the Senate Foreign Relations Committee.* May 26, 1999.

67. Vaughan D. *The Challenger Launch Decision: Risky Technology, Culture, and Deviance at NASA.* Chicago, IL: University of Chicago Press; 1997.

68. Amalberti R, Vincent C, Auroy Y. Violations and migrations in health care: a framework for understanding and management. *Qual Saf Health Care* 2006;15:166–171.

69. de Saint Maurice G, Auroy Y, Vincent C, Amalberti R. The natural lifespan of a safety policy: violations and system migration in anaesthesia. *Qual Saf Health Care* 2010; 19:327–331.

70. Scharf WR. Red rules: an error-reduction strategy in the culture of safety. *Focus Patient Saf* 2007;10:1–2.

71. Marx D. *Patient Safety and the "Just Culture": A Primer for Health Care Executives.* April 17, 2001. Available at: http://www.chpso.org/sites/main/files/file-attachments/marx_primer.pdf.

ADDITIONAL READINGS

Adler-Milstein JR, Singer SJ, Toffel MW. *Speaking Up Constructively: Managerial Practices that Elicit Solutions from Front-Line Employees.* Cambridge, MA: Harvard Business School; August 25, 2010. HBS Working Paper No. 11-005.

Bishop AC, Boyle TA. The role of safety culture in influencing provider perceptions of patient safety. *J Patient Saf* 2016;12:204–209.

Edmonson A, Reynolds S. *Building the Future: Big Teaming for Audacious Innovation.* Oakland, CA: Berrett-Koehler Publishers, Inc.; 2016.

Kotter JP. Leading change: why transformation efforts fail. *Harv Bus Rev* 1995;73:59–67.

Lucian Leape Institute at the National Patient Safety Foundation. *Unmet Needs: Teaching Physicians to Provide Safe Patient Care*. Boston, MA: Lucian Leape Institute at the National Patient Safety Foundation; March 2010.

Lyndon A, Sexton JB, Simpson KR, Rosenstein A, Lee KA, Wachter RM. Predictors of likelihood of speaking up about safety concerns in labour and delivery. *BMJ Qual Saf* 2012;21:791–799.

Sexton JB, Berenholtz SM, Goeschel CA, et al. Assessing and improving safety climate in a large cohort of intensive care units. *Crit Care Med* 2011;39:934–939.

Shortell SM, Singer SJ. Improving patient safety by taking systems seriously. *JAMA* 2008;299:445–447.

Sorokin R, Riggio JM, Moleski S, Sullivan J. Physicians-in-training attitudes on patient safety: 2003 to 2008. *J Patient Saf* 2011;7:132–137.

Spath PL, ed. *Error Reduction in Health Care: A Systems Approach to Improving Patient Safety*. 2nd ed. San Francisco, CA: Jossey-Bass; 2011.

Patankar MS, Brown JP, Sabin EJ, Bigda-Peyton TG. *Safety Culture: Building and Sustaining a Cultural Change in Aviation and Healthcare*. Burlington, VT: Ashgate; 2012.

Singer SJ, Molina G, Li Z, et al. Relationship between operating room teamwork, contextual factors, and safety checklist performance. *J Am Coll Surg* 2016;223:568–580.e2.

Verbakel NJ, Langelaan M, Verheij TJ, Wagner C, Zwart DL. Improving patient safety culture in primary care: a systematic review. *J Patient Saf* 2016;12:152–158.

WORKFORCE ISSUES | 16

OVERVIEW

In many discussions of patient safety, it is assumed that the workforce is up to the task—in training, competency, and numbers. In these formulations, a combination of the right processes, information technology, and culture is enough to ensure safe care.

However, as any frontline worker can tell you, neglecting issues of workforce sufficiency and competency omits an important part of the equation. For example, a nursing or physician staff that is overworked and demoralized will breed unsafe conditions, even if good communication, sound policies, and well-designed computer systems are in place.

In this chapter, we will discuss some key issues in workforce composition and organizational structure, including the nursing workforce, Rapid Response Teams, and trainee-related matters such as duty-hour restrictions and the so-called "July effect." We'll close with a discussion of the "second victim" phenomenon: the toll that errors take on caregivers themselves. In the next chapter, we'll discuss issues of training and competency.

NURSING WORKFORCE ISSUES

Much of our understanding of the interaction between workforce and patient outcomes and safety comes from studies of nursing, owing to a combination of pioneering research exploring these associations,[1-8] a nursing shortage that emerged in the late 1990s in the United States, and effective advocacy by nursing organizations. Because most hospital nurses in the United States are salaried and employed by the hospitals, they have a strong incentive to advocate for sensible workloads. This is in contrast to physicians, who (again in the United States) are mostly self-employed (although hospital employment of physicians is increasing) and therefore calibrate their own workload.

Substantial data suggest that medical errors increase with higher ratios of patients to nurses. One study found that surgical patients had a 31% greater chance of dying in hospitals when nurses cared for more than seven patients, on average. For every additional patient added to a nurse's average workload, patient mortality rose 7%, and nursing burnout and dissatisfaction increased 23% and 15%, respectively. The authors estimated that 20,000 annual deaths in the United States could be attributed to inadequate nurse-to-patient ratios.[1] One study, perhaps the most methodologically rigorous to date, confirmed the association between low nurse staffing and increased mortality. It also demonstrated that high rates of patient turnover were associated with mortality, even when average staffing was adequate.[4] A systematic review of the evidence supports the safety benefits of increased nurse staffing ratios.[9]

Unfortunately, the demand for nurses cannot be met by the existing supply. Despite some easing of the U.S. nursing shortage, projected nursing workforce needs remains a concern. One study looked at the nursing shortages in each of the 50 states and assigned a letter grade for nursing workforce shortages. The number of states receiving a poor grade (D or F) was projected to increase from 5 states in 2009 to 30 states by 2030. The authors cite a total shortage of almost one million nursing jobs.[10] While more young people have entered the nursing profession in recent years, nearly one million of the nation's nurses (approximately one in four) are over age 50, adding to the challenge.

Efforts to address the nursing shortage have centered on improved pay, benefits, and working conditions. In the future, technology could play an important role as well, particularly if it relieves nurses of some of their paperwork burden and allows them to spend more time with patients, or if robots or artificial intelligence can take over some tasks currently performed by nurses. In Chapter 13, we described the lunacy that results when a nurse takes a digital blood pressure reading and then begins an error-prone struggle to transcribe it in multiple places. Situations like this, which go on dozens of times during a typical shift, are one reason many nurses believe so much of their time and training are wasted.

Importantly, even as the nursing shortage has catalyzed efforts to improve pay, hours, staffing, and technology, it has also brought long-overdue attention to issues of nursing culture and satisfaction. Studies in this area often point to problematic relationships with physician colleagues. In one survey of more than 700 nurses, 96% said they had witnessed or experienced *disruptive behavior* by physicians. Nearly half pointed to "fear of retribution" as the primary reason that such acts were not reported to superiors. Thirty percent of the nurses also said they knew at least one nurse who had resigned as a result of boorish—or worse—physician behavior, while many others knew nurses who had changed shifts or clinical units to avoid interacting with particular doctors.[11–13] In addition, negative nurse–physician interactions may impact the quality and safety of care provided to patients, at least as perceived by nurses.[14] These concerns have been an important driver for the interdisciplinary training discussed in Chapter 15, and for increasing efforts to enforce acceptable behavioral standards among all healthcare professionals (Chapter 19).[15,16]

Driven by the strong association between nurse staffing and outcomes, several states have chosen to address nurse staffing in laws or regulations. Two of them (California and Massachusetts) mandate minimum nurse-to-patient ratios (usually 1:5 on medical-surgical wards and 1:2 in intensive care units). In addition, 16 states restrict mandatory overtime. The jury is out regarding whether these legislative solutions enhance safety. Some nurses complain that ancillary personnel (clerks, lifting teams) have been released in order to hire enough nurses to meet the ratios, resulting in little additional time for nurses to perform nursing-related tasks. Commentators have pointed out that the determination of adequate nurse staffing is complex and fluid, since it needs to take into account patient acuity, availability of adequate support staff, and a host of other factors that may vary shift-by-shift.[17,18]

In addition to these staffing standards, there has been an effort to develop quality and safety measures linked to the adequacy of nursing care. These *"nursing-sensitive" measures* include rates of falls, urinary tract infections, and decubitus ulcers.[19,20] While the Joint Commission assesses nurse staffing and working conditions in its accreditation process, many hospitals aspire to the even higher standards of the American Nurses Credentialing Center's *"magnet status."* Limited research suggests an association between magnet status and better patient outcomes.[21]

RAPID RESPONSE TEAMS

Analyses of deaths and unexpected cardiopulmonary arrests in hospitals often find signs of patient deterioration that went unnoticed for hours preceding the tragic turn of events. Measures of these so-called *failure to rescue* cases are included among the AHRQ Patient Safety Indicators (Appendix V).[22–24] Identifying warning signs may require better monitoring systems or improved nurse staffing.

Table 16-1   **REASONS FOR FAILURE TO RESCUE**
Monitoring technology is used only in the intensive care unit or step-down units
Hospital-ward monitoring is only intermittent (vital sign measurements)
Intervals between measurements can easily be eight hours or longer
Regular visits by a hospital-ward nurse vary in frequency and duration
Visits by a unit doctor may occur only once a day
When vital signs are measured, they are sometimes incomplete
When vital signs are abnormal, there may be no specific criteria for activating a higher-level intervention
Individual judgment is applied to a crucial decision
Individual judgment varies in accuracy according to training, experience, professional attitude, working environment, hierarchical position, and previous responses to alerts
If an alert is issued, the activation process goes through a long chain of command (e.g., nurse to charge nurse, charge nurse to intern, intern to resident, resident to fellow, fellow to attending physician)
Each step in the chain is associated with individual judgment and delays
In surgical wards, doctors are sometimes physically unavailable because they are performing operations
Modern hospitals provide care for patients with complex disorders and coexisting conditions, and unexpected clinical deterioration may occur while nurses and doctors are busy with other tasks

Reproduced with permission from Jones DA, DeVita MA, Bellomo R. Rapid-response teams. *N Engl J Med* 2011;365:139–146.

But such cases may also reflect a cultural problem: analyses of failure to rescue cases sometimes reveal that a nurse noticed that something was awry but was either unable to find an appropriate responder or reluctant to bypass the traditional hierarchy (i.e., the standard procedure to call the private physician at home before the in-house ICU physician, or the intern before the attending). Table 16-1 lists a variety of causes of failure to rescue.[24]

The concept of Rapid Response Teams (RRTs) was developed to address these problems. Now sometimes called "Rapid Response Systems" (RRSs) to emphasize the importance of both the monitoring and response phases, such teams have been widely promoted and adopted, particularly after they were included among the six "planks" of the Institute for Healthcare Improvement's "100,000 Lives Campaign" in 2005 (Table 20-2).[25,26]

Despite the face validity of RSSs, the evidence supporting them remains controversial. While several single-center, before-and-after comparisons found a reduction in hospital cardiac arrests,[24,27–29] a large randomized multi-site study demonstrated no impact.[30] Two meta-analyses have also questioned the benefit of RRSs,[31,32] while a more recent one found a general positive impact on mortality for both pediatric and adult patients.[33] Another recent study showed that delayed activation of a rapid response team was correlated with worse patient outcomes.[34] A pre-post study looking at implementation of RRSs across hospitals in the Netherlands found an association with improved patient outcomes, including decreased inpatient mortality, cardiac arrest and unplanned ICU admissions.[35] Overall, the weight of the evidence now seems to support the RRS concept.

At the present time, the optimal criteria to trigger an RRT response are unknown.[24] Some institutions use strict objective criteria, while others emphasize that anyone with concerns should feel free to activate the RRT. Some hospitals even allow patients and families to call the team.[36] One Australian hospital's poster illustrating its vital sign criteria for activating the Medical Emergency Team (another name for RRT) is shown in Figure 16-1.[24]

Similarly, the optimal composition of the responding team remains uncertain. Some hospitals have used physician-led teams, while other RRTs are led by nurses, often with respiratory therapists as partners.[37] RRTs have a positive impact on nursing satisfaction and perhaps retention, although the magnitude of this benefit has not been fully quanified.[38]

While the Joint Commission does not specifically require the presence of an RRT, it did spur adoption when, as part of its 2008 National Patient Safety Goals, it stipulated that accredited organizations select "a suitable method that enables healthcare staff members to directly request additional assistance from a specially trained individual(s) when the patient's condition appears to be worsening."[39] Ongoing research will hopefully answer the many questions surrounding RRTs, including the cost-effectiveness of the intervention. An RRT with round-the-clock dedicated staffing can easily cost a hospital hundreds of thousands of dollars per year.[40]

For now, RRTs remain attractive in theory, and their underlying rationale—that hospitals should have robust systems to monitor patients for deterioration as well as a structure and culture that ensure that appropriately qualified staff and necessary technology are available to care for deteriorating patients—seems unassailable. That said, the limited evidence of benefit is a concern, and RRTs have become Exhibit A in the debate among patient safety experts regarding the level of scientific evidence required before a so-called "safe practice" is required (Chapter 22).[41–43]

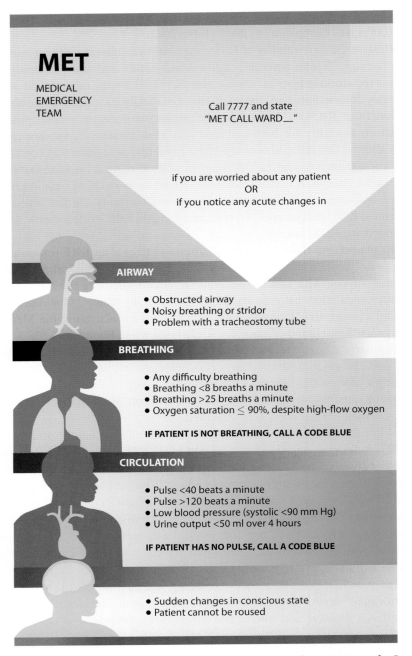

Figure 16-1 ▪ An Australian hospital poster listing criteria for activation of a Rapid Response Team. (Reproduced with permission from Jones DA, DeVita MA, Bellomo R. Rapid-response teams. *N Engl J Med* 2011;365:139–146.)

HOUSE STAFF DUTY HOURS

Amazingly, there is little research linking safety or patient outcomes to the workload of practicing (i.e., nontrainee) physicians. Dr. Michael DeBakey, the legendary Texas heart surgeon, was once said to have performed 18 cardiac bypass operations in a single day! The outcomes of the patients (particularly patient number 18) have not been reported. But the implicit message of such celebrated feats of endurance is that "real doctors" do not complain about their workload; they simply soldier on.

With little research to question this attitude and with the payment system in the United States continuing to reward productivity over safety, there have been few counterarguments to this machismo logic. And the evidence is far from ironclad. One recent study specifically sought to address impact of sleep loss on attending physician performance. Examining the outcomes of elective surgical procedures, it found no difference in mortality, complications, or readmissions between physicians who had sleep loss as compared to those who did not.[44]

Although attending physician fatigue has not typically been characterized as a patient safety issue, significant attention has been given to the workload and fatigue of physician trainees, particularly residents. At the core of residency training is the ritual of being "on call"—staying in the hospital overnight to care for sick patients. Bad as things are now, they have markedly improved since the mid-1900s, when many residents actually *lived* at the hospital (giving us the term "house officer") for months at a time. Even as recently as 30 years ago, some residents were on call every other night, accumulating as many as 120 weekly work hours—which is particularly remarkable when one considers that there are only 168 hours in a week.

Although resident call schedules became more reasonable over the past generation, until recently many residents continued to be on call every third night, with workweeks of more than 100 hours. But change has not come easily. As efforts to limit house staff shifts gained momentum, some physician leaders argued that traditional schedules were necessary to mint competent, committed physicians. For example, in 2002 the editor of the *New England Journal of Medicine* wrote that long hours:

> ... *have come with a cost, but they have allowed trainees to learn how the disease process modifies patients' lives and how they cope with illness. Long hours have also taught a central professional lesson about personal responsibility to one's patients, above and beyond work schedules and personal plans. Whether this method arose by design or was the fortuitous byproduct of an arduous training program designed primarily for economic reasons is not the point.*

Limits on hours on call will disrupt one of the ways we've taught young physicians these critical values …. We risk exchanging our sleep-deprived healers for a cadre of wide-awake technicians.[45]

Therein lies the tension: legitimate concerns that medical professionalism might be degraded by "shift work" and that excellence requires lots of practice and the ability to follow many patients from clinical presentation through work-up to denouement, balanced against worries regarding the effects of fatigue on performance and morale.[46–49] The latter concerns are well grounded. One study showed that 24 hours of sustained wakefulness results in performance equivalent to that of a person with a blood alcohol level of 0.1%—above the legal limit for driving in every state in the United States.[50]

Although early researchers felt that this kind of impairment occurred only after very long shifts, we now know that chronic sleep deprivation is just as harmful. Healthy volunteers performing math calculations were just as impaired after sleeping 5 hours per night for a week as they were after a single 24-hour wakefulness marathon.[51] The investigators in this study didn't check to see what happened when both these disruptions occurred in the *same* week, the norm for many residents operating under traditional training models.

Although it defies common sense to believe that sleep-deprived brains and bad medical decisions are not related, hard proof of this intuitive link has been surprisingly elusive. Most studies using surgical simulators or videotapes of surgeons during procedures show that sleep-deprived residents have problems with both precision and efficiency, yet studies of nonsurgical trainees are less conclusive. One showed that orthopedic residents were tired for almost 50% of their waking hours and experienced cognitive impairment over 25% of that time.[52] Another found that medical interns performed better on a simulated clinical scenario after a 16-hour shift than after a traditional extended dura-tion shift.[53] Yet other studies showed that tired radiology residents made no more mistakes reading x-rays than well-rested ones, and sleepy ER residents performed physical examinations and recorded patient histories with equal reliability in both tired and rested conditions.[54]

In 2003, the Accreditation Council for Graduate Medical Education (ACGME, the group that blesses the 10,000 residency and fellowship pro-grams in the United States, involving over 120,000 trainees) stepped into the breach, limiting residents to a maximum of 80 hours per week, with no shift lasting longer than 30 consecutive hours and at least one day off per week (Table 16-2).[55] Studies that followed these changes yielded surprisingly mixed results, with the weight of the evidence showing no significant change in patient safety or overall outcomes. The studies did, however, find improved quality of life for residents.[55–59]

Notwithstanding the ambiguous evidence, pressure on the ACGME to do more continued to mount, driven by public and professional advocacy and by the results of a prominent study that found that residents on ICU rotations who worked in shifts averaging 16 hours committed fewer errors than those working traditional overnight shifts.[55,60] In 2008, the Institute of Medicine (now the National Academy of Medicine) released a study recommending that overnight shifts for all residents be eliminated and that round-the-clock supervision be required.[61] In 2010, the ACGME responded by codifying the IOM's recommended supervision requirements, but prohibiting overnight shifts only for interns (first-year residents), not all residents (Table 16-2).[55,62]

The 2010 regulations went into effect in July 2011 and were immediately unpopular with training program directors, who feared that they would soon begin to graduate undertrained physicians.[49] Residents, interestingly, were conflicted—confident that the new rules would improve their own quality of life but skeptical that they would improve their training and patient safety.[59]

Several years into the 2011 duty hour changes, the literature does not support a positive impact on patient safety. One study showed no difference in surgical complication rates before and after the work hour changes,[63] and another showed no difference in mortality.[64] Another randomized trial examined the impact of 12-, 16-, and 24-hour shifts on patient safety and found no difference in patient outcomes, including mortality or adverse events, further suggesting that limiting duty hours by itself does not improve patient safety.[65] Another study, this of Medicare patients, found no difference in 30-day mortality rates or readmissions after the new duty hours.[66] Finally, Rajaram et al. looked at the outcomes of general surgery patients as well as resident performance on exams and found no difference in either, suggesting, in addition to their lack of impact on safety, the duty hour changes may not have adversely impacted education (as program directors had feared).[67] This is consistent with the findings from studies looking at the educational impact of the 2003 duty hour reforms.[68]

Interestingly, while one might have expected that residents would be supportive of the duty hour limits, the truth is more complex. In one survey, surgical interns reported decreased continuity of care, fewer hours in the operating room, and no improvement in their quality of life.[69] In a larger survey involving more than 6000 residents, researchers found that nearly half disapproved of the 2011 duty hour changes, a majority felt that they were less prepared to move forward in training, over 70% reported increased handoffs. Only first-year residents reported improved quality of life.[70] Based on these and other studies, some have advocated for a more flexible duty hour approach, and the ACGME endorsed a trial in which some surgical programs were allowed a less restrictive schedule. The resulting study, published in the *New England Journal of Medicine* in 2016, found no change in patient outcomes or resident

Table 16-2   COMPARISON OF THE 2010 ACGME RESIDENT DUTY-HOUR STANDARDS WITH THE 2008 IOM RECOMMENDATIONS AND THE 2003 ACGME REQUIREMENTS*

Standards	2003 ACGME Requirements	Institute of Medicine 2008 Recommendations	2010 ACGME Standards
Maximum hours of work per week	80-hour week, averaged over 4 weeks	No change	No change
Maximum shift length	30 hours (admitting patients up to 24 hours, and then 6 additional hours for transitional and educational activities)	■ 30 hours (admitting patients for up to 16 hours, plus 5-hour protected sleep period between 10 PM and 8 AM with the remaining hours for transition and educational activities) ■ 16 hours with no protected sleep period	■ Duty periods of PGY-1 residents must not exceed 16 hours in duration ■ Intermediate-level and senior residents may be scheduled to a maximum of 24 hours of continuous duty. Strategic napping, especially after 16 hours of continuous duty and between 10 PM and 8 AM, is strongly suggested
Maximum in-hospital on-call frequency	Every third night, on average	Every third night, no averaging	Intermediate-level and senior residents: every third night (no averaging)
Minimum time off between scheduled shifts	10 hours after shift	■ 10 hours after day shift ■ 12 hours after night shift ■ 14 hours after any extended duty period of 30 hours and not return until 6 AM the next day	■ PGY-1 residents should have 10 hours off and must have 8 hours free from duty between scheduled duty periods ■ Intermediate-level residents should have 10 hours off and must have 8 hours between duty periods and 14 hours free from duty after 24 hours of in-hospital duty ■ Residents in the final year of training should have 10 hours free from duty and must have 8 hours between scheduled duty periods
Maximum frequency of in-hospital night shifts	Not addressed	Four nights maximum; 48 hours off after three or four nights of consecutive duty	Residents must not be scheduled for more than six consecutive nights of night duty (night float)

(continued)

Table 16-2	COMPARISON OF THE 2010 ACGME RESIDENT DUTY-HOUR STANDARDS WITH THE 2008 IOM RECOMMENDATIONS AND THE 2003 ACGME REQUIREMENTS* *(continued)*		
Standards	**2003 ACGME Requirements**	**Institute of Medicine 2008 Recommendations**	**2010 ACGME Standards**
Mandatory time off-duty	■ 4 days off per month ■ 1 day (24 hours) off per week, averaged over 4 weeks	■ 5 days off per month ■ 1 day (24 hours) off per week, no averaging ■ One 48-hour period off per month	24 hours off per 7-day period when averaged over 4 weeks; home call cannot be assigned on these free days
Moonlighting	Internal moonlighting is counted against 80-hour weekly limit	■ Internal and external moonlighting is counted against 80-hour weekly limit ■ All other duty-hour limits apply to moonlighting in combination with scheduled work	■ Internal and external moonlighting count against 80-hour weekly limit ■ PGY-1 residents must not be permitted to moonlight, internally or externally
Limit on hours for exceptions	Maximum of 88 hours for individual programs with a sound educational rationale	No change	No change. Before submitting the request to review committee, the program director must obtain permission from the designated institutional official and the graduate medical education committee
Home call	■ Frequency of home call is not subject to the every-third-night, or 24 + 6 limitation ■ Residents on home call must have 1 day in 7 free from all responsibilities, averaged over 4 weeks ■ Hours logged when residents are called into the hospital are counted toward the 80-hour limit	Not addressed	■ Time on home call spent by residents in hospital must count toward the 80-hour maximum weekly limit ■ Frequency of home call is not subject to the every-third-night limitation ■ Residents are permitted to return to the hospital while on home call to care for new or established patients; each episode of this type of care, although it must be included in the 80-hour weekly maximum, will not initiate a new off-duty period

(continued)

Table 16-2	COMPARISON OF THE 2010 ACGME RESIDENT DUTY-HOUR STANDARDS WITH THE 2008 IOM RECOMMENDATIONS AND THE 2003 ACGME REQUIREMENTS* *(continued)*		
Standards	**2003 ACGME Requirements**	**Institute of Medicine 2008 Recommendations**	**2010 ACGME Standards**
Supervision	▪ Programs must ensure that qualified faculty provide appropriate supervision	▪ Residency review committee should establish measurable standards of supervision according to specialty and level of training ▪ Residents in the first year must have immediate access to in-house supervision	▪ Program-specific trainee supervising physician communication guidelines and policies will be required ▪ Faculty assignments to teaching services need to be of sufficient length

*The 2010 standards went into effect July 2011. ACGME, Accreditation Council for Graduation Medical Education; IOM, Institute of Medicine; PGY-1, first-year resident ("intern"). Reproduced with permission from Pastores SM, O'Connor MF, Kleinpell RM, et al. The Accreditation Council for Graduate Medical Education resident duty hour new standards: history, changes, and impact on staffing of intensive care units. *Crit Care Med* 2011;39:2540–2549.

satisfaction between the more flexible and less flexible general surgery residency programs.[71] Based on this trial and other evidence, in 2017 the ACGME announced that it would loosen some of its duty hours restrictions, most prominently the 16-hour limit on PGY-1s.[72]

The debate regarding duty hours, safety, education and resident quality of life is likely to continue, particularly since most other developed countries have duty-hour limits far more stringent than even the most recent 2011 U.S. standards, often in the range of 48 to 60 hours per week.

In discussions regarding duty hours and fatigue, analogies are often made to other industries that have far more severe limits on consecutive work hours. For example, U.S. commercial pilots cannot fly for more than eight hours straight without relief, and truck drivers must pull off the road for a mandatory break after 10 hours. But between these shifts, the machines either sit idle or are operated by another crew. Fumbles may occur in the handoffs of the machines but they are unusual, and no one hands over the reins in the middle of a critical function (such as an airport landing approach). In medicine, on the other hand, handoff errors are routine (Chapter 8). This means that the real patient safety question is not whether fatigued doctors make more mistakes (they probably do), but whether the errors caused by fumbled handoffs and more subtle information seepage will exceed those caused by fatigue.

The 2011 duty hour changes led to shortened shift length for first-year residents, and as a result, the number of patient handoffs has increased significantly, which of course poses increased opportunities for error. However, one prospective study found no impact of the increased discontinuity of care on adverse events.[73] This finding could in part be due to the heightened focus on safer handoffs that has accompanied the new duty hour reforms. (For a more detailed discussion on handoff errors and strategies to mitigate them, see Chapter 8.)

Moreover, a full accounting of the safety impact of duty-hour limits must also weigh the quality of care that physicians deliver *after* they enter full-time practice, and the substantial costs (well into the billions of dollars) to pay for new nonteaching services staffed by hospitalists, nurse practitioners, and physician assistants.[74] Finally, there is another, more subtle risk of the new standards: as the *New England Journal* editor feared, the new rules appear to be leading to a change in culture among some physicians, from a "do whatever it takes" mindset to a "shift work" mentality. Residents themselves remain torn by their understandable desire for more rest and their deeply felt commitment to their patients.[75,76]

Even as we ponder the implications and impact of the duty-hour changes, there can be little debate on one issue: 100-hour workweeks *must* be bad for young doctors (and older ones too, although no one is regulating their hours presently), their loved ones, and ultimately their patients. Because of this, some form of duty-hour limits are welcome, as long as they are accompanied by active efforts to make handoffs safer, to relieve residents of superfluous paperwork, to provide decent rest facilities in hospitals, to hire alternate providers to pick up the slack, and to promote professionalism among trainees. Moreover, these changes must be accompanied by rigorous research to assess both their benefits and harms.

THE "JULY EFFECT"

Though perhaps not as contentious as the debate over duty hours, another potential patient safety risk associated with trainees is the safety of patients cared for by new residents. Dubbed the "July effect" in the United States (since most new residents begin that month) and the more macabre "August killing season" in the United Kingdom,[77,78] the evidence supporting the association between new residents and harm has long been debated. However, a 2011 systematic review of 39 studies by Young et al. found that more methodologically rigorous studies did, in fact, find increased mortality (averaging about 8%) and decreased efficiency (longer lengths of stay).[79] Another retrospective cohort study looked at hospital-acquired conditions (cases of serious harm, including so-called "never events") and found that patient admitted in July were more likely to experience such conditions.[80] The July effect can probably be mitigated by a number of interventions, including improved supervision, a limitation on trainees' workload in the first few weeks, and staggered starting times for new residents, though this has not been proven.[81]

Young and his colleagues have also raised concerns about another trainee-related transition: the year-end handover of outpatients that occurs in teaching settings.[82] Residents typically accrue large ambulatory panels, and then abruptly hand these patients off to new interns at the completion of training. With this handoff, patients experience a vast drop in the experience level of their physicians—both clinical experience and practical knowledge regarding the inner workings of the healthcare organization. Estimates suggest that nearly 13,000 trainees hand their clinic populations off every July, so this handoff affects about 2 million unsuspecting patients. One study surveyed patients about this experience and found that over 40% could not correctly name their new primary care physician.[83]

The solutions to this problem are likely to be similar to those described above, including improved supervision and limited initial schedules. But here, the safety issues surrounding handoffs also assume great importance (Chapter 8). This means that fixes will also involve system changes such as Web-based ambulatory sign-out systems and mandatory discussions between outgoing residents and incoming interns, at least regarding the most active and challenging patients.

NIGHTS AND WEEKENDS

It is self-evident that hospitals are 24-7-365 enterprises, yet few hospitals staff the nights and weekends the way they do daytimes and weekdays. This is not completely without rationale: while the patients don't change, staffing needs partly relate to patients' requirements for transport or the intensity of testing and consultations. If more is being done to and for patients during the day or on weekdays because of the greater availability of personnel and equipment, richer staffing on these shifts may be appropriate.

That said, there are likely to be other explanations for lighter staffing on nights and weekends, relating to caregiver preferences or constrained hospital budgets. Such understaffing could easily put patients at risk on these "off hours." One hospital CEO, Dr. David Shulkin, put it well, after making a series of late-night administrative rounds.[84] "I've come to appreciate the fact that I work in two distinct places," Shulkin observed, a "day hospital" and a "night and weekend hospital." He continued:

> *The weekday hospital has a full administrative team, department chairs and service chiefs, experienced nurse managers, and a full complement of professional staff. The off-hours hospital, on the other*

hand, rarely, if ever, has senior managers present. Nurse-to-patient ratios are significantly lower. Even the number of residents is considerably lower—certainly lower than during my days of training— because of mandated work-hour restrictions.

Empirical data generally support Shulkin's concerns. The majority of studies that have scrutinized the outcomes of care on weekends and nights have documented higher death rates, higher readmission rates, and more surgical complications.[85–89] Moreover, survival rates after in-hospital cardiac arrest are lower, and medical mistakes are more common.[90,91] The evidence regarding the hazards of nights is slightly less robust than that of the weekends, but still of concern.[92,93]

The challenge will be to find the resources to provide adequate staffing on nights and weekends. In areas such as radiology or critical care, telemedicine may provide a partial answer by making physician expertise available without requiring on-site presence. In others, physicians will need to provide in-house coverage. Many hospitals have augmented their weekend and night staffing with a combination of hospitalists and intensivists. Selected groups of patients might benefit from being managed in specialized centers that offer adequate staffing at all times. For example, one study found that while stroke patients fared worse when admitted on weekends to general hospitals, this difference was eliminated when patients were admitted to specialized stroke centers.[94]

Some experts have argued for a more regulatory-based approach, and several states do in fact regulate nurse-to-patient ratios (see earlier discussion); these standards typically do not vary by time of day or day of the week. Ultimately, an integrated approach—including adequate staffing, appropriate oversight of trainees, and thoughtful use of technology, guided by evidence and supported by appropriate transparency and, when needed, regulatory or accreditation standards—will be needed to address the "two hospitals" problem.

"SECOND VICTIMS": SUPPORTING CAREGIVERS AFTER MAJOR ERRORS

While the healthcare system, correctly and understandably, focuses on the patient and family after a serious error, caregivers also require empathy and attention. In a 2000 article, Albert Wu of Johns Hopkins coined the term "second victim" to describe how caregivers themselves are affected after they commit an error.[95] In a 2011 interview, he expanded on this concept:

I think that there are two ways that healthcare workers are traumatized. The first are things we do to ourselves; these are self-inflicted wounds that result from internalized judgments .... we feel anxious, depressed, and demoralized. On the other hand, some healthcare workers are actively victimized by elements of the system or by other organizations. Those are people who work in places that still believe in shame-and-blame or crime-and-punishment, and they're sometimes official bodies like nursing boards and so forth. They actually punish people and, I think, add insult to those self-inflicted injuries …. Some people have persistent problems—the incidents go on to cause lasting harm. Some people are so depressed that they need to be hospitalized; some people are suicidal. People quit medicine or nursing because of what they did …. In our hospital … a boy with head trauma came in and was badly injured. He needed to be intubated, could not be intubated and could not be trached, and died in the emergency room. It was just a horrific incident and everyone felt unimaginably bad. But even though the emergency physician got some support, others were a little critical of his actions, and he quit clinical medicine within the year.[96]

Addressing the second victim issue is not easy. Colin West of the Mayo Clinic suggests that an opportunity be given to the caregiver to process the error, such as in an informal small group or a traditional M&M conference.[97–99] The Schwartz Center for Compassionate Healthcare has developed an approach called "Schwartz Rounds," which provides a space for caregivers to participate in a guided discussion focusing on the emotional and psychosocial aspects of patient care. Data from participating institutions suggests that these rounds enhance provider support.[100] Whichever forum is chosen, it is critical that participants model the importance of error acknowledgment and open discussion. Emotional support provided by a trusted colleague or a professional counselor is also helpful.

While such counseling can be obtained informally after an error, too often it is not, leaving caregivers to suffer in silence.[101,102] Because of this, some institutions have developed programs designed to sensitize all staff to the issues of second victims, including understanding that errors happen to every clinician and that perfection is not an attainable goal. Such educational programs should arm clinicians with coping strategies, and caution against maladaptive strategies that are often employed.

A few programs go even further. One of the most advanced is the second victim support team (the *forYOU Team*) developed by Susan Scott and colleagues at the University of Missouri.[103,104] Based on interviews with clinicians after adverse events, the Missouri investigators identified six stages in the second victim recovery process: (i) chaos and accident response, (ii) intrusive reflections, (iii) restoring personal integrity, (iv) enduring the inquisition, (v) obtaining emotional first aid, and (vi) moving on.[105] To support caregivers through these stages, after a serious adverse event a trained supervisor or peer is immediately dispatched to offer support (such trained individuals are embedded on every high-risk service). The goal is to prevent clinicians from going home before they receive initial counseling. From there, referrals are made for additional support. Any investigation of the incident (including a root cause analysis if appropriate) is conducted by different individuals than those on the support teams.

A few other institutions have instituted similar programs.[106-109] Early responses from clinicians to these programs are positive and the programs clearly fill an important gap. However, additional research is needed to determine the optimal structure, financing, and timing of second victim programs, and how to ensure that caregivers receive needed support while also allowing for rapid and effective incident investigations and responses (Chapter 14).

KEY POINTS

- Increasing attention is being paid to the importance of a well-trained, well-rested workforce to patient safety.
- In nursing, good studies have linked longer work hours, lower nurse-to-patient ratios, and higher patient turnover to poor outcomes.
- Many hospitals have organized specialized teams of caregivers available to respond to unexpected patient deteriorations (rapid response teams, RRTs). While the concept has face validity, studies of this strategy have yielded mixed results.
- Although research has linked long hours and fatigue in physicians to errors, it has not yet led to widespread efforts to regulate physician staffing. The exception is in residency training programs, where regulations now limit weekly hours and shift lengths. These limits (particularly the 80-hour work week) have improved resident well-being, but the impact on safety or education is less certain. Because of the surprising lack of evidence of benefit, the prohibition on overnight stays by interns was recently lifted.
- Attention is turning to the safety hazards of hospital care on nights and weekends, and to the risk of receiving care early in the training year in teaching hospitals.
- Clinicians involved in serious errors are often deeply affected by the experience. Several programs designed to support such "second victims" have been launched.

REFERENCES

1. Aiken LH, Clarke SP, Sloane DM, Sochalski J, Silber JH. Hospital nurse staffing and patient mortality, nurse burnout, and job dissatisfaction. *JAMA* 2002;288:1987–1993.

2. Aiken LH, Clarke SP, Cheung RB, Sloane DM, Silber JH. Educational levels of hospital nurses and surgical patient mortality. *JAMA* 2003;290:1617–1623.

3. Rogers AE, Hwang WT, Scott LD, Aiken LH, Dinges DF. The working hours of hospital staff nurses and patient safety. *Health Aff (Millwood)* 2004;23:202–212.

4. Needleman J, Buerhaus P, Pankratz VS, Leibson CL, Stevens SR, Harris M. Nurse staffing and inpatient hospital mortality. *N Engl J Med* 2011;364:1037–1045.

5. Aiken LH, Cimiotti JP, Sloane DM, Smith HL, Flynn L, Neff DF. Effects of nurse staffing and nurse education on patient deaths in hospitals with different nurse work environments. *Med Care* 2011;49:1047–1053.

6. Cimiotti JP, Aiken LH, Sloane DM, Wu ES. Nurse staffing, burnout, and health care-associated infection. *Am J Infect Control* 2012;40:486–490.

7. Aiken LH, Sloane DM, Bruyneel L, et al. Nurse staffing and education and hospital mortality in nine European countries: a retrospective observational study. *Lancet* 2014;383:1824–1830.

8. Dabney BW, Kalisch BJ. Nurse staffing levels and patient-reported missed nursing care. *J Nurs Care Qual* 2015;30:306–312.

9. Shekelle PG. Nurse-patient ratios as a patient safety strategy: a systematic review. *Ann Intern Med* 2013;158:404–409.

10. Juraschek SP, Zhang X, Ranganathan V, Lin VW. United States registered nurse workforce report card and shortage forecast. *Am J Med Qual* 2012;27:241–249.

11. Rosenstein AH, O'Daniel M. Disruptive behavior and clinical outcomes: perceptions of nurses and physicians. *Am J Nurs* 2005;105:54–64; [quiz 64–65].

12. Rosenstein AH, O'Daniel M. Impact and implications of disruptive behavior in the perioperative arena. *J Am Coll Surg* 2006;203:96–105.

13. Walrath JM, Dang D, Nyberg D. Hospital RNs' experiences with disruptive behavior: a qualitative study. *J Nurs Care Qual* 2010;25:105–116.

14. Laschinger HK. Impact of workplace mistreatment on patient safety risk and nurse-assessed patient outcomes. *J Nurs Adm* 2014;44:284–290.

15. Leape LL, Fromson JA. Problem doctors: is there a system-level solution? *Ann Intern Med* 2006;144:107–115.

16. The Joint Commission. Sentinel event alert. *Behaviors That Undermine a Culture of Safety.* July 9, 2008;(40):1–3.

17. Rich V. Nurse staffing ratios: the crucible of money, policy, research, and patient care. *AHRQ WebM&M* (serial online); August 2009. Available at: http://webmm.ahrq.gov/case.aspx?caseid=203.

18. Ball JE, Murrells T, Rafferty AM, Morrow E, Griffiths P. 'Care left undone' during nursing shifts: associations with workload and perceived quality of care. *BMJ Qual Saf* 2014;23:116–125.

19. Needleman J, Kurtzman ET, Kizer KW. Performance measurement of nursing care: state of the science and the current consensus. *Med Care Res Rev* 2007;64:10S–43S.

20. Kurtzman ET, O'Leary D, Sheingold BH, Devers KJ, Dawson EM, Johnson JE. Performance-based payment incentives increase burden and blame for hospital nurses. *Health Aff (Millwood)* 2011;30:211–218.

21. Kutney-Lee A, Stimpfel AW, Sloane DM, Cimiotti JP, Quinn LW, Aiken LH. Changes in patient and nurse outcomes associated with magnet hospital recognition. *Med Care* 2015;53:550–557.

22. Johnston M, Arora S, King D, Stroman L, Darzi A. Escalation of care and failure to rescue: a multicenter, multiprofessional qualitative study. *Surgery* 2014;155:989–994.

23. Taenzer AH, Pyke JB, McGrath SP. A review of current and emerging approaches to address failure-to-rescue. *Anesthesiology* 2011;115:421–431.

24. Jones DA, DeVita MA, Bellomo R. Rapid-response teams. *N Engl J Med* 2011;365:139–146.

25. Berwick DM, Calkins DR, McCannon CJ, Hackbarth AD. The 100,000 Lives Campaign: setting a goal and a deadline for improving health care quality. *JAMA* 2006;295:324–327.

26. Wachter RM, Pronovost PJ. The 100,000 Lives Campaign: a scientific and policy review. *Jt Comm J Qual Patient Saf* 2006;32:621–627.

27. Bellomo R, Goldsmith D, Uchino S, et al. A prospective before-and-after trial of a medical emergency team. *Med J Aust* 2003;179:283–287.

28. Sebat F, Musthafa AA, Johnson D, et al. Effect of a rapid response system for patients in shock on time to treatment and mortality during 5 years. *Crit Care Med* 2007;35:2568–2575.

29. Sharek PJ, Parast LM, Leong K, et al. Effect of a rapid response team on hospital-wide mortality and code rates outside the ICU in a children's hospital. *JAMA* 2007;298:2267–2274.

30. Hillman K, Chen J, Cretikos M, et al. Introduction of the medical emergency team (MET) system: a cluster-randomised controlled trial. *Lancet* 2005;365:2091–2097.

31. Chan PS, Jain R, Nallmothu BK, Berg RA, Sasson C. Rapid response teams: a systematic review and meta-analysis. *Arch Intern Med* 2010;170:18–26.

32. McGaughey J, Alderdice F, Fowler R, Kapila A, Mayhew A, Moutray M. Outreach and early warning systems (EWS) for the prevention of intensive care admission and death of critically ill adult patients on general hospital wards. *Cochrane Database Syst Rev* 2007;(3):CD005529–CD005529.

33. Maharaj R, Raffaele I, Wendon J. Rapid response systems: a systematic review and meta-analysis. *Crit Care* 2015;19:524.

34. Barwise A, Thongprayoon C, Gajic O, Jensen J, Herasevich V, Pickering BW. Delayed rapid response team activation is associated with increased hospital mortality, morbidity, and length of stay in a tertiary care institution. *Crit Care Med* 2016;44:54–63.

35. Ludikhuize J, Brunsveld-Reinders AH, Dijkgraaf MG, et al. Outcomes associated with the nationwide introduction of rapid response systems in the Netherlands. *Crit Care Med* 2015;43:2544–2551.

36. Vorwerk J, King L. Consumer participation in early detection of the deteriorating patient and call activation to rapid response systems: a literature review. *J Clin Nurs* 2016;25:38–52.

37. Stolldorf DP, Jones CB. Deployment of rapid response teams by 31 hospitals in a statewide collaborative. *J Qual Patient Saf* 2015;41:186–192.

38. Shapiro SE, Donaldson NE, Scott MB. Rapid response teams seen through the eyes of the nurse. *Am J Nurs* 2010;110:28–34.

39. The Joint Commission. *2009 National Patient Safety Goals*. Available at: http://www.jointcommission.org/standards_information/npsgs.aspx.

40. Bonafide CP, Localio AR, Song L, et al. Cost-benefit analysis of a medical emergency team in a children's hospital. *Pediatrics* 2014;134;235–241.

41. Winters BD, Pham J, Pronovost PJ. Rapid response teams—walk, don't run. *JAMA* 2006;296:1645–1647.

42. Auerbach AD, Landefeld CS, Shojania KG. The tension between needing to improve care and knowing how to do it. *N Engl J Med* 2007;357:608–613.

43. Berwick DM. The science of improvement. *JAMA* 2008;299:1182–1184.

44. Govindarajan A, Urbach DR, Kumar M, et al. Outcomes of daytime procedures performed by attending surgeons after night work. *N Engl J Med* 2015;373:845–853.

45. Drazen JM, Epstein AM. Rethinking medical training—the critical work ahead. *N Engl J Med* 2002;347:1271–1272.

46. Goitein L, Shanafelt TD, Wipf JE, Slatore CG, Back AL. The effects of work-hour limitations on resident well-being, patient care, and education in an internal medicine residency program. *Arch Intern Med* 2005;165:2601–2606.

47. Lockley SW, Landrigan CP, Barger LK, Czeisler CA; Harvard Work Hours Health and Safety Group. When policy meets physiology: the challenge of reducing resident work hours. *Clin Orthop Relat Res* 2006;449:116–127.

48. Hutter MM, Kellogg KC, Ferguson CM, Abbott WM, Warshaw AL. The impact of the 80-hour resident workweek on surgical residents and attending surgeons. *Ann Surg* 2006;243:864–871; [discussion 871–875].

49. Antiel RM, Thompson SM, Reed DA, et al. ACGME duty-hour recommendations—a national survey of residency program directors. *N Engl J Med* 2010;363:e12.

50. Dawson D, Reid K. Fatigue, alcohol and performance impairment. *Nature* 1997;388:235.

51. Linde L, Bergstrom M. The effect of one night without sleep on problem-solving and immediate recall. *Psychol Res* 1992;54:127–136.

52. McCormick F, Kadzielski J, Landrigan CP, Evans B, Herndon JH, Rubash HE. Surgeon fatigue: a prospective analysis of the incidence, risk and intervals of predicted fatigue-related impairment in residents. *Arch Surg* 2012;147:430–435.

53. Gordon JA, Alexander EK, Lockley SW, et al.; Harvard Work Hours, Health, and Safety Group (Boston, Massachusetts). Does simulator-based clinical performance correlate with actual hospital behavior? The effect of extended work hours on patient care provided by medical interns. *Acad Med* 2010;85:1583–1588.

54. Veasey S, Rosen R, Barzansky B, Rosen I, Owens J. Sleep loss and fatigue in residency training: a reappraisal. *JAMA* 2002;288:1116–1124.

55. Pastores SM, O'Connor MF, Kleinpell RM, et al. The Accreditation Council for Graduate Medical Education resident duty hour new standards: history, changes, and impact on staffing of intensive care units. *Crit Care Med* 2011;39:2540–2549.

56. Shetty KD, Bhattacharya J. Changes in hospital mortality associated with residency work-hour regulations. *Ann Intern Med* 2007;147:73–80.

57. Horwitz LI, Kosiborod M, Lin Z, Krumholz HM. Changes in outcomes for internal medicine inpatients after work-hour regulations. *Ann Intern Med* 2007;147:97–103.

58. Moonesinghe SR, Lowery J, Shahi N, Millen A, Beard JD. Impact of reduction in working hours for doctors in training on postgraduate medical education and patients' outcomes: systematic review. *BMJ* 2011;342:d1580.

59. Drolet BC, Spalluto LB, Fischer SA. Residents' perspectives on ACGME regulation of supervision and duty hours—a national survey. *N Engl J Med* 2010;363:e34.

60. Landrigan CP, Rothschild JM, Cronin JW, et al. Effect of reducing interns' work hours on serious medical errors in intensive care units. *N Engl J Med* 2004;351: 1838–1848.

61. Ulmer C, Wolman DM, Johns MME, eds. Committee on Optimizing Graduate Medical Trainee (Resident) Hours and Work Schedule to Improve Patient Safety. *Resident Duty Hours: Enhancing Sleep, Supervision, and Safety. Institute of Medicine*. Washington, DC: National Academies Press; 2008.

62. Iglehart JK. The ACGME's final duty-hour standards—special PGY-1 limits and strategic napping. *N Engl J Med* 2010;363:1589–1591.

63. Scally CP, Ryan AM, Thumma JR, Gauger PG, Dimick JB. Early impact of the 2011 ACGME duty hour regulations on surgical outcomes. *Surgery* 2015;158: 1453–1461.

64. Block L, Jarlenski M, Wu AW, et al. Inpatient safety outcomes following the 2011 residency work-hour reform. *J Hosp Med* 2014;9:347–352.

65. Parshuram CS, Amaral AC, Ferguson ND, et al. Patient safety, resident well-being and continuity of care with different resident duty schedules in the intensive care unit: a randomized trial. *CMAJ* 2015;187:321–329.

66. Patel MS, Volpp KG, Small DS, et al. Association of the 2011 ACGME resident duty hour reforms with mortality and readmissions among hospitalized Medicare patients. *JAMA* 2014;312:2364–2373.

67. Rajaram R, Chung JW, Jones AT, et al. Association of the 2011 ACGME resident duty hour reform with general surgery patient outcomes and with resident examination performance. *JAMA* 2014;312:2374–2384.

68. Jena AB, Schoemaker L, Bhattacharya J. Exposing physicians to reduced residency work hours did not adversely affect patient outcomes after residency. *Health Aff (Millwood)* 2014;33:1832–1840.

69. Antiel RM, Reed DA, Van Arendonk KJ, et al. Effect of duty hour restrictions on core competencies, education, quality of life, and burnout among general surgery interns. *JAMA Surg* 2013;148:448–455.

70. Drolet BC, Christopher DA, Fischer SA. Residents' response to duty-hour regulations—a follow-up national survey. *N Engl J Med* 2012;366:e35.

71. Bilimoria KY, Chung JW, Hedges LV, et al. National cluster-randomized trial of duty-hour flexibility in surgical training. *N Engl J Med* 2016;374:713–727.

72. Lowes R. ACGME won't extend resident shifts in 2016-2017. *Medscape Medical News* May 23, 2016. Available at: http://www.medscape.com/viewarticle/863642.

73. Fletcher KE, Singh S, Schapira MM, et al. Inpatient housestaff discontinuity of care and patient adverse events. *Am J Med* 2016;129:341–347.

74. Nuckols TK, Escarce JJ. Cost implications of ACGME's 2011 changes to resident duty hours and the training environment. *J Gen Intern Med* 2012;27:241–249.

75. Landrigan CP, Barger LK, Cade BE, Ayas NT, Czeisler CA. Interns' compliance with Accreditation Council for Graduate Medical Education work-hour limits. *JAMA* 2006;296:1063–1070.

76. Carpenter RO, Spooner J, Arbogast PG, Tarpley JL, Griffin MR, Lomis KD. Work hours restrictions as an ethical dilemma for residents: a descriptive survey of violation types and frequency. *Curr Surg* 2006;63:448–455.

77. Vaughan L, McAlister G, Bell D. 'August is always a nightmare': results of the Royal College of Physicians of Edinburgh and Society of Acute Medicine August transition survey. *Clin Med* 2011;11:322–326.

78. Levy K, Voit J, Gupta A, Petrilli CM, Chopra V. Examining the July Effect: a national survey of academic leaders in medicine. *Am J Med* 2016;129:754.e1–754.e5.

79. Young JQ, Ranji SR, Wachter RM, Lee CM, Niehaus B, Auerbach AD. "July Effect": impact of the academic year-end changeover on patient outcomes. A systematic review. *Ann Intern Med* 2011;155:309–315.

80. Wen T, Attenello FJ, Wu B, Ng A, Cen SY, Mack WJ. The July effect: an analysis of never events in the nationwide inpatient sample. *J Hosp Med* 2015;10:432–438.

81. Petrilli CM, Del Valle J, Chopra V. Why July matters. *Acad Med* 2016;91:910–912.

82. Young JQ, Wachter RM. Academic year-end transfers of outpatients from outgoing to incoming residents: an unaddressed patient safety issue. *JAMA* 2009;302:1327–1329.

83. Pincavage AT, Lee WW, Beiting KJ, Arora VM. What do patients think about year-end resident continuity clinic handoffs? A qualitative study. *J Gen Intern Med* 2013;28:999–1007.

84. Shulkin DJ. Like night and day—shedding light on off-hours care. *N Engl J Med* 2008;358:2091–2093.

85. Ricciardi R, Nelson J, Francone TD, et al. Do patient safety indicators explain increased weekend mortality? *J Surg Res* 2016;200:164–170.

86. Attenello FJ, Wen T, Cen SY, et al. Incidence of "never events" among weekend admissions versus weekday admissions to US hospitals: national analysis. *BMJ* 2015;350:h1460.

87. Aylin P, Yunus A, Bottle A, Majeed A, Bell D. Weekend mortality for emergency admissions. A large, multicentre study. *Qual Saf Health Care* 2010;19:213–217.

88. Kostis WJ, Demissie K, Marcella SW, Shao YH, Wilson AC, Moreyra AE; Myocardial Infarction Data Acquisition System (MIDAS 10) Study Group. Weekend versus weekday admission and mortality from myocardial infarction. *N Engl J Med* 2007;356:1099–1109.

89. Goldstein SD, Papandria DJ, Aboagye J, et al. The "weekend effect" in pediatric surgery—increased mortality for children undergoing urgent surgery during the weekend. *J Pediatric Surg* 2014;49:1087–1091.

90. Peberdy MA, Ornato JP, Larkin GL, et al.; for National Registry of Cardiopulmonary Resuscitation Investigators. Survival from in-hospital cardiac arrest during nights and weekends. *JAMA* 2008;299:785–792.

91. Hendey GW, Barth BE, Soliz T. Overnight and postcall errors in medication orders. *Acad Emerg Med* 2005;12:629–634.

92. Cavallazzi R, Marik PE, Hirani A, Pachinburavan M, Vasu TS, Leiby BE. Association between time of admission to the ICU and mortality: a systematic review and meta-analysis. *Chest* 2010;138:68–75.

93. Mourad M, Adler J. Safe, high quality care around the clock: what will it take to get us there? *J Gen Intern Med* 2011;26:948–950.

94. McKinney JS, Deng Y, Kasner SE, Kostis JB. Myocardial Infarction Data Acquisition System (MIDAS 15) Study Group. Comprehensive stroke centers overcome the weekend versus weekday gap in stroke treatment and mortality. *Stroke* 2011;42:2403–2409.

95. Wu AW. Medical error: the second victim. *BMJ* 2000;320:726–727.

96. In conversation with … Albert Wu, MD, MPH [Perspective]. *AHRQ PSNet* (serial online); May 2011. Available at: https://psnet.ahrq.gov/perspectives/perspective/61.

97. West CP, Huschka MM, Novotny PJ, et al. Association of perceived medical errors with resident distress and empathy: a prospective longitudinal study. *JAMA* 2006;296:1071–1078.

98. West CP. How do providers recover from errors? *AHRQ WebM&M* (serial online); January 2008. Available at: http://webmm.ahrq.gov/case.aspx?caseID=167.

99. Orlander JD, Barber TW, Fincke BG. The morbidity and mortality conference: the delicate nature of learning from error. *Acad Med* 2002;77:1001–1006.

100. Lown BA, Manning CF. The Schwartz Center Rounds: an evaluation of an interdisciplinary approach to enhancing patient-centered communication, teamwork, and provider support. *Acad Med* 2010;85:1073–1081.

101. Ullström S, Sachs MA, Hansson J, Øvretveit J, Brommels M. Suffering in silence: a qualitative study of second victims of adverse event. *BMJ Qual Saf* 2014;23:324–331.

102. Joesten L, Cipparrone N, Okuno-Jones S, DuBose ER. Assessing the perceived level of institutional support for the second victim after a patient safety event. *J Patient Saf* 2015;11:73–78.

103. Scott SD, Hirschinger LE, Cox KR, et al. Caring for our own: deployment of a second victim rapid response system. *Jt Comm J Qual Patient Saf* 2010;36:233–240.

104. Scott SD. The second victim phenomenon: a harsh reality of health care professions. *AHRQ WebM&M* (serial online); May 2011. Available at: http://webmm.ahrq.gov/perspective.aspx?perspectiveID=102.

105. Scott SD, Hirschinger LE, Cox KR, McCoig M, Brandt J, Hall LW. The natural history of recovery for the health care provider "second victim" after adverse patient events. *Qual Saf Health Care* 2009;18:325–330.

106. Shapiro J, Galowitz P. Peer support for clinicians: a programmatic approach. *Acad Med* 2016;91:1200–1204.

107. Shapiro J, Whittemore A, Tsen LC. Instituting a culture of professionalism: the establishment of a Center for Professionalism and Peer Support. *Jt Comm J Qual Patient Saf* 2014;40:168–177.

108. McDonald TB, Helmchen LA, Smith KM, et al. Responding to patient safety incidents: the "seven pillars". *Qual Saf Health Care* 2010;19:e11.

109. Edrees H, Connors C, Paine L, Norvell M, Taylor H, Wu AW. Implementing the RISE second victim support programme at the Johns Hopkins Hospital: a case study. *BMJ Open* 2016;6:e011708.

ADDITIONAL READINGS

Ahmed N, Devitt KS, Keshet I, et al. A systematic review of the effects of resident duty hour restrictions in surgery: impact on resident wellness, training, and patient outcomes. *Ann Surg* 2014;259:1041–1053.

Chen PW. The impossible workload for doctors in training. *New York Times*. April 18, 2013.

Christensen JF, Levinson W, Dunn PM. The heart of darkness: the impact of perceived mistakes on physicians. *J Gen Intern Med* 1992;7:424–431.

IOM (Institute of Medicine). *The Future of Nursing: Leading Change, Advancing Health.* Washington, DC: National Academies Press; 2011.

Jena AB, Prasad V. Duty hour reform in a shifting medical landscape. *J Gen Intern Med* 2013;28:1238–1240.

Rothschild JM, Gandara E, Woolf S, Williams DH, Bates DW. Single-parameter early warning criteria to predict life-threatening adverse events. *J Patient Saf* 2010;6:97–101.

Sanghavi D. The Phantom Menace of Sleep-Deprived Doctors. *New York Times Magazine*. August 5, 2011.

Sen S, Kranzler HR, Didwania AK, et al. Effects of the 2011 duty hour reforms on interns and their patients: a prospective longitudinal cohort study. *JAMA Intern Med* 2013;173:657–662.

West CP, Shanafelt TD, Kolars JC. Quality of life, burnout, educational debt, and medical knowledge among internal medicine residents. *JAMA* 2011;306:952–960.

EDUCATION AND TRAINING ISSUES | 17

OVERVIEW

Medicine has a unique problem when it comes to its trainees. Although all fields must allow trainees some opportunity to "practice" their craft before being granted a credential allowing them to work without supervision, legal, accounting, or architectural errors made by trainees generally have fewer consequences than medical errors do.

Moreover, the demands of medical practice (particularly the need for around-the-clock and weekend coverage; Chapter 16) have led to the use of trainees as cheap labor, placing them in situations in which the supervision provided is sometimes not sufficient given their skill level and experience. Although this early independence has been justified pedagogically as the need to allow "trainees to learn from their mistakes" and hone their clinical instincts, in truth much of it flowed from economic imperatives.

Yet the solution is not obvious. One can envision a training environment in which patients are protected from trainees—after all, who would *not* want the senior surgeon, rather than the second-year resident, performing his or her cholecystectomy? While such an environment might be safer initially, the downstream result would be more poorly trained physicians who lack the real-world, supervised experience needed to transform them from novices into experienced professionals. The problem would be similar for nurses and other caregivers.

These two fundamental tensions form the backdrop of any discussion of training issues in the context of patient safety. First, what is the appropriate balance between autonomy and supervision? Second, are there ways for trainees to traverse their learning curves more quickly without necessarily "learning from their mistakes" on real patients? This chapter will address these issues, closing with a short discussion about teaching patient safety. Other important training-related issues, such as teamwork training and duty-hour restrictions for residents, are covered elsewhere (Chapters 15 and 16, respectively).

AUTONOMY VERSUS OVERSIGHT

The third-year medical student was sent in to "preround" on a patient, a 71-year-old man who had undergone a hip replacement a few days earlier. The patient complained of new shortness of breath, and on exam was anxious and perspiring, with rapid, shallow respirations. The student, on his first clinical rotation, listened to the man's lungs, expecting to hear the crackles of pulmonary edema or pneumonia or perhaps the wheezes of asthma, yet they were clear as a bell.

The student was confused, and asked the patient what he thought was going on. "It's really hot in here, doc," said the patient, and, in fact, it was. The student reassured himself that the patient was just overheated, and resolved to discuss the case later that morning with his supervising resident. In his mind, calling the resident now would be both embarrassing and unnecessary—he had a good explanation for the patient's condition. An hour later, the patient was dead of a massive pulmonary embolism. The student never told anyone of his observations that morning, and felt shame about the case for decades afterwards.

In his terrific book, *Complications*, Harvard surgeon Atul Gawande describes the fundamental paradox of medical training:

In medicine, we have long faced a conflict between the imperative to give patients the best possible care and the need to provide novices with experience. Residencies attempt to mitigate potential harm through supervision and graduated responsibility.... But there is still no getting around those first few unsteady times a young physician tries to put in a central line, remove a breast cancer, or sew together two segments of colon. No matter how many protections we put in place, on average, these cases go less well with the novice than with someone experienced.

This is the uncomfortable truth about teaching. By traditional ethics and public insistence (not to mention court rulings), a patient's right to the best care possible must trump the objective of training

novices. We want perfection without practice. Yet everyone is harmed
if no one is trained for the future. So learning is hidden behind drapes
and anesthesia and the elisions of language.[1]

Traditionally, supervisors in medicine erred on the side of autonomy, in the belief that trainees needed to learn by doing—giving rise to the iconic mantra of medical training, "see one, do one, teach one." We now recognize this paradigm as being both ethically troubling and one more slice of the proverbial Swiss cheese, a constant threat to patient safety (Chapter 2).

Supervising physicians (the issue of supervision is also relevant to the training experience of other health professionals such as nurses, but the autonomy that novices in other fields can exercise and the potential for harm seem less than those of physicians) are terribly conflicted about all this.[2] Supervisors know that they could do many things better and more safely, but also recognize that trainees truly do need to learn by doing. Moreover, providing the degree of supervision necessary to ensure that trainees never get into trouble would create job descriptions for supervising attendings that might not be compatible with career longevity.

It is a scale that has, at one extreme, supervising physicians doing everything while trainees watch, and, at the other, trainees doing everything and calling their supervisors only when they are in trouble; until fairly recently most medical training systems were far too tilted toward autonomy. Prodded by some widely publicized cases of medical error that were due, at least in part, to inadequate supervision (the death of Libby Zion at New York Hospital in 1986 was the most vivid example[3]; Table 1-1), the traditional model of medical education—dominated by unfettered resident autonomy—is giving way to something safer. (As a side note, while the Libby Zion case is popularly attributed to long resident hours, the chair of the commission that investigated the case [Dr. Bertrand Bell] clearly saw the root cause more as inadequate supervision than sleepy residents.[4]) We now recognize that "learning from mistakes" is fundamentally unethical when it is built into the system, and that it is unreasonable to assume trainees will even know when they need help, particularly if they are thrust into the clinical arena with little or no practice and supervision.[5]

Our new appreciation of these issues has led not only to some system reforms (including the increased supervision requirements enacted by the Accreditation Council on Graduate Medical Education in 2011[6]; Table 16-2) but also to a crack in the dike of academic medical culture. For example, many attendings now stay late with their teams on admitting nights, a practice that would have been judged pathologically obsessive only 20 years ago (during the medical school days of the senior author

(RMW), one such attending picked up a nickname among the house staff of "the world's oldest intern").

In addition, the old culture of the "strong resident" or "strong student" (translated: one who never bothers or seems to need the supervising attending) is changing. Growing numbers of programs are building in expectations of oversight and creating structures to support it. For instance, around-the-clock attending presence (often with hospitalists and intensivists) to supervise trainees at night is increasingly common, although the impact on patient outcomes is not clear. One randomized trial concluded that staffing the ICU of an academic medical center at night with an in-hospital intensivist did not improve patient outcomes.[7] On the other hand, a recent systematic review concluded that there is good evidence that supervision is associated with safer surgery and invasive procedures.[8] Even here, though, the data are less clear-cut when it comes to emergency room or medical patients.[9,10]

At UCSF Medical Center, we now have hospitalists stay overnight with our residents. In addition to managing some patients independently, these faculty members supervise residents' care of critically ill patients and are available to help with more stable patients. Faculty who take on these "nocturnist" roles are advised that they should always ask the resident, "What would you be doing if I wasn't here?" before offering recommendations. These supervising physicians are also asked to emphasize to the residents that a call for help is a sign of strength and professionalism, not weakness.[11]

Ensuring appropriate communication is partly a cultural problem, but it also needs a scaffolding of thoughtfully developed guidelines. After analyzing a series of malpractice cases, the chiefs of surgical services at Harvard, working with the Harvard Risk Management Foundation, identified a series of "triggers" that should prompt direct communication between residents and attendings (Table 17-1).[12] A study at four of Harvard's teaching hospitals showed that, in one-third of cases, attendings were not notified after such trigger events.[13] The guidelines were subsequently codified, with promising results.[14]

Oversight is not a monolithic construct. Supervisors must modulate their degree of oversight based on their comfort with the trainee's level and demonstrated competency with the task at hand. After over 200 hours of ethnographic observation, as well as interviews with emergency department and general medicine teams, Kennedy et al. documented four types of oversight, each of which might be appropriate in different situations (Table 17-2).[15]

The challenge going forward will be to find the very narrow sweet spot between unfettered trainee autonomy and stifling attending oversight, varying the level of supervision to ensure patient safety while also permitting the

Table 17-1 EXPECTED COMMUNICATION PRACTICES FOR PATIENTS ADMITTED TO SURGICAL SERVICES OF HARVARD TEACHING HOSPITALS

1. **For all critical changes in a patient's condition, the attending will be notified promptly (generally within one hour following evaluation). These include:**
   - Admission to the hospital
   - Transfer to the intensive care unit (ICU)
   - Unplanned intubation or ventilatory support
   - Cardiac arrest
   - Hemodynamic instability (including arrhythmias)
   - Code blue
   - Development of significant neurological changes (suspected cerebrovascular accident/seizure/new-onset paralysis)
   - Development of major wound complications (dehiscence, evisceration)
   - Medication or treatment errors requiring clinical intervention (invasive procedure(s), increased monitoring, new medications except Narcan)
   - First blood transfusion without prior attending knowledge or instruction (before or after operation)
   - Development of any clinical problem requiring an invasive procedure or operation for treatment

2. **The following will be discussed with and approved by the attending before they occur:**
   - Discharge from the hospital or from the emergency department
   - Transfer out of ICU

3. **The attending should also be contacted if:**
   - Any trainee feels that a situation is more complicated than he or she can manage
   - Nursing or physician staff, or the patient, request that the attending surgeon be contacted

Reproduced with permission from ElBardissi AW, Regenbogen SE, Greenberg CC, et al. Communication practices on 4 Harvard surgical services. *Ann Surg* 2009;250:861–865.

graded independence that trainees need to become independent practitioners.[16,17] Thankfully, we are now much closer to finding the correct balance than we were even a decade ago.

We appreciate the importance of this issue in a very personal way. Both of us can cite examples that illustrate the tension between autonomy and oversight, and one of us (RMW) was the third-year medical student who missed the fatal pulmonary embolism in the case that began this section.[17]

Table 17-2	FOUR THEMES DRAWN FROM OBSERVING THE OVERSIGHT ACTIVITIES OF SUPERVISORS	
Theme	**Definition**	**Representative Transcript Excerpt**
Routine oversight	Clinical oversight activities that are planned in advance	"… each patient is always reviewed with the attending" (*a junior ED resident*) "At the end of the day we go over all the patients with either the senior resident or staff at some point, so we kind of go through what we have been doing so far … this happens on a daily basis" (*a junior general medicine resident*)
Responsive oversight	Clinical oversight activities that occur in response to trainee- or patient-specific issues (requested or not)	"I can recall working with a junior resident and, um, she had taken a history and there were a couple of things that were very important to confirm because it would affect your management, so I went back in and asked the patient the same questions. (I was) double-checking; I knew that she had asked them, she said she had asked them, but I needed to hear it myself to be sure" (*an ED attending physician*)
Direct patient care	Refers to instances when a supervisor moves beyond oversight to actively provide care for a trainee's patient	"If their patient is crashing I usually go there myself and do the acute management and I bring the clerk with me and I try to teach them how to observe …" (*a senior general medicine resident*)
Backstage oversight	Clinical oversight activities of which the trainee is not directly aware	"I go back to check the patients post-call when the students are not there" (*a general medicine attending physician*) "I read the nursing notes and I hear the nurses talking and so I know kind of what is going on. So in my mind I already have a picture of the patient" (*an ED attending physician*)

Reproduced with permission from Kennedy TJ, Lingard L, Baker GR, Kitchen L, Regehr G. Clinical oversight: conceptualizing the relationship between supervision and safety. *J Gen Intern Med* 2007;22:1080–1085.

SIMULATION TRAINING

Although many discussions about medical simulation emphasize the ability of simulators to create realistic situations in which participants "suspend disbelief" (including supporting role plays that focus on teamwork and communication skills; Chapter 15), another key use of simulation is to allow individuals to traverse their procedural learning curves without harming patients. Even if we tested for procedural aptitude, like the military, novices' first few operations or procedures would still be hazardous to patients' health. Recognizing this, new surgeons traditionally work under the close supervision of a veteran—but not for very long. The adage of "see one, do one, teach one" is not much of an exaggeration: after a couple of years' training, apprentice surgeons or other proceduralists are largely on their own for all but the most complex cases.

The problem does not end once formal training is completed. After the completion of residency or fellowship, practicing surgeons and other interventionalists are essentially left to their own devices to acquire new skills or keep up with the latest techniques. In *Complications*, Gawande writes that his father, a senior urologist in private practice, once estimated that three-quarters of the procedures he performed routinely did not exist when he was trained.[1] This means that acquiring new skills safely is a lifelong challenge for many clinicians, not just for trainees.

Consider the case of laparoscopic cholecystectomy, "lap choley" for short. Since being introduced more than two decades ago, this gallbladder removal technique has almost entirely replaced the much more invasive, and far more costly and risky, "open choley." Laparoscopic and other non-invasive techniques have revolutionized other surgeries as well, including joint repair, hysterectomy, splenectomy, and even some cardiac cases.

The problem is that few surgeons trained before 1990 learned laparoscopic technique during their supervised apprenticeship. Is that a problem? Well, yes. One early study of lap choleys showed that injuries to the common bile duct dropped almost 20-fold once surgeons had performed more than 12 cases. And the learning curve didn't end there: the rate of common bile duct injury on the 30th case was still 10 times higher than the rate after 50 cases.[18]

Until recently, the requirement that a surgeon certify his or her competency in any new procedure was nil—the system "trusted" that surgeons' professionalism would ensure adequate training before physicians began practicing on patients. Adding to the problem, there were few training models in which surgeons or other operators could efficiently learn new techniques without putting patients at risk. In earlier chapters (8, 9, and 15), we discussed what healthcare can learn from aviation when it comes to teamwork and communication. Here is yet another area in which aviation's approach to this problem—how to efficiently and safely achieve competency in high-risk situations using new equipment and procedures—seems far safer than medicine's.

In both commercial and military aviation, pilots prepare to fly new planes by first undergoing considerable formal training (in classrooms and in highly realistic simulators), followed by extensive, hands-on experience in the real thing, with an instructor pilot seated next to the pilot-in-training, manning a dual set of controls. After that, pilots must pass both written and flight tests to qualify in the new machine, and they are evaluated annually in "check rides" administered by senior instructors. If a pilot flunks a check ride, he or she is put back on training status until the deficiencies are eradicated. When pilots fail several of these checks or are involved in a serious incident or accident, they are evaluated by what the Air Force calls a "Flight Evaluation Board," which has the power to clip their wings.

Contrast this with medicine's laissez-faire attitude toward recertification. Until about 30 years ago, there was no requirement for recertification in any specialty in American medicine, no requirement for demonstrated competency in new procedures, and no formal, required apprenticeship in new techniques (although some individual hospitals have enforced more rigorous criteria, and most states require some form of continuing education). This situation has changed in recent years: all major specialty boards now require recertification ("*Maintenance of Certification*" [MOC]; Table 20-1) and a number of specialty societies have set minimum volume thresholds before allowing independent practice. Moreover, accrediting bodies (including the Accreditation Council for Graduate Medical Education and the Joint Commission) are beginning to enforce more stringent requirements for competency-based credentialing of trainees and practicing physicians (Chapter 20).[19]

Even before these more rigorous requirements were enacted, many physicians *did* receive some training before beginning to perform new procedures, driven by both individual professional integrity and the malpractice system. But the data are sobering: a 1991 survey found that 55% of 165 practicing surgeons who had participated in a two-day course on laparoscopic cholecystectomy felt the workshop had left them inadequately trained to start performing the procedure. Yet 74% of these surgeons admitted that they began performing lap choleys immediately after completing the course[20] (Chapter 5).

Now that the patient safety movement has convinced most observers that learning on patients is unethical when there are practical, safer alternatives, healthcare is increasingly looking to simulation. Procedural simulators have been around for decades in other industries. Military fliers used them even before World War II, although these "Link Trainers" were only crude approximations of the real thing. Static aircraft simulators (in which the cockpit is fixed to the floor while instruments give the impression of flight) became more sophisticated during the jet age, allowing new pilots not only to learn and practice normal instrument procedures but also to handle a wide variety of airborne emergencies. By the age of jumbo jets, supersonic airliners, and space shuttles, "full motion" simulators that gave the illusion of true flight became available—pilots could actually look out the window and "take off" and "land" at any airport in the world. And the U.S. military now uses sophisticated training simulators, with 10-channel sound effects, voice recognition

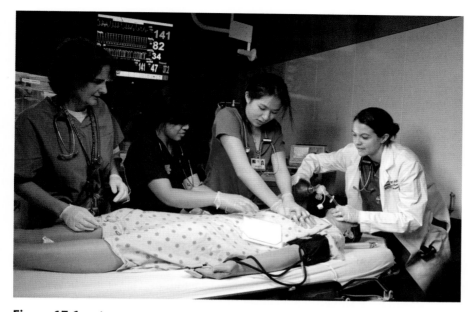

Figure 17-1 ▪ A team practicing its skills on a modern high-fidelity simulator. (Photo courtesy of the UCSF Kanbar Center for Simulation and Clinical Skills.)

software (including the languages of potential enemies and allies), and "battle smells" (burnt charcoal) to prepare troops for war.

Such training and performance evaluation aids—in which trainees interact with other human beings as well as with machinery and virtual displays—may hold the highest potential for medical simulations, which, until a decade or two ago, were pretty primitive. During medical school in the 1980s, it was common to learn how to give injections using oranges and suturing was often trialed on pig's feet. A somewhat lifelike mannequin (nicknamed "Annie," for unknown reasons) has been used for years to teach cardiopulmonary resuscitation (CPR). Recently, however, these models have become far more realistic, and they have advanced capabilities. Today's training mannequins allow students to deliver electric shocks with defibrillator paddles and note changes to heart rhythms, insert intravenous and intra-arterial lines, and perform intubations (Figure 17-1). Surgical simulators are now available to provide basic practice for medical students and residents and to help experienced surgeons learn new techniques. The major hurdle for these systems is simulating the feel of real flesh, but new technologies and materials are helping to overcome even that obstacle.

Increasingly, the literature supports the link between improved dexterity from simulator training and patient safety. For example, one systematic review looked at over 600 studies on technology-enhanced simulation training programs and concluded that simulation training leads to improved skills and knowledge.[21] Another review showed that improved competence and better patient outcomes were associated with procedural simulation training.[22] One study found that giving surgical trainees standardized feedback on simulated laparoscopic surgeries resulted in lower error rates.[23] Another demonstrated that anesthesia residents who underwent high-fidelity simulation training were more adept at weaning their patients off cardiopulmonary bypass than colleagues who received standard classroom-based training.[24]

A high-fidelity simulator program is expensive (some surgical simulators run over $100,000, and training practicing clinicians requires both paying for the instructors and covering provider "downtime") and logistically complex to administer. Lazzara et al. have identified eight principles and tips for a successful simulation program (Table 17-3).[25] Because of cost and complexity, the broad dissemination of simulator training will depend not only on evidence of effectiveness but also on regulatory requirements, cost sharing (e.g., some regions and professional societies have formed consortia to purchase simulators), and return-on-investment considerations. One study showed that, because novice surgeons are slower in the operating room (OR) and require substantial hand-holding by senior physicians, procedures involving a resident often take longer and incur increased costs.[26] In the end, the arguments for simulator training may hinge as much on clinical efficiency as on safety.

Although one clever experiment showed that trainees improved as much on a urologic simulator costing less than a dollar (rubber tubes standing in for the urethra, styrofoam cup for the bladder) as on a high-tech version costing tens of thousands of dollars,[27] today's trend is clearly toward more realistic, technologically sophisticated simulators. Modern virtual reality simulators are beginning to input actual human data, such as those drawn from an extraordinarily detailed digitized cadaver model known as the "Visible Human." Other simulators are being developed that, rather than using generic anatomical data, use real patients' anatomy drawn from computed tomography (CT) or magnetic resonance imaging (MRI) scans. The day may come when surgeons will practice their patient's operation virtually (based on actual anatomy) before scrubbing in for a complex procedure.

While it is easy to get breathless about this futuristic technology, simulators are unlikely to completely replace having a well-prepared young learner observing, then doing, and then being corrected by a seasoned veteran. The line between learning and doing will be further blurred as simulations become more realistic and real surgeries become less invasive and more like the simulations. As more and more surgeries and procedures become "virtual," it will be important to remember that simulators can help augment trainees' technical competence, but are highly unlikely to fully replace the need for trainees to learn their craft—as safely as possible—with real patients.

Table 17-3	EIGHT SUCCESS FACTORS AND TIPS FOR INCORPORATING THEM INTO SIMULATION PROGRAMS
Success Factor	**Tips for Incorporation**
1. Science	■ Utilize multidisciplinary collaborations of clinicians and training designers ■ Leverage available checklists to ensure that all facets of training have been accounted for ■ Use an in situ training location to foster attendance by having it conveniently located ■ Create a bulletin board to publicly announce desired behaviors ■ Provide impromptu drills to offer trainees more opportunity to practice
2. Staff	■ Recruit champions to promote the use of simulation for training ■ Demonstrate simulation in all departments to encourage interest and active participation ■ Capitalize on unique resources, such as college or high school volunteers, local theatrical students, and military medical personnel
3. Supplies	■ Procure supplies from surplus or expired equipment available in other units ■ Look to outside funding when obtaining from local facilities is not feasible
4. Space	■ Connect with the committee responsible for allocating facility space ■ Suggest temporary locations like a "time share" for the simulation laboratory when a permanent location is not possible ■ Seek off-site locations and consider community resources
5. Support	■ Offer simulation briefings and demonstrations to senior leadership to generate interest and support ■ Focus on the positives of simulation-based training and show its value ■ Consider publishing facility employee newsletter articles on simulation training to keep interest and awareness alive
6. Systems	■ Match the fidelity of the training with desired training objectives ■ Ensure that the network infrastructure/capabilities are sufficient ■ Consider upfront costs and recurring maintenance that is needed for simulation equipment
7. Success	■ Share success stories verbally and in newsletters or posters ■ Encourage sharing success stories
8. Sustainability	■ Hold contests for naming mannequins ■ Create simulation committees ■ Build a cadre of staff with new simulation champions and instructors

Reproduced with permission from Lazzara EH, Benishek LE, Dietz AS, Salas E, Adriansen DJ. Eight critical factors in creating and implementing a successful simulation program. *Jt Comm J Qual Saf* 2014;40:21–29.

TEACHING PATIENT SAFETY

Over the past decade, the central importance of teaching patient safety and its related competencies has come to be appreciated. Without high-quality and effective educational programs for health professionals, the progress we need to make in safety will be stunted. Of course, this book is one small part of many efforts to fill that gap.

While the needs are broad and encompass practicing clinicians as well as trainees in medicine, nursing, pharmacy, and healthcare administration, medical students have been a primary focus of efforts to transform education. In an influential 2010 white paper, the National Patient Safety Foundation's Lucian Leape Institute offered a series of thoughtful and ambitious recommendations, including the need to modify medical student selection criteria, provide foundational knowledge in patient safety and associated areas through a core curriculum, and alter trainees' clinical experiences to reinforce safety-related competencies (Table 17-4).[28] Importantly, the latter recommendation takes heed of the informal "hidden curriculum," which is closely linked to the overall safety culture (Chapter 15) and whose lessons can easily trump those of even the most well-intended formal programs.[29] For example, educating students about teamwork and professionalism in the classroom will mean little if they rotate onto the wards and see their supervising residents and attendings modeling noncollaborative and disrespectful behavior.

A number of key patient safety resources are listed in Appendix I. Individuals interested in learning more about patient safety can take advantage of many Web-based resources, such as *AHRQ WebM&M*,[30] a monthly case-based safety journal (Figure 14-1), and *AHRQ Patient Safety Network*,[31] a weekly update of studies, Web sites, conferences, and tools in patient safety (Figures 22-1 and 22-2). These free resources, along with additional sources of information for patient safety leaders, are described more fully in Chapter 22.

Prompted in part by the Accreditation Council for Graduate Medical Education's (ACGME) Clinical Learning Environment Review Program (CLER), which was launched in 2012 and aims to incorporate quality and safety into the accreditation process,[32] many residency training programs now offer training in patient safety. Through CLER, the ACGME evaluates academic training programs in six key areas: patient safety, quality improvement, care transitions, supervision, duty hours, and professionalism. The program aims to prompt engagement of trainees in quality and safety work in a meaningful way, with the hopes that they will incorporate associated skills and knowledge into their careers after training.

Several studies and systematic reviews of safety curricula have been published.[33–37] In addition, some larger organizations, such as the Institute for

Table 17-4 THE LUCIAN LEAPE INSTITUTE'S RECOMMENDATIONS FOR IMPROVING PATIENT SAFETY EDUCATION*

Recommendation 1. Medical school and teaching hospital leaders should place the highest priority on creating learning cultures that emphasize patient safety, model professionalism, enhance collaborative behavior, encourage transparency, and value the individual learner.

Recommendation 2. Medical school deans and teaching hospital CEOs should launch a broad effort to emphasize and promote the development and display of interpersonal skills, leadership, teamwork, and collaboration among faculty and staff.

Recommendation 3. As part of continuing education and ongoing performance improvement, medical school deans and teaching hospital CEOs should provide incentives and make available necessary resources to support the enhancement of faculty capabilities for teaching students how to diagnose patient safety problems, improve patient care processes, and deliver safe care.

Recommendation 4. The selection process for admission to medical school should place greater emphasis on selecting for attributes that reflect the concepts of professionalism and an orientation to patient safety.

Recommendation 5. Medical schools should conceptualize and treat patient safety as a science that encompasses knowledge of error causation and mitigation, human factors concepts, safety improvement science, systems theory and analysis, system design and redesign, teaming, and error disclosure and apology.

Recommendation 6. The medical school experience should emphasize the shaping of desired skills, attitudes, and behaviors in medical students that include, but are not limited to, the IOM and ACGME/ABMS core competencies—such as professionalism, interpersonal skills and communication, provision of patient-centered care, and working in interdisciplinary teams.

Recommendation 7. Medical schools, teaching hospitals, and residency training programs should ensure a coherent, continuing, and flexible educational experience that spans the four years of undergraduate medical education, residency and fellowship training, and lifelong continuing education.

Recommendation 8. The LCME should modify its accreditation standards to articulate expectations for the creation of learning cultures having the characteristics described in Recommendation 1, to establish patient safety education—having the characteristics described herein—as a curricular requirement, and to define specific terminal competencies for graduating medical students.

Recommendation 9. The ACGME should expand its Common Program Requirements to articulate expectations for the creation of learning cultures having the characteristics described in Recommendation 1 and to emphasize the importance of patient safety–related behavioral traits.

(*continued*)

Table 17-4 **THE LUCIAN LEAPE INSTITUTE'S RECOMMENDATIONS FOR IMPROVING PATIENT SAFETY EDUCATION* (*continued*)**
Recommendation 10. The LCME and the ACGME should direct particular attention to the adequacy of the patient safety–related preparation of graduating medical students for entry into residency training.
Recommendation 11. A survey of medical schools should be developed to evaluate school educational priorities for patient safety, the creation of school and teaching hospital cultures that support patient safety, and school effectiveness in shaping desired student skills, attitudes, and behaviors.
Recommendation 12. Financial, academic, and other incentives should be utilized to leverage desired changes in medical schools and teaching hospitals that will improve medical education and make it more relevant to the real world of patient care.

*ABMS, American Board of Medical Specialties; ACGME, Accreditation Council for Graduate Medical Education; CEO, chief executive officer; IOM, Institute of Medicine; LCME, Liaison Committee on Medical Education.Reproduced with permission from the Lucian Leape Institute at the National Patient Safety Foundation, *Unmet Needs: Teaching Physicians to Provide Safe Patient Care*. Boston, MA: Lucian Leape Institute at the National Patient Safety Foundation; March 2010.

Healthcare Improvement (IHI), the VA's National Center for Patient Safety, and the Risk Management Foundation of the Harvard Medical Institutions, have made their curricula available.[38–40] As one measure of trainees' hunger for patient safety education, at this writing more than 250,000 students and residents are registered on www.IHI.org and tens of thousands have taken courses through IHI's Open School for Health Professionals.[38]

Many other issues related to patient safety education, such as improving diagnostic reasoning (Chapter 6), computerized decision support (Chapter 13), teamwork training (Chapter 15), and using malpractice cases to teach patient safety (Chapter 18), are highlighted throughout this book.

KEY POINTS

- Medical training has always needed to balance autonomy and oversight, but has traditionally tipped this balance toward trainee autonomy, largely for economic reasons.
- Driven in large part by the patient safety movement, the pendulum has moved toward oversight, reflected in more available and involved supervisors and efforts to encourage trainees to admit their limitations and call for help.

- Particularly in procedural fields, the use of simulation will help trainees—and practicing clinicians who need to learn new procedures—traverse their learning curves with fewer risks to patients. Emerging data support the logical premise that simulation training leads to fewer errors and improved efficiency.
- Training the next generation of health professionals in patient safety–related competencies is crucial, and many curricula and resources have been developed for this purpose. Such training will need not only to provide foundational knowledge but also to pay attention to the "hidden curriculum" that trainees experience during their clinical rotations.

REFERENCES

1. Gawande AA. *Complications: A Surgeon's Notes on an Imperfect Science*. New York, NY: Henry Holt and Company; 2002.
2. Ranji SR. A piece of my mind. What gets measured gets (micro)managed. *JAMA* 2014;312:1637–1638.
3. Robins N. *The Girl Who Died Twice: Every Patient's Nightmare: The Libby Zion Case and the Hidden Hazards of Hospitals*. New York, NY: Delacorte Press; 1995.
4. Bell BM. Supervision, not regulation of hours, is the key to improving the quality of patient care. *JAMA* 1993;269:403–404.
5. Wu AW, Folkman S, McPhee SJ, Lo B. Do house officers learn from their mistakes? *JAMA* 1991;265:2089–2094.
6. Iglehart JK. The ACGME's final duty-hour standards—special PGY-1 limits and strategic napping. *N Engl J Med* 2010;363:1589–1591.
7. Kerlin MP, Small DS, Conney E, et al. A randomized trial of nighttime physician staffing in an intensive care unit. *N Engl J Med* 2013;368:2201–2209.
8. Snowdon DA, Hau R, Leggat SG, Taylor NF. Does clinical supervision of health professionals improve patient safety? A systematic review and meta-analysis. *Int J Qual Health Care* 2016;28:447–455.
9. Gonzalo JD, Kuperman EF, Chuang CH, Lehman E, Glasser F, Abendroth T. Impact of an overnight internal medicine academic hospitalist program on patient outcomes. *J Gen Intern Med* 2015;30:1795–1802.
10. Van Leer PE, Lavine EK, Rabrich JS, Wiener DE, Clark MA, Wong TYS. Resident supervision and patient safety: do different levels of resident supervision affect the rate of morbidity and mortality cases? *J Emerg Med* 2015;49:944–948.
11. Ross PT, McMyler ET, Anderson SG, et al. Trainees' perceptions of patient safety practices: recounting failures of supervision. *Jt Comm J Qual Patient Saf* 2011;37:88–95.
12. Manuel BM, McCarthy JL, Berry W, Dwyer K. Risk management and patient safety [Perspective]. *AHRQ WebM&M* (serial online); December 2010. Available at: https://psnet.ahrq.gov/perspectives/perspective/96.

13. ElBardissi AW, Regenbogen SE, Greenberg CC, et al. Communication practices on 4 Harvard surgical services: a surgical safety collaborative. *Ann Surg* 2009;250:861–865.

14. Arriaga AF, ElBardissi AW, Regenbogen SE, et al. A policy-based intervention for the reduction of communication breakdowns in inpatient surgical care: results from a Harvard surgical safety collaborative. *Ann Surg* 2011;253:849–854.

15. Kennedy TJ, Lingard L, Baker GR, Kitchen L, Regehr G. Clinical oversight: conceptualizing the relationship between supervision and safety. *J Gen Intern Med* 2007;22:1080–1085.

16. Tamuz M, Giardina TD, Thomas EJ, Menon S, Singh H. Rethinking resident supervision to improve safety: from hierarchical to interprofessional models. *J Hosp Med* 2011;6:448–456.

17. Ross PT, McMyler ET, Anderson SG, et al. Trainees' perceptions of patient safety practices: recounting failures of supervision. *J Qual Patient Saf* 2011;37:88–95.

18. Moore MJ, Bennett CL. The learning curve for laparoscopic cholecystectomy. The Southern Surgeons Club. *Am J Surg* 1995;170:55–59.

19. Holmboe ES, Sherbino J, Long DM, Swing SR, Frank JR. The role of assessment in competency-based medical education. *Med Teach* 2010;32:676–682.

20. Morino M, Festa V, Garrone C. Survey on Torino courses. The impact of a two-day practical course on apprenticeship and diffusion of laparoscopic cholecystectomy in Italy. *Surg Endosc* 1995;9:46–48.

21. Cook DA, Hatala R, Brydges R, et al. Technology-enhanced simulation for health professions education: a systematic review and meta-analysis. *JAMA* 2011;306:978–988.

22. Schmidt E, Goldhaber-Fiebert SN, Ho LA, McDonald KM. Simulation exercises as a patient safety strategy: a systematic review. *Ann Intern Med* 2013;158:426–432.

23. Boyle E, Al-Akash M, Gallagher AG, Traynor O, Hill AD, Neary PC. Optimising surgical training: use of feedback to reduce errors during a simulated surgical procedure. *Postgrad Med J* 2011;87:524–528.

24. Bruppacher HR, Alam SK, LeBlanc VR, et al. Simulation-based training improves physicians' performance in patient care in high-stakes clinical setting of cardiac surgery. *Anesthesiology* 2010;112:985–992.

25. Lazzara EH, Benishek LE, Dietz AS, Salas E, Adriansen DJ. Eight critical factors in creating and implementing a successful simulation program. *Jt Comm J Qual Patient Saf* 2014;40:21–29.

26. Allen RW, Pruitt M, Taaffe KM. Effect of resident involvement on operative time and operating room staffing costs. *J Surg Educ* 2016;73:979–985.

27. Matsumoto ED, Hamstra SJ, Radomski SB, Cusimano MD. The effect of bench model fidelity on endourological skills: a randomized controlled study. *J Urol* 2002; 167:2354–2357.

28. Lucian Leape Institute at the National Patient Safety Foundation. *Unmet Needs: Teaching Physicians to Provide Safe Patient Care*. Boston, MA: Lucian Leape Institute at the National Patient Safety Foundation; March 2010.

29. Pingleton SK, Davis DA, Dickler RM. Characteristics of quality and patient safety curricula in major teaching hospitals. *Am J Med Qual* 2010;25:305–311.

30. Available at: https://psnet.ahrq.gov/webmm.

31. Available at: https://psnet.ahrq.gov/.

32. Weiss KB, Wagner R, Bagian JP, Newton RC, Patow CA, Nasca TJ. Advances in the ACGME Clinical Learning Environment Review (CLER) Program. *J Grad Med Educ* 2013;5:718–721.

33. Wong BM, Etchells EE, Kuper A, Levinson W, Shojania KG. Teaching quality improvement and patient safety to trainees: a systematic review. *Acad Med* 2010:85;1425–1439.

34. Tregunno D, Ginsburg L, Clarke B, Norton P. Integrating patient safety into health professionals' curricula: a qualitative study of medical, nursing and pharmacy faculty perspectives. *BMJ Qual Saf* 2014;23:257–264.

35. Kirkman MA, Sevdalis N, Arora S, Baker P, Vincent C, Ahmed M. The outcomes of recent patient safety education interventions for trainee physicians and medical students: a systematic review. *BMJ Open* 2015;e007705.

36. Stahl K, Augenstein J, Schulman CI, Wilson K, McKenney M, Livingstone A. Assessing the impact of teaching patient safety principles to medical students during surgical clerkships. *J Surg Res* 2011;170:e29–e40.

37. Dudas RA, Bundy DG, Miller MR, Barone M. Can teaching medical students to investigate medication errors change their attitudes towards patient safety? *BMJ Qual Saf* 2011;20:319–325.

38. The IHI Open School. Institute for Healthcare Improvement. Available at: http://www.ihi.org/offerings/ihiopenschool/Pages/default.aspx.

39. U.S. Department of Veterans Affairs. *Patient Safety Curriculum*. Ann Arbor, MI: National Center for Patient Safety. Available at: http://www.patientsafety.va.gov/professionals/training/curriculum.asp.

40. *Core Curriculum for Patient Safety*. Risk Management Foundation of the Harvard Medical Institutions. Available at: https://www.rmf.harvard.edu/Clinician-Resources/.

ADDITIONAL READINGS

Cooper JB, Singer SJ, Hayes J, et al. Design and evaluation of simulation scenarios for a program introducing patient safety, teamwork, safety leadership, and simulation to healthcare leaders and managers. *Simul Healthc* 2011;6:231–238.

Gawande A. Personal best. *New Yorker*. October 3, 2011:44–53.

Howard JN. The missing link: dedicated patient safety education within top-ranked US nursing school curricula. *J Patient Saf* 2010;6:165–171.

Kneebone RL. Practice, rehearsal, and performance: an approach for simulation-based surgical and procedure training. *JAMA* 2009;302:1336–1338.

Myers JS, Nash DB. Graduate medical education's new focus on resident engagement in quality and safety: will it transform the culture of teaching hospitals? *Acad Med* 2014;89:1328–1330.

Voelker R. Medical simulation gets real. *JAMA* 2009;302:2190–2192.

Wong BM, Etchells EE, Kuper A, Levinson W, Shojania KG. Teaching quality improvement and patient safety to trainees: a systematic review. *Acad Med* 2010;85:1425–1439.

THE MALPRACTICE SYSTEM | 18

OVERVIEW

A middle-aged woman was admitted to the medical ward with a moderate case of pneumonia. After being started promptly on antibiotics and fluids, she stabilized for a few hours. But she deteriorated overnight, leading to symptoms and signs of severe hypoxemia and septic shock. The nurse paged a young physician working the overnight shift.

The doctor arrived within minutes. She found the patient confused, hypotensive, tachypneic, and hypoxic. Oxygen brought the patient's oxygen saturation up to the low 90s, and the doctor now had a difficult choice to make. The patient, confused and agitated, clearly had respiratory failure: the need for intubation and mechanical ventilation was obvious. But should the young doctor intubate the patient on the floor or quickly transport her to the ICU, a few floors below, where the experienced staff could perform the intubation more safely?

Part of this trade-off was the doctor's awareness of her own limitations. She had performed only a handful of intubations in her career, most under the guidance of an anesthesiologist in an unhurried setting, and the ward nurses also lacked experience in helping with the procedure. A third option was to call an ICU team to the ward, but that could take as long as transferring the patient downstairs.

After thinking about it for a moment, she made the decision to bring the patient promptly to the ICU. She called the unit to be ready. "In my mind it was a matter of what would be safest," she reflected later. And so the doctor, a floor nurse, and a respiratory therapist wheeled the patient's bed to the elevator, and then to the ICU.

Unfortunately, in the 10 minutes between notifying the ICU and arriving there, the patient's condition worsened markedly, and when she got to the unit she was in extremis. After an unsuccessful urgent intubation attempt, the patient became pulseless. Frantically, one doctor shocked the patient while another prepared to reattempt intubation. On the third shock, the patient's heart restarted and the intubation was completed. The patient survived, but was left with severe hypoxic brain damage.

The young physician apologized to the family, out of empathy rather than guilt. In her mind, despite the terrible outcome, she had made the decision that was in the best interest of the patient at the time.

Nearly two years later, the physician received notice that she was being sued. The patient's family was alleging negligence, citing a delay in intubation. The moment she received the news is forever seared into her memory, along with the horrible moments spent trying to save the patient whose family was now seeking to punish her. "I was sitting in the ICU," she said, "and my partner calls me up and says, 'You're being sued. This system is broken, and that's why I'm leaving medicine.'"[1]

▌TORT LAW AND THE MALPRACTICE SYSTEM

The need to compensate people for their injuries has long been recognized in most systems of law, and Western systems have traditionally done so by apportioning fault (*culpa*). *Tort law*, the general legal discipline that includes malpractice law (as well as product liability and personal injury law), takes these two principles—compensating the injured in an effort to "make them whole" and making the party "at fault" responsible for this restitution—and weaves them into a single system. The linking of compensation of the injured to the fault of the injurer is brilliant in its simplicity and works reasonably well when applied to many human endeavors.[2]

Unfortunately, medicine is not one of them. Most errors involve slips—glitches in automatic behaviors that can strike even the most conscientious practitioner (Chapter 2)—that are unintentional and therefore cannot be deterred by threat of lawsuits. Moreover, as we hope the rest of this book has made clear, for most adverse outcomes, the doctor or nurse holding the smoking gun is not truly "at fault," but simply the last link in a long error chain.

We are not referring here to the acts of unqualified, unmotivated, or reckless providers who fail to adhere to expected standards and whose mistakes are therefore deserving of blame. These situations will be discussed more fully in the next chapter, but the malpractice system (coupled with more vigorous efforts to hold the providers accountable and protect future patients) seems like an appropriate vehicle in dealing with such caregivers.

As an analogy, consider the difference between a driver who accidentally hits a child who darts into traffic chasing a ball and a drunk driver who hits a child on the sidewalk after losing control of his speeding car. Both accidents result in death, but the second driver is clearly more culpable. If the malpractice system confined its wrath to medicine's version of the drunk, speeding driver—particularly the repeat offender—it would be hard to criticize it. But that is far from the case.

Think about a doctor who performs a risky and difficult surgical procedure, and has done it safely thousands of time but finally slips. The injured patient sues, claiming that the doctor didn't adhere to the "standard of care." A defense argument that the surgeon normally *did* avoid the error, or that some errors are a statistical inevitability if you do a complex procedure often enough, holds little water in the malpractice system, which makes it fundamentally unfair to those whose jobs require frequent risky activities. As Alan Merry, a New Zealand anesthesiologist, and Alexander McCall Smith, Professor of Medical Law at the University of Edinburgh, observe, "All too often the yardstick is taken to be the person who is capable of meeting a high standard of competence, awareness, care, etc., *all the time*. Such a person is unlikely to be human."[2]

The malpractice system is also ill suited to dealing with judgment calls, such as the one the physician made in choosing to wheel her septic patient to the ICU prior to intubation. Such difficult decisions come up all the time. Because the tort system reviews them retrospectively, it creates a powerful instinct to assign blame (of course, we can never know what would have happened had the physician chosen to intubate the patient on the ward). "The tendency in such circumstances is to praise a decision if it proves successful and to call it 'an error of judgment' if not," write Merry and McCall Smith. "Success is its own justification; failure needs a great deal of explanation."

How can judges and juries (and patients and providers) avoid the distorting effects of hindsight and deal more fairly with caregivers doing their best under difficult conditions? Safety expert James Reason recommends the *Johnston substitution test*, which does not compare an act to an arbitrary standard of excellence, but asks only if a similarly qualified caregiver in the same situation would have behaved any differently. If the answer is "probably not," then, as the test's inventor Neil Johnston puts it, "Apportioning blame has no material role to play, other than to obscure systemic deficiencies and to blame one of the victims."[3,4]

Liability seems more justified when rules or principles have been violated, since these usually do involve conscious choices by caregivers. But—in healthcare at least—even rule violations may not automatically merit blame. For example, even generally rule-abiding physicians and nurses will periodically need to violate certain rules (e.g., proscriptions against verbal orders are often violated when compliance would cause unnecessary patient suffering, such as when a patient urgently requires analgesia, or patient harm, such as when a patient is seizing). That is not to condone healthcare anarchy—*routine rule violations* (Chapter 15) should cause us to rethink the rule in question, and some rules (such as "clean your hands before touching a patient" or "sign your site") should virtually never be broken.[5] But the malpractice system will seize upon evidence that a rule was broken when there is a bad outcome, ignoring the fact that some particular rules are broken by nearly everyone in the name of efficiency—or sometimes even quality and safety.

Tort law is fluid: every society must decide how to set the bar regarding fault and compensation. By marrying the recompense of the injured to the finding of fault, tort systems inevitably lower the fault-finding bar to allow for easier compensation of sympathetic victims. But this is not the only reason the bar tilts toward fault finding. Humans (particularly of the American variety) tend to be unsettled by vague "systems" explanations, and even more bothered by the possibility that a horrible outcome could have been "no one's fault." Moreover, the continuing erosion of professional privilege, a questioning of all things "expert," and sometimes unrealistic expectations of what modern medicine can provide (driven by the media, the Internet, and more) have further tipped the balance between plaintiff and defendant. But it was already an unfair match: faced with the heart-wrenching story of an injured patient or grieving family, who can possibly swallow an explanation that "things like this just happen" and that no one is to blame, especially when the potential source of compensation is a "rich doctor," or a faceless insurance company?[6]

The role of the expert witness further tips the already lopsided scales of malpractice justice. Almost by definition, expert witnesses are particularly well informed about their areas of expertise, which makes it exceptionally difficult for them to assume the mindset of "the reasonable practitioner," especially as the case becomes confrontational and experts gravitate to polarized positions.

Finally, adding to the confusion is the fact that doctors and nurses feel guilty when patients experience adverse outcomes (even when there was no true error or fault), often blaming ourselves because we failed to live up to our own expectation of perfection (Chapter 16). Just as naturally, what person would not instinctively lash out against a provider when faced with a brain-damaged child or dead spouse? It is to be expected that families or patients will blame the party holding the smoking gun, just as they would a driver who struck their child who ran into the street to chase a ball. Some bereaved families (and drivers and doctors) will ultimately move on to a deeper understanding that no one is to blame—that the tragedy is just that. But whether they do or do not, write Merry and McCall Smith, "It is essential that the law should do so."[2]

If the malpractice system unfairly assigns fault when there is none, what really is the harm, other than the payment of a few (or a few million) dollars

by physicians, hospitals, or insurance companies to injured patients and families? We believe that there *is* harm, particularly as we try to engage rank-
and-file clinicians in patient safety efforts. A 2011 study found that the vast
majority of physicians are sued at some point in their careers, and nearly one
in five physicians in the highest-risk fields (neurosurgery and cardiac surgery)
is sued *each year* (Figure 18-1).[7] Physicians, particularly in these fields, often

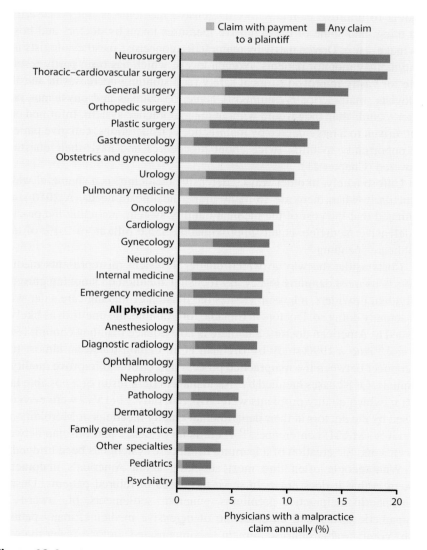

Figure 18-1 ■ Proportion of physicians facing a malpractice claim annually, according
to specialty. (Reprinted with permission from Jena AB, Seabury S, Lakdawalla D, Chandra A.
Malpractice risk according to physician specialty. *N Engl J Med* 2011;365:629–636.)

become demoralized, and depressed providers are not likely to be enthusiastic patient safety leaders. Tort law is adversarial by nature, while a culture of safety is collaborative (Chapter 15). In a safety-conscious culture, doctors and nurses willingly report their mistakes as opportunities to make themselves and the system better (Chapter 14), something they are unlikely to do in a litigious environment.

This is not to say—as some do—that the malpractice system has done nothing to improve patient safety. Defensive medicine is not necessarily a bad thing, and some of the defensive measures taken by doctors and hospitals make sense. Driven partly by malpractice concerns, anesthesiologists now continuously monitor patients' oxygen levels, which has been partly responsible for vastly improved surgical safety (and stunning decreases in anesthesiologists' malpractice premiums) (Chapter 5). Nurses and physicians keep better records than they would without the malpractice system. Informed consent, driven to a large degree by malpractice considerations, can give patients the opportunity to think twice about procedures and have their questions answered (Chapter 21).

Unfortunately, in other ways, "defensive medicine" is a shameful waste, particularly when there are so many unmet healthcare needs. A 2010 study estimated that the cost of the medical liability system, including the practice of defensive medicine, equals approximately $55.6 billion, or 2.4% of total healthcare spending.[8]

Costs aside, the way in which our legal system misrepresents medical errors is its most damning legacy. By focusing attention on smoking guns and individual providers, a lawsuit creates the illusion of making care safer without actually doing so. Doctors in Canada, for example, are one-fifth as likely to be sued as American doctors, and there is no evidence that they commit fewer errors.[1,9] And a 1990 study by Brennan et al. demonstrated an almost total disconnect between the malpractice process and efforts to improve quality in hospitals. Of 82 cases handled by risk managers (as a result of a possible lawsuit) in which quality problems were involved, only 12 (15%) were even discussed by the doctors at their departmental quality meetings or Morbidity and Mortality (M&M) conferences.[10] There is no evidence that this gap between lawsuits and the creation of a learning healthcare system has been bridged.

What people often find most shocking about America's malpractice system is that it does not even serve the needs of injured patients. Despite stratospheric malpractice premiums, generous settlements, big awards by sympathetic juries, and an epidemic of defensive medicine, many patients with "compensable injuries" remain uncompensated. In fact, fewer than 3% of patients who experience injuries associated with negligent care file claims. The reasons for this are varied, and include patients' unawareness that an error occurred, the fact that most cases are taken by attorneys on contingency (and thus will not be brought if the attorneys think that their investment in preparing the case is unlikely to be recouped), and the fact that many of the uncompensated or undercompensated claimants are on government assistance and lack the resources, personal initiative, or social clout to seek redress. Thus, some worthy malpractice claims go begging while others go forward for a host of reasons that have nothing to do with the presence or degree of negligence.

Even when injured patients' cases do make it through the malpractice system to a trial or settlement, it is remarkable how little money actually ends up in the hands of the victims and their families. After deducting legal fees and expenses, the average plaintiff sees about 40 cents of every dollar paid by the defendant. If the intent of the award is to help families care for a permanently disabled relative or to replace a deceased breadwinner's earnings, this 60% overhead makes the malpractice system a uniquely wasteful business.

ERROR DISCLOSURE, APOLOGIES, AND MALPRACTICE

For generations, physicians and health systems responded with silence after a medical error. This was a natural outgrowth of the shame that most providers feel after errors (driven, in part, by the traditional view of errors as stemming from individual failures rather than system problems) and by a malpractice system that nurtures confrontation and leads providers to fear that an apology will be taken as an admission of guilt, only to be used against them later.

The cycle played out time and time again: patients who believed they had possibly been victims of medical errors wanted to learn what really happened, but their caregivers and healthcare organizations frequently responded with defensiveness, sometimes even stonewalling. This, in turn, made patients and families angry, frustrated, and even more convinced that they were on the receiving end of a terrible mistake. Hickson et al. found that nearly half the families who sued their providers after perinatal injuries were motivated by their suspicion of a cover-up or a desire for revenge.[11]

But could this cycle be broken? Until the advent of the patient safety movement, most observers would have said no. Each side, after all, appeared to be acting in its own interests: patients seeking information and ultimately redress, and providers and hospitals trying to avoid painful conversations and payouts. Yet the results were so damaging to everyone that some began wondering whether there was a better way. Since the patient safety movement emphasized the role of improving systems, could a change in the system, and mental model, alter the toxic dynamics of malpractice?

After losing two large malpractice cases in the late 1980s, the Veterans Affairs Medical Center in Lexington, Kentucky, decided to adopt a policy of disclosure, apology, and early offer of a reasonable settlement, a policy it called "extreme honesty." Perhaps surprisingly, they found that their overall malpractice payouts were lower than those of comparable VA institutions.[12,13] While the study caught people's attention, the fact that it is challenging to sue a VA hospital (it *is* the federal government, after all) led many to question the generalizability of these results.

In 2007, Studdert et al. modeled the likely impact of policies to promote fuller disclosure. Full disclosure reveals errors to patients who knew or strongly suspected that they were victims of mistakes, and also to patients who did not suspect they were harmed by an error (and therefore had not considered suing). Because of this, Studdert et al.'s analysis revealed that even if fuller disclosure prevented some patients from suing, it would generate far *more* lawsuits overall because of new lawsuits filed by those patients previously unaware of an error. While affirming that from an ethical standpoint disclosure is "the right thing to do," Studdert et al. concluded that policies promoting it would be "an improbable risk management strategy."[14]

These concerns were put to rest, at least to a degree, in 2010, when the University of Michigan reported the results of its medical disclosure policy, built on the same principles as the Lexington VA's rapid disclosure of adverse events, apologies, and prompt and fair settlement offers when internal review found evidence of culpability.[15,16] (Importantly, the university vigorously defends cases when it believes there was no negligence.) While overall rates of malpractice payouts have been declining in the United States over the past decade (for reasons that are not entirely understood), Michigan's improvements far exceeded the secular trends: a 65% decrease in the rate of lawsuits, a 40% decrease in the time between a claim being made and its resolution, and a 60% decrease in total payouts (Figure 18-2).

It is important to acknowledge that the Michigan and Lexington findings do not entirely nullify Studdert's argument. In the medical literature, we often find early studies—conducted at atypical institutions with highly motivated leaders and investigators—that show breathtakingly positive effects that were not matched when the intervention was rolled out to other settings (We already discussed a similar experience with computerized provider order entry; Chapter 13). In fact, more recent literature examining the impact of disclosure and compensation programs has been somewhat mixed. While one recent study did show a decrease in malpractice costs associated with implementation of a disclosure program,[17] another survey study showed that error disclosure followed by full financial compensation was associated with more mistrust between patients (who became more likely to seek legal advice) and providers. The authors of the latter study suggest that institutions consider separating the disclosure and compensation processes and eliminating physicians from compensation discussions.[18] Despite some of the challenges, the

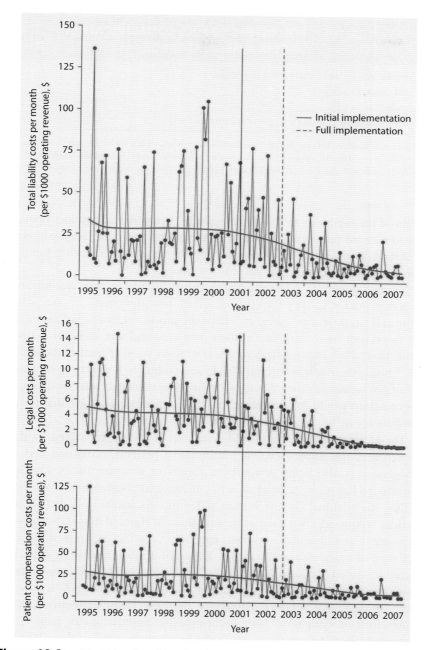

Figure 18-2 ▪ Monthly rates of legal and patient compensation costs before and after implementation of the University of Michigan Health System's disclosure-with-offer program. (Reprinted with permission from Kachalia A, Kaufman SR, Boothman R, et al. Liability claims and costs before and after implementation of a medical error disclosure program. *Ann Intern Med* 2010;153:213–221. © 2010 by American College of Physicians.)

Table 18-1	**FOUR STEPS TO FULL COMMUNICATION AFTER A MEDICAL ERROR**

- Tell the patient and family what happened
- Take responsibility
- Apologize
- Explain what will be done to prevent future events

Modified and reproduced with permission from the Massachusetts Coalition for the Prevention of Medical Errors. *When Things Go Wrong: Responding to Adverse Events.* Available at: http://www.macoalition.org/documents/respondingToAdverseEvents.pdf.

weight of the literature on this new approach is positive, and it does open the door to a broad rethinking of both the ethical and pragmatic implications of disclosure. The field of risk management has taken note, moving toward a more pro-disclosure stance in the past few years.[19]

Patients generally favor disclosure of all harmful errors, accompanied by an explanation of why the error occurred, how the error's impact will be minimized (in their own care), and steps the physician and organization will take to prevent its recurrence (in their own care and that of other patients) (Table 18-1).[20–23] Physicians favor disclosure as well, at least in theory, but they "choose their words carefully."[24] In responding to a variety of scenarios, 61% of physicians say they would tell their patient about an adverse event, but only one-third would fully disclose that the harm was caused by an error and apologize for it.[24]

The shifting of the tide toward disclosure has been prompted by these research findings and the evolving attitudes of patients, providers, and risk managers. It is also being driven by a variety of external forces. The Joint Commission has required disclosure of "unanticipated outcomes" since 2001. In 2006, the National Quality Forum added full disclosure to its list of "safe practices" (Appendix VII), the same year that the Harvard hospitals endorsed disclosure in an influential consensus paper.[23,25] Ten U.S. states now mandate disclosure of unanticipated outcomes, and as of 2008 a total of 36 states had enacted so-called "*apology laws*," excluding certain information contained in a caregiver's apology from being used in a malpractice lawsuit.[26] It is worth noting, though, that while the majority of these states explicitly exclude "expressions of sympathy," only eight prohibit "admissions of fault" from being admissible. As yet, there is no solid evidence that any of these laws are influencing the rates of malpractice suits.[27] In fact, some experts suggest that the flaws of some of these state laws may slow down full disclosure efforts.[28] A nongovernmental organization called "Sorry Works!" has been organized to promote disclosure.[29]

According to Tom Gallagher, a leading expert on disclosure, malpractice concerns are only one of several obstacles to effective disclosure. According to Gallagher[30]:

> Some people are trying to improve the practice of disclosure through what you might call moral exhortation. They try to remind healthcare workers that this is a professional and ethical duty, and then the implication is that we need to up our quotient of moral courage and just go do what we know is the right thing to do. But when you talk with healthcare workers … they really endorse the concept of disclosure, but struggle with its implementation. Among the key barriers we have encountered, one is clearly worry about the impact of disclosure on litigation. But that was not the only barrier, and for many clinicians it was not the most important barrier. Lots of clinicians really struggle with the concern that sometimes disclosure may not be beneficial to the patient …. The other barrier is the challenge of how awkward and uncomfortable these conversations are. Most physicians have told us that they haven't had any formal training in disclosure and are uncertain of just what to say.

Gallagher believes that the best disclosure training programs will combine some foundational knowledge, scenario-based training (probably using simulation; Chapter 17), and just-in-time coaching provided by experienced and trained medical directors or risk managers. Rathert and Phillips argue that training in disclosure will have additional benefits for organizations, in that it provides tangible evidence of an organization's "value-based ethics."[31] One review found that providing error disclosure training to clinicians led to improved comfort with the disclosure process.[32] Unsurprisingly, disclosure is more challenging if the error is made by another physician or occurred at a different institution; Gallagher et al. provide guidance to managing these difficult situations (Table 18-2).[33]

Some model language for telling a patient about a medication error is shown in Box 18-1.[23]

Clearly, the approach to patients after an error or an adverse event is evolving rapidly, after many years of stasis. The breadth of the rethinking—involving ethical imperatives, practical implications, training models, and laws and policies—is impressive, and ensures that this area will continue to change in coming years. McDonald et al., who have developed another widely praised disclosure program at the University of Illinois, describe seven pillars of an effective and comprehensive system of responding to adverse events in Table 18-3.[34]

Table 18-2	DISCLOSING HARMFUL ERRORS IN COMMON SITUATIONS INVOLVING OTHER CLINICIANS	
Clinical Situation	**Participants in Potential Disclosure**	**Rationale**
Error involving a clinician at your institution who is, or was, treating a patient with you (e.g., a consulting specialist or colleague on a different service who previously cared for the patient)	Joint responsibility, with both clinicians participating in disclosure conversation	A joint discussion ensures that key information is communicated to the patient and demonstrates teamwork.
Error involving a trainee or interprofessional colleague (e.g., a nurse or pharmacist) on a primary team caring for the patient	Attending physician, with the person who made the error encouraged to participate in disclosure planning and the conversation itself (if appropriate)	The attending physician leads the care team and probably has the most experience with disclosure. Errors involving solely an interprofessional colleague could be disclosed jointly by the attending physician and the relevant manager.
Error involving a clinician at your institution who lacks direct contact with the patient (e.g., a radiologist or pathologist)	Attending physician on primary service treating the patient, with the colleague invited to join discussion	An existing patient–provider relationship facilitates disclosure conversations.
Error unrelated to current care (e.g., a radiologist reviewing a chest radiograph of patient admitted for pneumonia notices a retained foreign body from previous abdominal surgery)	Medical director (or other senior leader) at the institution currently caring for the patient, after consultation with clinician involved in error, with the current attending physician invited to join the discussion	The current treating clinician may not be well suited to explain an error unrelated to the present care. A senior medical leader is better positioned to handle this complex situation.
Error involving a clinician at another institution	Medical director at the institution currently caring for the patient, after consultation with the outside institution, with the current attending physician invited to join the discussion	The medical director can provide the patient with clinical information (on the cause and implications of the error) as well as administrative perspective. A local medical society or malpractice insurer may provide support for physicians who do not have access to institutional or organizational resources.

Reproduced with permission from Gallagher TH, Mello MM, Levinson W, et al. Talking with patients about other clinicians' errors. *N Engl J Med* 2013;369:1752–1757.

Box 18-1   MODEL LANGUAGE FOR TELLING A PATIENT ABOUT A MEDICATION ERROR

"Let me tell you what happened. We gave you a chemotherapeutic agent, carboplatin, instead of the pamidronate you were supposed to receive.

I want to discuss with you what this means for your health, but first I'd like to apologize.

I'm sorry. This shouldn't have happened. Right now, I don't know exactly how this happened, but I promise you that we're going to find out what happened and do everything we can to make sure that it doesn't happen again. I will share with you what we find as soon as I know, but it may take some time to get to the bottom of it all.

Once again, let me say how sorry I am that this happened.

Now, what does this mean for your health? You received only a fraction of the usual dose of carboplatin, so it is unlikely you will have any adverse effects from the infusion. However, I would like to monitor you closely over the next weeks. In patients who receive a full dose, the side effects we expect include …. We usually monitor patients for these side effects by …. We treat these side effects by …. I want to see you in my clinic tomorrow so we can …."

_____

Modified and reproduced with permission from the Massachusetts Coalition for the Prevention of Medical Errors, November 18, 2011. *When Things Go Wrong: Responding to Adverse Events*. Available at: http://www.macoalition.org/documents/respondingToAdverseEvents.pdf.

NO-FAULT SYSTEMS AND "HEALTH COURTS": AN ALTERNATIVE TO TORT-BASED MALPRACTICE

A U.S. physician has a more than 1-in-100 chance of being sued after a patient has an adverse event, even when the doctor has done nothing wrong.[7,35] Although this may not sound like an excessive "risk" of a lawsuit, when you consider all the patients who suffer adverse events, this adds up to a lot of lawsuits. As noted earlier, recent research has shown that nearly all doctors will be sued at least once over the course of their career, and many will be sued multiple times.[7] There is tremendous variation across specialties in terms of the likelihood of facing a malpractice claim: among those in low-risk specialties, 36% will face a claim by age 45, as will 88% of physicians practicing in higher risk specialties. The risk is highest in neurosurgery: nearly 20% of these specialists are sued each year.[7]

Table 18-3   THE "SEVEN PILLARS" OF AN EFFECTIVE, COMPREHENSIVE SYSTEM OF RESPONDING TO ADVERSE EVENTS WITHIN A HEALTHCARE DELIVERY ORGANIZATION

"Pillar"	Explanation
1. Patient safety reporting system	Reports are "applauded"; can be made by phone, handwritten, online, or in person; clinical departments are penalized financially for failing to report incidents involving patient harm
2. Investigation	Risk manager performs preliminary investigation to ascertain harm. If yes, investigation and root cause analysis are commissioned. RCA to be completed within 72 hours of incident, including determination of whether "care was reasonable," using Reason's algorithm of unsafe acts (Chapter 19)[4,28]
3. Communication and disclosure	The "centerpiece of the process": ongoing communication with patient/family throughout process, including findings of "reasonableness" (#2). Third-party review offered if no consensus on whether care was reasonable. If "unreasonable," then full disclosure and apology follow—but this is "a process" that plays out over time and avoids premature disclosure before clear conclusions. A "Patient Communications Consult Service" is available to aid in disclosure process; a member of the service is present at all disclosures
4. Apology and remediation	Combines saying "we are sorry" with offer of a remedy, with rapid remediation (including waiving hospital bills) and early offer of compensation, if warranted
5. System improvement	Even after apology, the investigation continues to identify and implement system improvements. Patients and families are invited to participate in these efforts
6. Data tracking and performance evaluation	Data regarding all aspects of this process are tracked and fed back into system for subsequent improvements
7. Education and training	Staff required to participate in initial and continuing training requirement on this process, including disclosure practices. In addition, providers are made aware of availability of a caregiver support program ("second victim") for use after errors

Reproduced with permission from McDonald TB, Helmchen LA, Smith KM, et al. Responding to patient safety incidents: the "seven pillars". *Qual Saf Health Care* 2010;19:e11.

While claims are clearly associated with specialty risk, even within specialties there are substantial variations in risk. In fact, research suggests that a small fraction of physicians may account for a large fraction of paid malpractice claims.[36] Such studies help identify "high risk" physicians and, perhaps, identify actions (improving safety systems or offering education in physician–patient communication) that may lower the risk.

What types of cases trigger the most malpractice suits and yield the biggest awards? Research has shown that the magnitude of the patient's disability was by far a better predictor of victory and award size than was proof of a breach of "standard of care." In other words, the American malpractice system distributes compensation largely based on the degree of injury, not the degree of malpractice.

This is not altogether surprising, because malpractice cases are generally heard by juries composed of ordinary citizens who can see themselves in the plaintiff's shoes. "In a case like this," said the attorney who represented the physician in the case that began this chapter, "involving a patient who was already in the hospital, who has an arrest and anoxic [brain damage], one of the very significant perceptual issues we have to consider … is the fact that there was a catastrophic outcome, and to some jurors, catastrophic outcomes may equate with 'somebody must have messed up.'"[1] And so, despite expert testimony that the doctor's decision to postpone intubation was medically sound, the attorney advised his client to settle out of court, which she did. The frequency of this outcome—even when the physician believes she was anything but negligent—provides an incentive for more lawsuits.

Given the problems in the American malpractice system, *pain-and-suffering caps* (first implemented in California after a malpractice crisis in the 1980s) have been touted as a way of moderating insurance premiums.[37] Recent evidence suggests that such caps do in fact reduce malpractice payments.[38] However, such caps are politically charged, and at least one U.S. state (Illinois) has ruled them unconstitutional.[39,40] Moreover, caps don't solve the fundamental problem. Physicians worry more about the costs—both financial and psychological—of the process than the costs of the settlement. If a patient comes in with a headache and, after a conscientious work-up, we conclude it is almost certainly not a brain tumor, we reassure the patient and look for other diagnoses. However, if one out of every 5000 times a patient *does* have a brain tumor and we skipped the computed tomography (CT) scan, we can count on being sued. In that case, the expense and emotional costs—time lost to depositions, hand-wringing and demoralization, sleepless nights, and suppressed anger over the unfairness of it all—are essentially the same for the physician, whether the payout is $400,000 or $2 million. As doctors, our decision making is driven more by the potential for being sued than by the cost of losing a judgment.

In the early 2000s, Studdert, Brennan, and colleagues made a strong case for replacing the adversarial tort-based malpractice approach with a *no-fault system* modeled on workers' compensation.[1,41] It would function this way: a no-fault pool would be created from insurance premiums, from which awards would be made following the simple establishment that there was healthcare-associated harm. There would be no need to prove that the caregiver was negligent or the care was substandard. The proposed advantages of the system include more rapid adjudication of cases and far lower overhead (to lawyers, expert witnesses, and so on). In most no-fault proposals, institutions would be "experience rated" (i.e., their premiums would be set based on their payout histories), providing an incentive to create and maintain safe systems of care.

There are many concerns about the viability and political feasibility of a no-fault system in the United States, and setting the bar for compensation will be challenging. For instance, setting a low bar (such as compensation for a gastrointestinal bleed after appropriate use of a nonsteroidal anti-inflammatory agent) would cause the compensation pool to go broke. On the other hand, if compensation goes to only those patients who are the victims of horrible and dramatic events such as wrong-site surgery, then too many people suffering significant harm go uncompensated. Some experts also worry that a compensation pool approach would cause healthcare professionals to slacken their safety efforts. However, evidence supporting a deterrent effect of the current malpractice system is quite limited.[1]

In part because of political objections to the concept of—even the very words—"no fault," the discussion in recent years has tended to focus on so-called "*health courts*."[40,42] These build on the disclosure trend discussed earlier, but go further by informing patients at the time of disclosure that they can file a compensation claim. Such claims are heard by a panel of experts, which determines "avoidability" (a somewhat lower bar than negligence) and recommends a settlement: full recompense for economic losses and a pain and suffering award based on a predetermined compensation schedule that hinges on the severity of the injury. Enthusiasm for this model is growing, and some federal funding has been made available for pilot experiments.

The reports from other countries that have tried no-fault or health court systems have been mixed but generally favorable. New Zealand, for example, switched to a no-fault system for *all* personal injuries, including healthcare related ones, in 1972. The no-fault system is seen as a partial success, although there has been agitation for a more fault-based system to deal with egregious errors.[2,43] The Swedish no-fault system remains effective and popular after more than two decades. Sweden limits compensable events to medical injuries that were "avoidable," and eligible patients must have spent at least 10 days in the hospital or endured at least 30 sick days.[2,41,42]

These early experiences and international comparisons are helpful. Yet if there is one thing about the malpractice system that is clear, it is that the debate about the best way to handle patient injuries is driven more by political realities than policy arguments and data. For now, the American malpractice system remains highly unpopular, with few people believing that it fairly assesses blame or compensates victims.[44] From the standpoint of patient safety, the system's main problems are that it promotes an adversarial environment that encourages secrecy rather than the openness necessary for problem solving, and that it tends to point fingers at people rather than focus on system defects. In recent years, we have seen some impressive institutionally-based innovations, particularly around disclosure. But there seems little hope that the larger American malpractice system will give way to a better alternative any time in the foreseeable future, although Republican administrations tend to be more critical of the malpractice system than Democratic ones.

MEDICAL MALPRACTICE CASES AS A SOURCE OF SAFETY LESSONS

Before concluding our discussion of the malpractice system, it is worth recalling that it was a study of malpractice—the Harvard Medical Practice Study—that inspired the patient safety movement by generating the estimate of 44,000 to 98,000 yearly deaths from errors used by the Institute of Medicine in *To Err Is Human*.[45–47] Malpractice claims databases offer an important way of viewing patient safety, illustrating, for example, a far higher frequency of diagnostic errors (Chapter 6) than do other safety "lenses" such as incident reporting systems or administrative databases.[48] Many important safety insights have come from so-called *closed claim analyses*—analyses of malpractice cases that have already been settled.[49–54]

In addition, malpractice cases are a rich source of information for teaching about both patient safety content areas and the malpractice system itself. Hochberg et al. described a training intervention that used data from their own hospital's malpractice experience to educate surgical residents about both safety and malpractice.[55]

The fact that this intervention is considered an innovation points to yet another maddening aspect of the malpractice system: it is so politically charged that its potential as a rich font of patient safety knowledge and wisdom generally goes untapped. We live in a world of ever-increasing transparency, in which a hospital's mortality rates, readmission rates, financial health, and even what patients think of the food are all a click away on the Web. Yet information about malpractice cases remains the most cloistered in healthcare. It is time to begin tearing down this particular wall.[56] As we do, it will be vital for clinician-leaders, educators, and researchers to use this information prudently and effectively in the service of improving safety.[57]

KEY POINTS

- The medical malpractice system in the United States is governed by the rules of tort law, which compensates injury victims with the resources of at-fault providers.
- Among the criticisms of the malpractice system are its arbitrariness, its high administrative costs, and its tendency to assign individual blame rather than seek system solutions. The latter issue often places the malpractice system in conflict with the goals of the patient safety movement.
- An important recent trend has been to promote disclosure of adverse events and errors to patients. Emerging evidence is that disclosure and apology, when accompanied by rapid settlement offers where appropriate, may lower overall malpractice costs. Many states have passed laws protecting some portions of disclosures and accompanying apologies from being used in court.
- Pain and suffering award caps can help limit the size of awards and decrease the propensity of attorneys to accept cases on contingency, but do not improve the fundamental flaws in the system.
- No-fault or health court systems, in which patients are compensated based on their injuries without the need to assign fault, have been promoted in the United States. Early international experiences with such systems have been generally positive.

REFERENCES

1. Brennan TA, Mello MM. Patient safety and medical malpractice: a case study. *Ann Intern Med* 2003;139:267–273.
2. Merry A, McCall Smith A. *Errors, Medicine, and the Law*. Cambridge, UK: Cambridge University Press; 2001.
3. Johnston N. Do blame and punishment have a role in organizational risk management? *Flight Deck* 1995;Spring:33–36.
4. Reason JT. *Managing the Risks of Organizational Accidents*. Aldershot, Hampshire, UK: Ashgate Publishing Limited; 1997.
5. The National Patient Safety Foundation's Lucian Leape Institute Report of the Roundtable on Transparency. *Shining a Light: Safer Health Care Through Transparency*. Boston, MA: National Patient Safety Foundation; January 2015.
6. Wachter RM, Shojania KG. *Internal Bleeding: The Truth Behind America's Terrifying Epidemic of Medical Mistakes*. New York, NY: Rugged Land; 2004.
7. Jena AB, Seabury S, Lakdawalla D, Chandra A. Malpractice risk according to physician specialty. *N Engl J Med* 2011;365:629–636.

8. Mello MM, Chandra A, Gawande AA, Studdert DM. National costs of the medical liability system. *Health Aff (Millwood)* 2010;29:1569–1577.

9. Blendon RJ, Schoen C, DesRoches CM, Osborn R, Zapert K, Raleigh E. Confronting competing demands to improve quality: a five-country hospital survey. *Health Aff (Millwood)* 2004;23:119–135.

10. Brennan TA, Localio AR, Leape LL, et al. Identification of adverse events occurring during hospitalization. A cross-sectional study of litigation, quality assurance, and medical records at two teaching hospitals. *Ann Intern Med* 1990;112:221–226.

11. Hickson GB, Clayton EW, Githens PB, Sloan FA. Factors that prompted families to file medical malpractice claims following perinatal injuries. *JAMA* 1992;267:1359–1363.

12. Kraman SS, Hamm G. Risk management: extreme honesty may be the best policy. *Ann Intern Med* 1999;131:963–967.

13. Kraman SS, Cranfill L, Hamm G, Woodard T. John M. Eisenberg Patient Safety Awards. Advocacy: the Lexington Veterans Affairs Medical Center. *Jt Comm J Qual Improv* 2002;28:646–650.

14. Studdert DM, Mello MM, Gawande AA, Brennan TA, Wang YC. Disclosure of medical injury to patients: an improbable risk management strategy. *Health Aff (Millwood)* 2007;26:215–226.

15. Kachalia A, Kaufman SR, Boothman R, et al. Liability claims and costs before and after implementation of a medical error disclosure program. *Ann Intern Med* 2010;153:213–221.

16. Boothman RC, Blackwell AC, Campbell DA Jr, Commiskey E, Anderson S. A better approach to medical malpractice claims? The University of Michigan experience. *J Health Life Sci Law* 2009;2:125–159.

17. Lambert BL, Centomani NM, Smith KM, et al. The "Seven Pillars" response to patient safety incidents: effects on medical liability processes and outcomes. *Health Serv Res* 2016;51 Suppl 3:2491–2515.

18. Murtagh L, Gallagher TH, Andrew P, Mello MM. Disclosure-and-resolution programs that include generous compensation offers may prompt a complex patient response. *Health Aff (Millwood)* 2012;12:2681–2689.

19. Loren DJ, Garbutt J, Dunagan WC, et al. Risk managers, physicians, and disclosure of harmful medical errors. *Jt Comm J Qual Patient Saf* 2010;36:101–108.

20. Gallagher TH, Waterman AD, Ebers AG, Fraser VJ, Levinson W. Patients' and physicians' attitudes regarding the disclosure of medical errors. *JAMA* 2003;289:1001–1007.

21. Mazor KM, Reed GW, Yood RA, Fischer MA, Baril J, Gurwitz JH. Disclosure of medical errors: what factors influence how patients respond? *J Gen Intern Med* 2006;21:704–710.

22. Helmchen LA, Richards MR, McDonald TB. How does routine disclosure of medical error affect patients' propensity to sue and their assessment of provider quality? Evidence from survey data. *Med Care* 2010;48:955–961.

23. When Things Go Wrong: Responding to Adverse Events. *A Consensus Statement of the Harvard Hospitals*. Burlington, VT: Massachusetts Coalition for the Prevention of Medical Errors; 2006.

24. Gallagher TH, Garbutt JM, Waterman AD, et al. Choosing your words carefully: how physicians would disclose harmful medical errors to patients. *Arch Intern Med* 2006;166:1585–1593.

25. National Quality Forum. *Safe Practices for Better Healthcare: 2006 Update*. Washington, DC: National Quality Forum; 2007.

26. McDonnell WM, Guenther E. Narrative review: do state laws make it easier to say "I'm sorry?" *Ann Intern Med* 2008;149:811–815.

27. Perez B, DiDona T. Assessing legislative potential to institute error transparency: a state comparison of malpractice claims rates. *J Healthc Qual* 2010;32:36–41.

28. Mastroianni AC, Mello MM, Sommer S, Hardy M, Gallagher TH. The flaws in state 'apology' and 'disclosure' laws dilute their intended impact on malpractice suits. *Health Aff (Millwood)* 2010;29:1611–1619.

29. Available at: http://www.sorryworks.net/.

30. In Conversation with … Thomas H. Gallagher, MD [Perspective]. *AHRQ PSNet* (serial online); January 2009. Available at: https://psnet.ahrq.gov/perspectives/perspective/69.

31. Rathert C, Phillips W. Medical error disclosure training: evidence for values-based ethical environments. *J Bus Ethics* 2010;97:491–503.

32. Stroud L, Wong BM, Hollenberg E, Levinson W. Teaching medical error disclosure to physicians-in-training: a scoping review. *Acad Med* 2013;88:884–892.

33. Gallagher TH, Mello MM, Levinson W, et al. Talking with patients about other clinicians' errors. *N Engl J Med* 2013;369:1752–1757.

34. McDonald TB, Helmchen LA, Smith KM, et al. Responding to patient safety incidents: the "seven pillars". *Qual Saf Health Care* 2010;19:e11.

35. Studdert DM, Thomas EJ, Burstin HR, Zbar BI, Orav EJ, Brennan TA. Negligent care and malpractice claiming behavior in Utah and Colorado. *Med Care* 2000;38:250–260.

36. Studdert DM, Bismark MM, Mello MM, Singh H, Spittal MJ. Prevalence and characteristics of physicians prone to malpractice claims. *N Engl J Med* 2016;374:354–362.

37. Hellinger FJ, Encinosa WE. The impact of state laws limiting malpractice damage awards on health care expenditures. *Am J Public Health* 2006;96:1375–1381.

38. Seabury SA, Helland E, Jena AB. Medical malpractice reform: noneconomic damages caps reduced payments 15 percent, with varied effects by specialty. *Health Aff (Millwood)*. 2014;33:2048–2056.

39. Mello MM, Brennan TA. The role of medical liability reform in federal health care reform. *N Engl J Med* 2009;361:1–3.

40. Mello MM, Gallagher TH. Malpractice reform—opportunities for leadership by health care institutions and liability insurers. *N Engl J Med* 2010;362:1353–1356.

41. Studdert DM, Brennan TA. No-fault compensation for medical injuries: the prospect for error prevention. *JAMA* 2001;286:217–223.

42. Mello MM, Studdert DM, Kachalia AB, Brennan TA. "Health courts" and accountability for patient safety. *Milbank Q* 2006;84:459–492.

43. Bismark MM, Brennan TA, Patterson RJ, Davis PB, Studdert DM. Relationship between complaints and quality of care in New Zealand: a descriptive analysis of complainants and non-complainants following adverse events. *Qual Saf Health Care* 2006;15:17–22.

44. Gawande AA. The malpractice mess. *New Yorker*. 2005:62–71.

45. Brennan TA, Leape LL, Laird NM, et al. Incidence of adverse events and negligence in hospitalized patients. Results of the Harvard Medical Practice Study I. *N Engl J Med* 1991;324:370–376.

46. Leape LL, Brennan TA, Laird N, et al. The nature of adverse events and negligence in hospitalized patients. Results of the Harvard Medical Practice Study II. *N Engl J Med* 1991;324:377–384.

47. Kohn L, Corrigan J, Donaldson M, eds. *To Err Is Human: Building a Safer Health System*. Committee on Quality of Health Care in America, Institute of Medicine. Washington, DC: National Academies Press; 1999.

48. Levtzion-Korach O, Frankel A, Alcalai H, et al. Integrating incident data from five reporting systems to assess patient safety: making sense of the elephant. *Jt Comm J Qual Patient Saf* 2010;36:402–410.

49. Schiff GD, Puopolo AL, Huben-Kearney A, et al. Primary care closed claims experience of Massachusetts malpractice insurers. *JAMA Intern Med* 2013;173:2063–2068.

50. Gandhi TK, Kachalia A, Thomas EJ, et al. Missed and delayed diagnoses in the ambulatory setting: a study of closed malpractice claims. *Ann Intern Med* 2006;145:488–496.

51. Lee LA, Caplan RA, Stephens LS, et al. Posteroperative opioid-induced respiratory depression: a closed claims analysis. *Anesthesiology* 2015;122:659–665.

52. Goergen S, Schultz T, Deakin A, Runciman W. Investigating errors in medical imaging: lessons for practice from medicolegal closed claims. *J Am Coll Radiol* 2015;12:988–997.

53. Dutton RP, Lee LA, Stephens LS, Posner KL, Davies JM, Domino KB. Massive hemorrhage: a report from the anesthesia closed claims project. *Anesthesiology* 2014;121:450–458.

54. Bishop TF, Ryan AK, Casalino LP. Paid malpractice claims for adverse events in the inpatient and outpatient settings. *JAMA* 2011;305:2427–2431.

55. Hochberg MS, Seib CD, Berman RS, Kalet AL, Zabar SR, Pachter HL. Perspective: malpractice in an academic medical center: a frequently overlooked aspect of professionalism education. *Acad Med* 2011;86:365–368.

56. Alper EJ, Wachter RM. Commentary: medical malpractice and patient safety—tear down that wall. *Acad Med* 2011;86:282–284.

57. Mello MM, Studdert DM. Building a national surveillance system for malpractice claims. *Health Serv Res* 2016;51:2642–2648.

ADDITIONAL READINGS

Arlen J. *Economic Analysis of Medical Malpractice Liability and Its Reform*. New York, NY: New York University School of Law; May 9, 2013. Public Law Research Paper No. 13-25.

Gallagher TH, Farrell ML, Karson H, et al. Collaboration with regulators to support quality and accountability following medical errors: the communication and resolution program certification pilot. *Health Serv Res* 2016;51:2569–2582.

Gallagher TH. A 62-year-old woman with skin cancer who experienced wrong-site surgery: review of medical error. *JAMA* 2009;302:669–677.

Gallagher TH, Studdert D, Levinson W. Disclosing harmful medical errors to patients. *N Engl J Med* 2007;356:2713–2719.

Gawande A. *Complications: A Surgeon's Notes on an Imperfect Science*. New York, NY: Metropolitan Books; 2002.

Helmchen LA, Lambert BL, McDonald TB. Changes in physician practice patterns after implementation of a communication-and-resolution program. *Health Serv Res* 2016;51:2516–1536.

Mello MM, Studdert DM, Kachalia A. The medical liability climate and prospects for reform. *JAMA* 2014;312:2146–2155.

O'Reilly KB. "I'm sorry": why is that so hard for doctors to say? *American Medical News*. February 1, 2010.

Roland M, Rao SR, Sibbald B, et al. Professional values and reported behaviours of doctors in the USA and UK: quantitative survey. *BMJ Qual Saf* 2011;20:515–521.

Sage WM, Harding MC, Thomas EJ. Resolving malpractice claims after tort reform: experience in a self-insured Texas public academic health system. *Health Serv Res* 2016;51:2615–2633.

Thomas MO, Quinn CJ, Donohue GM. *Practicing Medicine in Difficult Times: Protecting Physicians from Malpractice Litigation*. Sudbury, MA: Jones Bartlett; 2009.

Youngberg BJ, ed. *Principles of Risk Management and Patient Safety*. Sudbury, MA: Jones Bartlett; 2011.

ACCOUNTABILITY | 19

OVERVIEW

As this book has emphasized, the fundamental underpinning of the modern patient safety field is "systems thinking"—the notion that most errors are made by competent, caring people, and that safe care therefore depends on embedding providers in systems that anticipate errors and block them from causing harm. That is an attractive viewpoint, and undoubtedly correct most of the time. But it risks causing us to avert our eyes from those providers or institutions who, for a variety of reasons, are not competent, or worse.

After last chapter's discussion of the malpractice system—the most visible, but often dysfunctional, incarnation of accountability in healthcare—this chapter focuses on more subtle issues, including "Just Culture," dealing with disruptive providers, and the role of the media in patient safety. At its heart, the chapter aims to address one of the most challenging questions in patient safety: can our desire for a "no blame" culture, with all its benefits, be reconciled with the need for accountability?[1]

ACCOUNTABILITY

Scott Torrence, a 36-year-old insurance broker, was struck in the head while going up for a rebound during his weekend basketball game. Over the next few hours, a mild headache escalated into a thunderclap, and he became lethargic and vertiginous. His girlfriend called an ambulance to take him to the emergency room in his local rural hospital, which lacked a CT or MRI scanner.

The ER physician, Dr. Jane Benamy, worried about brain bleeding, called neurologist Dr. Roy Jones at the regional referral hospital (a few hundred miles away) requesting that Torrence be transferred. Jones refused, reassuring Benamy that the case sounded like "benign positional vertigo." Benamy worried, but had no recourse. She sent Torrence home with medications for vertigo and headache.

The next morning, Benamy reevaluated Torrence, and he was markedly worse, with more headache and vertigo, now accompanied by vomiting and photophobia (bright lights hurt his eyes). She called neurologist Jones again, who again refused the request for transfer. Completely frustrated, she hospitalized Torrence for intravenous pain medications and close observation.

The next day, the patient was even worse. Literally begging, Benamy found another physician (an internist named Soloway) at Regional Medical Center to accept the transfer, and Torrence was sent there by air ambulance. The CT scan at Regional was read as unrevealing (in retrospect, a subtle but crucial abnormality was overlooked), and Soloway managed Torrence's symptoms with more pain medicines and sedation. Overnight, however, the patient deteriorated even further—"awake, moaning, yelling," according to the nursing notes—and needed to be physically restrained. Soloway called the neurologist, Dr. Jones, at home, who told him that he "was familiar with the case and … the non-focal neurological exam and the normal CT scan made urgent clinical problems unlikely." He went on to say that "he would evaluate the patient the next morning."

But by the next morning, Torrence was dead. An autopsy revealed that the head trauma had torn a small cerebellar artery, which led to a cerebellar stroke (an area of the brain poorly imaged by CT scan). Ultimately, the stroke caused enough swelling to trigger brainstem herniation—extrusion of the brain through one of the holes in the base of the skull, like toothpaste squeezing through a tube. This cascade of falling dominoes could have been stopped at any stage, but that would have required the expert neurologist to see the patient, recognize the signs of the cerebellar artery dissection, take a closer look at the CT scan, and order an MRI.[2]

Cases like this one—specifically Dr. Jones's refusal to personally evaluate a challenging and rapidly deteriorating patient when asked repeatedly by concerned colleagues to do so—demonstrate the tension between the "no-fault" stance embraced by the patient safety field and the importance of establishing and enforcing standards. That such cases occur should not surprise anyone. Despite years of training, doctors are as vulnerable as anyone to all the maladies that can beset professionals in high-demand, rapidly changing professions: not keeping up, drug and alcohol abuse, depression, burnout, or just failing to care enough.

But how can we reconcile the need for accountability with our desire to abandon our traditional "blame and shame" approach and embrace a new focus on system safety? As Dr. Lucian Leape, the Harvard surgeon and father of the modern patient safety movement, once said:

> *There is no accountability. When we identify doctors who harm patients, we need to try to be compassionate and help them. But in the end, if they are a danger to patients, they shouldn't be caring for them. A fundamental principle has to be the development and then the enforcement of procedures and standards. We can't make real progress without them. When a doctor doesn't follow them, something has to happen. Today, nothing does, and you have a vicious cycle in which people have no real incentive to follow the rules because they know there are no consequences if they don't. So there are bad doctors and bad nurses, but the fact that we tolerate them is just another systems problem.*[2]

One of the definitions of a profession is that it is self-policing: it sets its own standards and enforces them with its members (*"peer review"*). Despite this responsibility, it is undeniable that doctors and hospitals tend to protect their own, sometimes at the expense of patients. Hospital credentials committees, which certify and periodically recertify individual doctors, rarely limit a provider's privileges, even when there is stark evidence of failure to meet a reasonable standard of care. If alcohol or drug abuse is the problem, a physician may be ordered to enter a "diversion" program, a noble idea, but one that sometimes errs on the side of protecting the interests of the dangerous provider over an unwitting public. One survey study conservatively estimates that almost 10% of healthcare professionals may have encountered impaired or incompetent colleagues in the past year.[3] Another survey found that 70% of physicians believe it is their professional responsibility to report an impaired or incompetent colleague. However, of physicians familiar with just such a colleague, one-third admitted that they failed to report him or her to a relevant authority.[4]

Why has healthcare failed to live up to its ethical mandate to self-regulate? One reason is that it is difficult to sanction one's own peers, especially when the evidence of substandard practice is anecdotal and sometimes concerns issues of personality (i.e., the disruptive physician [an issue we'll return to below], or the physician who appears to be insufficiently responsive) rather than problems with "hard outcomes." A second issue is more practical: given the length of time that it takes to train physicians, credentials committees and licensing bodies are understandably reluctant to remove a physician's privileges after the community has invested so much money and effort in training.

A final reason is that physicians tend not to be strong organizational managers. Unlike fields like law and business, in which conflict and competition are commonplace, physicians are generally not accustomed to confronting colleagues, let alone managing the regulatory and legal consequences of such confrontations. This final point is important: because litigation often follows any challenges to a physician's clinical competence (and credentials committee members are only partially shielded from lawsuits), many physicians understandably will do backflips to avoid confrontation.

Unfortunately, the evidence that there *are* bad apples—and that they are not dealt with effectively—is reasonably strong. For example, from 2005 through 2014, just 1% of U.S. doctors were responsible for 32% of paid claims (66,426 claims in total) reported to the National Practitioner Data Bank, the confidential log of malpractice cases maintained by the federal government. During that period, among the 54,099 physicians with paid claims, 84% incurred only one claim, 16% had two claims and 4% had three or more claims. The risk of recurrent claims increased with the number of previously paid claims, leading the authors to conclude that a small number of physicians continue to be responsible for a significant fraction of paid claims.[5] Despite this data, there is little evidence to suggest that physicians who continue to practice inappropriately are adequately disciplined by state licensing boards; in fact, recent evidence suggests large state-to-state variations in disciplinary actions taken by medical licensure boards.[6]

Of course, in the group of oft-sued doctors[7] are some very busy obstetricians and neurosurgeons who take on tough cases (probably accompanied by poor bedside manner—there is a striking correlation between the number of patient complaints about a physician's personal style and the probability of lawsuits,[8] and a small fraction of physicians continue to account for a large number of complaints).[9] But this group undoubtedly also includes some very dangerous doctors. We simply must find better ways to measure whether doctors are meeting the relevant professional standards—the computerization of practice should help by making it easier to tell whether doctors are practicing high-quality, evidence-based medicine. Moreover, efforts at remediation (and discipline, if necessary) must begin early: one study found that evidence of unprofessional behavior in medical school was a powerful predictor of subsequent disciplinary action by medical boards, often decades later.[10]

While the above discussion has emphasized the quality of physician care, similar issues arise with other health professionals. In these other fields, however, there has been a stronger tradition of accountability, in part because nurses often work for institutions such as hospitals (and therefore can be more easily fired or disciplined) and because they have less power. But these judgments can also be arbitrary and ineffective, and the disparity with physicians creates its own problems. The bar for competence and performance should be set high for all healthcare professionals, and the consequences of failing to meet standards should be similar.[11] Nothing undermines an institution's claim to be committed to safety more than for frontline workers to see that there is one set of standards for nurses and a wholly different one for physicians.

In this regard, a major change over the past few years has been the development of critical safety rules and standards (see also Chapter 15). Whereas concerns about professional performance in the past largely centered on clinical competence (i.e., frequent diagnostic errors, poor surgical skill), they increasingly relate to failure to adhere to standards and regulations. For example, what should be done about the physician who chooses not to perform a "time out" prior to surgery (Chapter 5)? Or the nurse who habitually fails to clean her hands before patient contact (Chapter 10)? In the end, healthcare organizations must find the strength to enforce these rules and standards, recognizing that there is no conflict between this tough love stance and the "systems approach" to patient safety. As safety expert James Reason says of habitual rule benders:

> *Seeing them get away with it on a daily basis does little for morale or for the credibility of the disciplinary system. Watching them getting their "come-uppance" is not only satisfying, it also serves to reinforce where the boundaries of acceptable behavior lie .... Justice works two ways. Severe sanctions for the few can protect the innocence of the many.*[12]

Moreover, there are cases of such egregious deviations from professional norms that the perpetrators *must* be held accountable in the name of justice and patient protection. Take the case of the Saskatchewan anesthetist convicted of criminal negligence for leaving the operating room to make a phone call (after disconnecting the ventilator alarms), leading to permanent brain injury in a 17-year-old patient,[13] or the Boston surgeon who left his patient anesthetized on the table with a gaping incision in his back to go cash a check at his local bank.[14] And even these cases pale in comparison to those of psychopathic serial killers such as Dr. Michael Swango and Dr. Harold Shipman.[15,16] These cases cry out for justice and accountability, but they are overwhelmingly the exception, which is what makes the issue of exercising appropriate accountability so vexing. The more pressing issue is how to create and enforce a system of accountability in more common situations, such as when caregivers' behavior gets in the way of good patient care.

DISRUPTIVE PROVIDERS

Although TV physicians of yesteryear were usually kind, grandfatherly types (exemplified most famously by Robert Young as Marcus Welby, MD), the modern version is Dr. Gregory House: a brilliant diagnostician who is virtually impossible to work with. This stereotype, though both dramatic and amusing, can obscure the fact that disruptive and unprofessional behavior by clinicians is relatively common and can compromise patient safety.

While only 2% to 4% of caregivers regularly engage in disruptive behavior, those who do cause substantial problems.[17] In a 2008 survey of nearly 5000 nurses and physicians, 77% reported witnessing physicians engage in disruptive behavior (most commonly verbal abuse of a staff member), and 65% reported seeing disruptive behavior by nurses.[18] (This latter figure is an important reminder that this is not just a doctor issue.) Seventy-one percent of respondents believed that unprofessional behaviors increased the likelihood of medical errors, and more than one in four felt that they were associated with preventable deaths. Disruptive and disrespectful behavior by physicians has also been tied to nursing dissatisfaction and nurses leaving the profession (Chapter 16) and linked to adverse events in numerous clinical settings (Chapter 5).[19–21] Physicians in high-stakes and procedurally oriented specialties such as surgery, obstetrics, and cardiology are judged as the most prone to such behavior.[18]

Although disruptive behavior lacks a single, unifying definition, most experts include behaviors that show disrespect for others, or interpersonal interactions that impede the delivery of patient care. In terms of patient safety, one can easily see how disruptive behavior could impair efforts to create a safety culture (Chapter 15), buttress steep hierarchies and compromise teamwork (Chapter 9), and stand in the way of a "blame-free" environment.[22] In 2008, the Joint Commission drew attention to this issue in a sentinel event alert that called for facilities to institute a "zero tolerance" policy, offer educational programs, and enact robust processes for detecting, reporting, and addressing all instances of disruptive behavior.[23]

Unfortunately, there are few data to guide efforts to prevent and address disruptive behaviors. It is clear that eliminating such behaviors requires a clear and unwavering focus by organizational leaders (Chapter 22). Modeling good behaviors, maintaining a confidential incident reporting system with robust follow-up (Chapter 14), and training managers in conflict resolution seem like good ideas. Other interventions designed to improve safety culture (Chapter 15), such as teamwork training and structured communication protocols, also have the potential to reduce disruptive behaviors, or at least promote early identification and intervention.[24, 25]

Clearly, effective approaches need to harmonize the actions of a variety of stakeholders, including hospital accreditation organizations, and physician certifying boards (which have emphasized the importance of *professionalism* as a core physician competency[26]), medical licensing boards, and individual hospitals' credentialing committees and leadership bodies. One leader

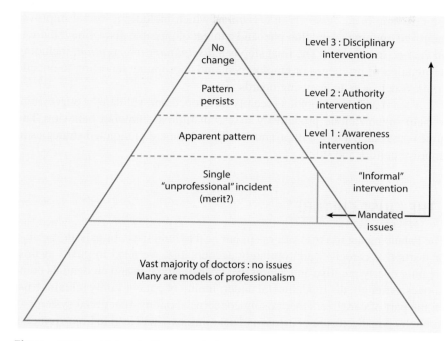

Figure 19-1 ■ Hickson's disruptive behavior pyramid for identifying, assessing, and dealing with unprofessional behavior. (Reproduced with permission from Hickson GB, Pichert JW, Webb LE, Gabbe SG. A complementary approach to promoting professionalism: identifying, measuring, and addressing unprofessional behaviors. *Acad Med* 2007;82:1040–1048.)

in this area, Dr. Gerald Hickson, has developed a "disruptive behaviors pyramid" (Figure 19-1), which has been used at his own institution (Vanderbilt University) and others to good effect.[27,28] It emphasizes the need for early identification and intervention, along with a strong and predictable escalation strategy for caregivers who fail to improve with counseling and support.

Following the pyramid from bottom to top, a single unprofessional incident should be assumed to be an isolated event and lead to an *informal intervention*, such as a "cup of coffee conversation." (Exceptions are those events for which laws or regulations mandate reporting, such as claims of sexual harassment, discrimination, or substance abuse.) For individuals who continue their unprofessional or disruptive behavior, the next step is an *awareness intervention*, in which an authority figure (or less commonly, a respected peer) shares aggregate data that demonstrate how the clinician's behavior varies from that of his or her peers. In Hickson's experience, many professionals improve after this intervention. For those caregivers who still fail to improve, the next step is an *authority intervention*, which includes a formal improvement and ongoing evaluation plan and a threat of possible discipline if there is no change in behavior. The final step is a *disciplinary intervention*, including termination of privileges or employment and appropriate reporting to outside entities such as state licensing boards.[27]

A team at Johns Hopkins recently developed and validated a survey tool to help organizations proactively assess disruptive clinician behavior. The hope is that such a tool will promote the development of targeted strategies to improve culture and safety.[29]

THE "JUST CULTURE"

The balancing act is a tricky one—in our zeal to hold the habitual rule-breaker or disruptive caregiver appropriately accountable, we need to guard against creating overly punitive and aggressive licensing boards and credentials committees. After all, the fundamental underpinning of patient safety remains trust on the part of caregivers that raising concerns about dysfunctional systems—through open disclosure of errors and near misses—will lead to improvements (Chapter 14). An overly punitive system will diminish this kind of open dialogue and exchange, and ultimately harm safety efforts.

How then to reconcile the tension between "no blame" and "blame?" In his classic book, *Managing the Risks of Organizational Accidents*, James Reason introduced the concept of Just Culture this way:

> *A 'no-blame' culture is neither feasible nor desirable. A small proportion of human unsafe acts are egregious … and warrant sanctions, severe ones in some cases. A blanket amnesty on all unsafe acts would lack credibility in the eyes of the workforce. More importantly, it would be seen to oppose natural justice. What is needed is a just culture, an atmosphere of trust in which people are encouraged, even rewarded, for providing essential safety-related information— but in which they are also clear about where the line must be drawn between acceptable and unacceptable behavior.[12]*

David Marx, an attorney and engineer, has popularized this concept over the past decade by helping to articulate where these behavioral boundaries lie. In Marx's model, Just Culture distinguishes between "human error," "at-risk behavior," and "reckless behavior." Only the latter category, defined as "acting in conscious disregard of substantial and unjustifiable risk," is blameworthy.[30,31] A simplified version of Marx's model is shown in Table 19-1.

Table 19-1 SIMPLIFIED VERSION OF MARX'S JUST CULTURE MODEL		
Mechanisms of Breach in Duty to Patient	Description	Appropriate Response by the System*
Human error	An inadvertent act by a caregiver (a "slip" or "mistake")	Console the provider
At-risk behavior	Taking shortcuts: conscious drift away from safe behaviors; caregiver violates a safety rule but doesn't perceive it as likely to cause harm (the equivalent of rolling through a stop sign)	Coach the provider
Reckless behavior	Conscious choice by caregiver to engage in behavior that he or she knows poses significant risk; ignoring required safety steps	Discipline the provider

*Importantly, Marx notes that these responses should be independent of the actual patient outcome.
  Adapted from Marx D. Patient safety and the "Just Culture": a primer for health care executives, April 17, 2001 and Marx D. *Whack-a-Mole: The Price We Pay for Expecting Perfection.* Plano, TX: By Your Side Studios; 2009.

Safety expert Allan Frankel has developed a useful algorithm, which combines several of the elements from Reason's, Marx's, and the NPSA's models (Figure 19-2).[32] Before approaching it in the context of a safety incident, Frankel asks us to reflect on several questions:

- Was the individual knowingly impaired?
- Did the individual consciously decide to engage in an unsafe act?
- Did the caregiver make a mistake that individuals of similar experience and training would be likely to make under the same circumstances ("substitution test")?
- Does the individual have a history of unsafe acts?

After having considered the answers to these questions, the algorithm guides the user through a series of steps, ultimately identifying the appropriate response for a given unsafe act.

1. Choose the column that best describes the caregiver's action. Read down the column for recommended responses.				
The caregiver's thinking was impaired by illegal or legal substances, cognitive impairment, or severe psychosocial stressors.	The caregiver wanted to cause harm.	The caregiver knowingly violated a rule and/or made a dangerous or unsafe choice. The decision appears to have been made with little or no concern about risk.	The caregiver made a potentially unsafe choice. Faulty or self-serving decision-making may be evident.	The caregiver makes or participates in an error while working appropriately and in the patient's best interest.
IMPAIRED JUDGEMENT	**MALICIOUS ACTION**	**RECKLESS ACTION**	**RISKY ACTION**	**UNINTENTIONAL ERROR**
• Discipline is warranted if illegal substances were used. • The caregiver's performance should be evaluated to determine whether a temporary work suspension would be helpful. • Help should be actively offered to the caregiver.	• Discipline and/or legal proceedings are warranted. • The caregiver's duties should be suspended immediately.	• Discipline may be warranted. • The caregiver is accountable and needs re-training. • The caregiver should participate in teaching others the lessons learned.	• The caregiver is accountable and should receive coaching. • The caregiver should participate in teaching others the lessons learned.	• The caregiver is not accountable. • The caregiver should participate in investigating why the error occured and teach others about the results of the investigation.

2. If three other caregivers with similar skills and knowledge would do the same in similar circumstances:		
The system supports reckless action and requires fixing. The caregiver is probably less accountable for the action, and system leaders share in the accountability.	The system supports risky action and requires fixing. The caregiver is probably less accountable for the action, and system leaders share in the accountability.	The system supports errors and requires fixing. The system's leaders are accountable and should apply error-proofing improvements.

3. If the caregiver has a history of repeatedly making mistakes, the caregiver may be in the wrong position. Evaluation is warranted, and coaching, transfer or termination should be considered. The corrective actions above should be modified accordingly.

Figure 19-2 ▪ Frankel's algorithm for analyzing caregivers' actions and recommended responses in analyzing risks. (Reproduced with permission from Leonard MW, Frankel A. The path to safe and reliable healthcare. *Patient Educ Couns* 2010;80:288–292.)

RECONCILING "NO BLAME" AND ACCOUNTABILITY

A prominent physician-executive once gave a lecture in which he quipped that he had three boxes on his corporate desk: his Inbox, his Outbox, and his "TooHard" box. During the first few years of the safety movement, enthusiasm for the "no blame" model led us to file the vital question of balancing "no blame" and accountability in our own TooHard box. The recent interest in these Just Culture models is a sign that we have finally dropped this issue into our collective Inboxes, where it belongs. Organizational leaders should study these models and then educate their providers and managers about the overall concept and at least one of the models. Formal training in the Just Culture concepts may help close the gap between leadership and frontline staff perceptions of safety culture.[33]

In a 2009 *New England Journal of Medicine* article, Wachter and Pronovost explore this issue more fully, focusing specifically on the need to include physicians in an accountability framework—one that does not shy away from blame and even penalties for those who fail to follow important evidence-based safety rules.[34] The authors use the example of hand hygiene to highlight a number of prerequisites that should be met before an accountability approach is applied (Table 19-2), and recommended actions once such conditions are met. They conclude the article this way:

> Part of the reason we must do this is that if we do not, other stakeholders, such as regulators and state legislatures, are likely to judge the reflexive invocation of the "no blame" approach as an example of guild behavior—of the medical profession circling its wagons to avoid confronting harsh realities, rather than as a thoughtful strategy for attacking the root causes of most errors. With that as their conclusion, they will be predisposed to further intrude on the practice of medicine, using the blunt and often politicized sticks of the legal, regulatory, and payment systems.
>
> Having our own profession unblinkingly deem some behaviors as unacceptable, with clear consequences, will serve as a vivid example of our professionalism and thus represent our best protection against such outside intrusions. But the main reason to find the right balance between "no blame" and individual accountability is that doing so will save lives.[34]

Before leaving the topic of accountability, it is worthwhile connecting the dots between the issues explored in this chapter and those highlighted in Chapter 2, when we discussed sharp-end and blunt-end errors. The kind of accountability that we have discussed in this chapter largely relates to sharp-end providers: the clinician who makes the diagnosis of aortic dissection, cuts out the lung tumor, reads the pathology specimen, or hangs the bag of dobutamine. Bell et al. emphasize the importance of *collective accountability*— accountability at the level of the individual clinician, the healthcare team, *and the institution*.[35] The increasing emphasis on public reporting (Chapter 14), disclosure of adverse events (Chapter 18), and regulatory and accreditation solutions (Chapter 20) are ways of promoting collective accountability. As you can see, even if we reach consensus that accountability and even blame are appropriate at times, trying to fairly identify the target for this accountability is yet another issue that has been in our "TooHard" box until recently. It will require a lot of thoughtful analysis and discussion to get this balance right as well.

Other issues surrounding safety and culture are covered, from a somewhat different perspective, in Chapter 15.

Table 19-2 PREREQUISITES FOR MAKING THE CHOICE TO PUNISH PROVIDERS FOR NOT ADHERING TO A PATIENT SAFETY PRACTICE, USING THE EXAMPLE OF HAND HYGIENE	
Prerequisite	**Example of Hand Hygiene**
The patient safety problem that is being addressed is important	Rates of healthcare-associated infections are unacceptably high, resulting in serious morbidity and mortality
The literature or expert consensus strongly supports adherence to the practice as an effective strategy to decrease the probability of harm	Many studies and long-standing expert consensus support the value of hand hygiene, and healthcare-associated infections are now reported publicly and are subject to "no pay" initiatives*
Clinicians have been educated about the importance of the practice and the evidence supporting it	Lectures, reminder systems, academic detailing, dissemination of literature, and other steps to educate caregivers have been completed
The system has been modified, if necessary, to make it as easy as possible to adhere to the practice without disrupting other crucial work or creating unanticipated negative consequences; concerns by providers regarding barriers to compliance have been addressed†	Hand gel dispensers have been placed in convenient locations throughout the building; dispensers are never empty and work well (e.g., they do not squirt gel onto providers' clothes)
Physicians, other providers, and leaders have reached a consensus on the value of the practice and the process by which it will be measured; physicians understand the behaviors for which they will be held accountable	Meetings have been held with relevant provider groups, including medical staff, to review the evidence behind hand hygiene, the rates of hospital-acquired infections, and the steps that have been taken to optimize the system
A fair and transparent auditing system has been developed, and clinicians are aware of its existence	Providers know that observers will periodically audit hand-hygiene practices; observers can determine whether providers adhere to the practices, even if hands are cleaned inside patients' rooms (including the use of video or systems that sound an alarm when providers approach patients' beds without using nearby hand-cleaning dispensers)
Clinicians who do not adhere to the practice once or perhaps twice have been counseled about the importance of the practice, about the steps that have been taken to make it easy to adhere, and about the fact that further transgressions will result in punishment; the consequences of failure to adhere have been described	A physician, for example, might receive a warning note or be counseled by a departmental chair after the first or second observed transgression

(continued)

Prerequisite	Example of Hand Hygiene
Table 19-2 **PREREQUISITES FOR MAKING THE CHOICE TO PUNISH PROVIDERS FOR NOT ADHERING TO A PATIENT SAFETY PRACTICE, USING THE EXAMPLE OF HAND HYGIENE (Continued)**	
The penalties for infractions are understood and applied fairly	Chronic failure to clean hands will result in a 1-week suspension from clinical practice, accompanied by completion of a 2-hour online educational module on infection prevention

*Because of the vigorous regulatory and reporting environment in patient safety, it is likely that if the first two criteria are met, the practice will be one that is mandated by an accrediting organization (such as the Joint Commission) or that adherence to the practice, or instances of the patient safety problem it addresses, are being publicly reported or are the subject of financial penalties (e.g., through Medicare's "no pay for errors" initiative). However, we do not believe that such external pressures should be the sole reason that a practice reaches the level of punishment, since some regulated or publicly reported safety standards are flawed. On the other hand, some safety practices may meet the first two criteria before they are regulated or reported publicly, and such practices should be candidates for the above approach.

†In light of the complexities of the healthcare workplace, it is important that staff members with training in systems engineering and human factors be involved in the creation of new systems of care wherever possible. Reproduced with permission from Wachter RM, Pronovost PJ. Balancing "no blame" with accountability in patient safety. *N Engl J Med* 2009;361:1401–1406.

THE ROLE OF THE MEDIA

Many people look to the media to shine a light on the problem of patient safety and to ensure accountability. The thinking goes that such transparency (sometimes driven by mandated public reporting of errors; see Chapters 3 and 14) will create a powerful business case for safety, drive hospitals and providers toward enforcing rules and standards, and generate the resources needed to catalyze systems change. And there is no doubt that such scrutiny can have precisely this effect—it is difficult to find hospitals or health systems as energized to improve safety as those that have been the subject of widespread media coverage after a major error (Table 1-1).

But while the patient safety efforts at institutions such as Johns Hopkins, Duke, Cedars-Sinai, and Dana-Farber were clearly turbocharged by mediagenic errors, media scrutiny can also tap into institutional and individual fear of public disclosure and spur an atmosphere of silence. Such a response increases the chance that providers and organizations will fail to discuss and learn from their own errors. Although this response is usually a reflection of organizational culture and leadership (Chapters 15 and 22), the way the media chooses to handle errors also influences the way organizations respond to the prospect of media attention. The more distorted the coverage (e.g., emphasizing bad apples over systems), the more harmful the effect is likely to be.[36]

And not all media coverage provides a balanced view. Lessons from media coverage of infection control lapses within the U.S. Veterans Health

Administration provides insight on how healthcare systems can achieve clarity on issues neglected by the media.[37] A 2015 analysis of news media coverage of sentinel events involving cancer patients concluded that the media tended to find fault with individual providers without analyzing events from a systems perspective.[38] Nevertheless, media reports of medical errors seem to increasingly (though far from uniformly) reflect a more sophisticated understanding of the issues, which increases the probability that such reports will help more than harm.

KEY POINTS

- Although the systems focus is the (correct) underpinning of the modern patient safety movement, incompetent or dangerous providers and institutions must also be held accountable.
- Healthcare tends to "protect its own," which undermines public trust in the medical professions.
- Some clinicians' behavior is sufficiently disruptive to create a patient safety risk. Organizations need a strategy to manage such behavior, which sabotages teamwork, communication, and job satisfaction among colleagues.
- Vehicles to determine and enforce accountability can be local (such as hospital credentials committees) or involve outside organizations (such as state licensing boards or national professional organizations).
- Several Just Culture algorithms have emerged to help organizations and managers determine which acts represent human errors, "at-risk" behaviors, or examples of negligence. Only the latter should lead to punishment.
- The media can play an important role in ensuring accountability, especially if reporting on errors is seen as fair and reflective of our modern understanding of patient safety.

REFERENCES

1. Wachter RM. Personal accountability in healthcare: searching for the right balance. *BMJ Qual Saf* 2013;22:176–180.
2. Wachter RM, Shojania KG. *Internal Bleeding: The Truth Behind America's Terrifying Epidemic of Medical Mistakes*. New York, NY: Rugged Land; 2004.
3. Weenink JW, Westert GP, Schoonhoven L, Wollersheim H, Kool RB. Am I my brother's keeper? A survey of 10 healthcare professions in the Netherlands about experiences with impaired and incompetent colleagues. *BMJ Qual Saf* 2015;24:56–64.

4. DesRoches CM, Rao SR, Fromson JA, et al. Physicians' perceptions, preparedness for reporting, and experiences related to impaired and incompetent colleagues. *JAMA* 2010;304:187–193.

5. Studdert DM, Bismark MM, Mello MM, Singh H, Spittal MJ. Prevalence and characteristics of physicians prone to malpractice claims. *N Engl J Med* 2016;374:354–362.

6. Harris JA, Byhoff E. Variations by state in physician disciplinary actions by US medical licensure boards. *BMJ Qual Saf* 2017;26:200–208.

7. Jena AB, Seabury S, Lakdawalla D, Chandra A. Malpractice risk according to physician specialty. *N Engl J Med* 2011;365:629–636.

8. Hickson GB, Federspiel CF, Pichert JW, Miller CS, Gauld-Jaeger J, Bost P. Patient complaints and malpractice risk. *JAMA* 2002;287:2951–2957.

9. Bismark MM, Spittal MJ, Gurrin LC, Ward M, Studdert DM. Identification of doctors at risk of recurrent complaints: a national study of healthcare complaints in Australia. *BMJ Qual Saf* 2013;22:532–540.

10. Papadakis MA, Teherani A, Banach MA, et al. Disciplinary action by medical boards and prior behavior in medical school. *N Engl J Med* 2005;353:2673–2682.

11. Johnstone MJ, Kanitsaki O. Processes for disciplining nurses for unprofessional conduct of a serious nature: a critique. *J Adv Nurs* 2005;50:363–371.

12. Reason JT. *Managing the Risks of Organizational Accidents.* Aldershot, Hampshire, England: Ashgate Publishing Limited; 1997.

13. Williams LS. Anesthetist receives jail sentence after patient left in vegetative state. *CMAJ* 1995;153:619–620.

14. Anonymous. Surgeon who left an operation to run an errand is suspended. *NY Times* (Print). 2002:A13.

15. Stewart J. *Blind Eye: The Terrifying Story of a Doctor who Got Away with Murder.* New York, NY: Simon and Schuster; 2000.

16. O'Neill B. Doctor as murderer. Death certification needs tightening up, but it still might not have stopped Shipman. *BMJ* 2000;320:329–330.

17. Rawson JV, Thompson N, Sostre G, Deitte L. The cost of disruptive and unprofessional behaviors in health care. *Acad Radiol* 2013;20:1074–1076.

18. Rosenstein AH, O'Daniel M. A survey of the impact of disruptive behaviors and communication defects on patient safety. *Jt Comm J Qual Patient Saf* 2008;34;464–471.

19. Saxton R, Hines T, Enriquez M. The negative impact of nurse–physician disruptive behavior on patient safety: a review of the literature. *J Patient Saf* 2009;5:180–183.

20. Rosenstein AH, Naylor B. Incidence and impact of physician and nurse disruptive behaviors in the emergency department. *J Emerg Med* 2012;43:139–148.

21. Cochran A, Elder WB. Effects of disruptive surgeon behavior in the operating room *Am J Surg* 2015;209:6–70.

22. Leape LL, Shore MF, Dienstag JL, et al. Perspective: a culture of respect—part 1 and part 2. *Acad Med* 2012;87:845–858.

23. The Joint Commission. *Sentinel event alert. Behaviors that undermine a culture of safety.* July 9, 2008;(40):1–3.

24. Saxton R. Communication skills training to address disruptive physician behavior. *AORN J* 2012;95:602–611.

25. Sanchez LT. Disruptive behaviors among physicians. *JAMA* 2014;312:2209–2210.

26. ABIM Foundation, ACP-ASIM Foundation, European Federation of Internal Medicine. Medical professionalism in the new millennium: a physician charter. *Ann Intern Med* 2002;136:243–246.

27. Hickson GB, Pichert JW, Webb LE, Gabbe SG. A complementary approach to promoting professionalism: identifying, measuring, and addressing unprofessional behaviors. *Acad Med* 2007;82:1040–1048.

28. In conversation with … Gerald Hickson [Perspective]. *AHRQ PSNet* (serial online); December 2009. Available at: https://psnet.ahrq.gov/perspectives/perspective/81.

29. Dang D, Nyberg D, Walrath JM, Kim MT. Development and validation of the Johns Hopkins Disruptive Clinician Behavior Survey. *Am J Med Qual* 2015;30:470–476.

30. Marx D. *Patient safety and the "Just Culture": a primer for health care executives.* Medical Event Reporting System for Transfusion Medicine, Columbia University, April 17, 2001.

31. Marx D. *Whack-a-Mole: The Price We Pay for Expecting Perfection.* Plano, TX: By Your Side Studios; 2009.

32. Leonard MW, Frankel A. The path to safe and reliable healthcare. *Patient Educ Couns* 2010;80:288–292.

33. Vogelsmeier A, Scott-Cawiezell J, Miller B, et al. Influencing leadership perceptions of patient safety through just culture training. *J Nurs Care Qual* 2010;25:288–294.

34. Wachter RM, Pronovost PJ. Balancing "no blame" with accountability in patient safety. *N Engl J Med* 2009;361:1401–1406.

35. Bell SK, Delbanco T, Anderson-Shaw L, McDonald TB, Gallagher TH. Accountability for medical error: moving beyond blame to advocacy. *Chest* 2011;140:519–526.

36. Dentzer S. Media mistakes in coverage of the Institute of Medicine's error report. *Eff Clin Pract* 2000;3:305–308.

37. Maguire EM, Bokhour BG, Asch SM, et al. Disclosing large scale adverse events in the US Veterans Health Administration: lessons from media responses. *Public Health* 2016;135:75–82.

38. Li JW, Morway L, Velasquez A, Weingart SN, Stuver SO. Perceptions of medical errors in cancer care: an analysis of how the news media describe sentinel events. *J Patient Saf* 2015;11:42–51.

| ADDITIONAL READINGS

Aveling EL, Parker M, Dixon-Woods M. What is the role of individual accountability in patient safety? A multi-site ethnographic study. *Sociol Health Illn* 2016;38:216–232.

Bosk CL. *Forgive and Remember: Managing Medical Failure.* 2nd ed. Chicago, IL: University of Chicago Press; 2003.

Chassin MR, Baker DW. Aiming higher to enhance professionalism: beyond accreditation and certification. *JAMA* 2015;313:1795–1796.

Dekker S. *Just Culture: Balancing Safety and Accountability.* 3rd ed. Boca Raton, FL: CRC Press; 2016.

Dekker S. *The Field Guide to Human Error Investigations.* 3rd ed. Aldershot, UK: Ashgate Publishing; 2014.

Dekker SWA, Breakey H. 'Just culture': improving safety by achieving substantive, procedural and restorative justice. *Saf Sci* 2016;85:187–193.

Driver TH, Katz PP, Trupin L, Wachter RM. Responding to clinicians who fail to follow patient safety practices: perceptions of physicians, nurses, trainees, and patients. *J Hosp Med* 2014;9:99–105.

McLaren K, Lord J, Murray S. Perspective: delivering effective and engaging continuing medical education on physicians' disruptive behavior. *Acad Med* 2011;86:612–617.

Pettker CM, Funai EF. Getting it right when things go wrong. *JAMA* 2010;303:977–978.

Shojania KG, Dixon-Woods M. 'Bad apples': time to redefine as a type of systems problem? *BMJ Qual Saf* 2013;22:528–531.

Wachter RM. The 'must do' list: certain patient safety practices should not be elective. *Health Aff (Millwood)* August 20, 2016. Available at: http://healthaffairs.org/blog/2015/08/20/the-must-do-list-certain-patient-safety-rules-should-not-be-elective/.

Webb LE, Dmochowski RR, Moore IN, et al. Using coworker observations to promote accountability for disrespectful and unsafe behaviors by physicians and advanced practice professionals. *Jt Comm J Qual Patient Saf* 2016;42:149–164.

Whittemore AD. The competent surgeon: individual accountability in the era of "systems" failure. *Ann Surg* 2009;250:357–362.

Viera A, Kramer R. *Management and Leadership Skills for Medical Faculty*. New York, NY: Springer; 2016.

ACCREDITATION AND REGULATIONS | 20

OVERVIEW

One might hope that professionalism and concern for patients would be sufficient incentive to motivate safe behaviors on the part of providers, as well as institutional investments in system safety. Sadly, experience has taught us that this is not the case. There are simply too many competing pressures for attention and resources, and the nature of safety is that individuals and organizations can often get away with bad behavior for long periods of time. Moreover, it is unlikely that all providers and institutions will or can keep up with best practices, given a rapidly evolving research base and the never-ending need to keep at least one eye on the bottom line.

These realities create a need for more prescriptive solutions to safety: standards set by external organizations, such as accreditors, regulatory bodies, payer representatives, and government. This chapter will examine some of these solutions, beginning with regulations and accreditation.

ACCREDITATION

Regulation is "an authoritative rule," while accreditation is a process by which an authoritative body formally recognizes that an organization or a person is competent to carry out specific tasks. Much of what we tend to call regulation is actually accreditation, but takes place in an environment in which a lack of accreditation has nearly the impact of failing to adhere to a regulatory mandate. For example, the *Accreditation Council for Graduate Medical Education* (ACGME), the body that blesses U.S. residency and fellowship programs, is not a regulator but an accreditor. Nevertheless, when the ACGME mandated that residents work less than 80 hours per week in 2003 and proscribed traditional overnight call shifts for first-year residents in 2011 (Chapter 16), these directives had the force of regulation, because ACGME has the power to shut down training programs for noncompliance.[1] It is worth noting that the ACGME relaxed the latter standards in 2017 based on the lack of evidence of safety benefit and increasing concerns about handoffs and threats to professionalism, an interesting case of a commonsense accreditation standard not achieving its desired effect.

The most important accreditor in the patient safety field (in the United States) is *the Joint Commission*. The Joint Commission, which began in 1951 as a joint program of the American College of Surgeons (which launched the first hospital inspections in 1918), the American College of Physicians, the American Hospital Association, the American Medical Association, and the Canadian Medical Association, has become an increasingly powerful force over the last 15 years by more aggressively exercising its mandate to improve the safety of American hospitals (and now, through its Joint Commission International subsidiary, hospitals around the world). A list of Joint Commission *National Patient Safety Goals*, one of the organization's key mechanisms for endorsing practices, highlighting safety problems, and generating action, is shown in Appendix IV.

Until the mid-2000s, Joint Commission visits to hospitals were announced years in advance and focused on hospitals' adherence to various policies and procedures. In 2006, the process became far more robust: the accreditor's visits now come unannounced and much of the visit centers around the *Tracer Methodology*, a process by which the inspectors follow a given patient's course throughout the hospital, checking documentation of care and speaking to caregivers about their actions and their understanding of safety principles and regulations. Indeed, this more vigorous approach has been an important force for improving safety.[2]

Beginning soon after Medicare was founded in 1965, the Joint Commission was granted an exclusive arrangement by the Centers for Medicare & Medicaid Services (CMS) to act as its inspection arm. Known as a *deeming authority*, CMS made the presumption that a hospital that passed a Joint Commission inspection was also in compliance with the CMS *Conditions of Participation*. In essence, this is what gives a Joint Commission inspection its teeth: failure puts an organization at risk of losing its Medicare payments, a significant portion of most U.S. hospitals' revenue. After a few high profile cases in which Joint Commission-accredited hospitals were later revealed to have major safety problems, in 2008 CMS announced that it would extend deeming authority to other organizations that met its requirements.[3] As of this writing (2017), only three other entities (DNV Healthcare, HFAP, and CIHQ) have been granted such authority; together they now accredit a few hundred U.S. hospitals (vs. several thousand for the Joint Commission).[4]

Although the Joint Commission does regulate some physicians' offices and ambulatory sites (such as surgery centers), most such sites are either unaccredited or accredited by another organization, such as the American Association for the Accreditation of Ambulatory Surgical Facilities (AAAASF).[5] As a result of concerns raised about the safety of ambulatory surgery, an increasingly forceful set of accreditation standards has been implemented in these environments.[6] Despite this change, the ambulatory environment continues to be affected far less by the pressures of regulation and accreditation, one of the key differences between patient safety in inpatient and office settings (Chapter 12).

Physicians are subject to both regulation and accreditation standards as well. In the United States, physicians require a license to practice; such licenses are issued by the individual states, and are not specialty specific. While physicians can lose their licenses for problems that include substance abuse, criminal convictions, and incompetence, they rarely do (Chapter 19). The process of license renewal has traditionally been relatively benign, often involving proving attendance at a certain number of continuing education conferences rather than showing evidence of ongoing competence. The Federation of State Medical Boards voted in 2010 to implement a *Maintenance of Licensure* (MOL) framework, which requires that physicians demonstrate ongoing competency and commitment to professional development to renew medical licensure. The specifics of this program are still being worked out, and it is likely that specialty board *Maintenance of Certification* (MOC) activities (see below) will be accepted as meeting MOL requirements.[7]

A higher bar for physicians is *board certification*, a voluntary process through which doctors participate in activities designed to show that they are currently competent in their own specialty. While board certification differs from licensure in many ways, a key difference is that board certification *is* specialty specific: one is board certified, for example, as an internist or a pediatric cardiologist, whereas licensure has traditionally been specialty agnostic. To become board certified, physicians complete training programs (either residencies, for initial training in areas such as internal medicine, surgery, or pediatrics, or fellowships, for specialized fields such as endocrinology or interventional radiology). They then "sit for the boards" to obtain their initial board certification. Approximately 750,000 U.S. physicians are board certified in at least one of 147 specialties and subspecialties. There is good evidence that board certification is associated with higher quality of care.[8–11]

Until the late 1980s, initial board certification lasted for an entire career for the vast majority of medical specialists. However, given healthcare's breakneck pace of change and the fact that other professionals (e.g., pilots and teachers) have to recertify every few years, the *American Board of Medical Specialties* (the umbrella organization for all 24 specialty boards) now requires that its diplomates participate in MOC programs.[12] The requirements for MOC include not only passing a specialty-specific test (Part III) but also

Table 20-1   THE STRUCTURE OF MAINTENANCE OF CERTIFICATION (MOC) PROGRAMS*
Part I: Professional Standing and Professionalism—Medical specialists must hold a valid, unrestricted medical license in at least one (1) state or jurisdiction in the United States, its territories, or Canada.
Part II: Lifelong Learning and Self-Assessment—Specialists participate in educational and self-assessment programs that meet specialty-specific standards that are set by their member board.
Part III: Assessment of Knowledge, Skills and Judgment—Specialists demonstrate, through formalized examination, that they have the fundamental, practice-related and practice environment–related knowledge to provide quality care in their specialty.
Part IV: Improvement in Medical Practice—Specialists are evaluated in their clinical practice according to specialty-specific standards for patient care. They are asked to demonstrate that they can assess the quality of care they provide compared to peers and national benchmarks, and then apply the best evidence or consensus recommendations to improve that care using follow-up assessments.

Source: American Board of Medical Specialties (ABMS). The individual "member boards" (such as the American Board of Internal Medicine) vary somewhat in how they apply these requirements. Most have traditionally required physicians to provide evidence of meeting the Part I requirement at the same time that they took the secure examination (Part III), approximately every 10 years. Diplomates were required to perform self-assessment (Part II) and complete a Practice Improvement Module (Part IV) periodically. In 2014, the ABMS refined the standards in the above four-part framework and articulated that the Program for MOC is designed to incorporate six ABMS/ACGME Core Competencies: Practice-based Learning & Improvement; Patient Care & Procedural Skills; Systems-based Practice; Medical Knowledge; Interpersonal & Communication Skills; and Professionalism.

engaging in activities to measure the quality of care in one's own practice, and demonstrating a commitment to improving quality and safety (Table 20-1).

While the bulk of the literature supports recertification, the evidence is not uniform. A 2014 study compared the performance of internists with time-unlimited internal medicine board certification with those who had time-limited certification and found no difference in patient outcomes across 10 primary care performance measures.[13] Another study found that the annual incidence of ambulatory care-sensitive hospitalizations (ACSHs) increased similarly across two cohorts of Medicare patients, one treated by physicians required to participate in MOC and the other by physicians who were grandfathered out of the requirements.[14] Over the past several years, MOC has been the subject of considerable criticism from some physician groups, and in 2015 the largest board, the American Board of Internal Medicine (ABIM), announced a suspension of key elements of the program pending a detailed review. This area is likely to evolve considerably in coming years.

While there are many other ways of measuring physician competence,[15] and a variety of other stakeholders (such as insurance companies and consumer-oriented Web sites) are trying to do so, the boards have some unique attributes. First, board certification is a voluntary process organized by the medical profession itself, giving it higher credibility among physicians than measures created by outside organizations. Second, because of the challenges in measuring diagnostic acumen (Chapter 6), the boards have a singular role in assessing physicians' knowledge and diagnostic abilities. Patients generally put a significant amount of stock in knowing that their doctor is board certified, rating it among their most highly valued measures of quality.[8] Increasingly, insurers and hospitals are requiring that their physicians be board certified and actively participate in MOC, although this is not invariable.[16]

REGULATIONS

Regulation is more potent than accreditation, in that compliance is mandatory (no hospital *has* to be accredited by the Joint Commission and no doctor *has* to be board certified, though the vast majority of both hospitals and physicians choose to be) and failure to comply generally carries stiff penalties. Today, the main U.S. regulatory authorities relevant to patient safety are state governments, although there are a few federal regulations and a handful of counties and cities have safety-related regulations. Unlike countries with national health systems (such as the UK's National Health Service), in the United States there is no single entity with the authority and mandate to regulate patient safety (although Medicare, as the main payer, is influential and is increasingly willing to flex its muscle), which explains why this function has largely been left to states.

For example, several states, including California, now regulate nurse-to-patient ratios (Chapter 16), more than half of the states now require reporting of certain types of errors to a state entity (Chapter 14), some states have passed laws mandating error disclosure (Chapter 18), and numerous states require that patients admitted to hospitals be screened for methicillin-resistant *Staphylococcus aureus* (Chapter 10). Pennsylvania and Virginia have even added requirements for a certain number of hours of patient safety–specific content within their overall continuing education requirements for license renewal.

OTHER LEVERS TO PROMOTE SAFETY

One of the most important organizations in the patient safety world is not a regulator or an accreditor, but rather a Washington, DC–based nonprofit organization called the *National Quality Forum* (NQF). The NQF was established in 1999 with a three-part mission: to set goals for performance improvement, to endorse standards for measuring and reporting on performance, and to promote educational and outreach programs. In the quality world (Chapter 3), the NQF is best known for its endorsement process: many organizations that are in the business of selecting measures for public reporting or payment changes now insist on using NQF-endorsed measures. Measures that receive such endorsement have survived a rigorous and multistakeholder process focusing on the strength of the evidence.

In the patient safety world, NQF has made two other major contributions. In 2002, the NQF published a list of serious adverse events, which NQF founding president Ken Kizer famously dubbed the *Never Events* list (Kizer described the items on the list as "things that should never happen" in healthcare).[17] While early items on the list included dramatic and iconic adverse events such as wrong-site surgery and retained foreign objects after surgery (Chapter 5), the list has grown (now to 29 items) and matured over the years (Appendix VI). Because many items are not known to be fully preventable even with perfect care, the name "Never Events" is now a misnomer (the list's actual name is *Serious Reportable Events*), though it is still frequently referred to by its original, more evocative name.[18] The SRE list has assumed great importance over the years, as it now provides a basis for several key safety policies, including Medicare's "no pay for errors" initiative and a wide variety of state-based adverse event reporting programs.[19,20]

In addition to the SRE list, NQF also endorses another list of "safe practices" (Appendix VII), originally based on the *Making Healthcare Safer* report produced for the U.S. Agency for Healthcare Research and Quality.[21] The safe practices list was last updated in 2010 (it now contains 34 items) and it is used by many stakeholders to focus their safety efforts.

Healthcare payers also have tremendous leverage to move the system, though they have not wielded it in the safety arena very aggressively. One exception has been the *Leapfrog Group*, a healthcare arm of many of America's largest employers (and thus the source of a significant amount of hospital and doctor payments), which was founded in 2000 in part to catalyze patient safety activities. Leapfrog uses its contracting power to promote safe practices, either through simple transparency or by steering patients toward institutions it deems to be better performers. In 2001, it recommended three "safe practices" (computerized provider order entry [CPOE], favoring high-volume providers when there was evidence linking higher volume to better outcomes (Table 5-1), and having full-time intensivists provide critical care). In 2006, Leapfrog endorsed the NQF list of serious reportable events (Appendix VI). The evidence that Leapfrog's activities have led to more widespread implementation of the endorsed practices is mixed,[22,23] as is the evidence that Leapfrog scores are associated with other measures of quality and safety.[24,25] In 2013, Leapfrog launched a Hospital Safety Score, which it updates and publicizes twice each year.

Table 20-2 THE "PLANKS" IN THE IHI'S 2005–2006 "100,000 LIVES CAMPAIGN" AND ITS 2006–2007 "CAMPAIGN TO PROTECT 5 MILLION LIVES FROM HARM"	
100,000 Lives Campaign	**5 Million Lives Campaign**
Prevent ventilator-associated pneumonia	Prevent pressure ulcers
Prevent catheter-related bloodstream infections	Reduce the incidence of methicillin-resistant *Staphylococcus aureus* (MRSA) infection
Prevent surgical site infections	Prevent harm from high-alert medications such as anticoagulants, sedatives, and insulins
Improve care for acute myocardial infarction	Reduce surgical complications
Prevent adverse drug reactions with medication reconciliation	Deliver reliable, evidence-based care for patients with heart failure
Deploy rapid response teams	Get healthcare system "boards on board"

Even softer influence has been exercised by professional societies and nonprofit safety-oriented organizations. For example, several professional physician and nursing societies have led campaigns to improve hand hygiene (Chapter 10) and discharge coordination (Chapter 8). In 2005, the *Institute for Healthcare Improvement* (IHI), a nonprofit support and consulting organization, launched a "campaign to save 100,000 lives" by promoting a set of six safety-oriented practices in American hospitals.[26] Although IHI lacks regulatory authority and is not a payer, its campaign succeeded in enrolling more than half the hospitals in the United States. This tremendous response was followed in late 2006 by another campaign to "prevent 5 million cases of harm" through six additional practices (Table 20-2).[27] Given the various forces promoting safety in American hospitals, it is difficult to isolate the effect of the IHI campaigns, but there is no doubt that they captured the attention of the American healthcare system and generated significant change.[28,29]

It is worth adding that funders—particularly the *Agency for Healthcare Research and Quality* (AHRQ) as well as foundations and other agencies in the United States and worldwide—have had a critical influence on safety extending well beyond the dollars they distribute. AHRQ, for example, has promoted education, disseminated best practices, commissioned evidence reviews, convened stakeholders, and engaged in myriad other activities that have made it an indispensable safety leader.

Increasingly, the U.S. healthcare system—led by CMS—is embracing transparency (e.g., public reporting of performance) and differential payments for better performance ("pay for performance" and "no pay for errors").[19,30-33] The idea behind these efforts is to create a *business case for quality and safety*—a set of incentives generated by patients choosing better and safer providers, or by providers receiving higher payments for better performance. These initiatives (such as *value-based purchasing* and *no pay for errors*) may ultimately become more important than both regulation and accreditation in driving safety efforts. They are described in considerable detail in Chapter 3. In 2011, CMS announced a billion dollar campaign (the "Partnership for Patients") to promote patient safety.[34] The fact that it drew many of its themes and strategies from the two IHI campaigns should have come as no great surprise: Dr. Don Berwick, the founding head of the IHI, became CMS director the prior year (he stepped down in December, 2011). The Partnership for Patients was associated with a 17% fall in hospital-related harms between 2010 and 2014.[35]

Finally, while patient-oriented and consumer groups have added an important voice to the patient safety field, they remain relatively small. None are influential enough yet to drive the national safety agenda by themselves, but they have made important contributions by working with more powerful organizations such as the IHI, the National Patient Safety Foundation (which merged with the IHI in 2017), and AHRQ (Chapter 21).

PROBLEMS WITH REGULATORY, ACCREDITATION, AND OTHER PRESCRIPTIVE SOLUTIONS

Since regulators and accreditors have the power to mandate change, why not use these levers more aggressively? Given the toll of medical errors, wouldn't we want to use our biggest, most prescriptive guns?

Perhaps, but regulation, accreditation, and laws are what policy experts call "blunt tools," because of their highly limited ability to take into account local circumstances or institutional culture and calibrate their mandates accordingly. Therefore, they are best used for "low-hanging fruit"—areas amenable to one-size-fits-all solutions, usually because they are not particularly complex and tend not to vary from institution to institution. Examples of such areas might be "sign-your-site" (Chapter 5) and abolition of high-risk abbreviations (Chapter 4): these standards are as applicable in a 600-bed academic medical center as in an 80-bed rural hospital.

But as regulation and accreditation inch into areas that are more nuanced and dependent on cultural changes, the risk of unforeseen consequences increases. For example, the Joint Commission's 2005 requirement for medication reconciliation, though based on legitimate concerns about medication errors at points of transition (Chapters 4 and 8), vexed hospitals around the United States because of implementation problems and the absence of established best practices.[36] Leapfrog's 2001 mandate that hospitals have CPOE seemed reasonable, but it was based on the experiences of only a few, highly atypical hospitals and it proved difficult for the coalition to distinguish between effective and ineffective CPOE (Chapter 13). ACGME's duty-hour limits (Chapter 16) have allowed residents to sleep but also created collateral damage by increasing handoffs (Chapter 8). And some nurses have complained that mandatory nurse-to-patient ratios have not enhanced safety, because some hospitals have replaced clerical staff or lifting teams to meet the ratios, leaving nurses with no more direct patient care time than they had before the law (Chapter 16).

Despite these limitations, regulation is vital in certain areas, particularly when providers and institutions fail to voluntarily adopt reasonable safety standards. For example, many take-out restaurants have long read back take-out orders to ensure accurate communication (by the way, they did this without a regulatory mandate—the business case to get your take-out order right is powerful enough to motivate the practice), but no healthcare organization required this practice until the Joint Commission did so in 2003 (Chapter 8).[37]

Regulation can also standardize practices that should be standardized. Prior to the Joint Commission regulations regarding "sign-your-site," many orthopedic surgeons had taken it upon themselves to begin signing limbs in an effort to prevent wrong-site surgery. The problem: some well-meaning surgeons marked the leg *to be operated on* with an X (as in, "cut here"), while others put an X on the leg *not to be operated on* (as in, "don't cut here").[37] Obviously, without a standard system for signing the site (the Joint Commission now mandates signing the site *to be operated on*), the opportunity for misunderstanding and errors is great (Chapter 5).

This chapter's discussion mostly pertains to the United States, where the relatively limited influence of regulations reflects the decentralized structure of the healthcare system and America's traditional discomfort with central authority. In more centralized healthcare systems, the role of national regulators tends to be more important. For example, early in the patient safety movement Britain created a *National Patient Safety Agency* (NPSA), charged with assessing the state of patient safety, conducting investigations, and issuing recommendations and regulations (in 2012, the NPSA's work was transferred to the NHS Commissioning Board Special Health Authority).[38] While such agencies have the virtue of efficiency, too much central control can hamper grassroots efforts and be insufficiently responsive to local circumstances.

The lessons of complex adaptive systems (Chapter 3) are worth heeding: one-size-fits-all solutions imposed by outside entities on frontline units in complex organizations are often surprisingly ineffective. With Medicare now demonstrating increased interest in using its vast market share to act more like a regulator of safety and quality than a "dumb payer," it will be important for the United States to learn what it can from other countries and organizations with long histories of centralized control.

In the end, prescriptive tools such as regulations, accreditation standards, and laws play an important role in ensuring patient safety. It is vital that they be used and enforced when they are the right instruments for the job, and that other vehicles (transparency, payment changes, market forces and competition, social marketing, changes in training, and appeals to professionalism) be employed when they are the more appropriate tools. A law or regulation can seem like the most straightforward way to fix an important safety problem, but we should never make the mistake of underestimating the messiness and complexity of our world.

KEY POINTS

- Regulation and accreditation are powerful tools to promote patient safety in that they can mandate (or nearly mandate) certain practices. In the United States, much of the regulation is state based, whereas other nations have more federally-based regulatory models. Medicare, though, now exerts more central authority through its dual position as regulator and dominant payer.
- Accreditation of hospitals (such as by the Joint Commission and other entities), physicians (through board certification), and training programs (via the ACGME) has been an extremely important vehicle for patient safety.
- Other organizations that lack regulatory or accreditation authority can also catalyze significant change, using levers such as the establishment of standards (the NQF), changing the payment system (the Leapfrog Group and other payers), promoting research (AHRQ), or taking advantage of well-established credibility and moral authority among caregivers and delivery organizations (the IHI).
- Regulation and accreditation are "blunt tools" that are best used for "low-hanging fruit": simple and relatively standardized processes whose effectiveness is independent of organizational size, complexity, and culture. They can be problematic when applied to more complex targets such as provider communication, leadership, computerization, and medication reconciliation.

REFERENCES

1. Pastores SM, O'Connor MF, Kleinpell RM, et al. The Accreditation Council for Graduate Medical Education resident duty hour new standards: history, changes, and impact on staffing of intensive care units. *Crit Care Med* 2011;39:2540–2549.

2. Schmaltz SP, Williams SC, Chassin MR, Loeb JM, Wachter RM. Hospital performance trends on national quality measures and the association with Joint Commission accreditation. *J Hosp Med* 2011;6:458–465.

3. Gaul G. Accreditors blamed for overlooking problems. *The Washington Post.* July 25, 2005:A01.

4. Fenner K. Accreditation options: A hospital CEO's strategic choice. *Becker's Hospital Review.* May 5, 2014. Available at: http://www.beckershospitalreview.com/quality/accreditation-options-a-hospital-ceo-s-strategic-choice.html.

5. Urman RD, Philip BK. Accreditation of ambulatory facilities. *Anesthesiol Clin* 2014;32:551–557.

6. Hartocollis A, Goodman JD. At surgery clinic, rush to save Joan Rivers's life. *New York Times.* September 9, 2014.

7. Chaudhry HJ, Talmage LA, Alguire PC, Cain FE, Waters S, Rhyne JA. Maintenance of licensure: supporting a physician's commitment to lifelong learning. *Ann Intern Med* 2012;157:287–289.

8. Brennan TA, Horwitz RI, Duffy FD, Cassel CK, Goode LD, Lipner RS. The role of physician specialty board certification status in the quality movement. *JAMA* 2004;292:1038–1043.

9. Lipner RS, Hess BJ, Phillips RL Jr. Specialty board certification in the United States: issues and evidence. *J Contin Educ Health Prof* 2013;33(suppl 1):S20–S35.

10. Holmboe ES, Wang Y, Meehan TP, et al. Association between maintenance of certification examination scores and quality of care for Medicare beneficiaries. *Arch Intern Med* 2008;168:1396–1403.

11. Chen J, Rathore SS, Wang Y, Radford MJ, Krumholz HM. Physician board certification and the care and outcomes of elderly patients with acute myocardial infarction. *J Gen Intern Med* 2006;21:238–244.

12. Weiss KB. Future of board certification in a new era of public accountability. *J Am Board Fam Med* 2010;23:S32–S39.

13. Hayes J, Jackson JL, McNutt GM, Hertz BJ, Ryan JJ, Pawlikowski SA. Association between physician time-unlimited vs time-limited internal medicine board certification and ambulatory patient care quality. *JAMA* 2014;312:2358–2363.

14. Gray BM, Vandergrift JL, Johnston MM, et al. Association between imposition of a Maintenance of Certification requirement and ambulatory care-sensitive hospitalizations and health care costs. *JAMA* 2014;312:2348–2357.

15. Horsley T, Lockyer J, Cogo E, Zeiter J, Bursey F, Campbell C. National programmes for validating physician competence and fitness for practice: a scoping review. *BMJ Open* 2016;6:e010368.

16. Freed GL, Dunham KM, Gebremariam A. Changes in hospitals' credentialing requirements for board certification 2005-2010. *J Hosp Med* 2013;8:298–303.

17. Vastag B. Kenneth W. Kizer, MD, MPH: health care quality evangelist. *JAMA* 2001;285:869–871.

18. Austin JM, Pronovost PJ. "Never events" and the quest to reduce preventable harm. *J Qual Patient Saf* 2015;41:279–288.

19. Wachter RM, Foster NE, Dudley RA. Medicare's decision to withhold payment for hospital errors: the devil is in the details. *Jt Comm J Qual Patient Saf* 2008;34:116–123.

20. Hanlon C, Sheedy K, Kniffin T, Rosenthal J. *2014 Guide to State Adverse Event Reporting Systems*. Portland, ME: National Academy for State Health Policy; 2015.

21. Shojania KG, Duncan BW, McDonald KM, Wachter RM, Markowitz AJ, eds. *Making Health Care Safer: A Critical Analysis of Patient Safety Practices*. Evidence Report/ Technology Assessment No. 43, AHRQ Publication No. 01-E058. Rockville, MD: Agency for Healthcare Research and Quality; July 2001.

22. Moran J, Scanlon D. Slow progress on meeting hospital safety standards: learning from the Leapfrog Group's efforts. *Health Aff (Millwood)* 2013;32:27–35.

23. Scanlon DP, Lindrooth RC, Christianson JB. Steering patients to safer hospitals? The effect of a tiered hospital network on hospital admissions. *Health Serv Res* 2008;43:1849–1868.

24. Austin JM, Jha AK, Romano PS, et al. National hospital ratings systems share few commons scores and may generate confusion instead of clarity. *Health Aff (Millwood)* 2015;34:423–430.

25. Qian F, Lustik SJ, Diachun CA, Wissler RN, Zollo RA, Glance LG. Association between Leapfrog safe practices score and hospital mortality in major surgery. *Med Care* 2011;49:1082–1088.

26. Berwick DM, Calkins DR, McCannon CJ, Hackbarth AD. The 100,000 Lives Campaign: setting a goal and a deadline for improving health care quality. *JAMA* 2006;295:324–327.

27. McCannon CJ, Hackbarth AD, Griffin FA. Miles to go: an introduction to the 5 Million Lives Campaign. *Jt Comm J Qual Patient Saf* 2007;33:477–484.

28. Wachter RM, Pronovost PJ. The 100,000 Lives Campaign: a scientific and policy review. *Jt Comm J Qual Patient Saf* 2006;32:621–627, 631–633.

29. Berwick DM, Hackbarth AD, McCannon CJ. IHI replies to "The 100,000 Lives Campaign: a scientific and policy review." *Jt Comm J Qual Patient Saf* 2006;32: 628–630 [discussion 631–633].

30. Lindenauer PK, Remus D, Roman S, et al. Public reporting and pay for performance in hospital quality improvement. *N Engl J Med* 2007;356:486–496.

31. Ferman JH. Value-based purchasing program here to stay: payments will be based on performance. *Health Exec* 2011;26:76, 78.

32. Lee GM, Kleinman K, Soumerai SB, et al. Effect of nonpayment for preventable infections in US hospitals. *N Engl J Med* 2012;367:1428–1437.

33. Minami CA, Dahlke A, Bilimoria KY. Public reporting in surgery: an emerging opportunity to improve care and inform patients. *Ann Surg* 2015;261:241–242.

34. McCannon J, Berwick DM. A new frontier in patient safety. *JAMA* 2011;305: 2221–2222.

35. Kronick R, Arnold S, Brady J. Improving safety for hospitalized patients: much progress but many challenges remain. *JAMA* 2016;316:489–490.

36. Anonymous. Practitioners agree on medication reconciliation value, but frustration and difficulties abound. Institute for Safe Medication Practices Newsletter. July 13, 2006. Available at: http://www.ismp.org/Newsletters/acutecare/articles/20060713.asp.

37. Wachter RM, Shojania KG. *Internal Bleeding: The Truth Behind America's Terrifying Epidemic of Medical Mistakes*. New York, NY: Rugged Land; 2004.
38. Scarpello J. After the abolition of the National Patient Safety Agency. *BMJ* 2010;341:c6076.

ADDITIONAL READINGS

Chassin MR, Baker DW. Aiming higher to enhance professionalism: beyond accreditation and certification. *JAMA* 2015;313:1795–1796.

Baron RJ, Braddock CH. Knowing what we don't know—improving maintenance of certification. *N Engl J Med* 2016;375:2516–1517.

The Joint Commission. *National Patient Safety Goals*. Available at: https://www.joint commission.org/standards_information/npsgs.aspx.

Langley GJ, Moen R, Nolan KM, Nolan TW, Norman CL, Provost LP. *The Improvement Guide: A Practical Approach to Enhancing Organizational Performance*. 2nd ed. San Francisco, CA: Jossey-Bass; 2009.

McClellan M, McKethan AN, Lewis JL, Roski J, Fisher ES. A national strategy to put accountable care into practice. *Health Aff (Millwood)* 2010;29:982–990.

Plsek P. Redesigning health care with insights from the science of complex adaptive systems. Appendix B. In: *Crossing the Quality Chasm: A New Health System for the 21st Century*. Committee on Quality Health Care in America, Institute of Medicine. Washington, DC: National Academies Press; 2001:309–322.

Rajaram R, Chung JW, Kinnier CV, et al. Hospital characteristics with penalties in the Centers for Medicare & Medicaid Services Hospital-Acquired Condition Reduction Program. *JAMA* 2015;314:375–383.

THE ROLE OF PATIENTS | 21

OVERVIEW

With increasing public attention to patient safety have come calls for more participation by patients and their advocates in the search for solutions. Some of these calls have focused on individual healthcare organizations, such as efforts to include patients on hospital safety committees. Most, however, have involved enlisting patients in efforts to improve their own individual safety—often framed as a version of the question: "What can patients do to protect themselves?" This chapter will explore some of the opportunities and challenges surrounding patient engagement in their own safety, including errors caused by patients themselves. The issues surrounding disclosure of errors to patients are covered in Chapter 18.

PATIENTS WITH LIMITED ENGLISH PROFICIENCY

A previously healthy 10-month-old girl was taken to a pediatrician's office by her monolingual Spanish-speaking parents, worried about their daughter's generalized weakness. The infant was diagnosed with iron-deficiency anemia. At the time of the clinic visit, no Spanish-speaking staff or interpreters were available. One of the nurses spoke broken Spanish and in general terms was able to explain that the girl had "low blood" and needed to take a medication. The parents nodded in understanding. The pediatrician wrote the following prescription in English:

Fer-Gen-Sol iron, 15 mg per 0.6 mL, 1.2 mL daily (3.5 mg/kg)

The parents took the prescription to the pharmacy. The local pharmacy did not have a Spanish-speaking pharmacist on staff, nor did they obtain an interpreter. The pharmacist attempted to demonstrate proper dosing and administration using the medication dropper

403

and the parents nodded their understanding. The prescription label on the bottle was written in English.

The parents administered the medication at home and, within 15 minutes, the baby vomited twice and appeared ill. They took her to the nearest emergency department, where the serum iron level one hour after ingestion was found to be 365 mcg/dL, twice the upper therapeutic limit. She was admitted to the hospital for intravenous hydration and observation. On questioning, the parents stated that they had given their child a tablespoon of the medication, a 12.5-fold overdose. Luckily, the baby rapidly improved and was discharged the next day.[1]

Any discussion of patient engagement needs to start from square one—do patients understand their care and the benefits and risks of various diagnostic and therapeutic strategies (i.e., *informed consent*)? If patients cannot understand the basics of their clinical care, it seems unlikely that they can advocate for themselves when it comes to safety.

Unfortunately, many patients are in no position to understand even the basics of their care, let alone serve as bulwarks against errors. First of all, just over 60 million Americans (almost 20% of the population) speak a primary language other than English at home, and about 25 million have limited English proficiency.[2] Few hospitals have adequate translation services[3]—translation frequently takes place on an ad hoc basis, often by untrained clerical personnel or even family members.[4]

Language barriers increase the chances of adverse events and compromise safety.[5] One UCSF study found that non-English-speaking patients had a 30% higher odds of 30-day readmission to the hospital than did English speakers.[6] Other studies have documented poorer adherence to treatment and follow-up, decreased satisfaction with care, decreased comprehension of diagnosis and treatment plans, increased length of stay and more adverse drug events.[7–10] The use of professional interpreters is associated with fewer communication errors, better patient comprehension, higher patient satisfaction, and improved clinical outcomes.[11]

Although state and federal legislation requires that adequate interpreting services be made available to limited English proficiency patients, the costs and scarcity of trained interpreters have made it difficult to ensure universal access to these services.[3] The increasingly widespread use of new communication technologies, including telephonic (Figure 21-1) and video interpreter services, and even Web-based voice recognition and translation services, represents a hopeful trend.[12,13]

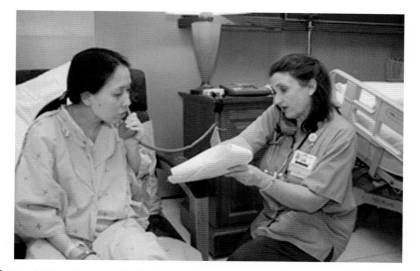

Figure 21-1 ■ The use of telephonic interpretation services in the care of hospitalized patients.

PATIENTS WITH LOW HEALTH LITERACY

Even when patients do speak English well, many are at risk because of low "health literacy," which is defined as "the degree to which individuals have the capacity to obtain, process, and understand basic health information and services needed to make appropriate health decisions."[14] It includes the skills that patients need to communicate with providers, read medical information, make decisions about treatments, carry out care regimens, and decide when and how to seek help.

In 2003, approximately 80 million U.S. adults (36%) had limited health literacy[15] (Figure 21-2); the problems are greater in patients with lower income, less education, and lower English language proficiency. Low health literacy is associated with poor communication between patients and clinicians and worse health outcomes.[15–17] Medication errors are a particular problem: studies have shown that patients with poor health literacy frequently misunderstand common dosing regimens ("Take one tablet by mouth twice daily") and auxiliary warnings (e.g., *Do not chew or crush; For external use only*).[18]

A number of strategies have been employed to mitigate the effects of low health literacy on safety. Many of them have focused on identifying patients with low literacy,[19,20] and then providing them with simplified health materials (such as brochures and medication labels), Web sites, and interactive

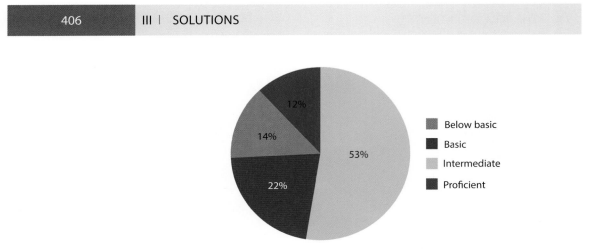

Figure 21-2 ▪ Health literacy of adults in the United States. *Below basic*: circle date on doctor's appointment slip. *Basic*: give two reasons a person with no symptoms should get tested for cancer based on a clearly written pamphlet. *Intermediate*: determine what time to take Rx medicine based on label. *Proficient*: calculate employee share of health insurance costs using table. (Reproduced with permission from National Assessment of Adult Literacy, National Center for Educational Statistics, U.S. Department of Education, 2003.)

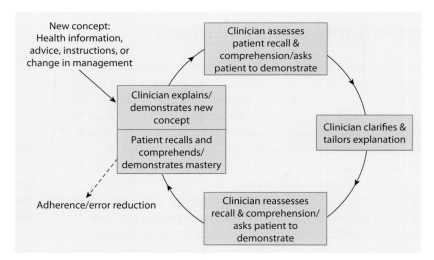

Figure 21-3 ▪ Example of a "teach back." (Reproduced with permission from Schillinger D, Piette J, Grumbach K, et al. Closing the loop: physician communication with diabetic patients who have low health literacy. *Arch Intern Med* 2003;163:83–90.)

videos.[21] Newer interventions focus on training providers to interact with low health literacy patients in appropriate ways. For example, the use of the "*teach back*" (patients are asked to restate to the provider their understanding of their condition or treatment plan) can help ensure that patients truly comprehend their situation (Figure 21-3).[22,23] An alternative strategy is the *Ask Me 3*, which prompts patients to ask their providers three questions: What is my main problem? What do I need to do? Why is it important for me to do this?[24] Patients who appear not to understand their care plan receive additional help.

In addition to these targeted interventions at the point of care, it will be important to embed education about health literacy into the training of physicians, nurses, and pharmacists. For example, a number of competencies for residents involve issues of doctor–patient communication and improving physicians' sensitivity to patients' varying communication styles and needs. Because so many of the problems surrounding health literacy revolve around medications,[15,22,25] the involvement of trained pharmacists can be crucial.[26]

ERRORS CAUSED BY PATIENTS THEMSELVES

Even when low health literacy or language differences are not at issue, patients may contribute to errors in their care. The causes are usually similar to those leading to provider-related errors: mostly competent humans interacting with a staggeringly complex system, sometime engaging in unsafe acts or violating safety rules. One group of New Zealand-based researchers divided patient errors into two groups: *action errors* (errors of patient behavior such as failing to attend an appointment or taking a medication with alcohol despite being advised not to do so) and *mental errors* (errors that involve patients' thought processes, such as "assuming I must be OK because I'm feeling good").[27] One study conducted within a large health maintenance organization found that nearly one in four adverse drug events (Chapter 4) was caused by patient error, such as the failure to take the medication at the proper dose or follow medication use instructions.[28]

The solutions to patient-generated errors are likely similar to those that address errors caused by clinicians: better communication and teamwork, more robust information systems, identification of at-risk individuals (such as those on multiple medications, and those with low health literacy and language differences) to trigger tailored interventions, and learning from past mistakes and experiences. The recognition that some errors are caused by patients is not an occasion to assign blame, since in the vast majority of circumstances the errors simply prove that the patients are humans who, as we know, err. The task for clinicians and healthcare systems will be to better understand these human frailties and design systems and approaches that make them less likely to cause harm.

PATIENT ENGAGEMENT AS A SAFETY STRATEGY

Obviously, patients who do not speak English (or whatever the dominant language is within the system in which they are seeking healthcare) or who have poor health literacy are in no position to advocate for their own safety, and are limited in their ability to participate meaningfully in clinical decision making and informed consent. This is a problem that needs to be tackled on its own merits.

But what about the patient who *is* competent and engaged, or who brings a family member to the clinical encounter able and willing to play an advocacy role? We have listed a number of questions that we would ask of a doctor or healthcare system in an effort to keep ourselves, or a family member, safe in Appendix IX. Responding to the public demand for answers to the "What can I do to stay safe?" question, several advocacy groups and professional organizations have launched campaigns—such as the Joint Commission's "Speak Up" campaign (Table 21-1)[29]—to address this issue.

However, as any healthcare provider who has been ill or has had a sick family member can attest, there are limits to what a layperson can do to protect against medical mistakes. These limitations were illustrated most vividly by Dr. Don Berwick, the founder of the Institute for Healthcare Improvement and former director of the U.S. Centers for Medicare & Medicaid Services. Berwick's poignant tale of his wife's series of hospitalizations (at several Harvard hospitals) for an obscure neurologic disease demonstrates the limitations of depending on patients or their families—even those with highly informed and engaged family members—to prevent medical errors:

> *The errors were not rare; they were the norm. During one admission, the neurologist told us in the morning, "By no means should you be getting anticholinergic agents [a medication that can cause neurological and muscle changes]," and a medication with profound anticholinergic side effects was given that afternoon. The attending neurologist in another admission told us by phone that a crucial and potentially toxic drug should be started immediately. He said, "Time is of the essence." That was on Thursday morning at 10:00 AM. The first dose was given 60 hours later—Saturday night at 10:00 PM. Nothing I could do, nothing I did, nothing I could think of made any difference. It nearly drove me mad. Colace [a stool softener] was discontinued by a physician's order on Day 1, and was nonetheless brought by the nurse every single evening throughout a 14-day admission. Ann was supposed to receive five intravenous doses of a very toxic chemotherapy agent, but dose #3 was labeled as "dose #2." For half a day, no record could be found that dose #2 had ever been given, even though I had watched it drip in myself. I tell you from my personal observation, no day passed—not one—without a medication error.[30]*

Before addressing the issue of patient engagement as a safety strategy, let's begin with core principles. The ethical virtues of an informed and participatory patient or family are unassailable, and the importance of

Table 21-1	THE JOINT COMMISSION'S "SPEAK UP" CAMPAIGN

Speak up if you have questions or concerns. If you still don't understand, ask again. It's your body and you have a right to know.

Pay attention to the care you get. Always make sure you're getting the right treatments and medicines by the right healthcare professionals. Don't assume anything.

Educate yourself about your illness. Learn about the medical tests you get, and your treatment plan.

Ask a trusted family member or friend to be your advocate (advisor or supporter).

Know what medicines you take and why you take them. Medicine errors are the most common healthcare mistakes.

Use a hospital, clinic, surgery center, or other type of healthcare organization that has been carefully checked out. For example, the Joint Commission visits hospitals to see if they are meeting Joint Commission quality standards.

Participate in all decisions about your treatment. You are the center of the healthcare team.

Available at: https://www.jointcommission.org/facts_about_speak_up/. © The Joint Commission, 2017. Reproduced with permission.

patient engagement has been emphasized by groups ranging from the Joint Commission to the Institute of Medicine, often under the broad umbrella of patient-centered care. And, shifting to a patient safety perspective, an extra set of eyes primed to notice hazards and empowered to point them out probably will prevent medical errors from time to time. In fact, one study found that patients identified twice as many adverse events as were identified by healthcare professionals reviewing medical records.[31] Another study demonstrated that parents were able to identify errors in the care of hospitalized children that were not captured in the medical record.[32]

Yet, we have reservations about the premise that patients and families can and should be central players in efforts to prevent medical mistakes. In fact, a 2014 systematic review suggests that more research is needed to better understand the best way to engage patients in promoting safety.[33]

The first source of our doubt is that it has not always worked, at least historically, and in some cases may increase the risk of harm. In the early days of "sign your site," before the process was standardized (Chapter 5), patients sometimes tried to be helpful by marking their own limbs before they dozed off from their anesthetic. Unfortunately, some patients marked the limb to be operated on, while others marked the limb to be avoided. As you might imagine, this kind of anarchy introduces new error possibilities.

Second, even if a well-informed, alert patient or loved one can help prevent some errors, too many patients don't have the resources to act as advocates for their own safety. Particularly in the hospital, many patients lack involved family members, are confused, anxious, or sedated, or—as we've seen—have language differences or problems with health literacy. Further, patients may not understand how to report safety issues and may not be able to distinguish between safety concerns and overall satisfaction with care.[34] Additionally, there may not be a system in place for collecting patient-identified concerns.[35] All of this means that relying on a strategy of patient engagement introduces an element of uncertainty, which creates its own problems. As British safety engineer Melinda Lyons observed:

> ... in safety engineering terms, ... patients are unlikely to provide a consistent and reliable contribution to the safety of the process of their own care. In a domain with a safety problem that is moving towards advocating the "systems approach," it seems nonsensical to also advocate a solution with apparently decreased reliability.[36]

Third, some patients and families, focused on doing what they can to prevent errors, will cross the thin line that separates being empowered and appropriately skeptical from being bellicose and confrontational. The latter attitude may lead providers to adopt a defensive stance or even generate outright avoidance. On the other hand, patients and families may be hesitant to challenge providers, perhaps fearing that confrontation will lead to a negative relationship. Such situations are not likely to promote safety.

Finally, we need to consider the sobering observation that patients and families often feel guilty about medical errors, which means that an emphasis on patients protecting themselves might amplify this guilt.[37] As a family member of a sickle cell patient who became critically ill after a medication error recalled:

> The feeling was impotence, because you can't stay with a patient 24 hours a day. That's why you rely on hospitals—you rely on nurses. You feel like you failed your family in terms of 'I should have been there.' That's a guilt that everyone shares.[37]

Even with these caveats, certain patient engagement strategies may be helpful. One study showed that patients who were willing to help monitor their providers' compliance with hand hygiene, were able to do so accurately, and did not feel that this would compromise the relationship with their caregivers.[38] (However, another study of Pennsylvania adults found that they were quite reluctant to challenge their providers.[39]) While researchers have found that patients often observe (and can report) errors that are missed through other ascertainment methods (Chapter 14),[40] barriers to patient engagement persist.[41]

Turning our attention to the policy sphere, the involvement of patients and their families has been a major force for change, as has been vividly illustrated by those patients and families that have channeled their sorrow over a devastating medical error into helping the system improve. For example, Sorrel King's grief over her daughter's death at Johns Hopkins Hospital was a major impetus for Hopkins' seminal contributions to the safety field.[42–44] And patient engagement at the organizational level, such as by having patients serve on key committees, may help keep systems focused and honest.

Both of us remain somewhat ambivalent regarding the role of patients in protecting themselves from mistakes, partly because of the paucity of evidence that it really works, and partly because of a more fundamental rejection of the premise itself: why *should* it fall to patients and family members to ensure their own safety?[45] When we board an airplane, we don't think about what we should be doing to keep ourselves safe. Instead, we try to relax, because we trust that the airlines and their regulators have done all they can to ensure our safety.

Patients encountering the healthcare system frequently lack this trust, which makes relaxation and passivity seem maladaptive, sometimes near-suicidal. That patients and families would want to do whatever they can to improve their odds of emerging unscathed is completely understandable. Unfortunately, research has not clearly established how well this strategy works or how to apply it most effectively.[46] Clearly, this should be the subject of ongoing studies.

In the meantime, while we should support efforts by patients and families to participate in their own safety when feasible, our primary focus should be on making such hypervigilance unnecessary. In our judgment, this problem is ours to fix, not theirs.

KEY POINTS

- Many patients have limited language proficiency and/or health literacy, which increases the risk that they will be victims of medical errors.
- Patients can cause errors in their own care; the solutions are likely to parallel those used for other kinds of errors.
- Patients and families can help promote safety, but (a) there are limitations to this strategy's effectiveness and (b) the responsibility to provide safe care should primarily be borne by providers, healthcare organizations, and policymakers, not patients.

▌REFERENCES

1. Flores G. Language barrier. *AHRQ WebM&M* (serial online); April 2006. Available at: https://psnet.ahrq.gov/webmm/case/123.

2. U.S. Census Bureau. Selected social characteristics: 2015. Available at: https://factfinder.census.gov/faces/nav/jsf/pages/index.xhtml.

3. Schiaffino MK, Nara A, Mao L. Language services in hospitals vary by ownership and location. *Health Aff (Millwood)* 2016;35:1399–1403.

4. Rice S. Hospitals often ignore policies on using qualified medical interpreters. *Mod Healthc* 2014;44:16–18, 20.

5. van Rosse F, de Bruijne M, Suurmond J, Essink-Bot ML, Wagner C. Language barriers and patient safety risks in hospital care. A mixed methods study. *Int J Nurs Stud* 2016;54:45–53.

6. Karliner LS, Kim SE, Meltzer DO, Auerbach AD. Influence of language barriers on outcomes of hospital care for general medicine inpatients. *J Hosp Med* 2010;5:276–282.

7. McCarthy DM, Waite KR, Curtis LM, Engel KG, Baker DW, Wolf MS. What did the doctor say? Health literacy and recall of medical instructions. *Med Care* 2012;50:277–282.

8. Lindholm M, Hargraves JL, Ferguson WJ, Reed G. Professional language interpretation and inpatient length of stay and readmission rate. *J Gen Intern Med* 2012;27:1294–1299.

9. Crane JA. Patient comprehension of doctor–patient communication on discharge from the emergency department. *J Emerg Med* 1997;16:1–7.

10. Gandhi TK, Burstin HR, Cook EF, et al. Drug complications in outpatients. *J Gen Intern Med* 2000;15:149–154.

11. Flores G, Abreau M, Barone CP, Bachur R, Lin H. Errors of medical interpretation and their potential clinical consequences: a comparison of professional versus ad hoc versus no interpreters. *Ann Emerg Med* 2012;60:545–553.

12. Masland MC, Lou C, Snowden L. Use of communication technologies to cost-effectively increase the availability of interpretation services in healthcare settings. *Telemed J E Health* 2010;16:739–745.

13. Standiford CJ, Nolan E, Harris M, Berstein SJ. Improving the provision of language services at an academic medical center: ensuring high-quality health communication for limited-English-proficient patients. *Acad Med* 2009;84:1693–1697.

14. Institute of Medicine. *Health Literacy: A Prescription to End Confusion*. Washington, DC: National Academies Press; 2004.

15. Berkman ND, Sheridan SL, Donahue KE, et al. *Health Literacy Interventions and Outcomes: An Updated Systematic Review*. Evidence Report/Technology Assessment: Number 199. Rockville, MD: Agency for Healthcare Research and Quality; March 2011. AHRQ Publication No. 11-E006.

16. Kripalani S, Jacobson TA, Mugalla IC, Cawthon CR, Niesner KJ, Vaccarino V. Health literacy and the quality of physician–patient communication during hospitalization. *J Hosp Med* 2010;5:269–275.

17. Omachi TA, Sarkar U, Yelin EH, Blanc PD, Katz PP. Lower health literacy is associated with poorer health status and outcomes in chronic obstructive pulmonary disease. *J Gen Intern Med* 2013;28:74–81.

18. Wolf MS, Bailey SC. The role of health literacy in patient safety [Perspective]. *AHRQ PSNet* (serial online); February/March 2009. Available at: https://psnet.ahrq.gov/perspectives/perspective/72.

19. Louis AJ, Arora VM, Matthiesen MI, Meltzer DO, Press VG. Screening hospitalized patients for low health literacy: beyond the REALM of possibility? *Health Educa Behav* 2017;44:360–364.

20. Baker DW. The meaning and the measure of health literacy. *J Gen Intern Med* 2006; 21:878–883.

21. Wolf MS, Curtis LM, Waite K, et al. Helping patients simplify and safely use complex prescription regimens. *Arch Intern Med* 2011;171:300–305.

22. Schillinger D, Piette J, Grumbach K, et al. Closing the loop: physician communication with diabetic patients who have low health literacy. *Arch Intern Med* 2003;163: 83–90.

23. Miller S, Lattanzio M, Cohen S. "Teach-back" from a patient's perspective. *Nursing* 2016;46:63–64.

24. Available at: http://www.npsf.org/?page=askme3.

25. Davis TC, Wolf MS, Bass PFIII, et al. Literacy and misunderstanding prescription drug labels. *Ann Intern Med* 2006;145:887–894.

26. Bell SP, Schnipper JL, Goggins K, et al. Effect of pharmacist counseling intervention on health care utilization following hospital discharge: a randomized control trial. *J Gen Intern Med* 2016;31:47–477.

27. Buetow S, Kiata L, Liew T, Kenealy T, Dovey S, Elwyn G. Patient error: a preliminary taxonomy. *Ann Fam Med* 2009;7:223–231.

28. Field TS, Mazor KM, Briesacher B, Debellis KR, Gurwitz JH. Adverse drug events resulting from patient errors in older adults. *J Am Geriatr Soc* 2007;55:271–276.

29. Available at: https://www.jointcommission.org/facts_about_speak_up/.

30. Berwick DM. *Escape Fire: Lessons for the Future of Health Care*. New York, NY: The Commonwealth Fund; 2002.

31. Weissman JS, Schneider EC, Weingart SN, et al. Comparing patient-reported hospital adverse events with medical record review: do patients know something that hospitals do not? *Ann Intern Med* 2008;149:100–108.

32. Khan A, Furtak SL, Melvin P, Rogers JE, Schuster MA, Landrigan CP. Parent-reported errors and adverse events in hospitalized children. *JAMA Pediatr* 2016;170:e154608.

33. Berger Z, Flickinger TE, Pfoh E, Martinez KA, Dy SM. Promoting engagement by patients and families to reduce adverse events in acute care settings: a systematic review. *BMJ Qual Saf* 2014;23:548–555.

34. De Brun A, Heavey E, Waring J, Dawson P, Scott J. PReSaFe: A model of barriers and facilitators to patients providing feedback on experiences of safety. *J Health Expect* November 16, 2016. [Epub ahead of print].

35. Mazor KM, Smith KM, Fisher KA, Gallagher TH. Speak up! Addressing the paradox plaguing patient-centered care. *Ann Intern Med* 2016;164:618–619.

36. Lyons M. Should patients have a role in patient safety? A safety engineering view. *Qual Saf Health Care* 2007;16:140–142.

37. Delbanco T, Bell SK. Guilty, afraid, and alone—struggling with medical error. *N Engl J Med* 2007;357:1682–1683.

38. Bittle MJ, LaMarche S. Engaging the patient as observer to promote hand hygiene compliance in ambulatory care. *Jt Comm J Qual Patient Saf* 2009;35:519–525, AP1–AP3.

39. Marella WM, Finley E, Thomas AD, Clarke JR. Health care consumers' inclination to engage in selected patient safety practices: a survey of adults in Pennsylvania. *J Patient Saf* 2007;3:184–189.

40. Weingart SN, Pagovich O, Sands DZ, et al. What can hospitalized patients tell us about adverse events? Learning from patient-reported incidents. *J Gen Intern Med* 2005;20:830–836.

41. Manias E, Rixon S, Williams A, Liew D, Braaf S. Barriers and enablers affecting patient engagement in managing medications within specialty hospital settings. *Health Expect* 2015;18:2787–2798.

42. In conversation with … Sorrel King [Perspective]. *AHRQ PSNet* (serial online); March 2007. Available at: https://psnet.ahrq.gov/perspectives/perspective/39.

43. King S. *Josie's Story: A Mother's Inspiring Crusade to Make Medical Care Safe*. New York, NY: Atlantic Monthly Press; 2009.

44. Pronovost P, Vohr E. *Safe Patients, Smart Hospitals: How One Doctor's Checklist can Help Us Change Health Care from the Inside Out*. New York, NY: Hudson Street Press; 2010.

45. Entwistle VA, Mello MM, Brennan TA. Advising patients about patient safety: current initiatives risk shifting responsibility. *Jt Comm J Qual Patient Saf* 2005;31:483–494.

46. Ocloo J, Matthews R. From tokenism to empowerment: progressing patient and public involvement in healthcare improvement. *BMJ Qual Saf* 2016;25:626–632.

ADDITIONAL READINGS

Alper J. *Health Literacy: Past, Present, and Future: Workshop Summary.* Institute of Medicine. Washington, DC: National Academies of Sciences, Engineering, and Medicine; 2015.

Flores G. Language barriers to health care in the United States. *N Engl J Med* 2006;355:229–231.

NPSF Lucian Leape Institute Roundtable on Consumer Engagement in Patient Safety. *Safety is Personal: Partnering with Patients and Families for the Safest Care.* Boston, MA: National Patient Safety Foundation; March 2014.

Ring DC, Herndon JH, Meyer GS. Case 34-2010: a 65-year-old woman with an incorrect operation on the left hand. *N Engl J Med* 2010;363:1950–1957.

Saha S, Fernandez A. Language barriers in health care. *J Gen Intern Med* 2007;22:281–282.

Schwappach DLB. Engaging patients as vigilant partners in safety: a systematic review. *Med Care Res Rev* 2010;67:119–148.

ORGANIZING A SAFETY PROGRAM 22

OVERVIEW

As the pressure to improve patient safety has grown, healthcare organizations, particularly hospitals but also larger healthcare systems, have struggled to create effective structures for their safety efforts. Although there are few studies comparing various organizational models, best practices for promoting organizational safety have begun to emerge.[1–6] This chapter will explore some of these issues. The organization of safety programs in ambulatory care is discussed in Chapter 12, and, of course, myriad issues relevant to organizing an effective safety program are addressed throughout this book.

STRUCTURE AND FUNCTION

Before the year 2000, few organizations had patient safety committees or officers. If there was any institutional focus on safety (in most institutions, there wasn't), it generally lived under the organization's physician leader (sometimes a Vice President for Medical Affairs or Chief Medical Officer [CMO], or perhaps the elected Chief of the Medical Staff) or nurse leader (Chief Nursing Officer). In academic medical centers, safety issues were usually handled through the academic departmental structure (e.g., chair of the department of medicine or surgery), promoting a fragmented, siloed approach. When an institutional nonphysician leader *did* become involved in safety issues, it was usually a hospital risk manager, whose primary role was to protect the institution from liability.[7] Although many risk managers considered preventing future errors to be part of their role, they rarely had the institutional clout or resources to make durable changes in processes, information technology, or culture. Larger institutions with quality committees or quality officers sometimes subsumed patient safety under these individuals or groups.

The latter structure is still common in small institutions that lack the resources to have independent safety operations, but many larger organizations have recognized the value of a separate structure and staff to focus on safety. The responsibilities of safety personnel include: monitoring and responding to the incident reporting system, educating providers and others about new safety practices (driven by the experience of others and the literature), measuring safety outcomes and developing programs to improve them, and supervising the approach to serious events (e.g., organizing root cause analyses [RCAs]) and to preventing future errors (e.g., implementing action plans after RCAs, performing failure mode and effects analyses [FMEA]) (Chapter 14).[8] In addition, such personnel must work collaboratively with other departments and personnel, such as those in information technology, infection prevention, quality, compliance, and risk management.

| MANAGING THE INCIDENT REPORTING SYSTEM

An organization interested in improving the quality of care (as opposed to patient safety) might not spend a huge amount of time and effort promoting reporting by caregivers to central administration. Why? To the extent that the quality issues of interest can be ascertained through outcome (e.g., mortality rates in patients with acute myocardial infarction, postoperative infection rates, readmission rates for patients with pneumonia) or process measures (did every patient with myocardial infarction for whom it was indicated receive a beta-blocker and aspirin?) (Chapter 3), performance assessment does not depend on the direct involvement of nurses and doctors. Instead, these data can be collected through chart review or, increasingly, by tapping into electronic data streams created in the course of care (Chapter 13). Obviously, when a quality leader identifies a "hot spot" through these measures, he or she cannot proceed without convening the relevant personnel to develop a complete understanding of the process and an action plan, but collecting the data can often be accomplished without provider participation.

Safety is different. In most cases, a safety officer or CMO will have no way of discovering errors or risky situations without receiving this information from frontline workers. Although other mechanisms (direct observation of practice, trigger tools) can identify some problems, clinicians are the best repository of the knowledge and wisdom needed to understand safety hazards, near misses, and true errors, and thus to create the system changes to prevent them. As described in Chapter 14, the institutional incident reporting system is the usual, albeit imperfect, vehicle for tapping this rich vein of experience.

The *patient safety officer (or manager)* will generally be charged with managing the incident reporting system. At small institutions, he or she may review every report, aggregate the data into meaningful categories (e.g., medication errors, falls), and triage the reports for further action. Based on the severity of the incidents, some reports will be simply noted, others will generate a limited analysis or an inquiry to a frontline manager, while still others will lead to a detailed investigation, usually in the form of an RCA. Many larger institutions have subdivided this task, selecting "category managers" to review incidents in a given domain (a pharmacist for medication errors, a nurse-leader for falls, the CMO for reports of unprofessional physician behavior; Table 14-2). The category managers are expected to review incidents within their categories, take appropriate action, and triage cases to the safety officer (or, at times, someone even higher in the organization) when the error is particularly serious or falls within an area that has regulatory or legal repercussions.

As with much of patient safety, results and culture are more important than structure. A technologically sophisticated incident reporting system will create little value if the frontline workers consider the approach to reports overly punitive, or if they see no evidence that reports are taken seriously or generate action.[9] So the safety officer is well advised to invest time and energy in making clear to caregivers that their reports result in important changes. Such an investment is every bit as important as one made in purchasing and maintaining a system that collects data and produces sophisticated pie charts. The RCA process is described in Chapter 14, including some of the changes we made at University of California, San Francisco (UCSF) Medical Center that markedly improved its value (Table 14-5).

DEALING WITH DATA

Although the safety officer will generally not be as data driven as the quality officer (for the reasons described above), he or she *will* have a steady stream of inputs that can be important sources of understanding and action. Some of these will be generated by the incident reporting system; here, it is important to use the information effectively while recognizing that voluntary reports capture only a small (and nonrandom) subset of errors, and that they cannot be used to determine rates of errors or harm.[10,11] An additional problem with incident reports is that nurses submit them far more frequently than physicians do, so they tend to underemphasize issues that physicians see (such as diagnostic errors, Chapter 6) and overemphasize nursing-related harms (e.g., falls).[12,13] Malpractice claims are an even more unpredictable and often flawed source of safety concerns (Chapter 18). Several studies have illuminated an

Table 22-1   **EXAMPLES OF TYPES OF INSTITUTIONAL DATA THAT SHOULD BE REGULARLY REVIEWED BY PATIENT SAFETY OFFICERS**

1. Data from the voluntary incident report system
2. Data drawn from trigger tools (and results of subsequent chart reviews)
3. Data drawn from real-time surveillance systems, such as those for certain healthcare-associated infections
4. Key outcome data such as risk-adjusted mortality and readmission rates
5. Key process and structural data (e.g., hand hygiene rates, appropriate use of checklists, use of computerized order entry, door-to-balloon time for patients with ST-segment elevation myocardial infarction)
6. Safety-related administrative and claims data, such as those used to produce the AHRQ Patient Safety Indicators (Appendix V)
7. Cases that qualify as National Quality Forum serious reportable events (Appendix VI)
8. Cases related to a Joint Commission National Patient Safety Goal (Appendix IV), or involve areas highlighted as concerns on a prior Joint Commission (or other important accreditation) local survey
9. Malpractice claims and payouts
10. Serious patient complaints
11. Data drawn from Executive Walk Rounds or other caregiver focus groups
12. Data drawn from Morbidity and Mortality conferences (or other sources of data from physicians)
13. Results of safety culture surveys completed by clinicians and managers
14. Results of patient experience surveys

important point: there is no one "right" way to view an organization's safety, and the safety leader must look for information from multiple sources to gain a complete view of the "elephant of patient safety" (Table 22-1).[14–16]

For safety problems that *can* be measured as rates (such as hospital-acquired infections, Chapter 10), the role of the safety officer (assuming this is his or her domain; in large institutions, an infection preventionist may be charged with this task) becomes more like the quality officer: studying the data to see when rates have spiked above prior baselines or above local, regional, or national norms (*benchmarks*). In these circumstances, the safety officer will complete an in-depth analysis of the problem and develop an action plan designed to improve the outcomes.

Increasingly, safety officers will need to audit areas that have been the subject of regulatory requirements or new institutional policies. Such audits are best done through direct observation, and backsliding should be expected. In fact, the safety officer should be skeptical if an audit six months after implementation of a new policy demonstrates 100% compliance with the practice: there is an excellent chance that these are biased data and more should be done to get a true snapshot of what is really happening.

Finally, as medical records become electronic (Chapter 13), innovative methods for screening caregiver notes, lab results and medication orders (such as via trigger tools, Chapter 14), operative reports, and discharge summaries will generate new and useful safety information.[17–19] More and more of this work will involve real-time surveillance systems, with automatic "just-in-time" feedback of information to providers rather than the traditional process of (retrospective) audit and (markedly delayed) feedback.[20]

Some of the most important safety data will be the results of *patient safety culture surveys*. There are several well-constructed, validated surveys that can be used for this purpose; a few have been used at hundreds, or even thousands, of institutions, meaning that an institution's results can be compared with those from like institutions or units (e.g., other academic medical centers, or other intensive care units [ICUs]).[21,22] As we discuss in Chapter 15, although it is appealing to think of institutions (such as hospitals or large healthcare delivery systems) as having organization-wide safety cultures (after all, humans like simple explanations, even when they're wrong), research repeatedly demonstrates that safety culture tends to be local: even within a single hospital, there will often be huge variations in culture between units down the hall from one another.[23,24]

The safety officer's job, then, is to ensure administration of the surveys and a reasonable response rate, that the results are thoughtfully analyzed, and—as always—that the data are converted into meaningful action. For clinical units with poor safety culture, it is critical to determine the nature of the problem. Is it poor leadership, and, if so, is leadership training or a new leader required? Is it poor teamwork, and, if so, should we consider a crew resource management or other teamwork training program (Chapter 15)? And, is there something to be learned from units with excellent culture that can be used to inform or stimulate change in the more problematic units?[25]

Finally, there is the challenge of integration and prioritization. The patient safety officer who monitors all of these data sources will have far more safety targets than he or she can possibly address in a year. This means that one crucial job is to help an organization prioritize among many worthwhile goals. It is natural that such prioritization will tend to elevate items required by regulators or accreditors over those that are not, measurable targets over softer ones, and efforts to change processes and structures over efforts to change culture and attitudes. The effective (and durably employed!) safety officer lives in the real world and addresses what needs to be addressed, but also works to counteract these biases when that is best for patients. For example, implementing a teamwork training initiative or an institution-wide program to prevent diagnostic errors may not be required, and the return on investment may be years away and hard to measure. The safety officer who believes that these activities are important for patients will—somehow—find the money, time, and political will to place them on the organization's agenda.

STRATEGIES TO CONNECT SENIOR LEADERSHIP WITH FRONTLINE PERSONNEL

Recognizing that an effective safety program depends on connecting the senior leadership (who control the bulk of the resources and key policies) with what is truly happening on the clinical units, and further appreciating that incident reporting systems paint a terribly incomplete picture of this frontline activity, many healthcare organizations have developed strategies to connect senior leaders with caregivers. The two most popular are Executive Walk Rounds and "Adopt-a-Unit."

Executive Walk Rounds are the healthcare version of the old business leadership strategy of "Managing by Walking Around" (MBWA).[26–29] At some interval (some institutions do Walk Rounds weekly, others monthly), the safety officer will accompany another member of the senior leadership team (e.g., CEO, COO, CMO) to a clinical unit—a medical floor, the emergency department, the labor and delivery suite, or perhaps an operating room. The visits are usually preannounced. Although the unit manager is generally present for the visit, the most important outcome is a frank discussion (with senior leadership spending more time listening than talking) about the problems and errors on the unit, and brainstorming solutions to these problems. Some institutions have formalized these visits with a script; a sample one is shown in Box 22-1.

Another strategy (not mutually exclusive, but institutions tend to favor one or the other) is *Adopt-a-Unit*.[30] Here, rather than executives visiting a variety of clinical areas around the hospital to get a broad picture of safety problems, one senior leader adopts a single unit and attends relevant meetings with staff there (perhaps monthly) for a long period (6–12 months). This method, pioneered at Johns Hopkins, has the advantage of more sustained engagement and automatic follow-through, and the disadvantage of providing each leader a more narrow view of the entire institution. Given that there are only so many senior leaders to go around, the *Adopt-a-Unit* strategy will generally mean that certain units will be neglected. For this reason, it is less popular than Executive Walk Rounds. However, for units experiencing important safety challenges or showing evidence of poor culture, this method, with its sustained focus, may have real value.

Box 22-1   SELECTED SCRIPTS FOR PATIENT SAFETY EXECUTIVE WALK ROUNDS

Opening statements:

"We are moving as an organization to open communication and a blame-free environment because we believe that by doing so we can make your work environment safer for you and your patients"

"We're interested in focusing on the system and not individuals (no names are necessary)"

"The questions are very general. To help you think of areas to which the questions might apply, consider medication errors, miscommunication between individuals (including arguments), distractions, inefficiencies, invasive treatments, falls, protocols not followed, and so on"

Questions to ask:

"Can you think of any events in the past day or few days that have resulted in prolonged hospitalization for a patient?"

Examples:

Appointments made but missed

Miscommunications

Delayed or omitted medications

"Have there been any near misses that almost caused patient harm but didn't?"

Examples:

Selecting a drug dose from the medications cart or pharmacy to administer to a patient and then realizing it's incorrect

Misprogramming a pump, but having an alert warn you

Incorrect orders by physicians or others caught by nurses or other staff

"What aspects of the environment are likely to lead to the next patient harm?"

Examples:

Consider all aspects of admission, hospital stay, and discharge

Consider movement within the hospital

Consider communication

Consider informatics and computer issues

"Is there anything we could do to prevent the next adverse event?"

Examples:

What information would be helpful to you?

Consider alterations in the interaction between clinicians

Consider teamwork

Consider environment and workflow

"What specific intervention from leadership would make the work you do safer for patients?"

Examples:

Organize interdisciplinary groups to evaluate a specific problem

Assist in changing the attitude of a particular group

Facilitate interaction between two specific groups

"How are we actively promoting a blame-free culture and working on the development of a blame-free reporting policy?"

Examples:

We do not penalize individuals for inadvertent errors

The institution grants immunity to individuals who report adverse events in a timely fashion (where criminal behavior is not an issue)

Closing comment:

"We're going to work on the information you've given us. In return, we would like you to tell two other people you work with about the concepts we've discussed in this conversation"

Reproduced with permission from Frankel A. *Patient Safety Leadership Walkrounds.* Institute for Healthcare Improvement (IHI); 2004. Available at: http://www.ihi.org/knowledge/Pages/Tools/PatientSafety LeadershipWalkRounds.aspx.

Whichever method is chosen, these efforts will be most useful if providers sense that senior leadership takes their concerns seriously, leaders demonstrate interest while being unafraid to show their ignorance about how things really work on the floor, and the frontline workers later learn about how their input led to meaningful changes.

STRATEGIES TO GENERATE FRONTLINE ACTIVITY TO IMPROVE SAFETY

Although connecting providers to senior leadership is vitally important, units must also have the capacity to act on their own. One of the dangers of an organizational "safety program" can be that individual clinical units will not be sufficiently active and independent—sharing stories of errors, problem solving, and doing the daily work of making care safer. Because many such efforts do not require major changes in policies or large infusions of resources, safety officers and programs need to create an environment and culture in which such unit-based problem solving is the norm, not the exception.

While some units will instinctively move in this direction (often as an outgrowth of strong local leadership and culture), others will need help. Many of the programs discussed previously (such as teamwork training) should leave behind an ongoing organizational structure that supports unit-based safety. Many healthcare systems, including ours, are adopting a version of unit-based leadership teams (UBLTs), in which a lead physician, nurse, and improvement specialist work together to identify problems and implement solutions.[31]

Developing this kind of unit-based safety enterprise requires training, leadership, and some resources (a small amount of compensation for the unit-based champions, time for the group to meet, and—of course—food). It is also important to sort out the "cross-walk" between the unit-based efforts and the larger institutional safety program. On the one hand, the unit-based team must be free to discuss errors, develop educational materials, and problem solve without being encumbered by the organizational bureaucracy. On the other hand, the unit-based program cannot completely bypass the institutional incident reporting system, and it is vital that central leadership rapidly learns of major errors that should generate broader investigations (i.e., RCAs) or mandatory reports to external organizations.

DEALING WITH MAJOR ERRORS AND SENTINEL EVENTS

The RCA process, including recent calls for its transformation, is described in Chapter 14. Whatever the exact version of RCA employed, the safety officer will often be charged with convening the RCA team, prepping senior leadership for the meetings, chairing the sessions, and converting the findings into meaningful action plans. Because many states and the Joint Commission now either encourage or require that sentinel events (and the results of subsequent RCAs) be reported promptly, the safety officer plays a key role in managing this process, often collaborating with the compliance officer (in larger institutions), or the institutional risk manager if there are potential legal ramifications.

In addition, major errors often raise knotty questions regarding the role of the media (Chapter 19).[32,33] While certainly not every error needs to be shared with local reporters, particularly bad errors should be discussed with the institution's media relations department, if there is one, to consider the plusses and minuses of a proactive media strategy. This is a delicate balance, but organizations that have cultivated an open, honest, and mutually respectful relationship with their local media sometimes find that early disclosure of serious errors works better than waiting for reporters to discover them on their own.

The issue of disclosing errors to patients is discussed in Chapter 18.

FAILURE MODE AND EFFECTS ANALYSES

The safety officer may also be charged with spearheading efforts to proactively assess and mitigate safety risks. The Joint Commission now requires that every healthcare organization carry out at least one failure mode and effects analysis (FMEA) yearly. The process of and rationale behind FMEA is discussed in Chapter 14. Just as with the results of RCAs, the safety officer will often be responsible for converting the results of the FMEA into changes in policies and practice. In complex organizations, this requires tremendous diplomatic and organizational skill, because the changes often require approval by multiple committees and buy-in from a wide variety of stakeholders who may not have participated in the analysis and lack a full understanding of patient safety or the issues at hand.

QUALIFICATIONS AND TRAINING OF THE PATIENT SAFETY OFFICER

The personal qualities of the patient safety officer are probably more important than his or her training and pedigree. Ideally, a safety officer will be a credible clinician with a strong interest in safety and specific training in many of the competencies described in this book, including human factors, information technology, data management, and culture change. He or she will be a team player—needing to constantly assemble and motivate interdisciplinary teams to problem solve. The officer must work collaboratively not only with front-line providers and senior leadership but also with armies of individuals with overlapping job descriptions: the quality officer, risk manager, information technology officer, compliance officer, and more.[8] The larger the institution, the more likely that these functions will be managed by separate individuals. In smaller institutions, these hats (perhaps with the exception of the information technology leader) may all be worn by the same person.

There are now a number of excellent courses to teach individuals the skills needed to be patient safety officers and leaders. Two of the most popular are the Certified Professional in Patient Safety (CPPS) pathway offered by the National Patient Safety Foundation (NPSF) and the training program offered by the Institute for Healthcare Improvement (IHI Patient Safety Executive Development Program). Other institutions including Johns Hopkins, Harvard Medical School, and the VA offer a variety of training programs focused on patient safety. Patient safety officers should also attend regional and national conferences on patient safety, and always be on the lookout for innovations and emerging best practices in the field.

Patient safety leaders also need to stay current on the literature, tools, and regulations in the field. The U.S. Agency for Healthcare Research and Quality (AHRQ) publishes *AHRQ Patient Safety Network* (http://psnet.ahrq.gov; Figure 22-1), a free Web site that posts 20 new resources each week in the field of patient safety, each with full annotations and rich links to related items (Figure 22-2). The site also hosts a searchable library of more than 20,000 safety resources, and offers a variety of other features, including advanced customizability ("My PSNet") and designated "Classics" in patient safety. It is an excellent resource for anyone interested in patient safety, and an indispensable one for the patient safety officer and his or her staff.

While AHRQ PSNet will deliver the week's most important safety resources to one's electronic doorstep, many people will want to also subscribe to key journals in the field, such as *BMJ Quality and Safety*, the *Joint Commission Journal of Quality and Patient Safety*, and the *Journal of Patient Safety*. In addition, several journals and textbooks focus on more specialized areas (informatics, device design, medication safety, cognitive errors, health policy) relevant to patient safety, and many clinical specialty journals (e.g., surgery, hospital medicine, critical care, nursing) now offer substantial safety content. Patient safety articles of interest to the broader healthcare community are often published in high-profile general journals such as the *New England Journal of Medicine*, *Annals of Internal Medicine*, *BMJ*, and *JAMA*. Finally, the patient safety officer should also be familiar with many of the key books and white papers in the field (Appendix I).

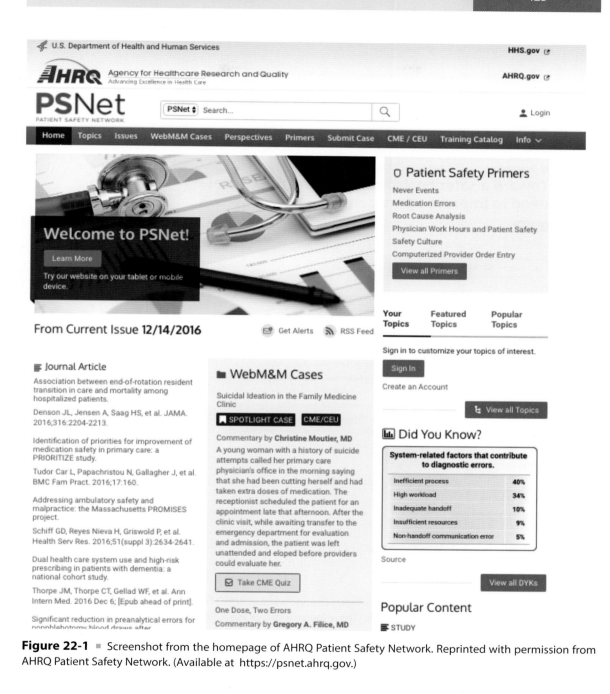

Figure 22-1 ▪ Screenshot from the homepage of AHRQ Patient Safety Network. Reprinted with permission from AHRQ Patient Safety Network. (Available at https://psnet.ahrq.gov.)

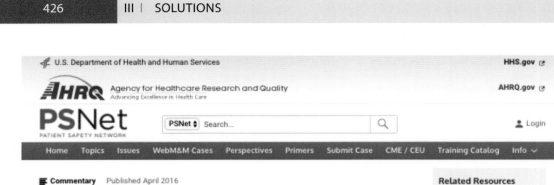

AHRQ Agency for Healthcare Research and Quality
Advancing Excellence in Health Care   AHRQ.gov

PSNet
PATIENT SAFETY NETWORK

PSNet ♦ Search...   👤 Login

Home   Topics   Issues   WebM&M Cases   Perspectives   Primers   Submit Case   CME / CEU   Training Catalog   Info ⌄

≡ Commentary   Published April 2016

Toward a safer health care system: the critical need to improve measurement.

CLASSIC

Jha A, Pronovost PJ. JAMA. 2016;315:1831-1832.

⊥ Topics ▾   66 Cite ▾   ↱ Share ▾   🖶 Print

In this call for better measurement and reporting, two patient safety experts lay out steps that federal policymakers can take to advance patient safety. The commentary emphasizes the need for valid patient safety measures and mentions the Surgeon Scorecard as an example of journalists and private companies stepping in to provide needed transparency. The authors suggest that the Centers for Medicare and Medicaid Services (CMS) focus on measures of the most common causes of iatrogenic harm to hospitalized patients, including adverse drug events, hospital-acquired conditions, and surgical complications. They recommend that CMS remove current metrics that rely on administrative data due to concerns about validity and accuracy of these measures. The commentary advocates for tasking an official agency with defining measurement standards and benchmarks. The authors also propose that Congress fund research on systems engineering. A recent PSNet interview discussed AHRQ's efforts to develop patient safety measures and improvement programs.

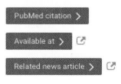

PubMed citation >

Available at > ⧉

Related news article > ⧉

Related Resources

≡ JOURNAL ARTICLE ›
REVIEW

From tokenism to empowerment: progressing patient and public involvement in healthcare improvement.
Ocloo J, Matthews R. BMJ Qual Saf. 2016;25:626-632.

≡ JOURNAL ARTICLE ›
COMMENTARY

An ethical framework for allocating scarce life-saving chemotherapy and supportive care drugs for childhood cancer.
Unguru Y, Fernandez CV, Bernhardt B, et al. J Natl Cancer Inst. 2016;108:djv392.

≡ JOURNAL ARTICLE ›
COMMENTARY

Rating the raters: the inconsistent quality of health care performance measurement.
Shahian DM, Normand ST, Friedberg MW, Hutter MM, Pronovost PJ. Ann Surg. 2016;264:36-38.

≡ JOURNAL ARTICLE ›
REVIEW

How safe is primary care? A systematic review.
Panesar SS, deSilva D, Carson-Stevens A, et al. BMJ Qual Saf. 2016;25:544-553.

Figure 22-2 ■ Screenshot from an individual resource annotation in AHRQ Patient Safety Network. Reprinted with permission from AHRQ Patient Safety Network. (The resource is that of Jha A, Pronovost PJ. Toward a safer health care system: the critical need to improve measurement. *JAMA* 2016;315:1831–1832. Available at: https://psnet.ahrq.gov/resources/resource/29975.)

Increasingly, the patient safety officer needs to face outward as well as inward, cultivating positive relationships with state regulators, regional and national accreditors, and colleagues with similar roles at other institutions. Many patient safety officers work at hospitals that are part of larger health systems. This can make available additional resources and sources of learning—a real plus—but it also adds complexity, as solutions or policies developed for a system may need to be "localized" to meet the needs of an individual hospital or clinic. A similar problem with a slightly different twist arises when the patient safety officer's institution becomes part of a broader *patient safety organization* (PSO, Chapter 14).

THE ROLE OF THE PATIENT SAFETY COMMITTEE

Whether or not there is a designated patient safety officer, most institutions now have a patient safety committee, often a committee of the medical staff. This committee reviews adverse events and incident reports, helps to set and endorse safety-related policies, develops new safety initiatives, and disseminates information about patient safety to providers. It generally will be made up of a diverse group of clinicians (physicians, nurses, pharmacists) and hospital administrators; a few institutions include lay members.

Patient safety committees need to address certain challenges. One is how the committee's activities will relate to those of other overlapping committees, such as risk management and quality improvement. This issue parallels the one the safety officer faces in interacting with his or her peers in these departments. And, like the safety officer, the correct answer involves combining appropriate amounts of overlap (some personnel should be shared across committees, so that each can know what the other is doing) with a clear mandate to focus on certain exclusive areas. For example, while the involvement of the risk manager on the patient safety committee can be quite helpful (and, in certain states, required to shield the committee's deliberations from being legally discoverable), it is crucial that the committee's focus remain on improving safety rather than reducing the organization's legal exposure.[7]

A second issue is making sure that the committee reserves some time and energy to focus on issues that are not regulatory mandates and are not generated from specific cases of harm—also a parallel issue to the patient safety officer's prioritization challenges mentioned earlier. The committee that explicitly sets a goal of completing one to two group-generated projects per year is more likely to "think outside the box" than the group that spends all its time in reactive and compliance mode.

A third and more recent issue flows from the fact that the vast majority of U.S. hospitals have gone from paper-based to digital in the past decade. This means that changes in the electronic health record or other enterprise technologies are often potential answers to safety problems. Making things far more complicated, at times the very same technologies are one of the root causes of safety problems! A strong relationship between the information technology leadership structure and the patient safety enterprise is increasingly crucial.

ENGAGING PHYSICIANS IN PATIENT SAFETY

Notwithstanding our emphasis on the role of teamwork and the vital contributions of all caregivers, the engagement of physicians is crucial in patient safety. In fact, the presence or absence of such engagement frequently predicts whether an organization's safety program is a smashing success or dismal failure.

Because so much of the accountability for patient safety (in the United States) is now being directed toward hospitals (Chapters 3, 14, and 20), cementing physician engagement tends to be comparatively (emphasis on "comparatively") easy in hospitals that either employ doctors (i.e., Veterans Affairs hospitals, many hospitals with hospitalists) or have physicians with strong links to the organization (i.e., Mayo and Cleveland Clinics, Kaiser Permanente, most academic health centers). In the thousands of hospitals in which physicians have weaker institutional links—members of the medical staff who use the hospital to provide care but receive no salary support and do not share in the organization's accountabilities—safety engagement tends to be more tenuous.

Taitz et al. conducted site visits and interviews at 10 high-performing teaching hospitals (mostly highly ranked academic medical centers) to highlight the best practices in engaging physicians in safety and quality.[34] Six themes emerging from this work are shown in Table 22-2, and major barriers to engagement are highlighted in Table 22-3. An important caveat is that these data come from medical centers that enjoy reasonably good physician–organizational alignment to begin with. The degree to which the results are applicable to community hospitals with lower baseline integration is unknown.

Table 22-2	SIX THEMES IN A FRAMEWORK FOR ENGAGING PHYSICIANS IN QUALITY AND SAFETY		
Theme	**Selected Interviewee Quotes**	**% Endorsing Theme**
1. Engaged leadership	"Leadership, that is, able to get physician buy-in to quality and safety, their commitment and belief in its value and the importance of making the final product better." "You need engaged leaders to have engaged physicians."	70
2. Physician compact	"The compact captures the focus on the patient. It also creates a common framework for why physicians are here, our relationship with the organizations, other physicians and our patients." "The compact is a living, breathing, dynamic reciprocal agreement that aligns expectations between the organization and our physicians."	15

(continued)

Theme	Selected Interviewee Quotes	% Endorsing Theme
	Table 22-2 **SIX THEMES IN A FRAMEWORK FOR ENGAGING PHYSICIANS IN QUALITY AND SAFETY (*Continued*)**	
3. Appropriate compensation	"Quality is not an add-on to busy physicians' schedules, otherwise you don't get full commitment."	50
4. Realignment of financial incentives		
Support financial incentives	"Have your professional values dominate and then align financial incentives around them." "Payment of incentives is important. Physicians are like everyone else, the monetary rewards are the power to drive behavior."	33
Oppose financial incentives	"Financial incentives are an insult to the professionalism of physicians." "We should rather reward value."	31
5. Data and enablers	"Physicians are data connoisseurs—it is imperative to get accurate data." "There is no greater force than peer pressure in a structured format." "Physicians don't just need data, they also need enablers or processes to improve their performance."	66
6. Data reporting		
Support internal transparency	"Need complete transparency internally to transform the culture of the organization." "Internal transparency is more a driver of change than external transparency."	95
Support external transparency	"We want to demystify the data and make it understandable to the public." "Data should be completely transparent so that patients know what we do well."	52
Oppose external transparency	"Be wary of publishing individual performance publically, external reporting should reflect system results." "Public reporting can be misleading."	26
7. Academic promotion*	"Tie academic promotion to outcomes and participation in quality-and-safety activities." "Quality-and-safety publications should be treated on a par with traditional research publications."	14

*Likely reflects study population: leaders at 10 teaching hospitals, mostly academic medical centers. Reproduced with permission from Taitz JM, Lee TH, Sequist TD. A framework for engaging physicians in quality and safety. *BMJ Qual Saf* 2012;21:722–728.

Table 22-3 BARRIERS TO PHYSICIANS' ENGAGEMENT IN QUALITY AND SAFETY	
Barrier	**% Reporting Barrier**
Lack of time	45
Institutional culture	31
Physician desire for autonomy	17
Lack of medical school training	17
Lack of trust in data	15
Lack of information system support	12
Lack of quality improvement skills	12

Reproduced with permission from Taitz JM, Lee TH, Sequist TD. A framework for engaging physicians in quality and safety. *BMJ Qual Saf* 2012;21:722–728.

BOARD ENGAGEMENT IN PATIENT SAFETY

Until recently, discussions about organizational leadership in safety tended to focus on the commitment of the CEO and physician and nursing leaders. But in many healthcare organizations, the role of the board can be decisive.

Traditionally, hospital boards have delegated quality and safety to the medical staff, focusing instead on their fiduciary responsibilities. Why? Most board members are lay people (often prominent business and community leaders) who felt that they did not—and perhaps could not—understand the clinical elements of quality and safety. Few board members or chairs were trained in quality and safety science,[35] and most boards lacked useful measures to help them judge the safety of their institutions.[36] A 2007–2008 survey of 722 board chairs found that fewer than half placed quality (and, by implication, safety) among the two most important priorities for evaluating their chief executive officers, and only slightly more than half considered quality to be one of their top two priorities for board oversight. Importantly, there was a strong association between the board chairs' stated priority for quality and the hospitals' actual quality performance (as assessed through publicly reported data [Figure 22-3]).[35] This is further supported by additional studies which conclude that the boards of higher performing hospitals tend to be more engaged in safety activities than the boards of hospitals that perform less well.[37,38]

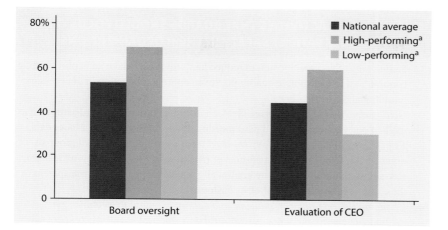

Figure 22-3 ■ Percentage of hospital board chairs reporting that quality of care is one of the top two priorities for board oversight or evaluation of chief executive officer (CEO) performance. The superscript "a" denotes statistical significance ($P < 0.001$) for comparisons of the difference between the highest- and lowest-performing hospitals. Rates are adjusted for the number of beds, region, location (urban vs. rural), teaching status, and ownership. (Reproduced with permission from Jha AK, Epstein AM. Hospital governance and the quality of care. *Health Aff (Millwood)* 2010;29:182–187. © 2010 by Project HOPE—The People-to-People Health Foundation, Inc.)

The safety movement has catapulted boards into action. While some of this undoubtedly flows from boards' new appreciation of their ethical obligations to patients, the emergence of a powerful business case for safety (Table 3-5) is undoubtedly playing a part as well.[39] There is no question that an engaged board can help promote safety, particularly when the board spends more than one-quarter of its time on safety and quality issues, the board regularly reviews quality and safety data, incentives for senior executives are partly based on quality and safety, and there is active dialogue between the board and the medical staff.[37,40,41] The IHI's 5 Million Lives Campaign (Table 20-2) included a plank called "boards on board," highlighting activities to promote board engagement in patient safety (Table 22-4).[42]

As with other parts of the organization, board members should be given data (culled from the various data streams described in Table 22-1, but summarized into an easy-to-read, high-level "dashboard") that help illuminate the key patient safety issues and the organization's performance in addressing them. That said, it is also crucial that each board meeting include at least one story of an actual patient harmed or killed while receiving care in the system. It is the drama and poignancy of the individual case—a person who was seriously injured by an error with a name, face, and family—that provides

Table 22-4   SIX ACTIVITIES THAT BOARDS SHOULD FOCUS ON TO PROMOTE PATIENT SAFETY IN THEIR ORGANIZATIONS

1. *Setting aims*: Set a specific aim to reduce harm this year. Make an explicit, public commitment to measurable quality improvement (e.g., reduction in unnecessary mortality and harm).
2. *Getting data and hearing stories*: Select and review progress toward safer care as the first agenda item at every board meeting. Put a "human face" on harm data.
3. *Establishing and monitoring system-level measures*: Identify a small group of organization-wide "roll-up" measures of patient safety (e.g., facility-wide harm, risk-adjusted mortality) that are continually updated and are made transparent to the entire organization and all of its customers.
4. *Changing the environment, policies, and culture*: Commit to establish and maintain an environment that is respectful, fair, and just for all who experience pain and loss as a result of avoidable harm and adverse outcomes: the patients, their families, and the staff at the sharp end of error.
5. *Learning—starting with the board*: Develop your capability as a board. Learn about how "best in the world" boards work with executive and MD leaders to reduce harm. Set an expectation for similar levels of education and training for all staff.
6. *Establishing executive accountability*: Oversee the effective execution of a plan to achieve your aims to reduce harm, including executive team accountability for clear quality improvement targets.

Reproduced with permission from Get Boards on Board. *How to Guide*. Institute for Healthcare Improvement (IHI). Available at: http://www.ihi.org/resources/Pages/Tools/HowtoGuideGovernanceLeadership.aspx.

the energy needed to inspire real action in safety. This energy can easily be sapped by a well-meaning recitation of bloodless statistics or the flashing of an endless series of PowerPoint graphs.

RESEARCH IN PATIENT SAFETY

Until a little more than a decade ago, there was scant research in patient safety. At the time, a simplistic understanding of errors (as individual failings rather than systems problems) led to little interest in empirical investigation. After all, if an error was a screwup by an individual doctor or nurse, what exactly needed to be studied? This mindset led to little funding for patient safety research, few faculty who devoted their careers to it, and few journals interested in publishing the fruits of this research.

This has changed drastically over the past 20 years. As we mentioned earlier, *AHRQ Patient Safety Network* now hosts approximately 20,000 resources, including 5000 research studies. The AHRQ PSNet list of "Classic" articles (articles of "enduring importance") now numbers more than 700.[43] (Another more immediate and tactile example: the number of references in the book you are holding has more than doubled since the first edition, which was written in 2008.) AHRQ's annual funding for patient safety–oriented work is now approximately $100 million, and substantial additional funding comes from other federal agencies (such as the Centers for Disease Control and Prevention and Medicare's Innovation Center), foundations, and other worldwide organizations. Hundreds of faculty members have made patient safety research the focus of their professional careers, and many have been successful in garnering grants, publications, and promotion.

One of the exciting things about patient safety research is that it is inherently interdisciplinary and eclectic. Studies of medication errors, for example, often involve collaboration among physicians, nurses, pharmacists, and informatics experts. Studying errors at the person-machine interface may require engineers and human factors researchers. Studies of mistakes related to communication and poor teamwork may include psychologists and experts from other industries such as aviation.

Because patient safety involves real-world work processes, studies tend to be messier than controlled trials of new medications or laboratory studies of physiologic systems. It is very difficult to isolate the effect of one intervention (e.g., computerized provider order entry or Rapid Response Teams) from scores of other interventions occurring simultaneously.[44,45] It is nearly impossible to randomize hospital floors or institutions to one complex, expensive intervention or another, and institutions that embrace interventions often differ from those that don't in fundamental (and confounding) ways. Moreover, safety research cannot be standardized ("1 g of vancomycin IV" is approximately the same thing when administered in a big hospital in San Francisco and a small one in Peoria, but "teamwork training" is decidedly not). Safety experts have emphasized the importance of "context" in safety research, since the environmental and other contextual factors are often precisely what explains how a safety intervention that worked spectacularly in one setting failed miserably in another.[46,47]

All of this makes patient safety research harder than, say, drug trials. But young safety researchers should take heart, for safety research also has some unique advantages. Small studies that isolate the effect of a single intervention often lead to deeper understanding and give rise to larger research projects. For example, the simple matter of introducing "goal cards" to a clinical unit led to important improvements in communications and outcomes,[48,49] setting the stage for more ambitious teamwork and communication interventions (Chapter 9). A study that randomized ICU residents to longer versus shorter shifts found far fewer errors in the latter group,[50] a finding that informed the debate over resident duty hours (Chapter 16). Small studies that demonstrated the value of process changes in preventing central line–associated bloodstream infections[51–53] ultimately led to a multifaceted set of interventions that slashed the number of bloodstream infections in more than 100 ICUs (Chapter 10).[54]

There is one more exciting aspect to patient safety research: in safety, unlike clinical medicine, the linkages to regulations, malpractice law, media scrutiny, and public pressure can lead to rapid dissemination of "safety practices." For example, laws, regulations, and accreditation requirements around nurse-to-patient ratios, medication reconciliation, and error disclosure all materialized after a relatively small number of studies demonstrated, or even hinted at, benefit. So too did a national, and even international, effort to use checklists to address error-prone systems of care. Because of this, well-designed and executed safety studies addressing important questions can rapidly lead to major changes in practice.

PATIENT SAFETY MEETS EVIDENCE-BASED MEDICINE

As research in safety has exploded, a fundamental question has arisen: what is the role of evidence in assessing patient safety practices? There are two schools of thought on this. One group points out that many safety practices have little downside, have substantial face validity, and are too complex to study effectively and efficiently. For these reasons, they have argued, traditional standards of evidence-based medicine should be relaxed for practices like Rapid Response Teams and computerized provider order entry.[55,56]

The other group posits that safety practices can be extremely expensive and disruptive, and they often have unforeseen consequences that only emerge over time. Accordingly, this group has argued that most safety practices should be studied, if feasible, before widespread implementation.[57–59] And, as the field of patient safety has matured, the evidence base for numerous patient safety strategies has grown.[60,61]

In 2013, AHRQ issued, *Making Health Care Safer II*,[62] an update on the evidence for patient safety practices (PSPs) since the publication of its 2001 report of the same name.[63] In this updated seminal report, the authors analyze the evidence supporting 41 distinct PSPs and derive a list of 10 practices they would strongly encourage healthcare institutions to adopt (Table 22-5).

The authors of MHCS II highlighted the growing evidence base in safety since the prior report). With the Federal investment in safety (under the "Partnership for Patients") of about $1 billion, and an investment of more than 20 times that amount in information technology implementation, we are on the cusp of an exploding database of research on safety practices.

Table 22-5	**STRONGLY ENCOURAGED PATIENT SAFETY PRACTICES**

1. Preoperative checklists and anesthesia checklists to prevent operative and postoperative events.
2. Bundles that include checklists to prevent central line-associated bloodstream infections.
3. Interventions to reduce urinary catheter use, including catheter reminders, stop orders, or nurse-initiated removal protocols.
4. Bundles that include head-of-bed elevation, sedation vacations, oral care with chlorhexidine, and subglottic-suctioning endotracheal tubes to prevent ventilator-associated pneumonia.
5. Hand hygiene.
6. "Do Not Use" list for hazardous abbreviations.
7. Multicomponent interventions to reduce pressure ulcers.
8. Barrier precautions to prevent healthcare-associated infections.
9. Use of real-time ultrasound for central line placement.
10. Interventions to improve prophylaxis for venous thromboembolisms.

Reproduced with permission from *Making Health Care Safer II: A Critical Analysis of Patient Safety Practices.* Agency for Healthcare Research and Quality; March 2013. AHRQ Publication No. 13-E001-EF. Available at: http://www.ahrq.gov/sites/default/files/wysiwyg/research/findings/evidence-based-reports/services/quality/ptsafetyII-full.pdf.

Yet recent studies of rates of harm have demonstrated how difficult improving safety really is and have caused policymakers and researchers to redouble their efforts to identify and implement safe practices in hospitals, nursing homes, and clinics. Individuals and institutions seeking to improve safety would do well to scrutinize the practices described in the MCHS II report—widespread implementation is likely to save hundreds, if not thousands, of lives. Even as we study the literature for evidence of effective practices, we must continue to refine our efforts to identify the factors associated with successful implementation of patient safety practices (PSPs), and to pinpoint, and hopefully prevent, any unintended consequences.[62]

KEY POINTS

- Because of the intense focus on patient safety and increasing regulatory and accreditation requirements, many organizations have begun safety programs, hired patient safety officers, and formed patient safety committees.
- The challenges of measuring safety mean that the inputs to safety programs will come from multiple sources, including voluntary reporting,

trigger tools, malpractice cases, patient and provider surveys, and structure, process, and outcome data relevant to patient safety.

- Safety officers and programs need to effectively collaborate with a variety of other personnel and programs: quality, risk management, information technology, and more.
- Effective safety programs blend elements of top-down management and bottom-up engagement and innovation. Boards and physicians must also be fully engaged for programs to be successful.
- Safety research is difficult to do, but its results can be highly influential, particularly when they lead to regulatory action or other broad-based mandates.
- In the early years of the safety field, there was debate regarding the degree to which traditional standards of evidence should be relaxed for patient safety practices. However, as patient safety research has matured, it is increasingly clear that rigorous studies are essential for understanding which interventions truly work, and the role of context in determining local effectiveness.

REFERENCES

1. In conversation with … Allan Frankel [Perspective]. *AHRQ PSNet* (serial online); July 2006. Available at: https://psnet.ahrq.gov/perspectives/perspective/26.
2. Tsai TC, Jha AK, Gawande AA, Huckman RS, Bloom N, Sadun R. Hospital board and management practices are strongly related to hospital performance on clinical quality metrics. *Health Aff (Millwood)* 2015;34:1304–1311.
3. Chassin MR, Loeb JM. High-reliability health care: getting there from here. *Millbank Q* 2013;92:459–490.
4. Brilli RJ, McClead RE Jr, Crandall WV, et al. A comprehensive patient safety program can significantly reduce preventable harm, associated costs, and hospital mortality. *J Pediatr* 2013;16:1638–1645.
5. Parand A, Dopson S, Renz A, Vincent C. The role of hospital managers in quality and patient safety: a systematic review. *BMJ Open* September 5, 2014;4:e005055.
6. Kenney C. *Transforming Health Care: Virginia Mason Medical Center's Pursuit of the Perfect Patient Experience*. New York, NY: Productivity Press; 2011.
7. In conversation with …Geri Amori, PhD [Perspective]. *AHRQ PSNet* (serial online); December 2010. Available at: https://psnet.ahrq.gov/perspectives/perspective/95.
8. Gandhi TK, Graydon-Baker E, Barnes JN, et al. Creating an integrated patient safety program. *Jt Comm J Qual Saf* 2003;29:383–390.
9. Macrae C. The problem with incident reporting. *BMJ Qual Saf* 2016;25:71–75.
10. Pham JC, Girard T, Pronovost PJ. What to do with healthcare incident reporting systems. *J Public Health Res* 2013;2:e27.

11. de Feijter JM, De Grave WS, Muijtjens AM, Scherpbier AJ, Kiipmans RP. A comprehensive overview of medical error in hospitals using incident-reporting systems, patient complaints and chart review of inpatient deaths. *PLoS One* 2012;7:e31125.

12. Bagenal J, Sahnan K, Shantikumar S. Comparing the attitudes and knowledge toward incident reporting in junior physicians and nurses in a district general hospital. *J Patient Saf* 2016;12:51–53.

13. In conversation with … Kaveh G. Shojania, MD [Perspective]. *AHRQ PSNet* (serial online); September 2011. Available at: https://psnet.ahrq.gov/perspectives/perspective/107.

14. Levtzion-Korach O, Frankel A, Alcalai H, et al. Integrating incident data from five reporting systems to assess patient safety: making sense of the elephant. *Jt Comm J Qual Patient Saf* 2010;36:402–410.

15. Shojania KG. The elephant of patient safety: what you see depends on how you look. *Jt Comm J Qual Patient Saf* 2010;36:399–401, AP1–AP3.

16. Vincent C, Burnett S, Carthey J. Safety measurement and monitoring in healthcare: a framework to guide clinical teams and healthcare organizations in maintaining safety. *BMJ Qual Saf* 2014;23:670–677.

17. McCoy THJr, Castro VM, Roberson AM, Snapper LA, Perlis RH. Improving prediction of suicide and accidental death after discharge from general hospitals with natural language processing. *JAMA Psychiatry* 2016;73:1064–1071.

18. Classen DC, Resar R, Griffin F, et al. "Global Trigger Tool" shows that adverse events in hospitals may be ten times greater than previously measured. *Health Aff (Millwood)* 2011;30:581–589.

19. FitzHenry F, Murff HJ, Matheny ME, et al. Exploring the frontier of electronic health record surveillance: the case of postoperative complications. *Med Care* 2013;51:509–516.

20. Michtalik HJ, Carolan HT, Haut ER, et al. Use of provider-level dashboards and pay-for-performance in venous thromboembolism prophylaxis. *J Hosp Med* 2015;10:172–178.

21. Colla JB, Bracken AC, Kinney LM, Weeks WB. Measuring patient safety climate: a review of surveys. *Qual Saf Health Care* 2005;14:364–366.

22. Agency for Healthcare Research and Quality. *Patient Safety Culture Surveys*. Rockville, MD: Agency for Healthcare Research and Quality; November 2010. Available at: http://www.ahrq.gov/qual/patientsafetyculture/.

23. Pronovost PJ, Sexton B. Assessing safety culture: guidelines and recommendations. *Qual Saf Health Care* 2005;14:231–233.

24. Schwendimann R, Zimmermann N, Küng K, Ausserhofer D, Sexton B. Variation in safety culture dimensions within and between US and Swiss Hospital units: an exploratory study. *BMJ Qual Saf* 2013;22:32–41.

25. Frankel A, Leonard M. Update on safety culture [Perspective]. *AHRQ PSNet* (serial online); July–August 2013. Available at: https://psnet.ahrq.gov/perspectives/perspective/144.

26. Peters TJ, Waterman RJ. *In Search of Excellence: Lessons from America's Best Run Companies*. New York, NY: HarperCollins; 2004.

27. Weaver SJ, Lubomski LH, Wilson RF, Pfoh ER, Martinez KA, Dy SM. Promoting a culture of safety as a patient safety strategy: a systematic review. *Ann Intern Med* 2013;158:369–374.

28. van Dusseldorp L, Huisman de Waal G, Hamers H, Westert G, Schoonhoven L. Feasibility and added value of executive walk rounds in long term care organizations in the Netherlands. *Jt Comm J Qual Patient Saf* 2016;42:545–557.

29. Ohrn A, Rutberg H, Nilsen P. Patient safety dialogue: evaluation of an intervention aimed at achieving an improved patient safety culture. *J Patient Saf* 2011;7:185–192.

30. Pronovost PJ. An interview with Peter Pronovost. *Jt Comm J Qual Saf* 2004;30:659–664.

31. Kim CS, King E, Stein J, Robinson E, Salameh M, O'Leary KJ. Unit-based interprofessional leadership models in six US hospitals. *J Hosp Med* 2014;9:545–550.

32. Wachter RM. The media: an essential, if sometimes arbitrary, promoter of patient safety [Perspective] *AHRQ PSNet* (serial online); October 2009. Available at: https://psnet.ahrq.gov/perspectives/perspective/80.

33. Maguire EM, Bokhour BG, Asch SM, et al. Disclosing large scale adverse events in the US Veterans Health Administration: lessons from media responses. *Public Health* 2016;135:75–82.

34. Taitz JM, Lee TH, Sequist TD. A framework for engaging physicians in quality and safety. *BMJ Qual Saf* 2012;21:722–728.

35. Jha AK, Epstein AM. Hospital governance and the quality of care. *Health Aff (Millwood)* 2010;29:182–187.

36. In conversation with ... James Reinertsen [Perspective]. *AHRQ PSNet* (serial online); July 2007. Available at: https://psnet.ahrq.gov/perspectives/perspective/45.

37. Millar R, Mannion R, Freeman T, Davies HTO. Hospital board oversight of quality and patient safety: a narrative review and synthesis of recent empirical research. *Milbank Q* 2013;91:738–770.

38. Tsai TC, Jha AK, Gawande AA, Huckman RS, Bloom N, Sadun R. Hospital board and management practices are strongly related to hospital performance on clinical quality metrics. *Health Aff (Millwood)* 2015;34:1304–1311.

39. Weeks WB, Bagian JP. Making the business case for patient safety. *Jt Comm J Qual Saf* 2003;29:51–54.

40. Millar R, Freeman T, Mannion R. Hospital board oversight of quality and safety: a stakeholder analysis exploring the role of trust and intelligence. *BMC Health Serv Res* 2015;15:196.

41. Goeschel CA, Berenholtz SM, Culbertson RA, Jin L, Pronovost PJ. Board quality scorecards: measuring improvement. *Am J Med Qual* 2011;26:254–160.

42. McCannon CJ, Hackbarth AD, Griffin FA. Miles to go: an introduction to the 5 Million Lives Campaign. *Jt Comm J Qual Patient Saf* 2007;33:477–484.

43. Available at: https://psnet.ahrq.gov/search?Site2Search=PSNet&q=&classic=true.

44. Brown C, Hofer T, Johal A, et al. An epistemology of patient safety research: a framework for study design and interpretation. *Qual Saf Health Care* 2008;17(3, pt 1, pt 2, pt 3, pt 4):158–181.

45. Whicher DM, Kass NE, Audera-Lopez C, et al. Ethical issues in patient safety research: a systematic review of the literature. *J Patient Saf* 2015;11:174–184.

46. Shekelle PG, Pronovost PJ, Wachter RM, et al. Advancing the science of patient safety. *Ann Intern Med* 2011;154:693–696.

47. Taylor SL, Dy S, Foy R, et al. What context features might be important determinants of the effectiveness of patient safety practice interventions? *BMJ Qual Saf* 2011;20:611–617.

48. Pronovost P, Berenholz S, Dorman T, Lipsett PA, Simmonds T, Haraden C. Improving communication in the ICU using daily goals. *J Crit Care* 2003;18:71–75.

49. Narasimhan M, Eisen LA, Mahoney CD, Acerra FL, Rosen MJ. Improving nurse–physician communication and satisfaction in the intensive care unit with a daily goals worksheet. *Am J Crit Care* 2006;15:217–222.

50. Landrigan CP, Rothschild JM, Cronin JW, et al. Effect of reducing interns' work hours on serious medical errors in intensive care units. *N Engl J Med* 2004;351:1838–1848.

51. Raad II, Hohn DC, Gilbreath BJ, et al. Prevention of central venous catheter-related infections by using maximal sterile barrier precautions during insertion. *Infect Control Hosp Epidemiol* 1994;15(4 pt 1):231–238.

52. Chaiyakunapruk N, Veenstra DL, Lipsky BA, Saint S. Chlorhexidine compared with povidone–iodine solution for vascular catheter-site care: a meta-analysis. *Ann Intern Med* 2002;136:792–801.

53. Deshpande KS, Hatem C, Ulrich HL, et al. The incidence of infectious complications of central venous catheters at the subclavian, internal jugular, and femoral sites in an intensive care unit population. *Crit Care Med* 2005;33:13–20 [discussion 234–235].

54. Pronovost P, Needham D, Berenholtz S, et al. An intervention to decrease catheter-related bloodstream infections in the ICU. *N Engl J Med* 2006;355:2725–2732.

55. Leape LL, Berwick DM, Bates DW. What practices will most improve safety? Evidence-based medicine meets patient safety. *JAMA* 2002;288:501–507.

56. Berwick DM. The science of improvement. *JAMA* 2008;299:1182–1184.

57. Shojania KG, Duncan BW, McDonald KM, Wachter RM. Safe but sound: patient safety meets evidence-based medicine. *JAMA* 2002;288:508–513.

58. Wachter RM. Expected and unanticipated consequences of the quality and information technology revolutions. *JAMA* 2006;295:2780–2783.

59. Auerbach AD, Landefeld CS, Shojania KG. The tension between needing to improve care and knowing how to do it. *N Engl J Med* 2007;357:608–613.

60. Shekelle PG, Pronovost PJ, Wachter RM, et al. The top patient safety strategies that can be encouraged for adoption now. *Ann Intern Med* 2013;158:365–368.

61. Wachter RM, Pronovost PJ, Shekelle PG. Strategies to improve patient safety: the evidence base matures. *Ann Intern Med* 2013;158:350–352.

62. Shekelle PG, Wachter RM, Pronovost PJ, eds. *Making Health Care Safer: A Critical Analysis of Patient Safety Practices*. Agency for Healthcare Research and Quality; March 2013. AHRQ Publication No. 13-E001-EF.

63. Shojania KG, Duncan BW, McDonald KM, et al. Drawing on safety practices from outside healthcare. In: Shojania KG, Duncan BW, McDonald KM, et al., eds. *Making Health Care Safer: A Critical Analysis of Patient Safety Practices*. Evidence Report/Technology Assessment No. 43, AHRQ Publication No. 01-E058. Rockville, MD: Agency for Healthcare Research and Quality; July 2001.

ADDITIONAL READINGS

Bohmer RMJ. The four habits of high-value healthcare organizations. *N Engl J Med* 2011;365:2045–2047.

Burnett S, Benn J, Pinto A, Parand A, Iskander S, Vincent C. Organisational readiness: exploring the preconditions for success in organisation-wide patient safety improvement programmes. *Qual Saf Health Care* 2010;19:313–317.

Leonard M, Frankel A, Federico F, Frush K, Haraden C, eds. *The Essential Guide for Patient Safety Officers*. 2nd ed. Oakbrook Terrace, IL: Joint Commission Resources, Institute for Healthcare Improvement; 2013.

Gandhi TK, Graydon-Baker E, Huber CN, Whittemore AD, Gustafson M. Closing the loop: follow-up and feedback in a patient safety program. *Jt Comm J Qual Patient Saf* 2005;31:614–621.

Ginsburg LR, Chuang YT, Berta WB, et al. The relationship between organizational leadership for safety and learning from patient safety events. *Health Serv Res* 2010;45:607–632.

Goeschel CA, Wachter RM, Pronovost PJ. Responsibility for quality improvement and patient safety: hospital board and medical staff leadership challenges. *Chest* 2010;138:171–178.

Mitchell I, Schuster A, Smith K, Wu A. Patient safety reporting: a qualitative study of thoughts and perceptions of experts 15 years after 'To Err Is Human'. *BMJ Qual Saf* 2016;25:92–99.

Parand A, Burnett S, Benn J, Pinto A, Iskander S, Vincent C. The disparity of frontline clinical staff and managers' perceptions of a quality and patient safety initiative. *J Eval Clin Pract* 2011;17:1184–1190.

Pronovost PJ. Learning accountability for patient outcomes. *JAMA* 2010;304:204–205.

Romig M, Goeschel C, Pronovost P, Berenholtz SM. Integrating CUSP and TRIP to improve patient safety. *Hosp Pract (Minneap)* 2010;38:114–121.

Singer SJ, Tucker AL. The evolving literature on safety walk rounds: emerging themes and practical messages. *BMJ Qual Saf* 2014;23:789–800.

Spath PL, ed. *Error Reduction in Health Care: A Systems Approach to Improving Patient Safety*. 2nd ed. San Francisco, CA: Jossey-Bass; 2011.

Wachter RM. Patient safety at ten: unmistakable progress, troubling gaps. *Health Aff (Millwood)* 2010;29:165–173.

Youngberg BJ, ed. *Principles of Risk Management and Patient Safety*. Sudbury, MA: Jones Bartlett; 2011.

CONCLUSION

The fireworks that accompanied the publication of *To Err Is Human* by the Institute of Medicine in late 1999 generated some magical thinking about how easy it would be to fix the problem of medical errors. A few computer systems here, some standard processes there (double checks, read-backs), and maybe just a sprinkling of culture change—and poof, patients would be safer.

We now know how naive this point of view was. The problem of medical errors is remarkably complex, and the solutions will need to be as varied as the problems. Do we need better information technology? Yes. Improved teamwork? Yes. Stronger rules and regulations? Yes. Checklists, simulation, decision support, forcing functions? Yes, yes, yes, and yes.

Organizationally, we have come to understand that solutions must be *both* top down and bottom up. Resources need to be made available from senior leadership and boards—for teamwork training, computers, and appropriate staffing. Yet much of the action in patient safety happens at the frontline: will a nurse simply work around a hazardous situation, leaving it unaddressed, or take the time and trouble to report it and help fix it? Will residents enthusiastically participate in teamwork training programs and M&M conferences? Will the senior surgeon welcome—truly welcome—input from the intern or the nurse who sees something that might put a patient at risk?

The analogies from other industries are extraordinarily helpful, but they take us only so far. Computerizing the hospital is far more challenging than computerizing the supermarket. Changing an operating room's culture is many times more complex than creating an environment in a hermetically sealed cockpit that allows two people—with similar training, expertise, and social status—to feel comfortable raising their concerns. Giving a patient a dozen medications safely is much more difficult than avoiding defects as a car slides down an assembly line. And yet there is much we can learn from all these settings, and that learning has truly begun.

And what is the proper role of patients in all of this? It is clear that patients should be involved in their care, and that patient engagement can be an important part of a comprehensive safety strategy. Moreover, being open and honest about our errors with patients and their families is undeniably right, independent of pragmatic considerations regarding whether such disclosures change the risk of a malpractice suit.

But why should a patient have to check into a hospital or enter a clinic and be worried—quite appropriately—that he or she will be injured by the medical system? We should be proud of the progress we have made in the relatively short time since *To Err Is Human* launched the modern patient safety movement. But we cannot rest until patients can approach the healthcare system free from fear and anxiety that they will be harmed or killed in the process of being helped. We still have much to do before we get there.

APPENDICES

APPENDICES

APPENDIX I. KEY BOOKS, REPORTS, SERIES, AND WEBSITES ON PATIENT SAFETY

Key Books and Reports on Medical Errors and Errors More Generally

1. Agency for Healthcare Research and Quality. *Advances in Patient Safety: From Research to Implementation*. Rockville, MD: Agency for Healthcare Research and Quality; February 2005. AHRQ Publication Nos. 050021 (1–4).

2. Agency for Healthcare Research and Quality. *Advances in Patient Safety: New Directions and Alternative Approaches*. Rockville, MD: Agency for Healthcare Research and Quality; July 2008. AHRQ Publication Nos. 080034 (1–4).

3. Agency for Healthcare Research and Quality. *Advancing Patient Safety: A Decade of Evidence, Design, and Implementation*. Rockville, MD: Agency for Healthcare Research and Quality; November 2009. AHRQ Publication No. 09(10)-0084.

4. Agency for Healthcare Research and Quality. *National Scorecard on Rates of Hospital-Acquired Conditions 2010 to 2015: Interim Data from National Efforts to Make Health Care Safer.* Rockville, MD: Agency for Healthcare Research and Quality; December 2016.

5. American Hospital Association, Health Research and Educational Trust, and Joint Commission Center for Transforming Healthcare. *Reducing the Risks of Wrong-Site Surgery: Safety Practices from the Joint Commission Center for Transforming Healthcare Project.* Chicago, IL: American Hospital Association, Health Research and Educational Trust, and Joint Commission Center for Transforming Healthcare; 2014.

6. Antonsen S. *Safety Culture: Theory, Method and Improvement*. Burlington, VT: Ashgate; 2009.

7. Berwick DM. *Escape Fire: Designs for the Future of Health Care*. San Francisco, CA: Jossey-Bass; 2003.

8. Betsy Lehman Center for Patient Safety and Error Reduction. *The Public's Views on Medical Error in Massachusetts*. Boston, MA: Harvard School of Public Health; December 2014.

9. Bosk CL. *Forgive and Remember: Managing Medical Failure*. 2nd ed. Chicago, IL: University of Chicago Press; 2003.

10. Bunting RF Jr, Schukman J, Wong WB. *A Comprehensive Guide to Managing Never Events and Hospital-Acquired Conditions.* Washington, DC: Atlantic Information Services Inc.; 2009.

11. Casey SM. *Set Phasers on Stun: And Other True Tales of Design, Technology, and Human Error.* 2nd ed. Santa Barbara, CA: Aegean Publishing Company; 1998.

12. Columbia Accident Investigation Board. *Report of the Columbia Accident Investigation Board;* August 2003.

13. Conway J, Federico F, Stewart K, Campbell MJ. *Respectful Management of Serious Clinical Adverse Events.* Cambridge, MA: Institute for Healthcare Improvement; 2010.

14. Cook RI, Woods DD, Miller C. *A Tale of Two Stories: Contrasting Views of Patient Safety.* National Patient Safety Foundation at the AMA: Annenberg Center for Health Sciences; 1998.

15. Dekker S. *The Field Guide to Human Error Investigations.* 3rd ed. Aldershot, UK: Ashgate Publishing; 2014.

16. Dekker S. *Just Culture: Balancing Safety and Accountability.* 3rd ed. Boca Raton, FL: CRC Press; 2016.

17. Donaldson L. *An Organisation with a Memory: Report of an Expert Group on Learning from Adverse Events in the NHS Chaired by the Chief Medical Officer.* London: The Stationery Office; 2000.

18. Farley DO, Ridgely MS, Mendel P, et al. *Assessing Patient Safety Practices and Outcomes in the U.S. Health Care System.* Santa Monica, CA: RAND Corporation; 2009.

19. Gawande A. *Complications: A Surgeon's Notes on an Imperfect Science.* New York, NY: Metropolitan Books; 2002.

20. Gawande A. *Better: A Surgeon's Notes on Performance.* New York, NY: Metropolitan Books; 2007.

21. Gawande A. *The Checklist Manifesto: How to Get Things Right.* New York, NY: Metropolitan Books; 2009.

22. Gibson R, Singh JP. *Wall of Silence: The Untold Story of the Medical Mistakes that Kill and Injure Millions of Americans.* Washington, DC: Lifeline; 2003.

23. Gosbee JW, Gosbee LL, eds. *Using Human Factors Engineering to Improve Patient Safety.* 2nd ed. Oakbrook Terrace, IL: Joint Commission Resources; 2010.

24. Griffin FA, Resar RK. *IHI Global Trigger Tool for Measuring Adverse Events.* 2nd ed. IHI Innovation Series White Paper. Cambridge, MA: Institute for Healthcare Improvement; 2009.

25. Groopman J. *How Doctors Think.* Boston, MA: Houghton Mifflin; 2007.

26. Helmreich RL, Merritt AC. *Culture at Work in Aviation and Medicine: National, Organizational, and Professional Influences.* Aldershot, Hampshire, UK: Ashgate; 1998.

27. Hollnagel E. *Safety-I and Safety-II: The Past and Future of Safety Management.* Aldershot, Hampshire, England: Ashgate; 2014.

28. Hughes RG, ed. *Patient Safety and Quality: An Evidence-Based Handbook for Nurses.* Rockville, MD: Agency for Healthcare Research and Quality; 2008. AHRQ Publication No. 08-0043.

29. Hurwitz B, Sheikh A, eds. *Health Care Errors and Patient Safety.* Hoboken, NJ: Wiley-Blackwell; 2009.

30. Joint Commission. *Getting the Board on Board: What Your Board Needs to Know About Quality and Safety, Third Edition.* Oakbrook, IL: Joint Commission; 2016.

31. Kahneman D, Slovic P, Tversky A. *Judgment Under Uncertainty: Heuristics and Biases.* Cambridge, England: Cambridge University Press; 1987.

32. Kahneman D. *Thinking Fast and Slow.* New York: Farrar, Strauss and Giroux; 2011.

33. King S. *Josie's Story.* New York, NY: Atlantic Monthly Press; 2009.

34. Krause TR, Hidley J. *Taking the Lead in Patient Safety: How Healthcare Leaders Influence Behavior and Create Culture.* Hoboken, NJ: Wiley; 2008.

35. Langley GJ, Moen R, Nolan KM, Nolan TW, Normal CL, Provost LP. *The Improvement Guide: A Practical Approach to Enhancing Organizational Performance.* 2nd ed. San Francisco, CA: Jossey-Bass; 2009.

36. Leonard M, Frankel A, Federico F, Frush K, Haraden C, eds. The Essential Guide for Patient Safety Officers, Second Edition. Oakbrook Terrace, IL: Joint Commission Resources, Institute for Healthcare Improvement; 2013.

37. Levinson DR. *Adverse Events in Hospitals: National Incidence Among Medicare Beneficiaries.* Washington, DC: US Department of Health and Human Services, Office of the Inspector General; November 2010. Report No. OEI-06-09-00090.

38. Lucian Leape Institute at the National Patient Safety Foundation. *Unmet Needs: Teaching Physicians to Provide Safe Patient Care.* Boston, MA: Lucian Leape Institute at the National Patient Safety Foundation; March 2010.

39. Lucian Leape Institute at the National Patient Safety Foundation Roundtable on Consumer Engagement in Patient Safety. *Safety is Personal: Partnering with Patients and Families for the Safest Care.* Boston, MA: National Patient Safety Foundation; March 2014.

40. Lucian Leape Institute at the National Patient Safety Foundation. *Shining a Light: Safer Health Care Through Transparency.* Boston, MA: National Patient Safety Foundation; January 2015.

41. Lucian Leape Institute at the National Patient Safety Foundation. *Transforming Health Care: A Compendium of Reports From the National Patient Safety Foundation's Lucian Leape Institute.* Boston, MA: Lucian Leape Institute at the National Patient Safety Foundation; May 2016.

42. Marx D. *Whack-a-Mole: The Price We Pay for Expecting Perfection.* Plano, TX: By Your Side Studios; 2009.

43. Massachusetts Coalition for the Prevention of Medical Errors. *When Things Go Wrong: Responding to Adverse Events.* A Consensus Statement of the Harvard Hospitals. Burlington, VT: Massachusetts Coalition for the Prevention of Medical Errors; 2006.

44. Merry A, Smith AM. *Errors, Medicine, and the Law.* Cambridge, England: Cambridge University Press; 2001.

45. Millenson ML. *Demanding Medical Excellence. Doctors and Accountability in the Information Age.* Chicago, IL: University of Chicago Press; 1997.

46. Morrow R. *Leading High-Reliability Organizations in Healthcare.* Boca Raton, FL: Productivity Press; 2016.

47. Nance JJ. *Why Hospitals Should Fly: The Ultimate Flight Plan to Patient Safety and Quality Care.* Boseman, MT: Second River Healthcare Press; 2008.

48. National Patient Safety Foundation. *Free From Harm: Accelerating Patient Safety Improvement Fifteen Years After To Err Is Human.* Boston, MA: National Patient Safety Foundation; 2015.

49. National Patient Safety Foundation. *RCA2: Improving Root Cause Analyses and Actions to Prevent Harm.* Boston, MA: National Patient Safety Foundation; 2015.

50. National Quality Forum. *Identification and Prioritization of Health IT Patient Safety Measures.* Washington, DC: National Quality Forum; February 2016.

51. National Quality Forum. *Safe Practices for Better Healthcare—2009 Update.* Washington, DC: National Quality Forum; 2009.

52. Nemeth CP, ed. *Improving Healthcare Team Communication: Building on Lessons from Aviation and Aerospace.* Burlington, VT: Ashgate Publishing; 2008.

53. Norman DA. *The Design of Everyday Things.* New York, NY: Basic Books; 2002.

54. Paget MA. *Unity of Mistakes: A Phenomenological Interpretation of Medical Work.* Philadelphia, PA: Temple University Press; 1993.

55. Perrow C. *Normal Accidents: Living with High-Risk Technologies. With a New Afterword and a Postscript on the Y2K Problem.* Princeton, NJ: Princeton University Press; 1999.

56. Pronovost P, Vohr E. *Safe Patients, Smart Hospitals: How One Doctor's Checklist can Help Us Change Health Care from the Inside Out.* New York, NY: Hudson Street Press; 2010.

57. Reason JT. *Human Error.* New York, NY: Cambridge University Press; 1990.

58. Reason JT. *Managing the Risks of Organizational Accidents.* Aldershot, Hampshire, UK: Ashgate; 1997.

59. Reason J. *The Human Contribution: Unsafe Acts, Accidents and Heroic Recoveries.* Farnham Surrey, UK: Ashgate; 2008.

60. Reynard J, Reynolds J, Stevenson P. *Practical Patient Safety.* Oxford, UK: Oxford University Press; 2009.

61. Robins NS. *The Girl who Died Twice: Every Patient's Nightmare: The Libby Zion Case and the Hidden Hazards of Hospitals.* New York, NY: Delacorte Press; 1995.

62. Rogers EM. *Diffusion of Innovation.* 5th ed. New York, NY: Free Press; 2003.

63. Rosenthal MM, Sutcliffe KM, eds. *Medical Error. What do We Know? What do We Do?* San Francisco, CA: John Wiley & Sons; 2002.

64. Rozovsky FA, Woods JR Jr, eds. *The Handbook of Patient Safety Compliance: A Practical Guide for Health Care Organizations.* San Francisco, CA: Jossey-Bass; 2005.

65. Sagan SD. *The Limits of Safety: Organizations, Accidents and Nuclear Weapons.* Princeton, NJ: Princeton University Press; 1993.

66. Sanders L. *Every Patient Tells A Story: Medical Mysteries and the Art of Diagnosis.* New York, NY: Broadway Books; 2009.

67. Schuster PM, Nykolyn L. *Communication for Nurses: How to Prevent Harmful Events and Promote Patient Safety.* Philadelphia, PA: F.A. Davis Company; 2010.

68. Sharpe VA, Faden AI. *Medical Harm: Historical, Conceptual, and Ethical Dimensions of Iatrogenic Illness.* New York, NY: Cambridge University Press; 1998.

69. Shekelle PG, Pronovost PJ, Wachter RM, et al.; PSP Technical Expert Panel. *Assessing the Evidence for Context-Sensitive Effectiveness and Safety of Patient Safety Practices:*

Developing Criteria. Rockville, MD: Agency for Healthcare Research and Quality; December 2010. AHRQ Publication No. 11-0006-EF.

70. Shojania KG, Duncan BW, McDonald KM, Wachter RM, eds. *Making Health Care Safer: A Critical Analysis of Patient Safety Practices*. Evidence Report/Technology Assessment No. 43 from the Agency for Healthcare Research and Quality: AHRQ Publication No. 01-E058. Rockville, MD: Agency for Healthcare Research and Quality; July 2001.

71. Spath PL. *Error Reduction in Health Care: A Systems Approach to Improving Patient Safety*. 2nd ed. San Francisco, CA: Jossey-Bass; 2011.

72. Stewart JB. *Blind Eye: How the Medical Establishment Let a Doctor Get Away with Murder*. New York, NY: Simon & Schuster; 1999.

73. Tenner E. *Why Things Bite Back: Technology and the Revenge of Unintended Consequences*. New York, NY: A.A. Knopf; 1996.

74. Truog RD, Browning DM, Johnson JA, Gallagher TH. *Talking with Patients and Families about Medical Error: A Guide for Education and Practice*. Baltimore, MD: Johns Hopkins University Press; 2011.

75. Ulmer C, Wolman DM, Johns MME, eds. *Resident Duty Hours: Enhancing Sleep, Supervision, and Safety*. Committee on Optimizing Graduate Medical Trainee (Resident) Hours and Work Schedule to Improve Patient Safety, Institute of Medicine. Washington, DC: National Academies Press; 2008.

76. Vance JE. *A Guide to Patient Safety in the Medical Practice*. Chicago, IL: American Medical Association; 2008.

77. Vaughan D. *The Challenger Launch Decision: Risky Technology, Culture, and Deviance at NASA*. Chicago, IL: University of Chicago Press; 1997.

78. Vincent C. *Patient Safety*. 2nd ed. West Sussex, UK: Wiley-Blackwell; 2010.

79. Vincent C, Amalberti R. *Safer Healthcare: Strategies for the Real World*. New York, NY: SpringerOpen; 2016.

80. Wachter RM, Shojania KG. *Internal Bleeding: The Truth Behind America's Terrifying Epidemic of Medical Mistakes*. New York, NY: Rugged Land; 2004.

81. Wachter R. *The Digital Doctor: Hope, Hype, and Harm at the Dawn of Medicine's Computer Age*. New York, NY: McGraw-Hill; 2015.

82. Weick KE. *Sensemaking in Organizations*. Thousand Oaks, CA: Sage Publications; 1995.

83. Weick KE, Sutcliffe KM. *Managing the Unexpected: Assuring High Performance in an Age of Complexity*. 2nd ed. San Francisco, CA: John Wiley & Sons; 2007.

84. Weick KE, Sutcliffe KM. *Managing the Unexpected: Sustained Performance in a Complex World, 3rd edition*. San Francisco, CA: John Wiley & Sons; 2015.

85. Wiener EL, Kanki BG, Helmreich RL. *Cockpit Resource Management*. San Diego, CA: Academic Press; 1993.

86. Woods DD, Dekker S, Cook R, Johannesen L, Sarter N. *Behind Human Error*. 2nd ed. Burlington, VT: Ashgate; 2010.

87. Wu AW, ed. *The Value of Close Calls in Improving Patient Safety*. Oakbrook Terrace, IL: Joint Commission Resources; 2011.

88. Wu HW, Nishimi RY, Page-Lopez CM, Kizer KW. *Improving Patient Safety Through Informed Consent for Patients with Limited Health Literacy*. Washington, DC: National Quality Forum; 2005.

89. Youngberg BJ, ed. *Principles of Risk Management and Patient Safety*. Sudbury, MA: Jones Bartlett; 2011.
90. Yu A, Flott K, Fontana G, Darzi A. *Patient Safety 2030*. London, UK: NIHR Imperial Patient Safety Translational Research Centre; 2016.

The National Academies of Sciences, Engineering, and Medicine (formerly the Institute of Medicine) Reports on Medical Errors and Healthcare Quality (From its "Quality Chasm" Series)

1. Kohn L, Corrigan J, Donaldson M, eds. *To Err Is Human: Building a Safer Health System*. Washington, DC: Committee on Quality of Health Care in America, Institute of Medicine: National Academies Press, 1999.
2. Committee on Quality of Health Care in America, IOM. *Crossing the Quality Chasm: A New Health System for the 21st Century*. Washington, DC: National Academies Press; 2001.
3. Page A, ed. *Keeping Patients Safe. Transforming the Work Environment of Nurses*. Committee on the Work Environment for Nurses and Patient Safety, Board on Health Care Services. Washington, DC: National Academies Press; 2004.
4. Aspden P, Corrigan JM, Wolcott J, Erickson SM, eds. *Patient Safety: Achieving a New Standard for Care*. Washington, DC: National Academies Press; 2004.
5. Nielsen-Bohlman L, Panzer AM, Kindig DA. Institute of Medicine Committee on Health Literacy. *Health Literacy: A Prescription to End Confusion*. Washington, DC: National Academies Press; 2004.
6. Aspden P, Wolcott J, Bootman JL, Cronenwett LR, eds. *Preventing Medication Errors*. Committee on Identifying and Preventing Medication Errors. Washington, DC: National Academies Press; 2007.
7. Balogh EP, Miller BT, Ball JR, eds. *Improving Diagnosis in Health Care*. Committee on Diagnostic Error in Health Care. Washington, DC: National Academies Press; 2015.

Quality Grand Rounds Series, Annals of Internal Medicine

1. Wachter RM, Shojania KG, Saint S, Markowitz AJ, Smith M. Learning from our mistakes: quality grand rounds, a new case-based series on medical errors and patient safety. *Ann Intern Med* 2002;136:850–852.
2. Chassin MR, Becher EC. The wrong patient. *Ann Intern Med* 2002;136:826–833.
3. Bates DW. Unexpected hypoglycemia in a critically ill patient. *Ann Intern Med* 2002;137:110–116.
4. Hofer TP, Hayward RA. Are bad outcomes from questionable clinical decisions preventable medical errors? A case of cascade iatrogenesis. *Ann Intern Med* 2002;137:327–333.
5. Gerberding JL. Hospital-onset infections: a patient safety issue. *Ann Intern Med* 2002;137:665–670.
6. Cleary PD. A hospitalization from hell: a patient's perspective on quality. *Ann Intern Med* 2003;138:33–39.

7. Lynn J, Goldstein NE. Advance care planning for fatal chronic illness: avoiding commonplace errors and unwarranted suffering. *Ann Intern Med* 2003;138:812–818.

8. Brennan TA, Mello MM. Patient safety and medical malpractice: a case study. *Ann Intern Med* 2003;139:267–273.

9. Goldman L, Kirtane AJ. Triage of patients with acute chest pain and possible cardiac ischemia: the elusive search for diagnostic perfection. *Ann Intern Med* 2003;139: 987–995.

10. Pronovost PJ, Wu AW, Sexton JB. Acute decompensation after removing a central line: practical approaches to increasing safety in the intensive care unit. *Ann Intern Med* 2004;140:1025–1033.

11. Redelmeier DA. Improving patient care. The cognitive psychology of missed diagnoses. *Ann Intern Med* 2005;142:115–120.

12. Gandhi TK. Fumbled hand-offs: one dropped ball after another. *Ann Intern Med* 2005;142:352–358.

13. McDonald CJ. Computerization can create safety hazards: a bar-coding near miss. *Ann Intern Med* 2006;144:510–516.

14. Shojania KG, Fletcher KE, Saint S. Graduate medical education and patient safety: a busy—and occasionally hazardous—intersection. *Ann Intern Med* 2006;145:592–598.

15. Wachter RM, Shojania KG, Markowitz AJ, Smith M, Saint S. Quality grand rounds: the case for patient safety. *Ann Intern Med* 2006;148:629–630.

Selected Theme Issues on Medical Errors

Focus on computerized provider order systems. *J Am Med Inform Assoc* 2007;14:25–75. Available at: http://www.jamia.org/content/vol14/issue1/.

Profiles in patient safety. Case-based series of articles. *Acad Emerg Med.* Available at: http://www.aemj.org/cgi/content/full/9/4/324.

Theme issue on medical error. *BMJ* 2000;320:7237. Available at: http://bmj.com/content/vol320/issue7237/.

Theme issue: contributions from ergonomics and human factors. *Qual Saf Health Care* 2010;19(suppl 3):i1–i79.

Theme issue: diagnostic error in medicine. Singh H, ed. *BMJ Qual Saf* 2013;22:ii1–ii72.

Theme issue: diagnostic error in medicine. Berner ES, Graber ML, eds. *Adv Health Sci Educ Theory Pract* 2009;14(suppl 1):1–112.

Theme issue: health information technology. *Am J Manag Care* 2014;20:492–554, e1–e31.

Theme issue: health information technology and clinical decision support systems. Ohno-Machado L, ed. *J Am Med Inform Assoc* 2014;21:e180–e375.

Theme issue: human factors and ergonomics in patient safety. Carayon P, Buckle P, eds. *App Ergon* 2010;41:643–718.

Theme issue: knowledge for improvement. *BMJ Qual Saf* 2011;20:1–105.

Theme issue: malpractice litigation alternatives. *Health Aff (Millwood)* 2014;33:6–66.

Theme issue: making healthcare safer. Shekelle PG, Pronovost PJ, Wachter RM, et al, eds. *Ann Intern Med* 2013;158:365–440.

Theme issue: medical liability and patient safety. Ridgely MS, Greenberg MD, Clancy CM, eds. *Health Serv Res* 2016;51:2395–2648.

Theme issue: medical malpractice and errors. *Health Aff (Millwood)* 2010;29:1564–1619.

Theme issue: new approaches to researching patient safety. Iedema R, ed. *Soc Sci Med* 2009;69:1701–1783.

Theme issue: nurses transforming care. *Am J Nurs* 2009;109(suppl 11):3–80, C3.

Theme issue: patient safety. Wagner VD, ed. *AORN* 2014;100:351–456.

Theme issue: patient safety. *J Health Serv Res Policy* 2015;20:S1–S60.

Theme issue: quality and safety in medicine. Nash DB, Goldfarb NI, Patow C, eds. *Acad Med* 2009;84:1641–1846.

Theme issue: safety by design. *Qual Saf Health Care* December 2006;15(suppl 1):i1–i90.

Theme issue: safety. Simmons D, ed. *Crit Care Nurs Clin North Am* 2010;22:161–290.

Theme issue: simulation. *BMJ Qual Saf* 2013;22:449–519.

Theme issue: special issue on health information technology. *J Gen Intern Med* 2008;23:353–507.

Theme issue: still crossing the quality chasm. *Health Aff (Millwood)* 2011;30:554–800.

Theme issue: teamwork. Salas E, Rosen MA, eds. *BMJ Qual Saf* 2013;22:369–448.

Selected Websites on Medical Errors

Agency for Healthcare Research and Quality (AHRQ). *Patient Safety & Medical Errors.* Available at: https://www.ahrq.gov/professionals/quality-patient-safety/index.html.

AHRQ Patient Safety Network (PSNet). Available at: https://psnet.ahrq.gov/.

AHRQ WebM&M: Morbidity and Mortality Rounds on the Web. Available at: https://psnet.ahrq.gov/webmm.

AHRQ Patient Safety Organizations. Available at: https://www.pso.ahrq.gov/listed.

AHRQ Health Care Innovations Exchange. Available at: https://innovations.ahrq.gov/.

American College of Surgeons. National Surgical Quality Improvement Program (NSQIP). Available at: https://www.facs.org/quality-programs/acs-nsqip.

American Hospital Association Patient Safety Center. Available at: http://www.aha.org/advocacy-issues/quality/index.shtml.

Association for Professionals in Infection Control and Epidemiology. Available at: http://www.apic.org/.

Institute for Healthcare Improvement (IHI). Available at: http://www.ihi.org.

Institute for Safe Medication Practices. Available at: http://www.ismp.org/.

Joint Commission. Available at: http://www.jointcommission.org.

Joint Commission Center for Transforming Healthcare. Available at: http://www.centerfor-transforminghealthcare.org/.

Joint Commission National Patient Safety Goals: Available at: http://www.jointcommission.org/standards_information/npsgs.aspx.

Leapfrog Group for Patient Safety. Available at: http://www.leapfroggroup.org/.

National Patient Safety Foundation. Available at: http://www.npsf.org/.

National Quality Forum. Available at: http://www.qualityforum.org.

US Department of Health and Human Services, Center for Medicare & Medicaid Services. *Partnership for Patients.* Available at: https://partnershipforpatients.cms.gov/.

World Health Organization (WHO) Patient Safety. Available at: http://www.who.int/patientsafety/en/.

WHO Patient Safety Human Factors Website. Available at: http://www.who.int/patientsafety/research/methods_measures/human_factors/en/.

APPENDIX II. THE AHRQ PATIENT SAFETY NETWORK (AHRQ PSNET) GLOSSARY OF SELECTED TERMS IN PATIENT SAFETY

Active error (or active failure)—The terms *active* and *latent* as applied to errors were coined by James Reason. Active errors occur at the point of contact between a human and some aspect of a larger system (e.g., a human–machine interface). They are generally readily apparent (e.g., pushing an incorrect button, ignoring a warning light) and almost always involve someone at the frontline. Active failures are sometimes referred to as errors at the sharp end, figuratively referring to a scalpel. In other words, errors at the sharp end are noticed first because they are committed by the person closest to the patient. This person may literally be holding a scalpel (e.g., an orthopedist operating on the wrong leg) or figuratively be administering any kind of therapy (e.g., a nurse programming an intravenous pump) or performing any aspect of care. Latent errors (or latent conditions), in contrast, refer to less apparent failures of organization or design that contributed to the occurrence of errors or allowed them to cause harm to patients. To complete the metaphor, latent errors are those at the other end of the scalpel—the blunt end—referring to the many layers of the healthcare system that affect the person "holding" the scalpel.

Adverse drug event (ADE)—An adverse event (i.e., injury resulting from medical care) involving medication use.

Examples:

- Anaphylaxis to penicillin
- Major hemorrhage from heparin
- Aminoglycoside-induced renal failure
- Agranulocytosis from chloramphenicol

As with the more general term adverse event, the occurrence of an ADE does not necessarily indicate an error or poor quality of care. ADEs that involve an element of error (of either omission or commission) are often referred to as *preventable* ADEs. Medication errors that reached the patient but by good fortune did not cause any harm are often called *potential* ADEs. For instance, a serious allergic reaction to penicillin in a patient with no prior such history is an ADE, but so is the same reaction in a patient who has a known allergy history but receives penicillin due to a prescribing oversight. The former occurrence would count as an adverse drug reaction or non-preventable ADE, while the latter would represent a preventable ADE. If a patient with a documented serious penicillin allergy received a penicillin-like antibiotic but happened not to react to it, this event would be characterized as a potential ADE.

An *ameliorable* ADE is one in which the patient experienced harm from a medication that, while not completely preventable, could have been mitigated. For instance, a patient taking a cholesterol-lowering agent (statin) may develop muscle pains and eventually progress to a more serious condition called rhabdomyolysis. Failure to periodically check a blood test that assesses muscle damage or failure to recognize this possible diagnosis in a patient taking statins who subsequently develops rhabdomyolysis would make this event an ameliorable ADE: harm from medical care that could have been lessened with earlier, appropriate management. Again, the initial development of some problem was not preventable, but the eventual harm that occurred need not have been so severe, hence the term ameliorable ADE.

Adverse drug reaction—Adverse effect produced by the use of a medication in the recommended manner—i.e., a drug side effect. These effects range from nuisance effects (e.g., dry mouth with anticholinergic medications) to severe reactions, such as anaphylaxis to penicillin. Adverse drug reactions represent a subset of the broad category of adverse drug events—specifically, they are non-preventable ADEs.

Adverse event—Any injury caused by medical care.

Examples:

- Pneumothorax from central venous catheter placement
- Anaphylaxis to penicillin
- Postoperative wound infection
- Hospital-acquired delirium (or "sundowning") in elderly patients

Identifying something as an adverse event does not imply "error," "negligence," or poor quality care. It simply indicates that an undesirable clinical outcome resulted from some aspect of diagnosis or therapy, not an underlying disease process. Thus, pneumothorax from central venous catheter placement counts as an adverse event regardless of insertion technique. Similarly, a postoperative wound infection counts as an adverse event even if the operation proceeded with optimal adherence to sterile procedures, the patient received appropriate antibiotic prophylaxis in the perioperative setting, and so on. (See also "iatrogenic").

Adverse events after hospital discharge—Being discharged from the hospital can be dangerous for patients. Nearly 20% of patients experience an adverse event in the first 3 weeks after discharge, including medication errors, healthcare-associated infections, and procedural complications.

Alert fatigue—Computerized warnings and alarms are used to improve safety by alerting clinicians of potentially unsafe situations. However, this proliferation of alerts may have negative implications for patient safety as well.

Anchoring error (or bias)—Refers to the common cognitive trap of allowing first impressions to exert undue influence on the diagnostic process.

Clinicians often latch on to features of a patient's presentation that suggest a specific diagnosis. Often, this initial diagnostic impression will prove correct, hence the use of the phrase *anchoring heuristic* in some contexts, as it can be a useful rule of thumb to "always trust your first impressions." However, in some cases, subsequent developments in the patient's course will prove inconsistent with the first impression. Anchoring bias refers to the tendency to hold on to the initial diagnosis, even in the face of disconfirming evidence.

APACHE—The Acute Physiologic and Chronic Health Evaluation (APACHE) scoring system has been widely used in the United States. APACHE II is the most widely studied version of this instrument (a more recent version, APACHE III, is proprietary, whereas APACHE II is publicly available); it derives a severity score from such factors as underlying disease and chronic health status. Other points are added for 12 physiologic variables (i.e., hematocrit, creatinine, Glasgow Coma Score, mean arterial pressure) measured within 24 hours of admission to the ICU. The APACHE II score has been validated in several studies involving tens of thousands of ICU patients.

Authority gradient—Refers to the balance of decision-making power or the steepness of command hierarchy in a given situation. Members of a crew or organization with a domineering, overbearing, or dictatorial team leader experience a steep authority gradient. Expressing concerns, questioning, or even simply clarifying instructions would require considerable determination on the part of team members who perceive their input as devalued or frankly unwelcome. Most teams require some degree of authority gradient; otherwise roles are blurred and decisions cannot be made in a timely fashion. However, effective team leaders consciously establish a command hierarchy appropriate to the training and experience of team members.

Authority gradients may occur even when the notion of a team is less well defined. For instance, a pharmacist calling a physician to clarify an order may encounter a steep authority gradient, based on the tone of the physician's voice or a lack of openness to input from the pharmacist. A confident, experienced pharmacist may nonetheless continue to raise legitimate concerns about an order, but other pharmacists might not.

Availability bias (or heuristic)—Refers to the tendency to assume, when judging probabilities or predicting outcomes, that the first possibility that comes to mind (i.e., the most cognitively "available" possibility) is also the most likely possibility. For instance, suppose a patient presents with intermittent episodes of very high blood pressure. Because episodic hypertension resembles textbook descriptions of pheochromocytoma, a memorable but uncommon endocrinologic tumor, this diagnosis may immediately come to mind. A clinician who infers from this immediate association that pheochromocytoma is the most likely diagnosis would be exhibiting availability bias. In addition to resemblance to classic descriptions of disease, personal experience can also trigger availability bias, as when the diagnosis underlying a recent patient's presentation immediately comes to mind when any subsequent patient presents with similar symptoms. Particularly memorable cases may similarly exert undue influence in shaping diagnostic impressions.

Bayesian approach—Probabilistic reasoning in which test results (not just laboratory investigations but also history, physical exam, or any aspect for the diagnostic process) are combined with prior beliefs about the probability of a particular disease. One way of recognizing the need for a Bayesian approach is to recognize the difference between the performance of a test in a population and that in an individual. At the population level, we can say that a test has a sensitivity and specificity of, say, 90%—that is, 90% of patients with the condition of interest have a positive result and 90% of patients without the condition have a negative result. In practice, however, a clinician needs to attempt to predict whether an individual patient with a positive or negative result does or does not have the condition of interest. This prediction requires combining the observed test result not just with the known sensitivity and specificity but also with the chance the patient could have had the disease in the first place (based on demographic factors, findings on exam, or general clinical gestalt).

Beers criteria—Beers criteria define medications that generally should be avoided in ambulatory elderly patients, doses or frequencies of administration that should not be exceeded, and medications that should be avoided in older persons known to have any of several common conditions. The criteria were originally developed using a formal consensus process for combining reviews of the evidence with expert input. The criteria for inappropriate use address commonly used categories of medications such as sedative-hypnotics, antidepressants, antipsychotics, antihypertensives, nonsteroidal anti-inflammatory agents, oral hypoglycemics, analgesics, dementia treatments, platelet inhibitors, histamine-2 blockers, antibiotics, decongestants, iron supplements, muscle relaxants, gastrointestinal antispasmodics, and antiemetics. The criteria were intended to guide clinical practice, but also to inform quality assurance review and health services research.

Most would agree that prescriptions for medications deemed inappropriate according to Beers criteria represent poor quality care. Unfortunately, harm does not only occur from receipt of these inappropriately prescribed medications. In one comprehensive national study of medication-related emergency department visits for elderly patients, most problems involved common and important medications not considered inappropriate according to the Beers criteria—principally, oral anticoagulants (e.g., warfarin), antidiabetic agents (e.g., insulin), and antiplatelet agents (aspirin and clopidogrel).

Benchmark—A benchmark in healthcare refers to an attribute or achievement that serves as a standard for other providers or institutions to emulate.

Benchmarks differ from other standard of care goals, in that they derive from empiric data—specifically, performance or outcomes data. For example, a statewide survey might produce risk-adjusted 30-day rates for death or other major adverse outcomes. After adjusting for relevant clinical factors, the top 10% of hospitals can be identified in terms of particular outcome measures. These institutions would then provide benchmark data on these outcomes. For instance, one might benchmark "door-to-balloon" time at 90 minutes, based on the observation that the top-performing hospitals all had door-to-balloon times in this range. In regard to infection control, benchmarks would typically be derived from national or regional data on the rates of relevant nosocomial infections. The lowest 10% of these rates might be regarded as benchmarks for other institutions to emulate.

Black Box Warnings—The prominent warning labels (generally printed inside black boxes) on packages for certain prescription medications in the United States. These warnings typically arise from post-market surveillance or post-approval clinical trials that bring to light serious adverse reactions. The U.S. Food and Drug Administration (FDA) subsequently may require a pharmaceutical company to place a black box warning on the labeling or packaging of the drug. Although medications with black box warnings often enjoy widespread use and, with cautious use, typically do not result in harm, these warnings remain important sources of safety information for patients and healthcare providers. They also emphasize the importance of continued, post-market surveillance for adverse drug reactions for all medications, especially relatively new ones.

Blunt end—The blunt end refers to the many layers of the healthcare system not in direct contact with patients, but which influence the personnel and equipment at the sharp end who do contact patients. The blunt end thus consists of those who set policy, manage healthcare institutions, and design medical devices, and other people and forces, which, though removed in time and space from direct patient care, nonetheless affect how care is delivered. Thus, an error programming an intravenous pump would represent a problem at the sharp end, while the institution's decision to use multiple different types of infusion pumps, making programming errors more likely, would represent a problem at the blunt end. The terminology of "sharp" and "blunt" ends corresponds roughly to active failures and latent conditions.

Checklist—Algorithmic listing of actions to be performed in a given clinical setting (e.g., advanced cardiac life support [ACLS] protocols for treating cardiac arrest) to ensure that, no matter how often performed by a given practitioner, no step will be forgotten. An analogy is often made to flight preparation in aviation, as pilots and air traffic controllers follow pre-takeoff checklists regardless of how many times they have carried out the tasks involved.

Clinical decision support system (CDSS)—Any system designed to improve clinical decision making related to diagnostic or therapeutic processes of care. Typically a decision support system responds to "triggers" or "flags"—specific diagnoses, laboratory results, medication choices, or complex combinations of such parameters—and provides information or recommendations directly relevant to a specific patient encounter.

CDSSs address activities ranging from the selection of drugs (e.g., the optimal antibiotic choice given specific microbiologic data) or diagnostic tests to detailed support for optimal drug dosing and support for resolving diagnostic dilemmas. Structured antibiotic order forms represent a common example of paper-based CDSSs. Although such systems are still commonly encountered, many people equate CDSSs with computerized systems in which software algorithms generate patient-specific recommendations by matching characteristics, such as age, renal function, or allergy history, with rules in a computerized knowledge base.

The distinction between decision support and simple reminders can be unclear, but usually reminder systems are included as decision support if they involve patient-specific information. For instance, a generic reminder (e.g., "Did you obtain an allergy history?") would not be considered decision support, but a warning (e.g., "This patient is allergic to codeine.") that appears at the time of entering an order for codeine would be.

Close call—An event or situation that did not produce patient injury, but only because of chance. This good fortune might reflect robustness of the patient (e.g., a patient with penicillin allergy receives penicillin, but has no reaction) or a fortuitous, timely intervention (e.g., a nurse happens to realize that a physician wrote an order in the wrong chart). Such events have also been termed near miss incidents.

Competency—Having the necessary knowledge or technical skill to perform a given procedure within the bounds of success and failure rates deemed compatible with acceptable care. The medical education literature often refers to core competencies, which include not just technical skills with respect to procedures or medical knowledge but also competencies with respect to communicating with patients, collaborating with other members of the healthcare team, and acting as a manager or agent for change in the health system.

Complexity science (or complexity theory)—Provides an approach to understanding the behavior of systems that exhibit nonlinear dynamics, or the ways in which some adaptive systems produce novel behavior not expected from the properties of their individual components. Such behaviors emerge as a result of interactions between agents at a local level in the complex system and between the system and its environment.

Complexity theory differs importantly from systems thinking in its emphasis on the interaction between local systems and their environment (such as the larger system in which a given hospital or clinic operates). It is often tempting to ignore the larger environment as unchangeable and therefore outside the scope of quality improvement or patient safety activities. According to complexity theory, however, behavior within a hospital or clinic (e.g., noncompliance with a national practice guideline) can often be understood only by identifying interactions between local attributes and environmental factors.

Computerized provider order entry or computerized physician order entry (CPOE)—Refers to a computer-based system of ordering medications and often other tests. Physicians (or other providers) directly enter orders into a computer system that can have varying levels of sophistication. Basic CPOE ensures standardized, legible, complete orders, and thus primarily reduces errors caused by poor handwriting and ambiguous abbreviations.

Almost all CPOE systems offer some additional capabilities, which fall under the general rubric of CDSS. Typical CDSS features involve suggested default values for drug doses, routes of administration, or frequency. More sophisticated CDSSs can perform drug allergy checks (e.g., the user orders ceftriaxone and a warning flashes that the patient has a documented penicillin allergy), drug-laboratory value checks (e.g., initiating an order for gentamicin prompts the system to alert you to the patient's last creatinine), drug–drug interaction checks, and so on. At the highest level of sophistication, CDSS prevents not only errors of commission (e.g., ordering a drug in excessive doses or in the setting of a serious allergy) but also errors of omission. For example, an alert may appear such as, "You have ordered heparin; would you like to order a partial thromboplastin time (PTT) in 6 hours?" Or, even more sophisticated: "The admitting diagnosis is hip fracture; would you like to order heparin for deep vein thrombosis (DVT) prophylaxis?" See also "Clinical decision support system."

Confirmation bias—Refers to the tendency to focus on evidence that supports a working hypothesis, such as a diagnosis in clinical medicine, rather than to look for evidence that refutes it or provides greater support to an alternative diagnosis. Suppose that a 65-year-old man with a past history of angina presents to the emergency department with acute onset of shortness of breath. The physician immediately considers the possibility of cardiac ischemia, so asks the patient if he has experienced any chest pain. The patient replies affirmatively. Because the physician perceives this answer as confirming his working diagnosis, he does not ask if the chest pain was pleuritic in nature, which would decrease the likelihood of an acute coronary syndrome and increase the likelihood of pulmonary embolism (a reasonable alternative diagnosis for acute shortness of breath accompanied by chest pain). The physician then orders an ECG and cardiac troponin. The ECG shows nonspecific ST changes and the troponin returns slightly elevated.

Of course, ordering an ECG and testing cardiac enzymes is appropriate in the work-up of acute shortness of breath, especially when it is accompanied by chest pain and in a patient with known angina. The problem is that these tests may be misleading, since positive results are consistent not only with acute coronary syndrome but also with pulmonary embolism. To avoid confirmation bias in this case, the physician might have obtained an arterial blood glass or a D-dimer level. Abnormal results for either of these tests would be relatively unlikely to occur in a patient with an acute coronary syndrome (unless complicated by pulmonary edema), but likely to occur with pulmonary embolism. These results could be followed up by more direct testing for pulmonary embolism (e.g., with a helical CT scan of the chest), while normal results would allow the clinician to proceed with greater confidence down the road of investigating and managing cardiac ischemia.

This vignette was presented as if information were sought in sequence. In many cases, especially in acute care medicine, clinicians have the results of numerous tests in hand when they first meet a patient. The results of these tests often do not all suggest the same diagnosis. The appeal of accentuating confirmatory test results and ignoring nonconfirmatory ones is that it minimizes cognitive dissonance.

A related cognitive trap that may accompany confirmation bias and compound the possibility of error is "anchoring bias"—the tendency to stick with one's first impressions, even in the face of significant disconfirming evidence.

Crew resource management (CRM)—Also called crisis resource management in some contexts (e.g., anesthesia), encompasses a range of approaches to training groups to function as teams, rather than as collections of individuals. Originally developed in aviation, CRM emphasizes the role of human factors—the effects of fatigue, expected or predictable perceptual errors (such as misreading monitors or mishearing instructions), as well as the impact of different management styles and organizational cultures in high-stress, high-risk environments. CRM training develops communication skills, fosters a more cohesive environment among team members, and creates an atmosphere in which junior personnel will feel free to speak up when they think that something is amiss. Some CRM programs emphasize education on the settings in which errors occur and the aspects of team decision making conducive to "trapping" errors before they cause harm. Other programs may provide more hands-on training involving simulated crisis scenarios followed by debriefing sessions in which participants assess their own and others' behavior.

Critical incidents—A term made famous by a classic human factors study by Jeffrey Cooper of "anesthetic mishaps," though the term had first been coined in the 1950s. Cooper and colleagues brought the technique of critical incident analysis to a wide audience in healthcare but followed the definition of the originator of the technique. They defined critical incidents as occurrences that are "significant or pivotal, in either a desirable or an undesirable way," though Cooper and colleagues (and most others since) chose to focus on incidents that had potentially undesirable consequences. This concept is best understood in the context of the type of investigation that follows, which is very much in the style of root cause analysis. Thus, *significant* or *pivotal* means that there was significant potential for harm (or actual harm), but also that the event has the potential to reveal important hazards in the organization. In many ways, it embodies the expression in quality improvement circles that "every defect is a treasure." In other words, these incidents, whether near misses or disasters in which significant harm occurred, provide valuable opportunities to learn about individual and organizational factors that can be remedied to prevent similar incidents in the future.

Decision support—Refers to any system for advising or providing guidance about a particular clinical decision at the point of care. For example, a copy of an algorithm for antibiotic selection in patients with community-acquired pneumonia would count as clinical decision support if made available at the point of care. Increasingly, decision support occurs via a computerized clinical information or order entry system. Computerized decision support includes any software employing a knowledge base designed to assist clinicians in decision making at the point of care.

Typically a decision support system responds to "triggers" or "flags"—specific diagnoses, laboratory results, medication choices, or complex combinations of such parameters—and provides information or recommendations directly relevant to a specific patient encounter. For instance, ordering an aminoglycoside for a patient with creatinine above a certain value might trigger a message suggesting a dose adjustment based on the patient's decreased renal function.

Diagnostic errors—Thousands of patients die every year due to diagnostic errors. While clinicians' cognitive biases play a role in many diagnostic errors, underlying healthcare system problems also contribute to missed and delayed diagnoses.

Disclosure, error disclosure—Many victims of medical errors never learn of the mistake, because the error is simply not disclosed. Physicians have traditionally shied away from discussing errors with patients, due to fear of precipitating a malpractice lawsuit and embarrassment and discomfort with the disclosure process.

Disruptive and unprofessional behavior—Popular media often depicts physicians as brilliant, intimidating, and condescending in equal measures. This stereotype, though undoubtedly dramatic and even amusing, obscures the fact that disruptive and unprofessional behavior by clinicians poses a definite threat to patient safety.

Duty hours—Long and unpredictable work hours have been a staple of medical training for centuries. In 2003, the Accreditation Council for Graduate Medical Education (ACGME) implemented new rules limiting duty hours for all residents to reduce fatigue. The implementation of resident duty-hour restrictions has been controversial, as evidence regarding its impact on patient safety has been mixed.

Error—An act of commission (doing something wrong) or omission (failing to do the right thing) that leads to an undesirable outcome or significant potential for such an outcome. For instance, ordering a medication for a patient with a documented allergy to that medication would be an act of commission. Failing to prescribe a proven medication with major benefits for an eligible patient (e.g., low-dose unfractionated heparin as venous thromboembolism prophylaxis for a patient after hip replacement surgery) would represent an error of omission.

Errors of omission are more difficult to recognize than errors of commission but likely represent a larger problem. In other words, there are likely many more instances in which the provision of additional diagnostic, therapeutic, or preventive modalities would have improved care than there are instances in which the care provided quite literally should not have been provided. In many ways, this point echoes the generally agreed-upon view in the healthcare quality literature that underuse far exceeds overuse, even though the latter historically received greater attention. (See definition for "Underuse, overuse, and misuse"). In addition to commission versus omission, three other dichotomies commonly appear in the literature on errors: active failures versus latent conditions, errors at the sharp end versus errors at the blunt end, and slips versus mistakes.

Error chain—Error chain generally refers to the series of events that led to a disastrous outcome, typically uncovered by a root cause analysis. Sometimes the chain metaphor carries the added sense of inexorability, as many of the causes are tightly coupled, such that one problem begets the next. A more specific meaning of error chain, especially when used in the phrase "break the error chain," relates to the common themes or categories of causes that emerge from root cause analyses. These categories go by different names in different settings, but they generally include (1) failure to follow standard operating procedures, (2) poor leadership, (3) breakdowns in communication or teamwork, (4) overlooking or ignoring individual fallibility, and (5) losing track of objectives. Used in this way, "break the error chain" is shorthand for an approach in which team members continually address these links as a crisis or routine situation unfolds. The checklists that are included in teamwork training programs have categories corresponding to these common links in the error chain (e.g., establish a team leader, assign roles and responsibilities, and monitor your teammates).

Evidence-based—Use of the phrase "evidence-based" in connection with an assertion about some aspect of medical care—a recommended treatment, the cause of some condition, or the best way to diagnose it—implies that the assertion reflects the results of medical research, as opposed to, for example, a personal opinion (plausible or widespread as that opinion might be). Given the volume of medical research and the not-infrequent occurrence of conflicting results from different studies addressing the same question, the phrase "reflects the results of medical research" should be clarified as "reflects the preponderance of results from relevant studies of good methodological quality."

The concept of evidence-based treatments has particular relevance to patient safety, because many recommended methods for measuring and improving safety problems have been drawn from other high-risk industries, without any studies to confirm that these strategies work well in healthcare (or, in many cases, that they work well in the original industry). The lack of evidence supporting widely recommended (sometimes even mandated) patient safety practices contrasts sharply with the rest of clinical medicine. While individual practitioners may employ diagnostic tests or administer treatments of unproven value, professional organizations typically do not endorse such aspects of care until well-designed studies demonstrate that these diagnostic or treatment strategies confer net benefit to patients (i.e., until they become evidence-based). Certainly, diagnostic and therapeutic processes do not become standard of care or in any way mandated until they have undergone rigorous evaluation in well-designed studies.

In patient safety, by contrast, patient safety goals established at state and national levels (sometimes even mandated by regulatory agencies or by law) often reflect ideas that have undergone little or no empiric evaluation. Just as in clinical medicine, promising safety strategies sometimes can turn out to confer no benefit or even create new problems—hence the need for rigorous evaluations of candidate patient safety strategies just as in other areas of medicine. That said, just how high to set the bar for the evidence required to justify actively disseminating patient safety and quality improvement strategies is a subject that has received considerable attention in recent years. Some leading thinkers in patient safety argue that an evidence bar comparable to that used in more traditional clinical medicine would be too high, given the difficulty of studying complex social systems such as hospitals and clinics, and the high costs of studying interventions such as rapid response teams or computerized order entry.

Face validity—The extent to which a technical concept, instrument, or study result is plausible, usually because its findings are consistent with prior assumptions and expectations.

Failure mode—Error analysis may involve retrospective investigations (as in Root Cause Analysis) or prospective attempts to predict "error modes."

Different frameworks exist for predicting possible errors. One commonly used approach is failure mode and effect analysis (FMEA), in which the likelihood of a particular process failure is combined with an estimate of the relative impact of that error to produce a "criticality index." By combining the probability of failure with the consequences of failure, this index allows for the prioritization of specific processes as quality improvement targets. For instance, an FMEA analysis of the medication dispensing process on a general hospital ward might break down all steps from receipt of orders in the central pharmacy to filling automated dispensing machines by pharmacy technicians. Each step in this process would be assigned a probability of failure and an impact score, so that all steps could be ranked according to the product of these two numbers. Steps ranked at the top (i.e., those with the highest "criticality indices") would be prioritized for error proofing.

Failure mode and effects analysis (FMEA)—A common process used to prospectively identify error risk within a particular process. FMEA begins with a complete process mapping that identifies all the steps that must occur for a given process to occur (e.g., programming an infusion pump or preparing an intravenous medication in the pharmacy). With the process mapped out, the FMEA then continues by identifying the ways in which each step can go wrong (i.e., the "failure modes" for each step), the probability that each error will be detected (i.e., so that it can be corrected before causing harm), and the consequences or impact of the error not being detected. The estimates of the likelihood of a particular process failure, the chance of detecting such failure, and its impact are combined numerically to produce a *criticality index*.

This criticality index provides a rough quantitative estimate of the magnitude of hazard posed by each step in a high-risk process. Assigning a criticality index to each step allows prioritization of targets for improvement. For instance, an FMEA analysis of the medication-dispensing process on a general hospital ward might break down all steps from receipt of orders in the central pharmacy to filling automated dispensing machines by pharmacy technicians. Each step in this process would be assigned a probability of failure and an impact score, so that all steps could be ranked according to the product of these two numbers. Steps ranked at the top (i.e., those with the highest criticality indices) would be prioritized for error proofing.

FMEA makes sense as a general approach and it (or similar prospective error-proofing techniques) has been used in other high-risk industries. However, the reliability of the technique is not clear. Different teams charged with analyzing the same process may identify different steps in the process, assign different risks to the steps, and consequently prioritize different targets for improvement.

Failure to rescue—Failure to rescue is shorthand for failure to rescue (i.e., prevent a clinically important deterioration, such as death or permanent disability) from a complication of an underlying illness (e.g., cardiac arrest in a patient with acute myocardial infarction) or a complication of medical care (e.g., major hemorrhage after thrombolysis for acute myocardial infarction). Failure to rescue thus provides a measure of the degree to which providers responded to adverse occurrences (e.g., hospital-acquired infections, cardiac arrest or shock) that developed on their watch. It may reflect the quality of monitoring, the effectiveness of actions taken once early complications are recognized, or both.

The technical motivation for using failure to rescue to evaluate the quality of care stems from the concern that some institutions might document adverse occurrences more assiduously than others. Therefore, using lower rates of in-hospital complications by themselves may simply reward hospitals with poor documentation. However, if the medical record indicates that a complication has occurred, the response to that complication should provide an indicator of the quality of care that is less susceptible to charting bias.

Forcing function—An aspect of a design that prevents a target action from being performed or allows its performance only if another specific action is performed first. For example, automobiles are now designed so that the driver cannot shift into reverse without first putting his or her foot on the brake pedal. Forcing functions need not involve device design. For instance, one of the first forcing functions identified in healthcare was the removal of concentrated potassium from general hospital wards. This action is intended to prevent the inadvertent preparation of intravenous solutions with concentrated potassium, an error that has produced small but consistent numbers of deaths for many years.

"Five Rights"—The "Five Rights"—administering the Right Medication, in the Right Dose, at the Right Time, by the Right Route, to the Right Patient—are the cornerstone of traditional nursing teaching about safe medication practice.

While the Five Rights represent goals of safe medication administration, they contain no procedural detail, and thus may inadvertently perpetuate the traditional focus on individual performance rather than system improvement. Procedures for ensuring each of the Five Rights must take into account human factor and systems design issues (such as workload, ambient distractions, poor lighting, problems with wristbands, ineffective double-check protocols, etc.) that can threaten or undermine even the most conscientious efforts to comply with the Five Rights. In the end, the Five Rights remain an important goal for safe medication practice, but one that may give the illusion of safety if not supported by strong policies and procedures, a system organized around modern principles of patient safety, and a robust safety culture.

Handoffs and handovers—Refer to the process when one healthcare professional updates another on the status of one or more patients for the purpose of taking over their care. Typical examples involve a physician who has been on call overnight telling an incoming physician about patients she has admitted so he can continue with their ongoing management, know what immediate issues to watch out for, and so on. Nurses similarly conduct a handover at the end of their shift, updating their colleagues about the status of the patients under their care and tasks that need to be performed. When the outgoing nurses return for their next duty period, they will in turn receive new updates during the change of shift handover.

Handovers in care have always carried risks: a professional who spent hours assessing and managing a patient, on completion of her work, provides a brief summary of the salient features of the case to an incoming professional who typically has other unfamiliar patients he must get to know. The summary may leave out key details due to oversight, exacerbated by an unstructured process and being rushed to finish work. Even structured, fairly thorough summaries during handovers may fail to capture nuances that could subsequently prove relevant.

Despite these long-recognized problems, handovers received relatively little attention until recent years, when they became more frequent. For instance, with reductions in duty hours for physician trainees, more handovers must occur in any given 24-hour period. And, with shorter lengths of stay in hospitals and other occupancy issues, patients more often move from one ward to another or from one institution to another (e.g., from an acute care hospital to a rehabilitation facility or skilled nursing facility).

Due to the increasing recognition of hazards associated with these transitions in care, the term "handovers" is often used to refer to the information transfer that occurs from one clinical setting to another (e.g., from hospital to nursing home), not just from one professional to another.

Healthcare-associated infections—Although long accepted by clinicians as an inevitable hazard of hospitalization, recent efforts demonstrate that relatively simple measures can prevent the majority of healthcare-associated infections. As a result, hospitals are under intense pressure to reduce the burden of these infections.

Health literacy—Individuals' ability to find, process, and comprehend the basic health information necessary to act on medical instructions and make decisions about their health. Numerous studies have documented the degree to which patients frequently do not understand basic information or instructions related to general aspects of their medical care, their medications, and procedures they will undergo. The limited ability to comprehend medical instructions or information in some cases reflects obvious language barriers (e.g., reviewing medication instructions in English with a patient who speaks very little English), but the scope of the problem reflects broader issues related to levels of education, cross-cultural differences, and overuse of technical terminology by clinicians.

Heuristic—Loosely defined or informal rules often arrived at through experience or trial and error that influence assessments and decisions (e.g., gastrointestinal complaints that wake patients up at night are unlikely to be benign in nature). Heuristics provide cognitive shortcuts in the face of complex situations, and thus serve an important purpose. Unfortunately, they can also turn out to be wrong, with frequently used heuristics often forming the basis for the many cognitive biases, such as anchoring bias, availability bias, confirmation bias, and others, that have received attention in the literature on diagnostic errors and medical decision making.

The Health Insurance Portability and Accountability Act (HIPAA)— HIPAA, passed by the U.S. Congress in 1996, was intended to increase privacy and security of patient information during electronic transmission or communication of "protected health information" (PHI) among providers or between providers and payers or other entities.

PHI includes all medical records and other individually identifiable health information. "Individually identifiable information" includes data explicitly linked to a patient, as well as health information with data items that carry a reasonable potential for allowing individual identification.

HIPAA also requires providers to offer patients certain rights with respect to their information, including the right to access and copy their records and the right to request amendments to the information contained in their records.

Administrative protections specified by HIPAA to promote the above regulations and rights include requirements for a Privacy Officer and staff training regarding the protection of patients' information.

High reliability organizations (HROs)—HROs refer to organizations or systems that operate in hazardous conditions but have fewer than their fair share of adverse events. Commonly discussed examples include air traffic control systems, nuclear power plants, and naval aircraft carriers. It is worth noting that, in the safety literature, organizations labeled as HROs are ones that operate with nearly failure-free performance records, not simply better than average ones. This shift in meaning is understandable given that the failure rates in these other industries are much lower than rates of errors and adverse events in healthcare. This comparison glosses over the difference in significance of a "failure" in the nuclear power industry compared with one in healthcare. The point remains, however, that some organizations achieve consistently safe and effective performance records despite unpredictable operating environments or intrinsically hazardous endeavors. Detailed case studies of specific HROs have identified some common features, which have been offered as models for other organizations to achieve substantial improvements in their safety records. These features include:

- Preoccupation with failure—the acknowledgment of the high-risk, error-prone nature of an organization's activities and the determination to achieve consistently safe operations.
- Commitment to resilience—the development of capacities to detect unexpected threats and contain them before they cause harm, or bounce back when they do.
- Sensitivity to operations—an attentiveness to the issues facing workers at the frontline. This feature comes into play when conducting analyses of specific events (e.g., frontline workers play a crucial role in root cause analysis by bringing up unrecognized latent threats in current operating procedures), but also in connection with organizational decision making.
- Decentralized decision making—management units at the frontline are given some autonomy in identifying and responding to threats, rather than adopting a rigid top-down approach.
- A culture of safety, in which individuals feel comfortable drawing attention to potential hazards or actual failures without fear of censure from management.

Hindsight bias—In a very general sense, hindsight bias relates to the common expression, "hindsight is 20/20." This expression captures the tendency for people to regard past events as expected or obvious, even when, in real time, the events perplexed those involved. More formally, one might say that after learning the outcome of a series of events—whether the outcome of the World Series or the steps leading to a war—people tend to exaggerate the extent to which they had foreseen the likelihood of its occurrence.

In the context of safety analysis, hindsight bias refers to the tendency to judge the events leading up to an accident as errors because the bad outcome is known. The more severe the outcome, the more likely that decisions leading up to this outcome will be judged as errors. Judging the antecedent decisions as errors implies that the outcome was preventable. In legal circles, one might use the phrase "but for," as in "but for these errors in judgment, this terrible outcome would not have occurred." Such judgments return us to the concept of "hindsight is 20/20." Those reviewing events after the fact see the outcome as more foreseeable and therefore more preventable than they would have appreciated in real time.

Human factors (or human factors engineering)—Refers to the study of human abilities and characteristics as they affect the design and smooth operation of equipment, systems, and jobs. The field concerns itself with considerations of the strengths and weaknesses of human physical and mental abilities and how these affect the systems design. Human factors analysis does not require designing or redesigning existing objects. For instance, the now generally accepted recommendation that hospitals standardize equipment such as ventilators, programmable IV pumps, and defibrillators (i.e., each hospital picks a single type, so that different floors do not have different defibrillators) is an example of a very basic application of a heuristic from human factors that equipment be standardized within a system wherever possible.

Iatrogenic—An adverse effect of medical care, rather than of the underlying disease (literally "brought forth by healer," from Greek *iatros*, for healer, and *gennan*, to bring forth); equivalent to adverse event.

Incident reporting—Refers to the identification of occurrences that could have led, or did lead, to an undesirable outcome. Reports usually come from personnel directly involved in the incident or events leading up to it (e.g., the nurse, pharmacist, or physician caring for a patient when a medication error occurred) rather than, say, floor managers. From the perspective of those collecting the data, incident reporting counts as a *passive* form of surveillance, relying on those involved in target incidents to provide the desired information. Compared with medical record review and direct observation (*active* methods), incident reporting captures only a fraction of incidents, but has the advantages of relatively low cost and the involvement of frontline personnel in the process of identifying important problems for the organization.

Informed consent—Refers to the process whereby a physician informs a patient about the risks and benefits of a proposed therapy or test. Informed consent aims to provide sufficient information about the proposed course and any reasonable alternatives that the patient can exercise autonomy in deciding whether to proceed.

Legislation governing the requirements of, and conditions under which, consent must be obtained varies by jurisdiction. Most general guidelines require patients to be informed of the nature of their condition, the proposed procedure, the purpose of the procedure, the risks and benefits of the proposed treatments, the probability of the anticipated risks and benefits, alternatives to the treatment and their associated risks and benefits, and the risks and benefits of not receiving the treatment or procedure.

Although the goals of informed consent are irrefutable, consent is often obtained in a haphazard, pro forma fashion, with patients having little true understanding of procedures to which they have consented. Evidence suggests that asking patients to restate the essence of the informed consent improves the quality of these discussions and makes it more likely that the consent is truly informed.

Just culture—The phrase "Just Culture" was popularized in the patient safety lexicon by David Marx, who outlined principles for achieving a culture in which frontline personnel feel comfortable disclosing errors—including their own—while maintaining professional accountability.

Traditionally, healthcare's culture has held individuals accountable for all errors or mishaps that befall patients under their care. By contrast, a Just Culture recognizes that individual practitioners should not be held accountable for system failings over which they have no control. It also recognizes many individual or "active" errors are the result of predictable interactions between human operators and the systems in which they work. However, in contrast to a culture that touts "no blame" as its governing principle, a Just Culture does not tolerate conscious disregard of clear risks to patients or gross misconduct (e.g., falsifying a record, performing professional duties while intoxicated).

In summary, a Just Culture recognizes that competent professionals make mistakes and acknowledges that even competent professionals will develop unhealthy norms (shortcuts, "routine rule violations"), but has zero tolerance for reckless behavior.

Latent error (or latent condition)—The terms *active* and *latent* as applied to errors were coined by James Reason. Latent errors (or latent conditions) refer to less apparent failures of organization or design that contributed to the occurrence of errors or allowed them to cause harm to patients. For instance, whereas the active failure in a particular adverse event may have been a mistake in programming an intravenous pump, a latent error might be that the institution uses multiple different types of infusion pumps, making programming errors more likely. Thus, latent errors are quite literally "accidents waiting to happen." Latent errors are sometimes referred to as errors at the blunt end, referring to the many layers of the healthcare system that affect the person "holding" the scalpel. Active failures, in contrast, are sometimes referred to as errors at the sharp end, or the personnel and parts of the healthcare system in direct contact with patients.

Learning curve—The acquisition of any new skill is associated with the potential for lower-than-expected success rates or higher-than-expected complication rates. This phenomenon is often known as a learning curve. In some cases, this learning curve can be quantified in terms of the number of procedures that must be performed before an operator can replicate the outcomes of more experienced operators or centers. While learning curves are almost inevitable when new procedures emerge or new providers are in training, minimizing their impact is a patient safety imperative. One option is to perform initial operations or procedures under the supervision of more experienced operators. Surgical and procedural simulators may play an increasingly important role in decreasing the impact of learning curves on patients, by allowing acquisition of relevant skills in laboratory settings.

Magnet hospital status—Refers to a designation by the Magnet Hospital Recognition Program administered by the American Nurses Credentialing

Center. The program has its genesis in a 1983 study conducted by the American Academy of Nursing that sought to identify hospitals that retained nurses for longer than average periods of time. The study identified institutional characteristics correlated with high retention rates, an important finding in light of a major nursing shortage at the time. These findings provided the basis for the concept of magnet hospital and led 10 years later to the formal Magnet Program.

Without taking anything away from the particular hospitals that have achieved magnet status, the program has its critics. Regardless of the particulars of the Magnet Recognition Program and the lack of persuasive evidence linking magnet status to quality, to many the term magnet hospital connotes a hospital that delivers superior patient care and, partly on this basis, attracts and retains high-quality nurses.

Medical Emergency Team—The concept of medical emergency teams (also known as rapid response teams) is that of a cardiac arrest team with more liberal calling criteria. Instead of just frank respiratory or cardiac arrest, medical emergency teams respond to a wide range of worrisome, acute changes in patients' clinical status, such as low blood pressure, difficulty breathing, or altered mental status. In addition to less stringent calling criteria, the concept of medical emergency teams de-emphasizes the traditional hierarchy in patient care in that anyone can initiate the call. Nurses, junior medical staff, or others involved in the care of patients can call for the assistance of the medical emergency team whenever they are worried about a patient's condition, without having to wait for more senior personnel to assess the patient and approve the decision to call for help.

Medication reconciliation—Patients admitted to a hospital commonly receive new medications or have changes made to their existing medications. As a result, the new medication regimen prescribed at the time of discharge may inadvertently omit needed medications that patients have been receiving for some time. Alternatively, new medications may unintentionally duplicate existing medications. Such unintended inconsistencies in medication regimens may occur at any point of transition in care (e.g., transfer from an intensive care unit [ICU] to a general ward), not just hospital admission or discharge. Medication reconciliation refers to the process of avoiding such inadvertent inconsistencies across transitions in care by reviewing the patient's complete medication regimen at the time of admission, transfer, and discharge and comparing it with the regimen being considered for the new setting of care.

Mental model—Mental models are psychological representations of real, hypothetical, or imaginary situations. Scottish psychologist Kenneth Craik (1943) first proposed mental models as the basis for anticipating events and explaining events (i.e., for reasoning). Though easiest to conceptualize in terms of mental pictures of objects (e.g., a DNA double helix or the inside of an internal combustion engine), mental models can also include "scripts" or processes and other properties beyond images. Mental models create differing expectations, which suggest different courses of action. For instance, when you walk into a fast-food restaurant, you are invoking a different mental model than when you enter a fancy restaurant. Based on this model, you automatically go to place your order at the counter, rather than sitting at a booth and expecting a waiter to take your order.

Metacognition—Metacognition refers to thinking about thinking—that is, reflecting on the thought processes that led to a particular diagnosis or decision to consider whether biases or cognitive short cuts may have had a detrimental effect. In some ways, metacognition amounts to playing devil's advocate with oneself when it comes to working diagnoses and important therapeutic decisions. However, the devil is often in the details—one must become familiar with the variety of specific biases that commonly affect medical reasoning. For instance, when discharging a patient with atypical chest pain from the emergency department, you might step back and consider how much the discharge diagnosis of musculoskeletal pain reflects the sign-out as a "soft rule out" you received from a colleague on the night shift. Or, you might mull over the degree to which your reaction to and assessment of a particular patient stemmed from his having been labeled a "frequent flyer." Another cognitive bias is that clinicians tend to assign more importance to pieces of information that required personal effort to obtain.

Mistakes—In some contexts, errors are dichotomized as slips or mistakes, based on the cognitive psychology of task-oriented behavior. Mistakes reflect failures during attentional behaviors—behavior that requires conscious thought, analysis, and planning, as in active problem solving. Rather than lapses in concentration (as with slips), mistakes typically involve insufficient knowledge, failure to correctly interpret available information, or application of the wrong cognitive heuristic or rule. Thus, choosing the wrong diagnostic test or ordering a suboptimal medication for a given condition represents a mistake. Mistakes often reflect lack of experience or insufficient training. Reducing the likelihood of mistakes typically requires more training, supervision, or occasionally disciplinary action (in the case of negligence).

Unfortunately, healthcare has typically responded to all errors as if they were mistakes, with remedial education and/or added layers of supervision. In point of fact, most errors are actually slips, which are failures of schematic behavior that occur due to fatigue, stress, or emotional distractions, and are prevented through sharply different mechanisms.

Near miss—An event or situation that did not produce patient injury, but only because of chance. This good fortune might reflect robustness of the patient (e.g., a patient with penicillin allergy receives penicillin, but has no reaction) or a fortuitous, timely intervention (e.g., a nurse happens to realize that a physician wrote an order in the wrong chart). This definition is identical to that for close call.

"Never Events" list—Nickname for a list launched and managed by the National Quality Forum, initially intended to be "things that should never happen in healthcare." The list, whose real name is the "Serious Reportable Events" list, has expanded over time to include adverse events that are unambiguous, serious, and to a reasonable degree preventable (Appendix VI). While most are rare, never events may be devastating to patients and indicate serious underlying organizational safety problems.

Normal accident theory—Though less often cited than high reliability theory in the healthcare literature, normal accident theory has played a prominent role in the study of complex organizations. In contrast to the optimism of high reliability theory, normal accident theory suggests that, at least in some settings, major accidents become inevitable and, thus, in a sense, "normal."

Safety expert Charles Perrow proposed two factors that create an environment in which a major accident becomes increasingly likely over time: complexity and tight coupling. The degree of complexity envisioned by Perrow occurs when no single operator can immediately foresee the consequences of a given action in the system. Tight coupling occurs when processes are intrinsically time dependent—once a process has been set in motion, it must be completed within a certain period of time. Importantly, normal accident theory contends that accidents become inevitable in complex, tightly coupled systems regardless of steps taken to increase safety. In fact, these steps sometimes increase the risk for future accidents through unintended collateral effects and general increases in system complexity.

Even if one does not believe the central contention of normal accident theory—that the potential for catastrophe emerges as an intrinsic property of certain complex systems—analyses informed by this theory's perspective have offered some fascinating insights into possible failure modes for high-risk organizations, including hospitals.

Normalization of deviance—The term "normalization of deviance" was coined by Diane Vaughan in her book *The Challenger Launch Decision*, in which she analyzes the interactions between various cultural forces within NASA that contributed to the Challenger disaster. Vaughn used this expression to describe the gradual shift in what is regarded as normal after repeated exposures to "deviant behavior" (behavior straying from correct [or safe] operating procedure). Corners get cut, safety checks bypassed, and alarms ignored or turned off, and these behaviors become *normal*—not just common but also stripped of their significance as warnings of impending danger. In their 2002 *Annals of Internal Medicine* discussion of a catastrophic error in healthcare, Chassin and Becher coined the phrase "a culture of low expectations." When a system routinely produces errors (paperwork in the wrong chart, major miscommunications between different members of a given healthcare team, patients in the dark about important aspects of the care), providers in the system become inured to malfunction. In such a system, what should be regarded as a major warning of impending danger is ignored as a *normal* operating procedure.

Onion—The *onion* model illustrates the multiple levels or layers of protection (as in the layers of an onion) in a complex, high-risk system such as any healthcare setting. These layers include external regulations (e.g., related to staffing levels or required organizational practices, such as medication reconciliation), organizational features such as a just culture, equipment and technology (e.g., computerized order entry), and education and training of personnel.

Patient safety—Fundamentally, patient safety refers to freedom from accidental or preventable injuries produced by medical care. Thus, practices or interventions that improve patient safety are those that reduce the occurrence of preventable adverse events.

Patient safety in ambulatory care—The vast majority of healthcare takes place in the outpatient, or ambulatory, setting, and a growing body of research has identified and characterized factors that influence safety in office practice, the types of errors commonly encountered in ambulatory care, and potential strategies for improving ambulatory safety.

Pay for performance ("P4P")—Refers to the general strategy of promoting quality improvement by rewarding providers (meaning individual clinicians or, more commonly, clinics or hospitals) who meet certain performance expectations with respect to healthcare quality or efficiency.

Performance can be defined in terms of patient outcomes but is more commonly defined in terms of processes of care (e.g., the percentage of eligible diabetics referred for annual retinal examinations, the percentage of children who received immunizations appropriate for their age, patients admitted to the hospital with pneumonia who receive antibiotics within six hours). P4P initiatives reflect the efforts of purchasers of healthcare—from the federal government to private insurers—to use their purchasing power to encourage providers to develop whatever specific quality improvement initiatives are required to achieve the specified targets. Thus, rather than committing to a specific quality improvement strategy, such as a new information system or a disease management program, which may have variable success in different institutions, P4P creates a climate in which provider groups will be strongly incentivized to find whatever solutions will work for them.

Physician work hours and patient safety—Long and unpredictable work hours have been a staple of medical training for centuries. However, little attention was paid to the patient safety effects of fatigue among residents until March 1984, when Libby Zion died due to a medication-prescribing error while under the care of residents in the midst of a 36-hour shift. In 2003, the Accreditation Council for Graduate Medical Education (ACGME) implemented new rules limiting work hours for all residents, with the key components being that residents should work no more than 80 hours per week or 24 consecutive hours on duty, should not be "on-call" more than every third night, and should have one day off per week.

Plan–do–study–act—Commonly referred to as PDSA, refers to the cycle of activities advocated for achieving process or system improvement. The cycle was first proposed by Walter Shewhart, one of the pioneers of statistical process control (see "run charts") and popularized by his student, quality expert W. Edwards Deming. The PDSA cycle represents one of the cornerstones of continuous quality improvement (CQI). The components of the cycle are briefly described as follows:

- Plan: Analyze the problem you intend to improve and devise a plan to correct the problem.
- Do: Carry out the plan (preferably as a pilot project to avoid major investments of time or money in unsuccessful efforts).
- Study: Did the planned action succeed in solving the problem? If not, what went wrong? If partial success was achieved, how could the plan be refined?
- Act: Adopt the change piloted above as is, abandon it as a complete failure, or modify it and run through the cycle again.

Regardless of which action is taken, the PDSA cycle continues, with either the same problem or a new one.

Potential ADE—A potential ADE is a medication error or other drug-related mishap that reached the patient but happened not to produce harm (e.g., a penicillin-allergic patient receives penicillin but happens not to have an adverse reaction). In some studies, potential ADEs refer to errors or other problems that, if not intercepted, would be expected to cause harm. Thus, in some studies, if a physician ordered penicillin for a patient with a documented serious penicillin allergy, the order would be characterized as a potential ADE, on the grounds that administration of the drug would carry a substantial risk of harm to the patient.

Production pressure—Represents the pressure to put quantity of output—for a product or a service—ahead of safety. This pressure is seen in its starkest form in the line speed of factory assembly lines, famously demonstrated by Charlie Chaplin in *Modern Times*, as he is carried away on a conveyor belt and into the giant gears of the factory by the rapidly moving assembly line.

In healthcare, production pressure refers to delivery of services—the pressure to run hospitals at 100% capacity, with each bed filled with the sickest possible patients who are discharged at the first sign that they are stable, or the pressure to leave no operating room unused and to keep moving through the schedule for each room as fast as possible. In a survey of anesthesiologists, half of respondents stated that they had witnessed at least one case in which production pressure resulted in what they regarded as unsafe care. Examples included elective surgery in patients without adequate preoperative evaluation and proceeding with surgery despite significant contraindications.

Production pressure produces an organizational culture in which frontline personnel (and often managers) are reluctant to suggest any course of action that compromises productivity, even temporarily. For instance, in the survey of anesthesiologists, respondents reported pressure by surgeons to avoid delaying cases through additional patient evaluation or canceling cases, even when patients had clear contraindications to surgery.

Rapid Response Team (RRT)—The concept of RRTs (also known as Medical Emergency Teams) is that of a Code Blue team with more liberal calling criteria. Instead of just frank respiratory or cardiac arrest, RRTs respond to a wide range of worrisome, acute changes in patients' clinical status, such as low blood pressure, difficulty breathing, or altered mental status. In addition to less stringent calling criteria, RRTs (now sometimes called "Rapid Response Systems," to highlight the importance of the activation criteria as well as the response) de-emphasize the traditional hierarchy in patient care in that anyone can initiate the call. Nurses, junior medical staff, or others involved in the care of patients (and, in some hospitals, patients or family members) can call for the assistance of the RRT whenever they are worried about a patient's condition, without having to wait for more senior personnel to assess the patient and approve the decision to call for help.

Read-backs—When information is conveyed verbally, miscommunication may occur in a variety of ways, especially when transmission may not occur clearly (e.g., by telephone or radio, or if communication occurs under stress). For names and numbers, the problem often is confusing the sound of one letter or number with another. To address this possibility, the military, civil aviation, and many high-risk industries use protocols for mandatory read-backs, in which the listener repeats the key information, so that the transmitter can confirm its correctness.

Because mistaken substitution or reversal of alphanumeric information is such a potential hazard, read-back protocols typically include the use of phonetic alphabets, such as the NATO system ("Alpha–Bravo–Charlie–Delta–Echo … X-ray–Yankee–Zulu") now familiar to many. In healthcare, traditionally, read-back has been mandatory only in the context of checking to ensure accurate identification of recipients of blood transfusions. However, there are many other circumstances in which healthcare teams could benefit from following such protocols, for example, when communicating key lab results or patient orders over the phone, and even when exchanging information in person (e.g., handoffs).

Red rules—Rules that must be followed to the letter. In the language of nonhealthcare industries, red rules "stop the line." In other words, any deviation from a red rule will bring work to a halt until compliance is achieved. Red rules, in addition to relating to important and risky processes, must also be simple and easy to remember.

An example of a red rule in healthcare might be the following: "No hospitalized patient can undergo a test of any kind, receive a medication or blood product, or undergo a procedure if they are not wearing an identification bracelet." The implication of designating this a red rule is that the moment a patient is identified as not meeting this condition, all activity must cease in order to verify the patient's identity and supply an identification band.

Healthcare organizations already have numerous rules and policies that call for strict adherence. The reason that some organizations are using red rules is that, unlike many standard rules, red rules will always be supported by the entire organization. In other words, when someone at the frontline calls for work to cease on the basis of a red rule, top management must always support this decision. Thus, when properly implemented, red rules should foster a culture of safety, as frontline workers will know that they can stop the line when they notice potential hazards, even when doing so may result in considerable inconvenience or be time consuming and costly, for their immediate supervisors or the organization as a whole.

Root cause analysis—A structured process for identifying the causal or contributing factors underlying adverse events or other critical incidents. The key advantage of RCA over traditional clinical case reviews is that it follows a predefined protocol for identifying specific contributing factors in various causal categories (e.g., personnel, training, equipment, protocols, scheduling) rather than attributing the incident to the first error one finds or to preconceived notions investigators might have about the case.

Rule of thumb—See "Heuristic." Loosely defined or informal rule often arrived at through experience or trial and error (e.g., gastrointestinal complaints that wake patients up at night are unlikely to be benign). Heuristics provide cognitive shortcuts in the face of complex situations, and thus serve an important purpose. Unfortunately, they can also turn out to be wrong.

The phrase "rule of thumb" probably has its origin with trades such as carpentry in which skilled workers could use the length of their thumb (roughly one inch from knuckle to tip) rather than more precise measuring instruments and still produce excellent results. In other words, they measured not using a "rule of wood" (old-fashioned way of saying ruler), but by a "rule of thumb."

Run charts—A type of statistical process control or quality control graph in which some observation (e.g., manufacturing defects or adverse outcomes) is plotted over time to see if there are "runs" of points above or below a center line, usually representing the average or median. In addition to the number of runs, the length of the runs conveys important information. For run charts with more than 20 useful observations, a run of 8 or more dots would count as a "shift" in the process of interest, suggesting some nonrandom variation. Other key tests applied to run charts include tests for "trends" (sequences of successive increases or decreases in the observation of interest) and "zigzags" (alternation in the direction—up or down—of the lines joining pairs of dots). If a nonrandom change for the better, or shift, occurs, it suggests that an intervention has succeeded. The expression "moving the dots" refers to this type of shift.

Safety culture—Safety culture refers to a commitment to safety that permeates all levels of an organization, from frontline personnel to executive management. More specifically, "safety culture" calls up a number of features identified in studies of high reliability organizations, organizations outside of healthcare with exemplary performance with respect to safety, including:

- Acknowledgment of the high-risk, error-prone nature of an organization's activities
- A blame-free environment where individuals are able to report errors or close calls without fear of reprimand or punishment
- An expectation of collaboration across ranks to seek solutions to vulnerabilities
- A willingness on the part of the organization to direct resources to addressing safety concerns

Sentinel event—An adverse event in which death or serious harm to a patient has occurred; usually used to refer to events that are not at all expected or acceptable—for example, an operation on the wrong patient or body part. The choice of the word *sentinel* reflects the egregiousness of the injury (e.g., amputation of the wrong leg) and the likelihood that investigation of such events will reveal serious problems in current policies or procedures.

Sensemaking—A term from organizational theory that refers to the processes by which an organization takes in information to make sense of its environment, to generate knowledge, and to make decisions. It is the organizational equivalent of what individuals do when they process information, interpret events in their environments, and make decisions based on these activities. More technically, organizational sensemaking constructs the shared meanings that define the organization's purpose and frame the perception of problems or opportunities that the organization needs to work on.

Sharp end—The sharp end refers to the personnel or parts of the healthcare system in direct contact with patients. Personnel operating at the sharp end may literally be holding a scalpel (e.g., an orthopedist who operates on the wrong leg) or figuratively be administering any kind of therapy (e.g., a nurse programming an intravenous pump) or performing any aspect of care. To complete the metaphor, the blunt end refers to the many layers of the healthcare system that affect the scalpels, pills, and medical devices, or the personnel wielding, administering, and operating them. Thus, an error in programming an intravenous pump would represent a problem at the sharp end, while the institution's decision to use multiple types of infusion pumps (making programming errors more likely) would represent a problem at the blunt end. The terminology of "sharp" and "blunt" ends corresponds roughly to active failures and latent conditions.

Signouts and signovers—The term "signout" is used to refer to the act of transmitting information about the patient. Handoffs and signouts have been linked to adverse clinical events in settings ranging from the emergency department to the intensive care unit.

Situational awareness—Situational awareness refers to the degree to which one's perception of a situation matches reality. In the context of crisis management, where the phrase is most often used, situational awareness includes awareness of fatigue and stress among team members (including oneself), environmental threats to safety, appropriate immediate goals, and the deteriorating status of the crisis (or patient). Failure to maintain situational awareness can result in various problems that compound the crisis. For instance, during a resuscitation, an individual or entire team may focus on a particular task, such as a difficult central line insertion or a particular medication to administer. Fixation on this problem can result in loss of situational awareness to the point that steps are not taken to address immediately life-threatening problems such as respiratory failure or a pulseless rhythm. In this context, maintaining situational awareness might be seen as equivalent to keeping the big picture in mind. Alternatively, in assigning tasks in a crisis, the leader may ignore signals from a team member, which may result in escalating anxiety for the team member, failure to perform the assigned task, or further patient deterioration.

Six sigma—Six sigma refers loosely to striving for near perfection in the performance of a process or production of a product. The name derives from the Greek letter sigma, often used to refer to the standard deviation of a normal distribution. By definition, 95% of a normally distributed population falls within 2 standard deviations of the average (or "2 sigma"). This leaves 5% of observations as "abnormal" or "unacceptable." Six Sigma targets a defect rate of 3.4 per million opportunities—6 standard deviations from the population average.

When it comes to industrial performance, having 5% of a product fall outside the desired specifications would represent an unacceptably high defect rate. What company could stay in business if 5% of its product did not perform well? For example, would we tolerate a pharmaceutical company that produced pills containing incorrect dosages 5% of the time? Certainly not. But when it comes to clinical performance—the number of patients who receive a proven medication, the number of patients who develop complications from a procedure—we routinely accept failure or defect rates in the 2% to 5% range, orders of magnitude below Six Sigma performance.

Not every process in healthcare requires such near-perfect performance. In fact, one of the lessons of Reason's Swiss cheese model is the extent to which low overall error rates are possible even when individual components have many "holes." However, many high-stakes processes are far less forgiving, since a single "defect" can lead to catastrophe (e.g., wrong-site surgery, accidental administration of concentrated potassium).

Slips (or lapses)—Errors can be dichotomized as slips or mistakes, based on the cognitive psychology of task-oriented behavior. Slips refer to failures of schematic behaviors, or lapses in concentration (e.g., overlooking a step in a routine task due to a lapse in memory, an experienced surgeon nicking an adjacent organ during an operation due to a momentary lapse in concentration).

Slips occur in the face of competing sensory or emotional distractions, fatigue, and stress. Reducing the risk of slips requires attention to the designs of protocols, devices, and work environments—using checklists so key steps will not be omitted, reducing fatigue among personnel (or shifting high-risk work away from personnel who have been working extended hours), removing unnecessary variation in the design of key devices, eliminating distractions (e.g., phones and pagers) from areas where work requires intense concentration, and other redesign strategies. Slips can be contrasted with mistakes, which are failures that occur in attentional behavior such as active problem solving.

Standard of care—What the average, prudent clinician would be expected to do under certain circumstances. The standard of care may vary by community (e.g., due to resource constraints). When the term is used in the clinical setting, the standard of care is generally felt not to vary by specialty or level of training. In other words, the standard of care for a condition may well be defined in terms of the standard expected of a specialist, in which case a generalist (or trainee) would be expected to deliver the same care or make a timely referral to the appropriate specialist (or supervisor, in the case of a trainee). Standard of care is also a term of art in malpractice law, and its definition varies from jurisdiction to jurisdiction. When used in this legal sense, often the standard of care is specific to a given specialty; it is often defined as the care expected of a reasonable practitioner with similar training practicing in the same location under the same circumstances.

Structure–process–outcome triad ("Donabedian Triad")—Most definitions of quality emphasize favorable patient outcomes as the gold standard for assessing quality. In practice, however, one would like to detect quality problems without waiting for poor outcomes to develop in such sufficient numbers that deviations from expected rates of morbidity and mortality can be detected. Donabedian first proposed that quality could be measured using aspects of care with proven relationships to desirable patient outcomes. For instance, if proven diagnostic and therapeutic strategies are monitored, quality problems can be detected long before demonstrable poor outcomes occur.

Aspects of care with proven connections to patient outcomes fall into two general categories: process and structure. Processes encompass all that is done to patients in terms of diagnosis, treatment, monitoring, and counseling. Cardiovascular care provides classic examples of the use of process measures to assess quality. Given the known benefits of aspirin and beta-blockers for patients with myocardial infarction, the quality of care for patients with myocardial infarction can be measured in terms of the rates at which eligible patients receive these proven therapies. The percentage of eligible women who undergo mammography at appropriate intervals would provide a process-based measure for quality of preventive care for women.

Structure refers to the setting in which care occurs and the capacity of that setting to produce quality. Traditional examples of structural measures related to quality include credentials, patient volume, and academic affiliation. More recent structural measures include the adoption of organizational models for inpatient care (e.g., closed ICUs and dedicated stroke units) and possibly the presence of sophisticated clinical information systems. Cardiovascular care provides another classic example of structural measures of quality. Numerous studies have shown that institutions that perform more cardiac surgeries and invasive cardiology procedures achieve better outcomes than institutions that see fewer patients. Given these data, patient volume represents a structural measure of quality of care for patients undergoing cardiac procedures.

Swiss cheese model—James Reason developed the "Swiss cheese model" (Figure 2-1) to illustrate how analyses of major accidents and catastrophic systems failures tend to reveal multiple, smaller failures leading up to the actual hazard.

In the model, each slice of cheese represents a safety barrier or precaution relevant to a particular hazard. For example, if the hazard were wrong-site surgery, slices of the cheese might include conventions for identifying sidedness on radiology tests, a protocol for signing the correct site when the surgeon and patient first meet, and a second protocol for reviewing the medical record and checking the previously marked site in the operating room. Many more layers exist. The point is that no single barrier is foolproof. They each have "holes," hence the Swiss cheese. For some serious events (e.g., operating on the wrong site or wrong person), even though the holes will align infrequently, even rare cases of harm (errors making it "through the cheese") will be unacceptable.

While the model may convey the impression that the slices of cheese and the location of their respective holes are independent, this may not be the case. For instance, in an emergency situation, all three of the surgical identification safety checks mentioned above may fail or be bypassed. The surgeon may meet the patient for the first time in the operating room. A hurried x-ray technologist might mislabel a film (or simply hang it backwards and a hurried surgeon may not notice it); "signing the site" may not take place at all (e.g., if the patient is unconscious), or, if it takes place, be rushed and offer no real protection. In the technical parlance of accident analysis, the different barriers may have a common failure mode, in which several protections are lost at once (i.e., the holes in several layers of the cheese line up).

In healthcare, such failure modes, in which slices of the cheese line up more often than one would expect if the location of their holes were independent of each other (and certainly more often than wings fall off airplanes), occur distressingly commonly. In fact, many of the systems problems discussed by Reason and others—poorly designed work schedules, lack of teamwork, and variations in the design of important equipment between and even within institutions—are sufficiently common that many of the slices of cheese already have their holes aligned. In such cases, one slice of cheese may be all that is left between the patient and significant hazard.

Systems approach—Medicine has traditionally treated quality problems and errors as failings on the part of individual providers, perhaps reflecting inadequate knowledge or skill levels. The systems approach, by contrast, takes the view that most errors reflect predictable human failings in the context of poorly designed systems (e.g., expected lapses in human vigilance in the face of long work hours or predictable mistakes on the part of relatively inexperienced personnel faced with cognitively complex situations). Rather than focusing corrective efforts on reprimanding individuals or pursuing remedial education, the systems approach seeks to identify situations or factors likely to give rise to human error and implement systems changes that will reduce their occurrence or minimize their impact on patients. This view holds that efforts to catch human errors before they occur or block them from causing harm will ultimately be more fruitful than ones that seek to somehow create flawless providers.

This systems focus includes paying attention to human factors engineering (or ergonomics), including the design of protocols, schedules, and other factors that are routinely addressed in other high-risk industries but have traditionally been ignored in medicine.

"Time outs"—Refer to planned periods of quiet and/or interdisciplinary discussion focused on ensuring that key procedural details have been addressed. For instance, protocols for ensuring correct site surgery often recommend a time out to confirm the identification of the patient, the surgical procedure, site, and other key aspects, often stating them aloud for double-checking by other team members. In addition to avoiding major misidentification errors involving the patient or surgical site, such a time out ensures that all team members share the same "game plan," so to speak. Taking the time to focus on listening and communicating the plans as a team can rectify miscommunications and misunderstandings before a procedure gets underway.

Teamwork Training—Providing safe healthcare depends on highly trained individuals with disparate roles and responsibilities acting together in the best interests of the patient. The need for improved teamwork has led to the application of teamwork training principles, originally developed in aviation, to a variety of healthcare settings.

Triggers—Refer to signals for detecting likely adverse events. Triggers alert providers involved in patient safety activities to probable adverse events so they can review the medical record to determine if an actual or potential adverse event has occurred. For instance, if a hospitalized patient received naloxone (a drug used to reverse the effects of narcotics), the patient probably received an excessive dose of morphine or some other opiate. In the emergency department, the use of naloxone would more likely represent treatment of a self-inflected opiate overdose, so the trigger would have little value in that setting. But, among patients already admitted to hospital, a pharmacy could use the administration of naloxone as a "trigger" to investigate possible ADEs.

In cases in which the trigger correctly identified an adverse event, causative factors can be identified and, over time, interventions developed to reduce the frequency of particularly common causes of adverse events. The traditional use of triggers has been to efficiently identify adverse events after the fact. However, using triggers in real time has tremendous potential as a patient safety tool. In a study of real-time triggers in a single community hospital, for example, more than 1000 triggers were generated in six months, and approximately 25% led to physician action and would not have been recognized without the trigger.

As with any alert or alarm system, the threshold for generating triggers has to balance true and false positives. The system will lose its value if too many triggers prove to be false alarms. This concern is less relevant when triggers are used as chart review tools. In such cases, the tolerance of false alarms depends only on the availability of sufficient resources for medical record review. Reviewing four false alarms for every true adverse event might be quite reasonable in the context of an institutional safety program, but frontline providers would balk at (and eventually ignore) a trigger system that generated four false alarms for every true one.

Underuse, overuse, and misuse—For process of care, quality problems can arise in one of the three ways: underuse, overuse, and misuse.

Underuse refers to the failure to provide a healthcare service when it would have produced a favorable outcome for a patient. Standard examples include failures to provide appropriate preventive services to eligible patients (e.g., Pap smears, flu shots for elderly patients, screening for hypertension) and proven medications for chronic illnesses (steroid inhalers for asthmatics; aspirin, beta-blockers, and lipid-lowering agents for patients who have suffered a recent myocardial infarction).

Overuse refers to providing a process of care in circumstances where the potential for harm exceeds the potential for benefit. Prescribing an antibiotic for a viral infection such as a cold, for which antibiotics are ineffective, constitutes overuse. The potential for harm includes adverse reactions to the antibiotics and increases in antibiotic resistance among bacteria in the community. Overuse can also apply to diagnostic tests and surgical procedures.

Misuse occurs when an appropriate process of care has been selected but a preventable complication occurs and the patient does not receive the full potential benefit of the service. Avoidable complications of surgery or medication use are misuse problems. A patient who suffers a rash after receiving penicillin for strep throat, despite having a known allergy to that antibiotic, is an example of misuse. A patient who develops a pneumothorax after an inexperienced operator attempted to insert a subclavian line would represent another example of misuse.

Voluntary patient safety event reporting—See incident reporting. Patient safety event reporting systems are ubiquitous in hospitals and are a mainstay of efforts to detect safety and quality problems. However, while event reports may highlight specific safety concerns, they do not provide insights into the epidemiology of safety problems.

Workaround—From the perspective of frontline personnel trying to accomplish their work, the design of equipment or the policies governing work tasks can seem counterproductive. When frontline personnel adopt consistent patterns of bypassing safety features of medical equipment, these patterns and actions are referred to as workarounds. Although workarounds "fix the problem," the system remains unaltered and thus continues to present potential safety hazards for future patients.

From a definitional point of view, it does not matter if frontline users are justified in working around a given policy or equipment design feature. What does matter is that the motivation for a workaround lies in getting work done, not laziness or whim. Thus, the appropriate response by managers to the existence of a workaround should not consist of reflexively reminding staff about the policy and restating the importance of following it. Rather, workarounds should trigger assessment of workflow and the various competing demands for the time of frontline personnel. In busy clinical areas where efficiency is paramount, managers can expect workarounds to arise whenever policies create added tasks for frontline personnel, especially when the extra work is perceived to be out of proportion to the importance of the safety goal.

Wrong-site, wrong-procedure, and wrong-patient surgery—Few medical errors are as terrifying as those that involve patients who have undergone surgery on the wrong body part, undergone the incorrect procedure, or had a procedure intended for another patient. These "wrong-site, wrong-procedure, wrong-patient errors" (WSPEs) are rightly termed never events.

Reprinted with permission from AHRQ Patient Safety Network: Shojania KG, Wachter RM, Hartman EE. AHRQ Patient Safety Network Glossary. Available at: https://psnet .ahrq.gov/glossary.

APPENDIX III. SELECTED MILESTONES IN THE FIELD OF PATIENT SAFETY

Year	Event
Fourth century BC	Hippocrates writes, "I will never do harm to anyone," which is later translated (and changed) into "Primum non nocere," or "first do no harm."
1857	Ignaz Semmelweiss publishes his findings, demonstrating that hand disinfection leads to fewer infections (puerperal fever).
1863	Florence Nightingale, in *Notes on Hospitals*, writes, "It may seem a strange principle to enunciate as the very first requirement in a Hospital that it should do the sick no harm."
1911	Ernest Codman, a Boston surgeon, establishes his "End Result" hospital—with a goal of following and learning from patient outcomes, include errors in treatment.
1917	The first specialty board (ophthalmology) is formed. Ultimately, 24 boards are founded to certify physicians in the United States.
1918	The American College of Surgeons begins the first program of hospital inspection and certification. In 1951, the program becomes the Joint Commission on Accreditation of Healthcare Organizations (JCAHO), now the Joint Commission.
1959	Robert Moser, an Army physician, publishes *Diseases of Medical Progress*, arguing that iatrogenic disease is common and preventable.
1964	Elihu Schimmel, a Yale physician, publishes one of the first studies of iatrogenic illness, finding that 20% of patients admitted to a university hospital experienced an "untoward episode."
1977	Ivan Illich publishes *Limits of Medicine. Medical Nemesis: the Expropriation of Health*, arguing that healthcare is actually a threat to health.
1985	The Anesthesia Patient Safety Foundation (APSF) is founded, a year after Jeffrey Cooper's seminal paper analyzing failures in anesthesia machines. Twelve years later, the National Patient Safety Foundation is founded, modeled on the APSF.
1990	James Reason publishes *Human Error* (and, seven years later, *Managing the Risks of Organisational Accidents*), describing his new theory of error as systems failure. His work will go undiscovered by healthcare until Leape's 1994 *JAMA* article.
1991	Publication of Harvard Medical Practice studies (from which the IOM later derives its 44,000 to 98,000 deaths/year estimate).

(continued)

Year	Event
1994	Lucian Leape publishes *Error in Medicine* in *JAMA*, the first mainstream article in the healthcare literature arguing for a systems approach to safety.
1999	The release of the IOM report, *To Err Is Human*, creates a media sensation and begins the modern patient safety movement.
2000	Following the IOM report, the UK's National Health Service releases another major report, *An Organisation with a Memory*.
2001	The IOM releases its *Quality Chasm* report.
2001	The Agency for Healthcare Research and Quality (AHRQ) receives $50 million from Congress to begin an aggressive patient safety research and improvement program.
2002	The Joint Commission releases its first National Patient Safety Goals.
2002	The National Quality Forum launches its list of Serious Reportable Events (the "Never Events" list), which later becomes the scaffolding for public reporting and "no pay" programs.
2003	The Accreditation Council on Graduate Medical Education (ACGME) institutes duty-hour regulations, limiting residents to 80 hours/week.
2004	The U.S. government creates the Office of the National Coordinator for Healthcare IT (ONCHIT), the first federal initiative to computerize healthcare.
2005–2006	The Institute for Healthcare Improvement launches its 100,000 Lives Campaign, followed a year later by its 5 Million Lives Campaign.
2005	The U.S. Congress passes the Patient Safety Act, paving the way for the creation of patient safety organizations beginning in 2009.
2006	Pronovost and colleagues report the results of the Keystone project, which slashed the rate of central line–associated bloodstream infections in Michigan intensive care units, and highlights the role of checklists in patient safety.
2008	Medicare launches its "no pay for errors" initiative.
2009	As part of the American Recovery and Reinvestment Act of 2009 (commonly known as "the stimulus package"), Congress allocates about $30 billion to be distributed to eligible clinicians and hospitals which implement electronic health records that meet criteria for "meaningful use."
2010	Patient safety leader Don Berwick becomes director of the U.S. Centers for Medicare & Medicaid Services (CMS). A year later, he announces the "Partnership for Patients," with nearly $1 billion in support of patient safety and quality activities. Over the next five years, studies confirm a significant (approximately 20%) reduction in hospital-acquired conditions.
2010	President Obama signs into law the Affordable Care Act. In addition to its expansion and reform of the health insurance market, it also contains many provisions that aim to improve safety and quality, including penalties for hospital-associated conditions, a push for value-based purchasing, and the establishment of a Medicare innovation center to test new models of care.

(continued)

Year	Event
2011	The U.S. government begins distributing incentive payments to hospitals and doctors for implementing healthcare information technology (HIT) systems that meet certain "meaningful use" criteria.
2011	ACGME further tightens its residency duty-hour and supervision requirements. In 2017, the work-hour restrictions were loosened slightly, after studies failed to confirm safety gains associated with the 2011 changes.
2012	Medicare launches Value Based Purchasing.
2014	Medicare launches Hospital-Acquired Condition Reduction Program.
2015	The NAS releases its report on improving diagnosis in medicine, highlighting diagnostic error as a central patient safety issue.

Adapted from various sources and authors' own analysis.

APPENDIX IV. THE JOINT COMMISSION'S NATIONAL PATIENT SAFETY GOALS (HOSPITAL VERSION, 2017)

NPSG.01.01.01

Use at least two patient identifiers when providing care, treatment, and services.

NPSG.01.03.01

Eliminate transfusion errors related to patient misidentification.

NPSG.02.03.01

Report critical results of tests and diagnostic procedures to the right staff person on a timely basis.

NPSG.03.04.01

Before a procedure, label medicines that are not labeled. *Note:* medication containers include syringes, medicine cups, and basins.

NPSG.03.05.01

Reduce the likelihood of patient harm associated with the use of anticoagulant therapy.

NPSG.03.06.01

Maintain and communicate accurate information about patients' medications.

NPSG.06.01.01

Ensure that medical equipment alarms are audible and responded to on time.

NPSG.07.01.01

Comply with either the current Centers for Disease Control and Prevention (CDC) hand hygiene guidelines or the current World Health Organization (WHO) hand hygiene guidelines.

NPSG.07.03.01

Implement evidence-based practices to prevent healthcare-associated infections due to multidrug-resistant organisms in acute care hospitals. *Note*: This requirement applies to, but is not limited to, epidemiologically important organisms such as methicillin-resistant *Staphylococcus aureus* (MRSA), *Clostridium difficile* (CDI), vancomycin-resistant enterococci (VRE), and multidrug-resistant gram-negative bacteria.

NPSG.07.04.01

Implement evidence-based practices to prevent central line–associated bloodstream infections. *Note*: This requirement covers short- and long-term central venous catheters and peripherally inserted central catheter (PICC) lines.

NPSG.07.05.01

Implement evidence-based practices for preventing surgical site infections.

NPSG.07.06.01

Implement evidence-based practices to prevent indwelling catheter-associated urinary tract infections (CAUTI).

NPSG.15.01.01

Identify patients at risk for suicide. *Note*: This requirement applies only to psychiatric hospitals and patients being treated for emotional or behavioral disorders in general hospitals.

UP.01.01.01

Conduct a preprocedure verification process to ensure that the correct procedure is done on the correct patient at the correct site on the body.

UP.01.02.01

Mark the procedure site.

UP.01.03.01

A time out is performed before the procedure.

© The Joint Commission, 2017. Reprinted with permission. Available at: https://www.joint commission.org/assets/1/6/2017_NPSG_HAP_ER.pdf.

Skipped numbers represent retired Goals (the numbers are not replaced).

NPSG, National Patient Safety Goal; UP, Universal Protocol.

APPENDIX V. AGENCY FOR HEALTHCARE RESEARCH AND QUALITY'S (AHRQ) PATIENT SAFETY INDICATORS (PSIS)

Provider (hospital)-level PSIs (n = 19)

- Death in low-mortality diagnosis-related groups (PSI 02)
- Pressure ulcer rate (PSI 03)
- Death among surgical inpatients with treatable serious complications (PSI 04)

- Foreign body left in during procedure (PSI 05)
- Iatrogenic pneumothorax rate (PSI 06)
- Central venous catheter-related bloodstream infection rate (PSI 07)
- Postoperative hip fracture rate (PSI 08)
- Perioperative hemorrhage or hematoma rate (PSI 09)
- Postoperative physiologic and metabolic derangements (PSI 10)
- Postoperative respiratory failure rate (PSI 11)
- Postoperative pulmonary embolism or deep vein thrombosis rate (PSI 12)
- Postoperative sepsis rate (PSI 13)
- Postoperative wound dehiscence rate (PSI 14)
- Accidental puncture or laceration rate (PSI 15)
- Transfusion reaction count (PSI 16)
- Birth trauma rate—injury to neonate (PSI 17)
- Obstetric trauma rate—vaginal delivery with instrument (PSI 18)
- Obstetric trauma rate—vaginal delivery without instrument (PSI 19)
- Patient safety for selected indicators (PSI 90)

Area-level indicators (e.g., county, state) (n = 7)

- Foreign body left in during procedure (PSI 21)
- Iatrogenic pneumothorax rate (PSI 22)
- Central venous catheter-related bloodstream infection rate (PSI 23)
- Postoperative wound dehiscence rate (PSI 24)
- Accidental puncture or laceration rate (PSI 25)
- Transfusion reaction rate (PSI 26)
- Postoperative hemorrhage or hematoma rate (PSI 27)

Reprinted from *Patient Safety Indicators. A Tool to Help Assess Quality and Safety of Care to Adults in the Hospital* [brochure]. AHRQ Publication No. 15-M053-4-EF. Rockville, MD: Agency for Healthcare Research and Quality; September 2015. Available at: http://www.qualityindicators.ahrq.gov/Downloads/Modules/PSI/V50/PSI_Brochure.pdf.

APPENDIX VI. THE NATIONAL QUALITY FORUM'S LIST OF SERIOUS REPORTABLE EVENTS, 2011

1. **Surgical or invasive procedure events (*n* = 5)**
   - Surgery or other invasive procedure performed on the wrong site
   - Surgery or other invasive procedure performed on the wrong patient
   - Wrong surgical or other invasive procedure performed on a patient
   - Unintended retention of a foreign object in a patient after surgery or other invasive procedure
   - Intraoperative or immediately postoperative/postprocedure death in an ASA Class 1 patient

2. **Product or device events** (*n* = 3)
   - Patient death or serious injury associated with the use of contaminated drugs, devices, or biologics provided by the healthcare setting
   - Patient death or serious injury associated with the use or function of a device in patient care, in which the device is used for functions other than as intended
   - Patient death or serious injury associated with intravascular air embolism that occurs while being cared for in a healthcare setting

3. **Patient protection events** (*n* = 3)
   - Discharge or release of a patient/resident of any age, who is unable to make decisions, to other than an authorized person
   - Patient death or serious injury associated with patient elopement (disappearance)
   - Patient suicide, attempted suicide, or self-harm that results in serious injury, while being cared for in a healthcare setting

4. **Care management events** (*n* = 9)
   - Patient death or serious injury associated with a medication error (e.g., errors involving the wrong drug, wrong dose, wrong patient, wrong time, wrong rate, wrong preparation, or wrong route of administration)
   - Patient death or serious injury associated with unsafe administration of blood products
   - Maternal death or serious injury associated with labor or delivery in a low-risk pregnancy while being cared for in a healthcare setting
   - Death or serious injury of a neonate associated with labor or delivery in a low-risk pregnancy (*new in 2011*)
   - Patient death or serious injury associated with a fall while being cared for in a healthcare setting
   - Any Stage 3, Stage 4, and unstageable pressure ulcers acquired after admission/presentation to a healthcare setting
   - Artificial insemination with the wrong donor sperm or wrong egg
   - Patient death or serious injury resulting from the irretrievable loss of an irreplaceable biological specimen (*new in 2011*)
   - Patient death or serious injury resulting from failure to follow up or communicate laboratory, pathology, or radiology test results (*new in 2011*)

5. **Environmental events** (*n* = 4)
   - Patient or staff death or serious injury associated with an electric shock in the course of a patient care process in a healthcare setting
   - Any incident in which systems designated for oxygen or other gas to be delivered to a patient contain no gas, the wrong gas, or are contaminated by toxic substances

■ Patient or staff death or serious injury associated with a burn incurred from any source in the course of a patient care process in a healthcare setting

■ Patient death or serious injury associated with the use of physical restraints or bedrails while being cared for in a healthcare setting

6. **Radiologic events ($n = 1$)**

■ Death or serious injury of a patient or staff associated with the introduction of a metallic object into the MRI area (*new in 2011*)

7. **Potential criminal events ($n = 4$)**

■ Any instance of care ordered by or provided by someone impersonating a physician, nurse, pharmacist, or other licensed healthcare provider

■ Abduction of a patient/resident of any age

■ Sexual abuse/assault on a patient or staff member within or on the grounds of a healthcare setting

■ Death or serious injury of a patient or staff member resulting from a physical assault (i.e., battery) that occurs within or on the grounds of a healthcare setting

Reproduced with permission from The National Quality Forum. Available at: http://www.qualityforum.org/Topics/SREs/List_of_SREs.aspx. This list is still commonly known as the "Never Events" list.

APPENDIX VII. THE NATIONAL QUALITY FORUM'S LIST OF "SAFE PRACTICES FOR BETTER HEALTHCARE—2010 UPDATE"

Safe Practice	Practice Statement
1. Leadership structures and systems	Leadership structures and systems must be established to ensure that there is organization-wide awareness of patient safety performance gaps, leaders are directly accountable for those gaps and there is adequate investment in performance improvement abilities, and actions are taken to ensure safe care of every patient served.
2. Culture measurement, feedback, and intervention	Healthcare organizations must measure their culture, provide feedback to the leadership and staff, and undertake interventions that will reduce patient safety risk.
3. Teamwork training and skill building	Healthcare organizations must establish a proactive, systematic, organization-wide approach to developing team-based care through teamwork training, skill building, and team-led performance improvement interventions that reduce preventable harm to patients.

(continued)

Safe Practice	Practice Statement
4. Identification and mitigation of risks and hazards	Healthcare organizations must systematically identify and mitigate patient safety risks and hazards with an integrated approach in order to continuously drive down preventable patient harm.
5. Informed consent	Ask every patient or legal surrogate to "teach back," in his or her own words, key information about the proposed treatments or procedures for which he or she is being asked to provide informed consent.
6. Life-sustaining treatment	Ensure that written documentation of the patient's preferences for life-sustaining treatment is prominently displayed in his or her chart.
7. Disclosure	Following serious unanticipated outcomes, including those that are clearly caused by systems failures, the patient and, as appropriate, the family should receive timely, transparent, and clear communication concerning what is known about the event.
8. Care of the caregiver	Following serious unintentional harm due to systems failures and/or errors that resulted from human performance failures, the involved caregivers should receive timely and systematic care—and the opportunity to fully participate in event investigation and risk identification and mitigation activities that will prevent future events.
9. Nursing workforce	Implement critical components of a well-designed nursing workforce, including (a) an adequate nursing plan, (b) senior nurse administrative leaders as part of the hospital's senior management team, (c) governance board engagement in nurse staffing decisions, and (d) budget to support nursing education and skill building.
10. Direct caregivers	Ensure that non-nursing direct care staffing levels are adequate, that staff are competent, and that they have had adequate orientation, training, and education.
11. Intensive care unit care	All patients in general ICUs should be managed by physicians who have specific training and certification in critical care medicine.
12. Patient care information	Ensure that care information is transmitted and appropriately documented in a timely manner and in a clearly understandable form to patients and to all relevant caregivers.
13. Order read-back and abbreviations	Incorporate a safe, effective communication strategy, structure, and systems to include (a) record and "read-backs" for verbal orders and critical test results; (b) use of a standard "do not use" abbreviation list.
14. Labeling of diagnostic studies	Implement standardized policies, processes, and systems to ensure accurate labeling of radiographs, lab specimens, and other studies to ensure accuracy.
15. Discharge systems	A "discharge plan" must be prepared for each patient at the time of hospital discharge, and a concise discharge summary must be relayed to the caregiver accepting responsibility for postdischarge care in a timely manner. Organizations should confirm receipt of this communication.

(continued)

Safe Practice	Practice Statement
16. Safe adoption of computerized provider order entry	Implement a CPOE system built on the requisite foundation of reengineered evidence-based care, an assurance of healthcare organization staff and independent practitioner readiness, and an integrated information technology infrastructure.
17. Medication reconciliation	The healthcare organization must develop, reconcile, and communicate an accurate patient medication list throughout the continuum of care.
18. Pharmacist leadership structures and systems	Pharmacy leaders should have an active role on the administrative leadership team that reflects their authority and accountability for medication management systems performance across the organization.
19. Hand hygiene	Comply with current Centers for Disease Control and Prevention (CDC) Hand Hygiene guidelines.
20. Influenza prevention	Comply with current CDC guidelines regarding influenza vaccination and prevention/control.
21. Central line–associated bloodstream infection prevention	Take actions to prevent central line–associated bloodstream infections by implementing evidence-based intervention practices.
22. Surgical site infection prevention	Take actions to prevent surgical site infections by implementing evidence-based intervention practices.
23. Care of the ventilated patient	Take actions to prevent complications associated with ventilated patients: ventilator-associated pneumonia, venous thromboembolism, peptic ulcer disease, dental complications, and pressure ulcers.
24. Multidrug-resistant organism prevention	Implement a systematic multidrug-resistant organization prevention program.
25. Catheter-associated urinary tract infection prevention	Take actions to prevent catheter-associated urinary tract infections by implementing evidence-based intervention practices.
26. Wrong-site, wrong-procedure, wrong-person surgery prevention	Implement the Universal Protocol for preventing wrong-site, wrong-procedure, wrong-person surgery for all procedures.
27. Pressure ulcer prevention	Take actions to prevent pressure ulcers by implementing evidence-based intervention practices.
28. Venous thromboembolism prevention	Evaluate each patient on admission and regularly thereafter for the risk of developing venous thromboembolism. Utilize clinically appropriate evidence-based prophylaxis methods.
29. Anticoagulation practice	Organizations should implement practices to prevent harm due to anticoagulant therapy.
30. Contrast media–induced renal failure prevention	Utilize validated protocols to evaluate patients who are at risk for contrast media–induced renal failure and gadolinium-associated nephrogenic systemic fibrosis.

(continued)

Safe Practice	Practice Statement
31. Organ donation	Hospital policies that are consistent with applicable law and regulations should be in place and should address patient and family preferences for organ donations.
32. Glycemic control	Take actions to improve glycemic control by implementing evidence-based intervention practices that prevent hypoglycemia and optimize the care of patients with hyperglycemia and diabetes.
33. Fall prevention	Take actions to prevent patient falls and to reduce fall-related injuries by implementing evidence-based intervention practices.
34. Pediatric imaging	When CT imaging studies are undertaken on children, "child-size" techniques should be used to reduce unnecessary exposure to ionizing radiation.

Adapted with permission from National Quality Forum. *Safe Practice for Better Healthcare—2010 Update. A Consensus Report.* Available at www.qualityforum.org.

APPENDIX VIII. MEDICARE'S "NO PAY FOR ERRORS" LIST*

- Stage III and IV pressure ulcers
- Fall or trauma resulting in serious injury
- Vascular catheter-associated infection
- Catheter-associated urinary tract infection
- Foreign object retained after surgery
- Certain surgical site infections (following coronary artery bypass graft, bariatric surgery for obesity, certain orthopedic procedures, implantation of cardiac electronic devices)
- Iatrogenic pneumothorax with venous catheter placement
- Air embolism
- Blood incompatibility
- Certain manifestations of poor blood sugar control
- Certain deep vein thromboses or pulmonary embolisms (following certain orthopedic procedures such as total knee replacement and total hip replacement)

Source: Centers for Medicare & Medicaid Services.

---

*The policy works this way: if under the old payment system an item on this list would have increased the reimbursement for a given hospitalization under Medicare's system of diagnosis-related groups (DRGs), the hospital no longer receives that additional reimbursement under this policy. However, if there are any other so-called "complicating conditions," the hospital still does receive the higher reimbursement, which mutes the financial impact of the policy. List is current as of August 2015.

APPENDIX IX. THINGS PATIENTS AND FAMILIES CAN DO, AND QUESTIONS THEY CAN ASK, TO IMPROVE THEIR CHANCES OF REMAINING SAFE IN THE HOSPITAL

What to Do or Check	Discussion or Recommendation
Make friends with your nurses, phlebotomists, and other hospital personnel. Make sure they address you by name at least once each shift.	
Before you are given a medication, ask what it is and what it's for.	
Before you are given a medication, a transfusion, an x-ray, or a procedure, make sure the nurse confirms your name by both asking you and checking your wristband.	Some hospitals may supplement this through the use of bar coding, for example, checking that the bar code on your wristband and the bar code on a medication bottle match.
Before being taken off the floor for a procedure, ask what it is and be sure you understand where you are going and why.	
Be sure your family members' contact information is available to the hospital or nursing home personnel.	It is not a bad idea to place a card with your family members' contact information by your bedside (in addition to being sure that this information is in the chart).
Before being transferred from floor to floor in a hospital (such as from the ICU to the general medical or surgical floor) or from one institution to another, check to be sure all catheters and other paraphernalia that should be removed have been.	Sometimes (particularly when there are no checklists), caregivers will forget to remove an IV line or urinary catheter before a transfer, which creates an unnecessary risk of infections. Believe it or not, doctors (one out of three in one study) will often forget whether their patient even has a urinary catheter in place. Don't be reluctant to ask your doctors or nurses whether you still need your catheters after the urgent need for them has passed.
Ask your caregivers whether they have washed (or cleaned) their hands.	Increasingly, you won't see them wash their hands, because they will be rubbing their hands with an antiseptic hand gel placed in a dispenser outside your room. We'd also want to know the hospital's overall hand hygiene rate, which should be above 80%.
What is the hospital's rate of central line–associated bloodstream infections?	Most hospitals with strong safety and infection prevention programs have driven this rate down to less than 1.5 per 1000 catheter-days. Similar benchmark rates for adverse events such as falls are likely to emerge in the next few years.

(continued)

What to Do or Check	Discussion or Recommendation
If you have an advance directive (and you should), keep a copy with you, make sure your family has one, give one to your nurse or doctor to place on your chart, and be certain it is transferred from site to site with you.	
Does the hospital have CPOE, an electronic medical record, and bar coding? If not, when do they plan to have them?	It would be great if they had them and they were up and running. If they have CPOE, ask what percent of physicians' orders are written on the computerized system (if it is less than half, then the doctors are still kicking the tires and the system is not really implemented). If CPOE is not in place, we'd worry—more than 90% of American hospitals and 80% of physician offices now have it.
Is there a functioning, preferably computerized, incident reporting system, on which hospital personnel can report errors and near misses?	The computerized systems make reporting, and dissemination of the information, much easier. So it would be good to hear, "yes we do." Unfortunately, there is no guarantee that the hospital is using the reports productively to improve safety.
How many incident reports are logged each month?	Although it might seem counterintuitive, this is probably a case of the more the better. If a midsized hospital (approximately 300 beds) doesn't receive a few hundred reports a month, then it may be that workers aren't sharing errors and near misses because either they are worried about blame or they are convinced that it isn't worth reporting because reports enter a black hole.
What is done with these reports?	You'd like to know that they go to the relevant managers in the area (the catheterization lab, the OR), who are expected to respond to them. Also, there should be an uber manager who watches for trends (e.g., an uptick in patient falls, bed ulcers, or medication administration errors).
How many detailed root cause analyses have been done in the past year?	Like the incident reports, you might think that "zero" would be a great answer because it would mean there were no major errors. But you can be sure that there were. So we'd expect that the average hospital will have done at least 20 full-blown RCAs in the past year.
Is there a Patient Safety Officer who is compensated for this role? What are his or her qualifications?	Some small hospitals will not have a paid Patient Safety Officer, but all midsized and large hospitals should have one. This guarantees that it is someone's job to be concerned about safety. It should be a respected physician, nurse, or pharmacist with additional training in human factors, systems engineering, quality improvement, and similar areas.

(continued)

What to Do or Check	Discussion or Recommendation
Is there an active Patient Safety Committee that meets at least monthly?	The answer must be yes.
Are there trained intensivists in the critical care units (ICUs) and hospitalists on the medical wards?	There is strong evidence that the on-site presence of intensivists, at least during the day, is associated with better ICU outcomes. For small hospitals without intensivists, linking the ICU electronically to trained intensivists who remotely monitor the patients also may improve outcomes. The evidence supporting the value of hospitalists caring for general medical and surgical patients is not quite as strong, but two studies did show lower death rates. I believe that the on-site presence of physicians who specialize in overseeing and coordinating patients' hospital care is likely to improve safety.
Which physicians are "in house" overnight?	We'd like to know that there is at least one senior attending physician in the building overnight to deal with acute issues, even if there are also residents.
Are the physicians who will care for you board certified in their specialty?	All else being equal, board certification indicates that your physician has demonstrated a certain level of knowledge and competence, and is keeping up in his or her field.
What is the nurse-to-patient ratio, and what percentage of the nurses are registered nurses (RNs)?	Ratios of more than 6–7:1 on the medical and surgical wards are associated with higher rates of errors (it should be much lower, such as 2:1, in the ICUs). Error rates also seem to be higher when more than about 30% of total nursing care is delivered by non-RNs (i.e., licensed practical nurses or nurses' aides).
Are there clinical pharmacists on the hospital wards who can help you understand and organize your medications?	There is good evidence that the involvement of clinical pharmacists, particularly in the discharge process, improves safety.
What is the hospital's system to prevent readmissions?	Good hospitals now have organized programs to do this, including robust discharge counseling, some type of postdischarge follow-up (phone call or visit), a prompt discharge summary, and a well-organized and rapid visit to the follow-up provider.
Does the hospital run simulator or other specific teamwork training?	Ideally, the hospital would require simulator training for people working in high-risk areas such as the OR, ER, and on Code Blue teams. In addition, specific teamwork training (CRM) is helpful, and a hospital that has an organized simulator and CRM program is probably ahead of the patient safety curve.

(*continued*)

What to Do or Check	Discussion or Recommendation
What does the hospital do to prevent handoff errors?	I would want to know that, at very least, there are read-backs of verbal orders and checklists before patients move from one unit to another (such as the ICU to the floor or from the floor to a nursing home).
What patient safety initiatives has the hospital undertaken in the past year?	They should have several that they can describe proudly, preferably with measurable results they can cite.

Reproduced and updated with permission from Wachter RM, Shojania KG. *Internal Bleeding: The Truth Behind America's Terrifying Epidemic of Medical Mistakes*. New York, NY: Rugged Land; 2004.

Index